NEUROSURGICAL
CLASSICS

NEUROSURGICAL CLASSICS

Compiled by

•Robert H. Wilkins, M.D.
Division of Neurosurgery
Duke University Medical Center
Durham, North Carolina

Under the auspices of

The Harvey Cushing Society
Paul C. Bucy, M.D.
Director of Publications
and
The Journal of Neurosurgery
Louise Eisenhardt, M.D.
Managing Editor

Editorial Board:
Bronson S. Ray, M.D., Chairman
Eben Alexander, Jr., M.D.
Donald D. Matson, M.D.
David L. Reeves, M.D.
Henry G. Schwartz, M.D.
Arthur A. Ward, Jr., M.D.

JOHNSON REPRINT CORPORATION
NEW YORK AND LONDON
1965

Printed in the United States of America

This work is dedicated to

Barnes Woodhall, M. D.

A man of broad vision whose efforts as a surgeon, teacher, investigator and administrator
have had an equally broad influence on the
recent development of neurological surgery

Preface

The idea for this book was conceived in 1960 when I was a resident in surgery at the Duke University Medical Center. A short time before, after a stimulating clinical and research experience with Dr. Barnes Woodhall and Dr. Guy L. Odom, I had decided on a career in neurological surgery. Then at Christmas, Dr. Blaine S. Nashold, Jr. initiated my interest in the history of the specialty by giving me a copy of *The Torch* that was autographed by Dr. Wilder Penfield. As this interest grew, I began to think about collecting the classical works in neurosurgery for my library. It also occurred to me that such a collection, especially if it were accompanied by commentaries and lists of related references, might be of value to other students of neurosurgery as well. I approached Dr. Woodhall, at that time a member of the Editorial Board of the Journal of Neurosurgery, with this idea, and with his direction and support the project was begun.

In the selection of the Classics, an effort was made to include only works published before 1940. Areas in neurosurgery that have been developed since that time, such as isotope scanning, have not been included. In addition, many of the outstanding contributions made before 1940 were omitted for various reasons. Works relating to the development of anesthesia, antisepsis and asepsis were excluded because they are not unique to neurosurgery. Other contributions of prime importance were not included because of their length. A number of books were omitted for this reason, as well as the papers on electroencephalography by Hans Berger.

Many pioneering neurosurgeons are not represented in the collection of Classics because their major contributions were not made in written form. In addition, biographical material has been minimized in the present volume.

In some areas of neurosurgery it proved difficult to find single outstanding works suitable for reproduction. To correct this deficiency in part, a list of references in these areas has been included in the Appendix, which also contains a number of other supplementary references. In most part the references chosen for the appendix are in English, which is a reflection of my deficiencies in other languages.

The collection and synthesis of the material was carried out with the encouragement of Dr. Alfred S. Ketcham during my tenure as a Clinical Associate in the Surgery Branch of the National Cancer Institute, Bethesda, Maryland, from 1961 to 1963. In this undertaking I was given a great deal of assistance by Mrs. Thelma P. Robinson, Mrs. Everlyne K. Murdock, Mrs. Irene O. Jacobs, Mrs. Virginia L. Hudson, Mr. Redrick Rice, and Mr. William H. Everhardy of the Library Branch, and Mr. Roy Perry of the Medical Arts and Photography Branch of the Division of Research Services, National Institutes of Health. The personnel of the National Library of Medicine were also very helpful, and a large portion of my work was carried out in that fine library. The picture for the dust cover, for example, was obtained through the efforts of Dr. Peter D. Olch, from *Chirurgiae universalis opus absolutum*, Venice, Robertus Meietus, 1596, by Giovanni Andrea della Croce.

As it was completed, each of the Neurosurgical Classics was reviewed by Dr. Barnes Woodhall, Dr. Bronson S. Ray, Dr. David L. Reeves, Dr. Henry G. Schwartz, Dr. Eben Alexander, Jr., and Dr. Arthur A. Ward, Jr. of the Editorial Board of the JOURNAL OF NEUROSURGERY. Then with its acceptance, each was edited carefully by Dr. Louise Eisenhardt with the aid of Mrs. D. Harold Dennis. Dr. Eisenhardt spent many hours, in addition to those devoted to her usual responsibilities, in smoothing over the rough sentences, correcting the errors, verifying the many references, and preparing the manuscripts and photographs for the printer. Without her ability and personal interest this volume would not exist.

The printing of the separate Classics has been performed with skill and efficiency through the efforts of Mr. C. A. Wiese of the George Banta Company, Inc. of Menasha, Wisconsin. The present volume is the work of the Johnson Reprint Corporation of New York City. From the beginning, the collection, synthesis, editorial correction and publication of the material have been supervised by Dr. Paul C. Bucy. His wise advice has been appreciated greatly.

Finally, I am indebted to my wife, Gloria, for her interest, encouragement, and tolerance.

Robert H. Wilkins, M. D.
Durham, North Carolina
January, 1965

CONTENTS

NEUROSURGERY IN ANTIQUITY

The Edwin Smith surgical papyrus. *James Henry Breasted*...................... 1

On injuries of the head. *Hippocrates*.. 6

BASIC EXPERIMENTAL AND CLINICAL INVESTIGATIONS

The electrical excitability of the cerebrum. (Ueber die elektrische Erregbarkeit des Grosshirns). *G. Fritsch and E. Hitzig*.................................... 15

The basophil adenomas of the pituitary body and their clinical manifestations (pituitary basophilism). *Harvey Cushing*.................................... 28

Loss of speech, chronic softening and partial destruction of the left anterior lobe of the brain. (Perte de la parole, ramollissement chronique et destruction partielle du lobe antérieur gauche du cerveau). [*P.*] *Broca*........................... 61

New observation of aphemia produced by a lesion of the posterior half of the second and third frontal convolutions. (Nouvelle observation d'aphémie produite par une lésion de la moitié postérieure des deuxième et troisième circonvolutions frontales). *Paul Broca*.. 64

Internal hydrocephalus. An experimental, clinical and pathological study. *Walter E. Dandy and Kenneth D. Blackfan*.. 69

Discussion on the localization of function in the cortex cerebri. [*D.*] *Ferrier*........ 119

The dermatomes in man. *O. Foerster*.. 129

Decerebrate rigidity, and reflex coordination of movements. *C. S. Sherrington*.... 154

The structure and functions of the cerebellum examined by a new method. *Victor Horsley and R. H. Clarke*.. 162

Experimental alteration of brain bulk. *Lewis H. Weed and Paul S. McKibben*...... 186

Oligodendrogliomas of the brain. *Percival Bailey and Paul C. Bucy*............... 202

The cerebral cortex and consciousness. *Wilder Penfield*......................... 224

DIAGNOSTIC PROCEDURES AND TECHNIQUES

Ventriculography following the injection of air into the cerebral ventricles. *Walter E. Dandy*.. 242

Röntgenography of the brain after the injection of air into the spinal canal. *Walter E. Dandy*.. 251

General method of radiological exploration by iodized oil (lipiodol). [Méthode générale d'exploration radiologique par l'huile iodée (lipiodol)]. [*J.-A.*] *Sicard and* [*J.*] *Forestier*... 257

Iodinated organic compounds as contrast media for radiographic diagnoses. III. Experimental and clinical myelography with ethyl iodophenylundecylate (Pantopaque). *Theodore B. Steinhausen, Clarence E. Dungan, Joseph B. Furst, John T. Plati, S. Willard Smith, A. Perry Darling, E. Clinton Wolcott, Jr., Stafford L. Warren, and William H. Strain*.................................. 259

Arterial encephalography, its importance in the localization of cerebral tumors. (L'encéphalographie artérielle, son importance dans la localisation des tumeurs cérébrales). *Egas Moniz* 264

The description of an ophthalmoscope. (Beschreibung eines Augen-Spiegels zur Untersuchung der Netzhaut im lebenden Auge). *H. Helmholtz* 277

About the complication of inflammation of the optic nerve with diseases of the brain. (Ueber Complication von Sehnervenentzündung mit Gehirnkrankheiten). *A. v. Gräfe* 293

About hydrocephalus. (Ueber Hydrocephalus). *H. Quincke* 298

An aid to the diagnosis of spinal cord compression. (Zur Diagnose der Rückenmarks-kompression). [*H. H. G.*] *Queckenstedt* 309

A method for the localization of brain tumors—the pineal shift. *Howard C. Naffziger* 313

SURGICAL PROCEDURES AND TECHNIQUES—BASIC

Antiseptic wax. *Victor Horsley* 318

Note on haemostasis by application of living tissue. *Victor Horsley* 318

The control of bleeding in operations for brain tumors. With the description of silver "clips" for the occlusion of vessels inaccessible to the ligature. *Harvey Cushing* .. 319

Electro-surgery as an aid to the removal of intracranial tumors. With a preliminary note on a new surgical-current generator. *Harvey Cushing and W. T. Bovie* 329

SURGICAL PROCEDURES AND TECHNIQUES—CRANIOCEREBRAL

Case of cerebral tumour. *A. Hughes Bennett and Rickman J. Godlee* 361

Case of cerebral tumour. [Abst.] With discussion by Hughlings Jackson, David Ferrier, William Macewen, and Victor Horsley. *A. Hughes Bennett and Rickman J. Godlee* 372

Intra-cranial lesions, illustrating some points in connexion with the localisation of cerebral affections and the advantages of antiseptic trephining. III. Tumour of dura mater. *William Macewen* 374

Contribution to endocranial surgery. *F. Durante* 375

The temporary resection of the calvarium instead of trepanation. (Die temporäre Resektion des Schädeldaches an Stelle der Trepanation). *W. Wagner* 377

On the method of temporary cranial resection by means of my wire saw. (Zur Technik der temporären Schädelresektion mit meiner Drahtsäge). *Leonardo Gigli* 380

Technical methods of performing certain cranial operations. *Harvey Cushing* 383

A method of combining exploration and decompression for cerebral tumors which prove to be inoperable. *Harvey Cushing* 389

Pyogenic infective diseases of the brain and spinal cord. Meningitis, abscess of brain, infective sinus thrombosis. *William Macewen* 391

Remarks on the various surgical procedures devised for the relief or cure of trigeminal neuralgia (tic douloureux). *Victor Horsley, James Taylor, and Walter S. Colman* .. 404

Intracranial neurectomy of the second and third divisions of the fifth nerve. A new method. *Frank Hartley* 410

Excision of the gasserian ganglion and of the trigeminal trunk situated centrally from it. (Entfernung des Ganglion Gasseri und des central davon gelegenen Trigeminus-stammes). *Fedor Krause*.. 412

The division of the sensory root of the trigeminus for the relief of tic douloureux; an experimental, pathological and clinical study, with a preliminary report of one surgically successful case. *William G. Spiller and Charles H. Frazier*............ 418

Intracranial aneurysms: cerebral arterio-radiography: surgical treatment. *Norman M. Dott*.. 428

Intracranial aneurysm of the internal carotid artery. Cured by operation. *Walter E. Dandy*.. 437

Attempt at surgical treatment of certain psychoses. (Essai d'un traitement chirurgical de certaines psychoses). *Egas Moniz*.................................... 442

An operation for the total removal of cerebellopontile (acoustic) tumors. *Walter E. Dandy*.. 449

The surgical-mortality percentages pertaining to a series of two thousand verified intracranial tumours. *Harvey Cushing*..................................... 469

SURGICAL PROCEDURES AND TECHNIQUES—SPINAL

The treatment of persistent pain of organic origin in the lower part of the body by division of the anterolateral column of the spinal cord. *William G. Spiller and Edward Martin*.. 477

Experimental work on the function of the anterolateral column of the spinal cord. *Williams B. Cadwalader and J. E. Sweet*................................... 480

A case of tumour of the spinal cord. Removal; recovery. *W. R. Gowers and Victor Horsley*.. 484

Rupture of the intervertebral disc with involvement of the spinal canal. *William Jason Mixter and Joseph S. Barr*.. 495

A case in which acute spasmodic pain in the left lower extremity was completely relieved by sub-dural division of the posterior roots of certain spinal nerves, all other treatment having proved useless. Death from sudden collapse and cerebral haemorrhage on the twelfth day after the operation, at the commencement of apparent convalescence. *William H. Bennett*............................... 504

A contribution to the surgery of the spine. *Robert Abbe*....................... 512

APPENDIX OF ADDITIONAL REFERENCES............................. 516

INDEX.. 522

Neurosurgical Classic—1

THE Edwin Smith Surgical Papyrus, dating from the seventeenth century B.C., is one of the oldest of all known medical papyri.[1–12] Its differs fundamentally from the others in the following ways:

"1. The seventeen columns on the *recto* comprise part of a *surgical* treatise, the first thus far discovered in the ancient Orient, whether in Egypt or Asia. It is therefore the oldest known surgical treatise.

"2. This surgical treatise consists exclusively of *cases*, not recipes.

"3. The treatise is systematically organized in an arrangement of cases, which begin with injuries of the head and proceed downward through the body, like a modern treatise on anatomy.

"4. The treatment of these injuries is rational and chiefly surgical; there is resort to magic in only one case out of the forty-eight cases preserved.

"5. Each case is classified by one of three different verdicts: (1) favorable, (2) uncertain, or (3) unfavorable. The third verdict, expressed in the words, 'an ailment not to be treated,' is found in no other Egyptian medical treatise.

"6. This unfavorable verdict occurring fourteen times in the Edwin Smith Papyrus marks a group of cases (besides one more case) which the surgeon cannot cure and which he is led to discuss by his scientific interest in the phenomena disclosed by his examination."[1]

It is of special interest to the neurosurgeon because it contains the first descriptions of the cranial sutures, the meninges, the external surface of the brain, the cerebrospinal fluid, and the intracranial pulsations. It also contains the first accounts of surgical stitching and of various types of dressings. Brain injuries are noticed to be associated with changes in the function of other parts of the body, especially the lower limbs, and hemiplegic contractures are described in Case 8. Changes in bodily functions are also described in association with injuries of the cervical spine. Case 31 contains the first description of quadriplegia, urinary incontinence, priapism, and seminal emission following cervical vertebral dislocation.

The Egyptologist who brought this manuscript to light, Edwin Smith, was born in Connecticut in 1822, the year that Egyptian hieroglyphic was first deciphered. In Luxor, Egypt, in 1862, Smith bought an ancient manuscript roll which lacked some of its outer portions. Two months later the same vandals sold him the remaining fragments glued onto a dummy roll. Although Smith recognized the fraud, pieced the two together, and made an attempt at translation, it was not until 1930 that James H. Breasted translated the treatise and established its importance. Breasted was then Director of the University of Chicago Oriental Institute, and had been requested by the New York Historical Society to translate the papyrus, which the Society had received in 1906 from Edwin Smith's daughter.

According to Breasted, the Edwin Smith Papyrus is a copy of an ancient composite manuscript which contained, in addition to the original author's text (3000–2500 B.C.), a commentary added a few hundred years later in the form of 69 explanatory notes (glosses). It contains 48 systematically arranged case histories, beginning with injuries of the head and proceeding downward to the thorax and spine, where the document unfortunately breaks off. These cases are typical rather than individual, and each presentation of a case is divided into title, examination, diagnosis, and treatment. There is a definite differentiation between rational surgical treatments and the much less employed medico-magical measures. Significantly, trepanation is not mentioned.

The scribe who copied the Edwin Smith Papyrus from the earlier document in the seventeenth century B.C. made many errors some of which he corrected in the margins.

...ning and end of the original document are missing from the copy, and the name of the author is not present.

"The scribe of over 3,500 years ago, to whom we owe our present manuscript, could have had little consciousness of the momentous decision he, or possibly some one for him, was making when he pushed aside the ancient Surgical Treatise, then already a thousand years old, while his own copy was still incomplete. He had copied at least eighteen columns of the venerable treatise and had reached the bottom of a column when, pausing in the middle of a line, in the middle of a sentence, in the middle of a word, he . . . laid down his pen and pushed aside forever the great Surgical Treatise he had been copying, leaving 15½ inches (39 cm.) bare and unwritten at the end of his roll."[1]

Of the 48 cases described in the Edwin Smith Papyrus, 27 concern head trauma and 6 deal with spine trauma.[3] Of the 27 head injuries, 4 are deep scalp wounds exposing the skull, and 11 are skull fractures.

"The latter, according to our present day terminology would be classified as follows: two compound linear fractures; four compound depressed fractures; four compound comminuted fractures; and one comminuted fracture without external wound. The symptoms and signs of head injury are given in considerable detail. Feeble pulse and fever are associated with hopeless injuries and deafness as well as aphasia are recognized in fractures of the temporal region."[5]

The following thirteen cases are reproduced, in part, from Breasted's classic translation:[1]*

Case Two

Title: Instructions concerning a [gaping] wound [in his head], penetrating to the bone.

Examination: If thou examinest a man having a [gaping] wound [in] his [head], penetrating to the bone, thou shouldst lay thy hand upon it (and) [thou shouldst] pal[pate hi]s [wound]. If thou findest his skull [uninjured, not hav]ing a perforation in it . . .

Diagnosis: Thou shouldst say regarding [him]: "One hav[ing a gaping wou]nd in his head. An ailment which I will treat."

Treatment: [Thou] shouldst bind [fresh meat upon it the first day; thou shouldst apply for him two strips of linen, and treat afterward

* Reprinted in part from *The Edwin Smith Surgical Papyrus*. By James H. Breasted. *Chicago: Univ. Chicago Press*, 1930, 2 vols. With the kind permission of the University of Chicago Press.

with grease, honey, (and) lin]t every day until he recovers.

Gloss: As for: "Two strips of linen," [it means] two bands [of linen which one applies upon the two lips of the gaping wound in order to cause that one join] to the other.

Case Three

Title: [Instructions concerning] a gaping [wo]und in his head, penetrating to the bone (and) perforating his [skull].

Examination: [If thou examinest a man having a gaping wound in] his [head], penetrating to the bone, (and) perforating his skull; thou shouldst palpate his wound; [shouldst thou find him unable to look at his two shoulders] and his [br]east, (and) suffering with stiffness in his neck . . .

Diagnosis: Thou shouldst say [regarding] him: "One having [a gaping wound in his head, penetrating to the bone, (and) per]forating his skull, while he suffers with stiffness in his neck. An ailment which I will treat."

Treatment: Now [after thou has stitched it, thou shouldst lay] fresh [meat] upon his wound the first day. Thou shouldst not bind it. Moor (him) [at his mooring stakes until the period of his injury passes by]. Thou shouldst [tre]at it afterward with grease, honey, and lint every day, until he recovers . . .

Gloss: As for: "Moor (him) at his mooring stakes," it means putting him on his customary diet, without administering to him a prescription.

Case Four

Title: Instructions concerning a gaping wound in his head, penetrating to the bone, (and) splitting his skull.

Examination: If thou examinest a man having a gaping wound in his head, penetrating to the bone, (and) splitting his skull, thou shouldst palpate his wound. Shouldst thou find something disturbing therein under thy fingers, (and) he shudders exceedingly, while the swelling which is over it protrudes, he discharges blood from both his nostrils (and) from both his ears, he suffers with stiffness in his neck, so that he is unable to look at his two shoulders and his breast . . .

Diagnosis: Thou shouldst say regarding him: "One having a gaping wound in his head, penetrating to the bone, (and) splitting his skull; while he discharges blood from both his nostrils (and) from both his ears, (and) he suffers with stiffness in his neck. An ailment with which I will contend."

Treatment: Now when thou findest that the skull of that man is split, thou shouldst not bind him, (but) moor (him) at his mooring stakes until the period of his injury passes by. His treatment is sitting. Make for him two supports of brick, until thou knowest he has reached a decisive point. Thou shouldst apply grease to his head, (and) soften his neck therewith and both his shoulders. Thou shouldst do likewise for every man whom thou findest having a split skull . . .

Gloss: As for "(Until) thou knowest he has reached a decisive point," it means (until thou knowest whether he will die or he will live; for he is (a case of) "an ailment with which I will contend."

Case Five

Title: Instructions concerning a gaping wound in his head, smashing his skull.

Examination: If thou examinest a man having a gaping wound in his head, penetrating to the bone, (and) smashing his skull; thou shouldst palpate his wound. Shouldst thou find that smash which is in his skull deep (and) sunken under thy fingers, while the swelling which is over it protrudes, he discharges blood from both his nostrils (and) both his ears, (and) he suffers with stiffness in his neck, so that he is unable to look at his two shoulders and his breast . . .

Diagnosis: Thou shouldst say regarding him: "One having a gaping wound in his head, penetrating to the bone, (and) smashing his skull, while he suffers with stiffness in his neck. An ailment not to be treated."

Treatment: Thou shalt not bind him (but) moor (him) at his mooring stakes, until the period of his injury passes by . . .

Case Six

Title: Instructions concerning a gaping wound in his head, penetrating to the bone, smashing his skull, (and) rending open the brain of his skull.

Examination: If thou examinest a man having a gaping wound in his head, penetrating to the bone, smashing his skull, (and) rending open the brain of his skull, thou shouldst palpate his wound. Shouldst thou find that smash which is in his skull [like] those corrugations which form in molten copper, (and) something therein throbbing (and) fluttering under thy fingers, like the weak place of an infant's crown before it becomes whole—when it has happened there is no throbbing (and) fluttering under thy fingers until the brain of his (the patient's) skull is rent open—(and) he discharges blood from both his nostrils, (and) he suffers with stiffness in his neck . . .

Diagnosis: [Thou shouldst say concerning him]: "An ailment not to be treated."

Treatment: Thou shouldst anoint that wound with grease. Thou shalt not bind it; thou shalt not apply two strips upon it: until thou know-

est that he has reached a decisive point.

Gloss: As for: "Smashing his skull, (and) rending open the brain of his skull," (it means) the smash is large, opening to the interior of his skull, (to) the membrane enveloping his brain, so that it breaks open his fluid in the interior of his head. . . .

Case Eight

Title: Instructions concerning a smash in his skull under the skin of his head.

Examination: If thou examinest a man having a smash of his skull, under the skin of his head, while there is nothing at all upon it, thou shouldst palpate his wound. Shouldst thou find that there is a swelling protruding on the outside of that smash which is in his skull, while his eye is askew because of it, on the side of him having that injury which is in his skull; (and) he walks shuffling with his sole, on the side of him having that injury which is in his skull . . .

Diagnosis: Thou shouldst account him one whom something entering from outside has smitten, as one who does not release the head of his shoulder-fork, and one who does not fall with his nails in the middle of his palm; while he discharges blood from both his nostrils (and) from both his ears, (and) he suffers with stiffness in his neck. An ailment not to be treated.

Treatment: His treatment is sitting, until he [gains color], (and) until thou knowest he has reached the decisive point. . . .

Gloss: As for: "He walks shuffling with his sole," he (the surgeon) is speaking about his walking with his sole dragging, so that it is not easy for him to walk, when it (the sole) is feeble and turned over, while the tips of his toes are contracted to the ball of his sole, and they (the toes) walk fumbling the ground. He (the surgeon) says: "He shuffles," concerning it . . .

Case Twenty

Title: Instructions concerning a wound in his temple, penetrating to the bone, (and) perforating his temporal bone.

Examination: If thou examinest a man having a wound in his temple, penetrating to the bone, (and) perforating his temporal bone, while his two eyes are blood-shot, he discharges blood from both his nostrils, and a little drops; if thou puttest thy fingers on the mouth of that wound (and) he shudder exceedingly; if thou ask of him concerning his malady and he speak not to thee; while copious tears fall from both his eyes, so that he thrusts his hand often to his face that he may wipe both his eyes with the back of his hand as a child does, and knows not that he does so . . .

Diagnosis: Thou shouldst say concerning him: "One having a wound in his temple, penetrating to the bone, (and) perforating his temporal bone; while he discharges blood from both his nostrils, he suffers with stiffness in his neck, (and) he is speechless. An ailment not to be treated."

Treatment: Now when thou findest that man speechless, his [relief] shall be sitting; soften his head with grease, (and) pour [milk] into both his ears.

Case Twenty-two

Title: Instructions concerning a smash in his temple.

Examination: If thou examinest a man having a smash in his temple, thou shouldst place thy thumb upon his chin (and) thy finger upon the end of his ramus, so that the blood will flow from his two nostrils (and) from the interior of his ear having that smash. Cleanse (it) for him with a swab of linen until thou seest its fragments (of bone) in the interior of his ear. If thou callest to him (and) he is speechless (and) cannot speak . . .

Diagnosis: Thou shouldst say concerning him: "One having a smash in his temple; he discharges blood from his two nostrils and from his ear; he is speechless; (and) he suffers with stiffness in his neck. An ailment not to be treated." . . .

Gloss: As for: "Thou seest its fragments in the interior of his ear," it means that some of the fragments of the bone come away to adhere to the swab which was introduced to cleanse the interior of his ear.

Case Twenty-nine

Title: Instructions concerning a gaping wound in a vertebra of his neck.

Examination: If thou examinest a man having a gaping wound in a vertebra of his neck, penetrating to the bone, (and) perforating a vertebra of his neck; if thou examinest that wound, (and) he shudders exceedingly, (and) he is unable to look at his two shoulders and his breast . . .

Diagnosis: Thou shouldst say concerning him: "[One having] a wound in his neck, penetrating to the bone, perforating a vertebra of his neck, (and) he suffers with stiffness in his neck. An ailment with which I will contend."

Treatment: Thou shouldst bind it with fresh meat the first day. Now afterward moor (him) at his mooring stakes until the period of his injury passes by.

Case Thirty

Title: Instructions concerning a sprain in a vertebra of his neck.

Examination: If thou examinest a man having a sprain in a vertebra of his neck, thou shouldst say to him: "Look at thy two shoulders and thy breast." When he does so, the seeing possible to him is painful.

Diagnosis: Thou shouldst say concerning him: "One having a sprain in a vertebra of his neck. An ailment which I will treat."

Treatment: Thou shouldst bind it with fresh meat the first day. Now afterward thou shouldst treat [with] *ymrw* (and) honey every day until he recovers.

Gloss: As for: "A sprain," he is speaking of a rending of two members (although) it (=each) is (still) in its place.

Case Thirty-one

Title: Instructions concerning a dislocation in a vertebra of [his] neck.

Examination: If thou examinest a man having a dislocation in a vertebra of his neck, shouldst thou find him unconscious of his two arms (and) his two legs on account of it, while his phallus is erected on account of it, (and) urine drops from his member without his knowing it; his flesh has received wind; his two eyes are blood-shot; it is a dislocation of a vertebra of his neck extending to his backbone which causes him to be unconscious of his two arms (and) his two legs. If, however, the middle vertebra of his neck is dislocated, it is an *emissio seminis* which befalls his phallus.

Diagnosis: Thou shouldst say concerning him: "One having a dislocation in a vertebra of his neck, while he is unconscious of his two legs and his two arms, and his urine dribbles. An ailment not to be treated."

Gloss: As for: "A dislocation in a vertebra of his neck," he is speaking of a separation of one vertebra of his neck from another, the flesh which is over it being uninjured; as one says, "It is *wnh*," concerning things which had been joined together, when one has been severed from another.

Case Thirty-three

Title: Instructions concerning a crushed vertebra in his neck.

Examination: If thou examinest a man having a crushed vertebra in his neck (and) thou findest that one vertebra has fallen into the next one, while he is voiceless and cannot speak; his falling head downward has caused that one vertebra crush into the next one; (and) shouldst thou find that he is unconscious of his two arms and his two legs because of it . . .

Diagnosis: Thou shouldst say concerning him: "One having a crushed vertebra in his neck; he is unconscious of his two arms (and) his two legs, (and) he is speechless. An ailment not to be treated." . . .

Gloss: As for: "His falling head downward has

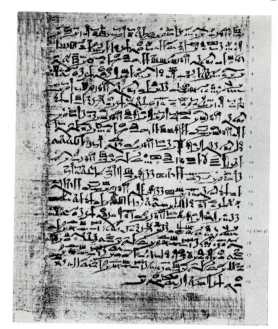

FIG. 1. Cases 47 and 48 in the Edwin Smith Surgical Papyrus. (Plate XVII from Breasted.[1])

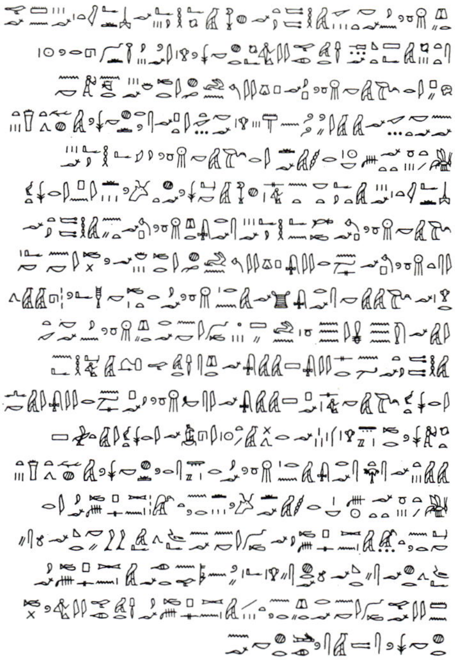

FIG. 2. Hieroglyphic interpretation of Cases 47 and 48. (Plate XVIIA from Breasted.[1])

caused that one vertebra crush into the next," it means that he has fallen head downward upon his head, driving one vertebra of his neck into the next.

Case Forty-eight

Title: Instructions concerning a sprain of a vertebra [in] his spinal column.

Examination: If thou examinest [a man having] a sprain in a vertebra of his spinal column, thou shouldst say to him: "Extend now thy two legs (and) contract them both (again)." When he extends them both he contracts them both immediately because of the pain he causes in the vertebra of his spinal column in which he suffers.

Diagnosis: Thou shouldst say concerning him: "One having a sprain in a vertebra of his spinal column. An ailment which I will treat."

Treatment: Thou shouldst place him prostrate on his back; thou shouldst make for him. . . .

References

1. BREASTED, J. H. The Edwin Smith surgical papyrus. Chicago: Univ. Chicago Press, 1930, 2 vols. (see 1: pp. xvi, 6, 430–435, 437–439, 446–448, 451–454, 466; 2: pl. XVII, XVIIA).
2. CASTIGLIONI, A. A history of medicine. E. B. Krumbhaar, Transl. New York: A. A. Knopf, 1947, 2nd ed., xxx, 1192, lxi pp. (see pp. 55–57).
3. ELSBERG, C. A. The Edwin Smith surgical papyrus and the diagnosis and treatment of injuries to the skull and spine 5000 years ago. Ann. med. Hist., 1931, n.s. 3: 271–279.
4. ELSBERG, C. A. The anatomy and surgery of the Edwin Smith surgical papyrus. J. Mt. Sinai Hosp., 1945, 12: 141–151.
5. HORRAX, G. Neurosurgery. An historical sketch. Springfield, Ill.: Charles C Thomas, 1952, xi, 135 pp. (see pp. 12–16).
6. KHARADLY, M. E. A. Surgery in ancient Egypt. J. int. Coll. Surg., 1957, 28: 491–500.
7. METTLER, C. C. History of medicine. A correlative text, arranged according to subjects. F. A. Mettler, Ed. Philadelphia: Blakiston Co., 1947, xxix, 1215 pp. (see pp. 795–797).
8. O'CONNOR, D. C., and WALKER, A. E. Prologue. In: A history of neurological surgery. A. E. Walker, Ed. Baltimore: Williams & Wilkins Co., 1951, xii, 583 pp. (see pp. 1–22).
9. POWER, D'A. Some early surgical cases. I. The Edwin Smith papyrus. Brit. J. Surg., 1933, 21: 1–4.
10. POWER, D'A. Some early surgical cases. II. The Edwin Smith papyrus. Brit. J. Surg., 1934, 21: 385–387.
11. SACHS, E. The history and development of neurological surgery. New York: P. B. Hoeber, Inc., 1952, 158 pp. (see pp. 21–23).
12. WILSON, J. A. Medicine in ancient Egypt. Bull. Hist. Med., 1962, 36: 114–123.

Neurosurgical Classic—2

OR more than twenty centuries the writings of Hippocrates have exerted an influence on the practice of medicine. Few other individuals have added so significantly to medical knowledge. However, little is known about the personal life of Hippocrates, and his influence has been due mainly to the inherent worth of the writings attributed to him.[7,24,28,40]

"The number of writings that are ascribed to Hippocrates differs considerably according to the criteria used. Littré, who certainly was the most authoritative of the students and interpreters of Hippocrates, counts 53 subjects in 72 books. . . . The definitive editing and combination of all these writings under the name of Hippocrates dates from the third century B.C., when, at the command of the Egyptian *diadochi*, they were collected for the Library of Alexandria. . . .

"There is no doubt whatever that in this collection there are works coming from authors of different periods and schools. In the editing and style there are manifest divergences and even opposite statements about the same subject in different Hippocratic texts. It is evident, then, . . . that, as has happened with many classical texts of antiquity, the books of Hippocrates, collected and codified at Alexandria, represent in reality an agglomeration of works coming from various sources, most of which reflect the direct influence of the individuality of Hippocrates and his school. . . . "[5]

"English translations of Hippocrates were incomplete and unsatisfactory until The Sydenham Society of England commissioned Francis Adams, a Scottish surgeon, in the early nineteenth century, to make a translation. His book was first published in 1849, again in 1886 and in 1929. It is a scholarly work with numerous and extensive foot-notes. . . . "[17]

In his various writings, Hippocrates dealt with several subjects of neurosurgical interest. Among other things, he discussed epilepsy,[2,16,18—20,25,29—31] the coexistence of spinal deformity with pulmonary tubercles,[11] and the functional effects of compression of the spinal cord.[20] He devised a method of reducing vertebral dislocations,[20] and mentioned trephining as a cure for blindness without

evident ocular disease.[3] He also described permanent and transient facial paralyses, sciatica, the condition later known as Raynaud's disease, and the complex of headache, visual disturbance, and vomiting.[20]

"Judged by modern standards, the Hippocratic writers were surprisingly ignorant of all but surface anatomy. This was the natural result of the fact that Hippocratic medicine was based upon humoral rather than structural pathology. Indeed, no urgent need for anatomic information was perceived until the influence of the humoral theory had been dissipated. The anatomy of the Hippocratic treatise *On head injuries*, which contains most of the information of the early Greeks upon this subject, is no exception to this rule and reveals at best an approximate, and often incorrect, knowledge of the skull and its contents. While parts of the initial passage, which deals with the arrangement of the sutures, are admissible the passage as a whole is excessively vague and did more to confuse the subsequent literature than to clarify treatment. It states . . . that if the head shows a frontal prominence the sutures take the form of the letter T, with the long limb running down the neck. If an occipital protuberance presents itself, the long limb of the T is reversed and runs down to the brow, as in the metopic suture. If both occipital and frontal protuberances are present the sutures are arranged in the form of the letter H and, if no prominence occurs, in the form of X. Aristotle, Pliny, Galen, Avicenna, Vesalius and Paré were all disposed to accept this strange version which may have been the result of examination of fractured and weather-beaten enemy skulls on the battlefields of Greece. . . . "[21]

Despite their anatomical errors, the writings of Hippocrates dealing with head injuries greatly influenced the treatment of these injuries until the nineteenth century.[4,36] The ability of Hippocrates as an observer is well demonstrated by his descriptions of aphasia, unconsciousness, respiratory and cardiac irregularity, carphologia, hippus, pupillary inequality, and ophthalmoplegia associated with cerebral disease.[20] He realized that a blow on one side of the head occasionally is followed by convulsions or paralysis of the contralateral side of the body,[3,10,32] and he recognized the poor prognosis of a patient with a head injury complicated by a dural laceration.[27] Hippocrates also was aware of the danger of an initial period of unconsciousness following a head injury.[20]

"... To Hippocrates ... the presence of a skull fracture was a matter of great seriousness and required immediate attention. For untreated, the condition would result in fever in seven days in summer or fourteen days in winter, followed by local changes in the wound, convulsions and death. ...

"In the discussion of wounds of the head, the emphasis was upon fractures which were classified as fissured, contused, depressed, dinted (hedra) and contrecoup fractures. Of these, the fissured, dinted and contused required trephining, rarely the depressed fractures. If a fracture was not evident upon inspection, Hippocrates advised applying a cataplasm and a sooty oil to the area. If, on the following day, the black line of the fracture was visible, a raspatory was to be used to scrape away the bone until it was no longer visible.[36]

"... Hippocrates recommended the operation of perforating the cranium, in cases of simple fractures and contusions, whenever he apprehended that these would be followed by serious consequences, such as inflammation, extravasation of blood, and the effusion of matter ... Hippocrates operated in these cases during the first three days, before any serious symptoms had come on. ...'[1]

"... His instructions for the use of the trepan were most precise. The opening should not be made over the cranial sutures, for the membranes, being adherent, were likely to be damaged. The temporal region was to be avoided also for fear of damaging the vessel (middle meningeal artery?) which might lead to convulsions on the opposite side of the body. Hippocrates warned that the trephine should be repeatedly removed from the skull and cooled with water during the procedure and the incision examined to be sure the dura mater was not reached. He believed that a thin shell of inner table should be left to protect the membrane. The bone would later extrude itself as suppuration developed."[22]

A large number of the observations by Hippocrates on head injuries and their treatment are contained in his work, *On Injuries of the Head*,[1,12,13] which is judged today as genuinely Hippocratic.[5,40] Although certain of these observations were not original,[38] and despite the fact that forms of trephination had been carried out since prehistoric times,[6,8,9,14,15,21–23,26,27,33–35,37,39] Hippocrates performed a valuable service. He added his

many original observations to this preexisting knowledge and organized it into a meaningful whole.[3] This work was a beacon to surgeons for over 2000 years, until the development of anesthesia, asepsis, and cerebral localization in the nineteenth century established the foundation of modern neurosurgery.

References

1. ADAMS, F. On injuries of the head. The argument. In: Hippocrates[12] (see *1*: 353–370).
2. ADAMS, F. On the sacred disease. The argument. In: Hippocrates[12] (see *2*: 327–334).
3. BALLANCE, C. The Thomas Vicary lecture: a glimpse into the history of the surgery of the brain. *Lancet*, 1922, *1*: 111–116; 165–172.
4. BOWMAN, A. K. The life and teaching of Sir William Macewen. A chapter in the history of surgery. *London: W. Hodge & Co., Ltd.*, 1942, x, 425 pp. (see pp. 250–251).
5. CASTIGLIONI, A. A history of medicine. E. B. Krumbhaar, Transl. *New York: A. A. Knopf*, 1941, xxviii, 1013, xl pp. (see pp. 151–153).
6. CHIPAULT, A. Chirurgie opératoire du système nerveux. *Paris: Rueff & Cie*, 1894–1895, 2 vols. (see *1*: 1–38).
7. CLENDENING, L. Source book of medical history. *New York: P. B. Hoeber, Inc.*, 1942, xiv, 685 pp. (see pp. 13–14).
8. DALAND, J. Depressed fracture and trephining of the skull by the Incas of Peru. *Ann. med. Hist.*, 1935, n.s. *7*: 550–558.
9. ENGLAND, I. A. Trephining through the ages. *Radiography*, 1962, *28*: 301–314.
10. GARRISON, F. H. History of neurology. In: *Textbook of nervous diseases for the use of students and practitioners of medicine.* C. L. Dana, Ed. New York: W. Wood & Co., 1925, 10th ed., lvi, 667 pp. (see pp. xv–lvi).
11. GARRISON, F. H. An introduction to the history of medicine with medical chronology, suggestions for study and bibliographic data. *Philadelphia: W. B. Saunders Co.*, 1929, 4th ed., 996 pp. (see pp. 92–101).
12. HIPPOCRATES. The genuine works of Hippocrates. Translated from the Greek with a preliminary discourse and annotations by Francis Adams. *New York: W. Wood & Co.*, 1886, 2 vols. in one (see *1*: 370–390; *2*: 334–346).
13. HIPPOCRATES. On injuries of the head. *Med. Classics*, 1938, *3*: 145–160.
14. HORRAX, G. Neurosurgery. An historical sketch. *Springfield, Ill.: Charles C Thomas*, 1952, xi, 135 pp. (see pp. 5–16).
15. HORSLEY, V. Brain surgery in the stone age. *Brit. med. J.*, 1887, *1*: 582.
16. KANNER, L. The folklore and cultural history of epilepsy. *Med. Life*, 1930, *37*: 167–214.
17. KELLY, E. C., Compiler. Works of Hippocrates. Introduction. *Med. Classics*, 1938, *3*: iii–vi.
18. LENNOX, W. G. Epilepsy. In: The history and conquest of common diseases. W. R. Bett, Ed. *Norman, Okla.: Univ. of Oklahoma Press*, 1954, ix, 334 pp. (see pp. 243–259).

19. Marshall, C. Surgery of epilepsy and motor disorders. In: *A history of neurological surgery.* A. E. Walker, Ed. Baltimore: Williams & Wilkins Co., 1951, xii, 583 pp. (see pp. 288–305).

20. Mettler, C. C. History of medicine. A correlative text, arranged according to subjects. F. A. Mettler, Ed. *Philadelphia: Blakiston Co.,* 1947, xxix, 1215 pp. (see pp. 490–493; 801–802).

21. Mettler, F. A., and Mettler, C. C. Historic development of knowledge relating to cranial trauma. *Res. Publ. Ass. nerv. ment. Dis.,* 1945, *24:* 1–47.

22. O'Connor, D. C., and Walker, A. E. Prologue. In: *A history of neurological surgery.* A. E. Walker, Ed. Baltimore: Williams & Wilkins Co., 1951, xii, 583 pp. (see pp. 1–22).

23. Parry, T. W. Trephination of the living human skull in prehistoric times. *Brit. med. J.,* 1923, *1:* 457–460.

24. Penfield, W. The torch. *Boston: Little, Brown & Co.,* 1960, xiv, 370 pp.

25. Riese, W. A history of neurology. *New York: MD Publications, Inc.,* 1959, 223 pp. (see pp. 78–79).

26. Rogers, L. The history of craniotomy: an account of the methods which have been practiced and the instruments used for opening the human skull during life. *Ann. med. Hist.,* 1930, n.s. *2:* 495–514.

27. Sachs, E. The history and development of neurological surgery. *New York: P. B. Hoeber, Inc.,* 1952, 158 pp. (see pp. 17–28).

28. Sigerist, H. E. On Hippocrates. *Bull. Inst. Hist. Med.,* 1934, *2:* 190–214.

29. von Storch, T. C. An essay on the history of epilepsy. *Ann. med. Hist.,* 1930, n.s. *2:* 614–650.

30. Streeter, E. C. A note on the history of the convulsive state prior to Boerhaave. *Res. Publ. Ass. nerv. ment. Dis.,* 1931, *7:* 5–29.

31. Temkin, O. The falling sickness. A history of epilepsy from the Greeks to the beginnings of modern neurology. *Baltimore: Johns Hopkins Press,* 1945, xv, 380 pp.

32. Thomas, H. M. Decussation of the pyramids—an historical inquiry. *Johns Hopk. Hosp. Bull.,* 1910, *21:* 304–311.

33. Thompson, C. J. S. The history and evolution of surgical instruments. *New York: Schuman's,* 1942, 113 pp.

34. Torkildsen, A. Trekk av hjernekirurgiens historie. *Tidsskr. norske Laegeforen.,* 1948, *68:* 328–332.

35. Trelles, J. O. Cranial trepanation in ancient Peru. *World Neurol.,* 1962, *3:* 538–545.

36. Walker, A. E. Surgery of craniocerebral trauma. In: *A history of neurological surgery.* A. E. Walker, Ed. Baltimore: Williams & Wilkins Co., 1951, xii, 583 pp. (see pp. 216–247).

37. Walker, A. E. The dawn of neurosurgery. *Clin. Neurosurg.,* 1959, *6:* 1–38.

38. Wilkins, R. H. Neurosurgical classic—XVII. *J. Neurosurg.,* 1964, *21:* 240–244.

39. Young, A. The limitations of surgery, past and present. *Glasg. med. J.,* 1924, *102:* 273–313.

40. Zimmerman, L. M., and Veith, I. Great ideas in the history of surgery. *Baltimore: Williams & Wilkins Co.,* 1961, xii, 587 pp. (see pp. 14–27).

On Injuries of the Head*

 EN'S heads are by no means all like to one another, nor are the sutures of the head of all men constructed in the same form. Thus, whoever has a prominence in the anterior part of the head (by prominence is meant the round protuberant part of the bone which projects beyond the rest of it), in him the sutures of the head take the form of the Greek letter *tau*, T; for the head has the shorter line running transverse before the prominence, while the other line runs through the middle of the head, all the way to the neck. But whoever has the prominence in the back part of the head, in him the sutures are constructed in quite the opposite form to the former; for in this case the shorter line runs in front of the prominence, while the longer runs through the middle all along to the forehead. But whoever has a prominence of the head both before and behind, in him the sutures resemble the Greek letter *êta* H; for the long lines of the letter run transverse before each prominence while the short one runs through the middle and terminates in the long lines. But whoever has no prominence on either part he has the sutures of the head resembling the Greek letter χ; for the one line comes transverse to the temple while the other passes along the middle of the head. The bone at the middle of the head is double, the hardest and most compact part being the upper portion, where it is connected with the skin, and the lowest, where it is connected with the meninx (dura mater); and from the uppermost and lowermost parts the bone gradually becomes softer and less compact, till you come to the *diploe.* The diploe is the most porous, the softest, and most cavernous part. But the whole bone of the head, with the exception of a small portion of the uppermost and lowermost portions of it, is like a sponge; and the bone has in it many juicy substances, like caruncles; and if one will rub them with the fingers, some blood will issue from them. There are also in the bone certain very slender and hollow vessels full of blood. So it is with regard to hardness, softness, and porosity.

* Reprinted from *Medical Classics,* 1938, *3:* 145–160, with the kind permission of the Williams & Wilkins Company.

2. In respect to thickness and thinness; the thinnest and weakest part of the whole head is the part about the bregma; and the bone there has the smallest and thinnest covering of flesh upon it, and the largest proportion of brain is situated in that region of the head. And hence it happens that from similar or even smaller wounds and instruments, when a person is wounded to the same or a less degree, the bone of the head there is more contused, fractured, and depressed; and that injuries there are more deadly and more difficult to cure; and it is more difficult to save one's life in injuries there than in any other part of the head; that from having sustained a similar or even a less wound a man will die, and that, too, in a shorter space of time than from a wound in any other part of the head. For the brain about the bregma feels more quickly and strongly any mischief that may occur to the flesh or the bone; for the brain about the bregma is in largest quantity, and is covered by the thinnest bone and the least flesh. Of the other portions, the weakest is that about the temples; for it is the conjunction of the lower jaw with the cranium, and there is motion there up and down as at a joint; and the organ of hearing is near it; and further, a hollow and important vein runs along the temple. But the whole bone of the head behind the vertex and the ear is stronger than the whole anterior part, and the bone itself has a larger and deeper covering of flesh upon it. And hence it follows, that when exposed to the same or even greater injuries from instruments of the same or greater size, the bone is less liable to be fractured and depressed than elsewhere; and that in a fatal accident the patient will live longer when the wound is in the posterior part of the head than when elsewhere; and that pus takes longer time to form and penetrate through the bone to the brain, owing to the thickness of the bone; and moreover, as there is less brain in that part of the head, more persons who are wounded in the back part of the head escape than of those who are wounded in the anterior part. And in fatal cases, a man will survive longer in winter than in summer, whatever be the part of the head in which the wound is situated.

3. As to the *hœdræ* (dints *or* marks?) of sharp and light weapons, when they take place in the bone without fissure, contusion, or depression inwards (and these take place equally in the anterior and posterior part of the head), death, when it does occur, does not properly result from them. A suture appearing in a wound, when the bone is laid bare, on whatever part of the head the wound may have been inflicted, is the weakest point of the head to resist a blow or a weapon, when the weapon happens to be impinged into the suture itself; but more especially when this occurs in the bregma at the weakest part of the head, and the sutures happen to be situated near the wound,

and the weapon has hit the sutures themselves.

4. The bone in the head is liable to be wounded in the following modes, and there are many varieties in each of these modes of fracture: When a wounded bone breaks, in the bone comprehending the fissure, contusion necessarily takes place where the bone is broken; for an instrument that breaks the bone occasions a contusion thereof more or less, both at the fracture and in the parts of the bone surrounding the fracture. This is the first mode. But there are all possible varieties of fissures; for some of them are fine, and so very fine that they cannot be discovered, either immediately after the injury, or during the period in which it would be of use to the patient if this could be ascertained. And some of these fissures are thicker and wider, certain of them being very wide. And some of them extend to a greater, and some to a smaller, distance. And some are more straight, nay, completely straight; and some are more curved, and that in a remarkable degree. And some are deep, so as to extend downwards and through the whole bone; and some are less so, and do not penetrate through the whole bone.

5. But a bone may be contused, and yet remain in its natural condition without any fracture in it; this is the second mode. And there are many varieties of contusion; for they occur to a greater and less degree, and to a greater depth, so as sometimes to extend through the whole bone; or to a less depth, so as not to extend through the whole bone; and to a greater and smaller length and breadth. But it is not possible to recognize any of these varieties by the sight, so as to determine their form and extent; neither, indeed, is it visible to the eyes when any mischief of this kind takes place, and immediately after the injury, whether or not the bone has been actually bruised, as is likewise the case with certain fractures at a distance from the seat of injury.

6. And the bone being fractured, is sometimes depressed inwards from its natural level along with the fractures, otherwise there would be no depression; for the depressed portion being fractured and broken off, is pushed inwards, while the rest of the bone remains in its natural position; and in this manner a fracture is combined with the depression. This is the third mode. There are many varieties of depression, for it may comprehend a greater and a small extent of bone, and may either be to a greater depth, or less so, and more superficial.

7. When a *hedra*, or dint of a weapon, takes place in a bone, there may be a fracture combined with it; and provided there be a fracture, contusion must necessarily be joined, to a greater or less extent, in the seat of the dint and fracture, and in the bone which comprehends them. This is the fourth mode. And there may be a *hedra*, or indentation of the bone, along with contusion of the

surrounding bone, but without any fracture either in the *hedra* or in the contusion inflicted by the weapon. But the indentation of a weapon takes place in a bone, and is called *hedra*, when the bone remaining in its natural state, the weapon which struck against the bone leaves its impression on the part which it struck. In each of these modes there are many varieties, with regard to the contusion and fracture, if both these be combined with the *hedra*, or if contusion alone, as it has been already stated that there are many varieties of contusion and fracture. And the *hedra*, *or* dint, of itself may be longer and shorter, crooked, straight, and circular; and there are many varieties of this mode, according to the shape of the weapon; and they may be more or less deep, and narrower or broader, and extremely broad. When a part is cleft, the cleft or notch which occurs in the bone, to whatever length or breadth, is a *hedra*, if the other bones comprehending the cleft remain in their natural position, and be not driven inwards; for in this case it would be a depression, and no longer a *hedra*.

8. A bone may be injured in a different part of the head from that on which the person has received the wound, and the bone has been laid bare. This is the fifth mode. And for this misfortune, when it occurs, there is no remedy; for when this mischief takes place, there is no means of ascertaining by any examination whether or not it has occurred, or on what part of the head.

9. Of these modes of fracture, the following require trepanning: the contusion, whether the bone be laid bare or not; and the fissure, whether apparent or not. And if, when an indentation (*hedra*) by a weapon takes place in a bone it be attended with fracture and contusion, and even if contusion alone, without fracture, be combined with the indentation, it requires trepanning. A bone depressed from its natural position rarely requires trepanning; and those which are most pressed and broken require trepanning the least; neither does an indentation (*hedra*) without fracture and contusion require trepanning; nor does a notch, provided it is large and wide; for a notch and a *hedra* are the same.

10. In the first place, one must examine the wounded person, in what part of the head the wound is situated, whether in the stronger or weaker parts; and ascertain respecting the hairs about the wound, whether they have been cut off by the instrument, and have gone into the wound; and if so, one should declare that the bone runs the risk of being denuded of flesh, and of having sustained some injury from the weapon. These things one should say from a distant inspection, and before laying a hand on the man; but on a close examination one should endeavor to ascertain clearly whether the bone be denuded of flesh or not; and if the denuded bone be visible to the

eyes, this will be enough; but otherwise an examination must be made with the sound. And if you find the bone denuded of the flesh, and not safe from the wound, you must first ascertain the state of the bone, and the extent of the mischief, and what assistance it stands in need of. One should also inquire of the wounded person how and in what way he sustained the injury; and if it be not apparent whether the bone has sustained an injury or not, it will be still more necessary, provided the bone be denuded, to make inquiry how the wound occurred, and in what manner; for when contusions and fractures exist in the bone, but are not apparent, we must ascertain, in the first place from the patient's answers, whether or not the bone has sustained any such injuries, and then find out the nature of the case by word and deed, with the exception of sounding. For sounding does not discover to us whether the bone has sustained any of these injuries or not; but sounding discovers to us an identation inflicted by a weapon, and whether a bone be depressed from its natural position, and whether the bone be strongly fractured; all which may also be ascertained visibly with the eyes.

11. And a bone sustains fractures, either so fine as to escape the sight, or such as are apparent, and contusions which are not apparent, and depression from its natural position, especially when one person is intentionally wounded by another, or when, whether intentionally or not, a blow or stroke is received from an elevated place, and if the instrument in the hand, whether used in throwing or striking, be of a powerful nature, and if a stronger person wound a weaker. Of those who are wounded in the parts about the bone, or in the bone itself, by a fall, he who falls from a very high place upon a very hard and blunt object is in most danger of sustaining a fracture and contusion of the bone, and of having it depressed from its natural position; whereas he that falls upon more level ground, and upon a softer object, is likely to suffer less injury in the bone, or it may not be injured at all. Of those instruments which, falling upon the head, wound the parts about the bone, or the bone itself, that which falls from a very high place, and the least on a level with the person struck, and which is at the same time very hard, very blunt, and very heavy, and which is the least light, sharp, and soft, such an instrument would occasion a fracture and contusion of the bone. And there is most danger that the bone may sustain these injuries, under such circumstances, when the wound is direct and perpendicular to the bone, whether struck from the hand or from a throw, or when any object falls upon the person, or when he is wounded by falling, or in whatever way the bone sustains a direct wound from this instrument. Those weapons which graze the bone obliquely are less apt to fracture, con-

tuse, or depress the bone, even when the bone is denuded of flesh; for in some of those wounds thus inflicted the bone is not laid bare of the flesh. Those instruments more especially produce fractures in the bone, whether apparent or not, and contusions, and inward depression of the bone, which are rounded, globular, smooth on all sides, blunt, heavy, and hard; and such weapons bruise, compress, and pound the flesh; and the wounds inflicted by such instruments, whether obliquely or circularly, are round, and are more disposed to suppurate, and to have a discharge, and take longer time to become clean; for the flesh which has been bruised and pounded must necessarily suppurate and slough away. But weapons of an oblong form, being, for the most part, slender, sharp, and light, penetrate the flesh rather than bruise it, and the bone in like manner; and such an instrument may occasion a *hedra* and a cut (for a *hedra* and a cut are same thing); but weapons of this description do not produce contusions, nor fractures, nor depressions inwardly. And in addition to the appearances in the bone, which you can detect by the sight, you should make inquiry as to all these particulars (for they are symptoms of a greater or less injury), whether the wounded person was stunned, and whether darkness was diffused over his eyes, and whether he had vertigo, and fell to the ground.

12. When the bone happens to be denuded of flesh by the weapon, and when the wound occurs upon the sutures, it is difficult to distinguish the indentation (*hedra*) of a weapon which is clearly recognized in other parts of the bone, whether it exist or not, and especially if the *hedra* be seated in the sutures themselves. For the suture being rougher than the rest of the bone occasions confusion, and it is not clear which is the suture, and which the mark inflicted by the instrument, unless the latter (*hedra*) be large. Fracture also for the most part is combined with the indentation when it occurs in the sutures; and this fracture is more difficult to discern when the bone is broken, on this account, that if there be a fracture, it is situated for the most part in the suture. For the bone is liable to be broken and slackened there, owing to the natural weakness of the bone there, and to its porosity, and from the suture being readily ruptured and slackened: but the other bones which surround the suture remain unbroken, because they are stronger than the suture. For the fracture which occurs at the suture is also a slackening of the suture, and it is not easy to detect whether the bone be broken and slackened by the indentation of a weapon occurring in the suture, or from a contusion of the bone at the sutures; but it is still more difficult to detect a fracture connected with contusion. For the sutures, having the appearance of fissures, elude the discernment and sight of the physician, as being rougher than the rest of the bone, unless the bone be strongly cut and slackened, (for a cut and a *hedra* are the same thing). But it is necessary, if the wound has occurred at the sutures, and the weapon has impinged on the bone or the parts about it, to pay attention and find out what injury the bone has sustained. For a person wounded to the same, or a much smaller, extent, and by weapons of the same size and quality, and even much less, will sustain a much greater injury, provided he has received the blow at the sutures, than if it was elsewhere. And many of these require trepanning, but you must not apply the trepan to the sutures themselves, but on the adjoining bone.

13. And with regard to the cure of wounds in the head, and the mode of detecting injuries in the bone which are not apparent, the following is my opinion:—In a wound of the head, you must not apply anything liquid, not even wine, but as little as possible, nor a cataplasm, nor conduct the treatment with tents, nor apply a bandage to an ulcer on the head, unless it be situated on the forehead, in the part which is bare of hairs, or about the eyebrow and eye, for wounds occurring there require cataplasms and bandages more than upon any other part of the head. For the rest of the head surrounds the whole forehead, and the wounds wherever situated become inflamed and swelled, owing to an influx of blood from the surrounding parts. And neither must you apply cataplasms and bandages to the forehead at all times; but when the inflammation is stopped and the swelling has subsided, you must give up the cataplasms and bandages. A wound in any other part of the head must not be treated with tents, bandages, or cataplasms, unless it also requires incision. You must perform incision on wounds situated on the head and forehead, whenever the bone is denuded of flesh, and appears to have sustained some injury from the blow, but the wound has not sufficient length and breadth for the inspection of the bone, so that it may be seen whether it has received any mischief from the blow, and of what nature the injury is, and to what extent the flesh has been contused, and whether the bone has sustained any injury, or whether it be uninjured by the blow, and has suffered no mischief; and with regard to the treatment, what the wound, and the flesh, and the injury of the bone stand in need of. Ulcers of this description stand in need of incision; and, if the bone be denuded of the flesh, and if it be hollow, and extend far obliquely, we cut up the cavity wherever the medicine cannot penetrate readily, whatever medicine it may be; and wounds which are more inclined to be circular and hollow, and for the most part others of the like shape, are cut up by making a double incision in the circle lengthways, according to the figure of the man, so as to make the wound of a long form. Incisions may be practiced with impunity on other parts of

the head, with the exception of the temple and the parts above it, where there is a vein that runs across the temple, in which region an incision is not to be made. For convulsions seize on a person who has been thus treated; and if the incision be on the left temple, the convulsions seize on the right side; and if the incision be on the right side, the convulsions take place on the left side.

14. When, then, you lay open a wound in the head on account of the bones having been denuded of the flesh, as wishing to ascertain whether or not the bone has received an injury from the blow, you must make an incision proportionate to the size of the wound, and as much as shall be judged necessary. And in making the incision you must separate the flesh from the bone where it is united to the membrane (*pericranium?*) and to the bone, and then fill the whole wound with a tent, which will expand the wound very wide next day with as little pain as possible; and along with the tents apply a cataplasm, consisting of a mass (*maza*) of fine flour pounded in vinegar, or boiled so as to render it as glutinous as possible. On the next day, when you remove the tent, having examined the bone to see what injury it has sustained, if the wound in the bone be not right seen by you, nor can you discover what mischief the bone itself has sustained, but the instrument seems to have penetrated to the bone so as to have injured it, you must scrape the bone with a raspatory to a depth and length proportionate to the suture of the patient, and again in a transverse direction, for the sake of the fractures which are not seen, and of the contusions which are not discovered, as not being accompanied with depression of the bone from its natural position. For the scraping discovers the mischief, if the injuries in the bone be not otherwise manifest. And if you perceive an indentation (*hedra*) left in the bone by the blow, you must scrape the dint itself and the surrounding bones, lest, as often happens, there should be a fracture and contusion, or a contusion alone, combined with the dint, and escape observation. And when you scrape the bone with the raspatory, and it appears that the wound in the bone requires the operation, you must not postpone it for three days, but do it during this period, more especially if the weather be hot, and you have had the management of the treatment from the commencement. If you suspect that the bone is broken or contused, or has sustained both these injuries, having formed your judgment from the severity of the wound, and from the information of the patient, as that the person who inflicted the wound, provided it was done by another person, was remarkably strong, and that the weapon by which he was wounded was of a dangerous description, and then that the man had been seized with vertigo, dimness of vision, and stupor, and fell to the ground,—under these circumstances, if

you cannot discover whether the bone be broke, contused, or both the one and the other, nor can see the truth of the matter, you must dissolve the jet-black ointment, and fill the wound with it when this dissolved, and apply a linen rag smeared with oil, and then a cataplasm of the maza with a bandage; and on the next day, having cleaned out the wound, scrape the bone with the raspatory. And if the bone is not sound, but fractured and contused, the rest of it which is scraped will be white; but the fracture and contusion, having imbibed the preparation, will appear black, while the rest of the bone is white. And you must again scrape more deeply the fracture where it appears black; and, if you thus remove the fissure, and cause it to disappear, you may conclude that there has been a contusion of the bone to a greater or less extent, which has occasioned the fracture that has disappeared under the raspatory; but it is less dangerous, and a matter of less consequence, when the fissure has been effaced. But if the fracture extend deep, and do not seem likely to disappear when scraped, such an accident requires trepanning. But having performed this operation, you must apply the other treatment to the wound.

15. You must be upon your guard lest the bone sustain any injury from the fleshy parts if not properly treated. When the bone has been sawed and otherwise denuded, whether it be actually sound, or only appears to be so, but has sustained some injury from the blow, there may be danger of its suppurating (although it would not otherwise have done so), if the flesh which surrounds the bone be ill cured, and become inflamed and strangled; for it gets into a febrile state, and becomes much inflamed. For the bone acquires heat and inflammation from the surrounding flesh, along with irritation and throbbing, and the other mischiefs which are in the flesh itself, and from these it gets into a state of suppuration. It is a bad thing for the flesh (*granulations?*) in an ulcer to be moist and mouldy, and to require a long time to become clean. But the wound should be made to suppurate as quickly as possible; for, thus the parts surrounding the wound would be the least disposed to inflammation, and would become the soonest clean; for the flesh which has been chopped and bruised by the blow, must necessarily suppurate and slough away. But when cleaned the wound must be dried, for thus the wound will most speedily become whole, when flesh devoid of humors grows up, and thus there will be no fungous flesh in the sore. The same thing applies to the membrane which surrounds the brain: for when, by sawing the bone, and removing it from the meninx, you lay the latter bare, you must make it clean and dry as quickly as possible, lest being in a moist state for a considerable time, it become soaked therewith and

swelled; for when these things occur, there is danger of its mortifying.

16. A piece of bone that must separate from the rest of the bone, in consequence of a wound in the head, either from the indentation (*hedra*) of a blow in the bone, or from the bone being otherwise denuded for a long time, separates mostly by becoming exsanguous. For the bone becomes dried up and loses its blood by time and a multiplicity of medicines which are used; and the separation will take place most quickly, if one having cleaned the wound as quickly as possible will next dry it, and the piece of bone, whether larger or smaller. For a piece of bone which is quickly dried and converted, as it were, into a shell, is most readily separated from the rest of the bone which retains its blood and vitality; for, the part having become exsanguous and dry, more readily drops off from that which retains its blood and is alive.

17. Such pieces of bone as are depressed from their natural position, either being broken off or chopped off to a considerable extent, are attended with less danger, provided the membrane be safe; and bones which are broken by numerous and broader fractures are still less dangerous and more easily extracted. And you must not trepan any of them, nor run any risks in attempting to extract the pieces of bone, until they rise up of their own accord, upon the subsidence of the swelling. They rise up when the flesh (*granulations*) grows below, and it grows from the diploe of the bone, and from the sound portion, provided the upper table alone be in a state of necrosis. And the flesh will shoot up and grow below the more quickly, and the pieces of bone ascend, if one will get the wound to suppurate and make it clean as quickly as possible. And when both the tables of the bone are driven in upon the membrane, I mean the upper and lower, the wound, if treated in the same way, will very soon get well, and the depressed bones will quickly rise up.

18. The bones of children are thinner and softer, for this reason, that they contain more blood [than those of adults]; and they are porous and spongy, and neither dense nor hard. And when wounded to a similar or inferior degree by weapons of the same or even of an inferior power, the bone of a young person more readily and quickly suppurates, and that in less time than the bone of an older person; and in accidents, which are to prove fatal, the younger person will die sooner than the elder. But if the bone is laid bare of flesh, one must attend and try to find out, what even is not obvious to the sight, and discover whether the bone be broken and contused, or only contused; and if, when there is an indentation in the bone, whether contusion, or fracture, or both be joined to it; and if the bone has sustained any of these injuries, we must give issue to the blood by perforating the bone with a small trepan, ob-

serving the greatest precautions, for the bone of young persons is thinner and more superficial than that of elder persons.

19. When a person has sustained a mortal wound on the head, which cannot be cured, nor his life preserved, you may form an opinion of his approaching dissolution, and foretell what is to happen from the following symptoms which such a person experiences. When a bone is broken, or cleft, or contused, or otherwise injured, and when by mistake it has not been discovered, and neither the raspatory nor trepan has been applied as required, but the case has been neglected as if the bone were sound, fever will generally come on before the fourteenth day if in winter, and in summer the fever usually seizes after seven days. And when this happens, the wound loses its color, and the inflammation dies in it; and it becomes glutinous, and appears like a pickle, being of a tawny and somewhat livid color; and the bone then begins to sphacelate, and turns black where it was white before, and at last becomes pale and blanched. But when suppuration is fairly established in it, small blisters form on the tongue and he dies delirious. And, for the most part, convulsions seize the other side of the body; for, if the wound be situated on the left side, the convulsions will seize the right side of the body; or if the wound be on the right side of the head, the convulsion attacks the left side of the body. And some become apoplectic. And thus they die before the end of seven days, if in summer; and before fourteen, if in winter. And these symptoms indicate, in the same manner, whether the wound be older or more recent. But if you perceive that fever is coming on, and that any of these symptoms accompany it, you must not put off, but having sawed the bone to the membrane (*meninx*), or scraped it with a raspatory, (and it is then easily sawed or scraped,) you must apply the other treatment as may seem proper, attention being paid to circumstances.

20. When in any wound of the head, whether the man has been trepanned or not, but the bone has been laid bare, a red and erysipelatous swelling supervenes in the face, and in both eyes, or in either of them, and if the swelling be painful to the touch, and if fever and rigor come on, and if the wound look well, whether as regards the flesh or the bone, and if the parts surrounding the wound be well, except the swelling in the face, and if the swelling be not connected with any error in the regimen, you must purge the bowels in such a case with a medicine which will evacuate bile; and when thus purged the fever goes off, the swelling subsides, and the patient gets well. In giving the medicine you must pay attention to the strength of the patient.

21. With regard to trepanning, when there is a necessity for it, the following particular should be

known. If you have had the management of the case from the first, you must not at once saw the bone down to the meninx; for it is not proper that the membrane should be laid bare and exposed to injuries for a length of time, as in the end it may become fungous. And there is another danger if you saw the bone down to the meninx and remove it at once, lest in the act of sawing you should wound the meninx. But in trepanning, when only a very little of the bone remains to be sawed through, and the bone can be moved, you must desist from sawing, and leave the bone to fall out of itself. For to a bone not sawed through, and where a portion is left of the sawing, no mischief can happen; for the portion now left is sufficiently thin. In other respects you must conduct the treatment as may appear suitable to the wound. And in trepanning you must frequently remove the trepan, on account of the heat in the bone, and plunge it in cold water. For the trepan being heated by running round, and heating and drying the bone, burns it and makes a larger piece of bone around the sawing to drop off, than would otherwise do. And if you wish to saw at once down to the membrane, and then remove the bone, you must also, in like manner, frequently take out the trepan and dip it in cold water. But if you have not charge of the treatment from the first, but undertake it from another after a time,

you must saw the bone at once down to the meninx with a serrated trepan, and in doing so must frequently take out the trepan and examine with a sound (specillum), and otherwise along the tract of the instrument. For the bone is much sooner sawn through, provided there be matter below it and in it, and it often happens that the bone is more superficial, especially if the wound is situated in that part of the head where the bone is rather thinner than in other parts. But you must take care where you apply the trepan, and see that you do so only where it appears to be particularly thick, and having fixed the instrument there, that you frequently make examinations and endeavor by moving the bone to bring it up. Having removed it, you must apply the other suitable remedies to the wound. And if, when you have the management of the treatment from the first, you wish to saw through the bone at once, and remove it from the membrane, you must, in like manner, examine the tract of the instrument frequently with the sound, and see that it is fixed on the thickest part of the bone, and endeavor to remove the bone by moving it about. But if you use a perforator (*trepan?*), you must not penetrate to the membrane, if you operate on a case which you have had the charge of from the first, but must leave a thin scale of bone, as described in the process of sawing.

Neurosurgical Classic—3

THE initiation of modern neurological surgery was made possible by three discoveries in the nineteenth century. The introduction of two of these, anesthesia and antisepsis, vastly increased the scope of surgery in general, and made brain surgery feasible technically. Such operations were performed rarely, however, because there was no way to locate lesions that did not involve the skull. The problem was solved when it was discovered that in the brain there is focal representation of bodily function. This third fundamental concept—cerebral localization—became an important part of the foundation on which modern neurosurgery was built.[14]

Since the dawn of recorded surgery it has been recognized that brain injuries are sometimes accompanied by localized losses of bodily function. In the fifth century B. C., Hippocrates noticed the association between brain damage and aphasia, ophthalmoplegia, and anisocoria.[10] He also recognized that unilateral brain injury occasionally is followed by convulsions or paralysis of the opposite side of the body.[1] However, for twenty-three centuries there were no scientific theories advanced to explain these associations. Instead, interest in cerebral physiology centered around philosophical discussions of the seat of the soul.[9,12,17]

In the early nineteenth century Franz Joseph Gall and Johann Caspar Spurzheim advanced a pseudoscientific theory of brain localization known as phrenology.[7,9,15,17] These men believed that various subdivisions of the brain governed various intellectual activities, and that the relative development of the subdivisions could be assessed by examination of the overlying cranium. Although certain aspects of their theory were correct, most of their ideas were so absurd that the entire theory was rejected by most scientists. Especially opposed to the concepts

of cerebral localization and phrenology was Pierre Flourens, whose studies on animals indicated to him that cerebral gray matter was homogeneous and equipotential. Flourens was an established physiologist, and his authoritative views were accepted for half a century.[13,16,17]

However, clinical evidence to the contrary was accumulated. For example, Jean Bouillaud and Paul Broca found that injuries to the third left frontal convolution resulted in motor aphasia, and Hughlings Jackson defined the relationship between convulsions on one side of the body and disease of the opposite hemisphere.[3,9,11,13,17] Related experimental studies did not support these clinical observations immediately, probably because of the crude laboratory apparatus then in use. In the early nineteenth century Luigi Rolando had observed muscular contractions during the electrical stimulation of the cerebral hemispheres of a pig.[17] But it was not until 1870 that the doctrine of cerebral localization was placed on a firm basis by experimentation.

In that year, two young Berlin physicians, Gustav Fritsch and Eduard Hitzig, published the results of cerebral stimulation and ablation in dogs.[2] Because there had been no suitable laboratories available to them, they did their first experiments in Hitzig's home, operating on Frau Hitzig's dressing table.[8] Despite these modest facilities, Fritsch and Hitzig produced a classical work which opposed the prevailing concepts of cerebral function. Their experiments were confirmed by David Ferrier, and initiated a series of similar studies which made possible the first modern operations for localized cerebral lesions.[17]

Fritsch produced no scientific contributions of note after 1870, but Hitzig continued to contribute to the understanding of cerebral localization for 35 years.[4-6,8]

References

1. BALLANCE, C. A glimpse into the history of the surgery of the brain. *Lancet*, 1922, *1*: 111–116; 165–172 (see p. 114).
2. FRITSCH, G., and HITZIG, E. Ueber die elektrische Erregbarkeit des Grosshirns. *Arch. Anat. Physiol. wiss. Med.*, 1870, *37*: 300–332.
3. HEAD, H. Aphasia: an historical review. *Brain*, 1921, *43*: 390–411.
4. HITZIG, E. Untersuchungen über das Gehirn. Abhandlungen physiologischen und pathologischen Inhalts. *Berlin: A. Hirschwald*, 1874, xiii, 276 pp.
5. HITZIG, E. Hughlings Jackson und die motorischen Rindencentren im Lichte physiologischer Forschung. *Berlin: A. Hirschwald*, 1901, 39 pp.
6. HITZIG, E. Welt und Gehirn. *Berlin: A. Hirschwald*, 1905, viii, 67 pp.
7. HOLLANDER, B. The centenary of Francis Joseph Gall, 1758–1828. *Med. Life*, 1928, *35*: 373–380.
8. KUNTZ, A. Eduard Hitzig (1838–1907). In: *The founders of neurology*. W. Haymaker, Ed. Springfield, Ill.: Charles C Thomas, 1953, xxvii, 479 pp. (see pp. 138–142).
9. LEVINSON, A. Early studies of cerebral function. *Bull. Soc. med. Hist., Chicago*, 1923, *3*: 116–121.
10. METTLER, C. C. History of medicine. A correlative text, arranged according to subjects. F. A. Mettler, Ed. *Philadelphia: Blakiston Co.*, 1947, xxix, 1215 pp. (see p. 490).
11. RIESE, W. The early history of aphasia. *Bull. Hist. Med.*, 1947, *21*: 322–334.
12. RIESE, W., and HOFF, E. C. A history of the doctrine of cerebral localization. Sources, anticipations, and basic reasoning. *J. Hist. Med.*, 1950, *5*: 50–71.
13. RIESE, W., and HOFF, E. C. A history of the doctrine of cerebral localization. Second part: Methods and main results. *J. Hist. Med.*, 1951, *6*: 439–470.
14. SCARFF, J. E. Fifty years of neurosurgery, 1905–1955. *Int. Abstr. Surg.*, 1955, *101*: 417–513 (see p. 418).
15. TEMKIN, O. Gall and the phrenological movement. *Bull. Hist. Med.*, 1947, *21*: 275–321.
16. TIZARD, B. Theories of brain localization from Flourens to Lashley. *Med. Hist.*, 1959, *3*: 132–145.
17. WALKER, A. E. The development of the concept of cerebral localization in the nineteenth century. *Bull. Hist. Med.*, 1957, *31*: 99–121.

The Electrical Excitability of the Cerebrum[*]

G. FRITSCH AND E. HITZIG

Physiology ascribes to all nerves, as a necessary condition of the concept, the characteristic of excitability, i.e. the capability of responding with their specific energy to all the influences by which their state is changed at a certain rate. But for the central part of the nervous system other ideas exist, though to be sure certain aspects of these are not accepted generally. It would be too long a process and it would also not serve the special purpose of the present work if we wanted to mention from the enormous relevant literature only the results that seem to us reliable and that were obtained by stimulative experiments on all the separate parts of the central nervous system. However, while with regard to the excitability of the organs composing the brain stem there exists a very great difference of opinion regarding stimulations other than organic ones, while very recently a violent dispute broke out about the excitability of the spinal cord, the conviction generally has been held since the beginning of the century that the hemispheres of the cerebrum are absolutely not excitable by any stimuli familiar to physiologists.

Haller and Zinn[1] alleged that they saw convulsive movements when the medullary substance of the cerebrum was injured. However, at that time people were too little accustomed to a strict limitation of the stimuli used, which meet almost insurmountable obstacles in the brain, to pay much attention to these data later. As Longet remarked, it is probable that those experimenters had penetrated up to the medulla oblongata with their instruments.

But Longet[2] himself says the following on the subject:

"On dogs, rabbits, and on some kids, we have stimulated the white substance of the cerebral lobes with the scalpel; we have cauterized it with potassium, nitric acid, etc., we have passed galvanic currents in every direction through it, without succeeding in initiating involuntary muscular contractions or developing convulsive twitchings; the same negative result was obtained by directing the same agents toward the gray or cortical substance."

Magendie's vivisections[3] led to the same results. Later we shall deal with the rather similar conclusions of Flourens which are based upon results of bisections and denudations.

Matteucci[4] also found the cerebrum and cerebellum of the rabbit to be entirely nonexcitable by electrical stimuli.

Van Deen,[5] with whose name the theory of non-

* Translation of: Ueber die elektrische Erregbarkeit des Grosshirns, by G. Fritsch and E. Hitzig, *Archiv für Anatomie, Physiologie und wissenschaftliche Medizin*, 1870, *37*: 300–332. Printed with the kind permission of Springer-Verlag, Berlin, Göttingen and Heidelberg, Germany.

[1] Mémoires sur la nature sensible et irritable du corps animal. Lausanne 1756, vol. I, p. 201, ff.

[2] Anatomie et physiologie du système nerveux de l'homme et des animaux vertébrés. Paris 1842, vol. I, p. 644, ff.

[3] Leçons sur les fonctions et les maladies du système nerveux. Paris 1839, vol. I, p. 175, ff.

[4] Traité des phénomènes électrophysiologiques des animaux. Paris 1843, p. 242.

[5] Moleschott's Untersuchungen u.s.w. vol. VII, no. IV, p. 381.

excitability of the cerebrospinal centers was connected recently, went even considerably farther in his conclusions than all the experimenters before him and most of those after him. While previously, besides the spinal cord, at least some basal portions of the brain were still regarded as being excitable, he stated positively, on the basis of his experiments on the rabbit, which moreover were very poorly described, that the entire central nervous system was not excitable.

Likewise, Eduard Weber[6] in experiments with the rotation apparatus in the cerebrum of frogs, saw no muscular spasms occur.

Budge,[7] who also sacrificed an extremely large number of animals, expresses himself, apart from many other similar points, as follows:

"If, according to the present standpoint of science, we are permitted to conclude that no motor fibers exist in nervous tissue in which no spasms occur after a stimulation, then we can assert with the greatest certainty that not a single fiber of such nerves, which proceed into voluntary muscles, runs in the hemispheres of the cerebrum. Not a single observer has ever seen a movement of such muscles after stimulation of the above-mentioned central parts."

Finally, we also mention the opinion of Schiff,[8] one of the most experienced vivisectors:

"In accordance with the declaration of many investigators, I can confirm that the stimulation of the cerebral lobes, of the corpora striata and of the cerebellum does not produce any trace of spasm in any of the free muscles of the body. Even the intestines remained motionless when these parts were stimulated while I had maintained the circulation, which is absolutely necessary in such experiments."

It can be seen that in any science other than physiology there was hardly a question about which the opinions agreed so well, and which appeared as completely settled, as the question of excitability of the cerebral hemispheres. Moreover, it would be easy to collect additional similar citations if this would be of some benefit.

So far as we know, only one author besides Haller and Zinn has seen something different, and his information aroused in Eckhard,[9] who mentions the fact, so little belief that Eckhard conceals the name and the source. The statement in question reads: "It has been reported that, in disk-like ablation of the frontal lobes of the brain, lively movements were seen in the anterior legs."

[6] R. Wagner's Handwörterbuch der Physiologie, vol. III, part II, p. 16.
[7] Untersuchungen über das Nervensystem. Frankfurt a. M. 1842, no. II, p. 84.
[8] Lehrbuch der Physiologie des Menschen. Lahr. 1858–59. vol. I, p. 362.
[9] Experimentalphysiol. d. Nervensystems. Giessen 1867, p. 157.

To be sure, this in itself is not much, for one cannot see from it how the experiment was performed. However, if it was performed with the necessary precautions, it would prove an important principle, namely, the principle that by some kind of stimulus, either that of the scalpel, or of the oxygen or blood, movements of voluntary muscles can be produced from the frontal lobes. In any case, it seems that this isolated observation has not been followed up by anybody, for this report by Eckhard was the only trace left.

Before we turn to our own experiments, it is necessary to present the opinion concerning the motor processes in the central organs which was formed in consequence of the above-mentioned experiments and of the famous cerebral ablations by Flourens.[10]

This ingenious and successful investigator was able, by using at least purer methods, to arrive at results that deserve to be regarded as a basis for almost all the knowledge obtained later on this subject.

After numerous ablations of the cerebrum, most of which were performed on birds but also on mammals, Flourens saw all signs of volition and consciousness of sensation disappear; however, at the same time, in all the muscles of the body, movements could be incited by outside stimuli. Such animals can stand very well on their feet, they run when they are hit; birds fly when they are tossed into the air, they defend themselves when they are tested, they swallow objects which are placed in their mouths, and even the iris contracts because of light stimulus. But never do such movements occur without the influence of an external stimulus. Animals deprived of their cerebrum always sit in a sunken position, as if sleeping, and this state of theirs cannot be changed even when—although starving—they are placed on a mountain of foodstuffs.

Flourens concluded therefrom that the cerebral hemispheres are not the site of the immediate principle of muscular movements, but are only the site of the volition and of the sensations.[11]

Although this series of experiments and the conclusions drawn from it seem to be quite satisfactory, the additional results and conclusions of Flourens cannot be reconciled with results obtained by other means.

When Flourens ablated only one hemisphere from animals, they became blind on the opposite side, but they retained their full control of volition over all the voluntary muscles, and after overcoming a weakness of the opposite half of the body, which did not always occur, they did not

[10] Recherches expérimentales sur les propriétés et les fonctions du système nerveux dan les animaux vertébrés. 2nd edit. Paris, 1842.
[11] In the place cited, p. 35.

differ in anything from nonmutilated animals. When he progressively ablated disks of the cerebrum of other animals, either from the front backward or from the back forward, or from above downward or from the outside inward, he noticed under all these conditions a regular gradual decrease of the sensory perceptions and of volition. But if he went beyond a certain limit, then all these characteristics attributed to the mind were suddenly extinguished, and the animal sank into the described dreaming state.

Furthermore, if he kept the ablation at that limit, the animal regained within a few days the previously lost faculties and was able to continue to exist for a long time with the same psychic characteristics as if nothing was taken away from its cerebral substance. Flourens concluded from that[12] that the cerebral lobes exercise their functions with their entire mass, and that there is no separate site either for the various faculties or for the various perceptions. He also concluded—in contradiction to the first conclusion—that a remaining part of the hemispheres can recover the full use of all functions.

In any case, the most striking of all the reported experiments is the one described in the book mentioned, part II, page 101. In this experiment Flourens had ablated from a pigeon the entire attainable cortex of the cerebrum on both sides, therefore the ganglionic part, i.e., the part that still was regarded as the essential portion that shelters the first tools of the psyche. Nevertheless this pigeon began as early as the 3rd day to again exercise its psychic functions, and on the 6th day it had regained everything that seemed to have been entirely taken away from it through the operation. However, these experiments or their applicability were hardly or not yet tried on higher animals, and Schiff[13] states the same thing about that, although this investigator calls attention to the evident differences in structure and function between animal and human brain.

Therefore, according to these and later expanded investigations, the following approximate opinion was formed about the central locations of muscular movement:

In most parts of the brain stem, also downward to the spinal cord, there are a number of preformed mechanisms, which are capable of a normal total excitation on two paths. One of them runs from the periphery—the path of the reflex; the other radiates from the center—the path of volition, of the psychic impulses. This center lies presumably in the ganglionic substance of the cerebral hemispheres, but the individual parts of the psychic center are not localized on the individual parts of the organic center. However, its

discovery, the discovery of the probable site, or of the nearest tools of the psyche, remains closed to us, because the substrate does not respond to the stimuli familiar to us with any apparent reaction.[14]—Whatever objections could be raised with regard to clinical observation, were soon eliminated by the not unjustified reference to the imperfection and ambiguity of autopsy sections and the simplicity and clarity of these vivisections. Finally, cases of congenital or acquired defects of individual cerebral parts without corresponding disturbances of cerebral functions were mentioned to prove how unessential the brain is for life.

These views were gradually modified in limited areas by a series of well ascertained facts indicating other conditions. Through Bouillaud it had become known a long time ago (1825) that the symptom complex, which is now called aphasia, can be caused by destruction of a small eccentric part of the cerebrum. Recently, numerous authors have contributed to a more precise definition of this sentence. There also exist in the literature a certain number of cases which showed paralysis of an arm or leg during life, and small disorganizations of the cerebrum at autopsy. Unfortunately, from Andral's compilation[15] it cannot be seen how many such cases refer to the cerebrum itself and how many to its large ganglia. However, we must completely agree with what he states at the end of this observation:

"How can one fail to conclude from these facts that in the present state of science a distinct site in the brain can be assumed for the movements of the upper and lower limbs? Undoubtedly this distinct site exists, because each of these limbs can be paralyzed separately, but we do not yet know it."

To this statement we can only add that the cases concerning the corpus striatum and the optic thalamus must be excluded when these statistics are used for the determination of the place of origin of movement, because in these two large ganglia conducting paths from the hemispheres to the periphery already exist. Such facts indicated that the origin of at least individual psychic functions is tied to circumscribed parts of the brain. Goltz also came to the same conclusion when he was able to demonstrate in frogs, whose cerebrum he had extirpated, a residue of intelligence still existing in the optic lobe.

The only investigator who, on the basis of anatomic examinations, the possibility of which was doubted by some, assumed a quite decisive viewpoint which deviated considerably from the prevailing opinion, was Meynert. According to him,

[12] In the place cited, pages 99 and 101.
[13] In the same book, page 336.

[14] See the newest textbooks of physiology, for example, Ranke, Grundzüge etc., page 750, ff.—L. Hermann, Grundriss, 3 ed., 1870, p. 426 and 436, ff.
[15] Clinique médicale Paris 1834, vol. V, p. 357, ff.

the cerebral cortex, which must be regarded as the center of concepts, is divided into many much less circumscribed areas, whose significance for the individual kinds of concepts is produced by the nerve fibers of the so-called projection system which inosculate in the ganglion cells.

Meanwhile the premises for many conclusions to be drawn from the fundamental characteristics of the cerebrum were changed by the results of our own examinations.

The starting point for these studies arose from observations which one of us had the opportunity to make on man,[16] and which concern the first movements of voluntary muscles that were brought about by direct stimulation of the cerebral organs and observed on man. He found out that, by conduction of constant galvanic currents through the posterior part of the head, movements of the eyes could be easily obtained which, according to their nature, could have been incited only by direct stimulation of cerebral centers. Since these movements occurred only by galvanization of that region of the head, it could be assumed that they were caused by stimulation of the corpora quadrigemina, as indicated by some things, or of adjoining parts. However, since such ocular movements also appeared when the temporal region was galvanized and certain techniques were used which increased the stimulation, the question arose whether in the latter method, loops of current, which penetrated up to the base, caused the movements of the eyes or whether the cerebrum, in contradiction to the general opinion, possesses electrical excitability.

After a preliminary experiment by one of us had given a generally positive result with regard to the rabbit, we pursued the following course for the definite solution of the latter question.

The skulls of dogs, which were not narcotized in the first experiments but were later narcotized, were opened by a crown trephine at a flat spot. Then, with cutting, rounded bone pincers, either the entire half of the vault of the cranium or only the portion covering the anterior lobe was removed. In most cases, after using one hemisphere, we proceeded in exactly the same manner with the other half of the vault of the cranium. In all these cases, however, after a dog bled to death because of a slight injury to the longitudinal sinus, we left completely intact a median bone bridge protecting this sinus. Then the hitherto uninjured dura was slightly incised, seized with the pincers, and completely removed up to the edges of the bone. During this maneuver the dogs expressed severe pain by crying out and by char-

acteristic reflex movements. But later, when the stimulus of air had acted for a long time, the remaining hard cerebral membranes became much more sensitive, a fact which we were very careful to take into consideration when we arranged the stimulative experiment. We were able to insult the pia to various degrees by mechanical or other stimuli, without the animal showing any sign of sensation.

The devices for the electrical stimulation were arranged as follows: the poles of a chain of 10 daniells went over a commutator to two terminals of a Pohl tumbler switch, from which the cross was removed. The conducting wires supplying the current of a secondary induction coil ended at the two opposite terminals. From the middle pair of terminals, two wires led to a rheostat of 0-2100 Siemens-unit resistance, which was inserted as shunt. The main circuit continued over a DuBois switch to two small insulated cylindrical terminals which, on the other side, carried the electrodes in the form of very fine platinum wires, which were each provided in the front with a very small knob. These platinum wires ran through two small pieces of cork, the front of which they perforated, not parallel, but in a small angle, so that the little knobs could quickly change their distance from each other by a slight displacement. As a rule, this distance was about 2–3 mm. It was necessary to give to the platinum wires only a small mechanical resistance and the little knobs, because otherwise any uncertainty of the hand, even the respiratory movements of the brain, led immediately to injuries of the soft mass of the central organs.

The chains we used consisted of Siemens-Halske cardboard elements which, according to a previous test, did not possess the full electromotor force of a daniell, and each had a resistance of about 5 Siemens units. As a rule, the resistance of the shunt circuit was low, namely, at 30–40 Siemens units. The strength of the current was so small that metallic closing of the circuit just produced a sensation on the tongue touched with the little knob. Considerably higher strengths of current, as well as the elimination of the shunt circuit, were used only for control experiments. In the stimulative experiments with the induction current, which were instituted much more infrequently, the resistance of the shunt naturally depended each time on the arrangement of the coils. In most of the experiments we also used a current which just produced a sensation on the tongue.

By using this method, we obtained the following results which we present as the product of a very large number of experiments that agree up to the smallest details for the brain of the dog, without describing all these experiments. Since the method is precisely described and the factors to be mentioned in the following discussion are

---

[16] Hitzig: Ueber die galvanischen Schwindelempfindungen und eine neue Methode galvanischer Reizung der Augenmuskeln. Verhandl. der Berl. med. Gesellsch. vom 19. Jan. 1870 in Berl. klin. Wochenschrift 1870, Nr. 11. A comprehensive work will soon follow.

considered, the repetition of our experiments is so
easy that one will not have to wait a long time for
confirmations.

One part of the convexity of the cerebrum of
the dog is motor (this expression is used in the
sense of Schiff), another part is not motor.

In general, the motor part lies more to the front,
the nonmotor part lies to the rear. By electrical
stimulation of the motor part, combined contractions of muscles of the opposite half of the body
are obtained.

When weak currents are used, these contractions of muscles can be localized on certain, limited groups of muscles. When stronger currents
are used, other muscles and even muscles of the
corresponding half of the body, also participate
in the stimulation of the same or adjoining places.
However, the possibility of isolated stimulation of
a limited group of muscles is reduced when very
weak currents are used on very small places which
we want to call centers for short. As a rule, a very
small shifting of the electrodes sets the same extremity into motion; however, if, for example,
extension occurs, then the shifting causes flexion
or rotation. We found the parts of the cerebral
surface lying between the centers designated by
us, to be nonexcitable by the above-described
method of stimulation when the minimal strength
of current was used. However, when we increased
either the distance between the two electrodes or
the strength of the current, then twitchings could
be produced; but these contractions of muscles
seized the entire body in such a manner that it
was not possible to distinguish whether they were
individual or bilateral.

In the dog the location of the centers, which
soon will be designated further, is very constant.
The precise ascertainment of this fact encountered, at first, some difficulties. However, we removed these difficulties by finding out first the
place which gave the strongest spasm of the
group concerned when the stimulating current
was weakest. Then we introduced a pin between
the two electrodes into the brain of the still-living
animal and compared, after taking the brain out,
the individually marked spots with those of the
alcohol preparations of previous experiments.
How constantly the same centers are localized is
best indicated by the fact that we have repeatedly
been able to find the desired center in the central
point of a single crown-trephine opening without
any other opening of the skull. After removal of
the dura, the muscles controlled by it twitched
with the same certainty as if the entire hemisphere
had been exposed. To be sure, in the beginning
we had greater difficulties even in a quite free
field of operation. For, although the individual
convolutions of the brain are quite constant,
their development in their individual parts and
location to one another shows considerable differ-

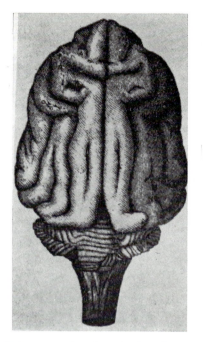

ences. It is even rather the rule than the exception
that the corresponding gyri of the two hemispheres of the same animal are differently built
in separate parts. Besides, one time the middle
portion of the convexity is more developed, another time the portions situated in the front or in
the rear are more developed.[17] If one also takes
into consideration the necessity of leaving intact
a certain portion of the meninges of the brain,
and the darkening of the picture by the varied
vascular distribution which make the gyri very
indistinct, one will not be surprised about the
difficulties we found in the beginning.

In order to make the repetition of our experiments still easier, we give below more accurate
data concerning the location of the individual
motor centers and we follow the nomenclature
of Owen.[18]

The center of the cervical muscles (see △ of the
figure) lies in the middle of the prefrontal gyrus,
where the surface of this convolution drops
sharply. The extreme end of the postfrontal gyrus
shelters in the region of the end of the frontal fissure (see + of the figure) the center for the extensors and adductors of the foreleg. Somewhat to
the rear from that and nearer the coronal fissure
(see + of the figure) lie the central regions controlling the flexion and rotation of the limb. The
place for the hind leg (see # of the figure) is also
in the postfrontal gyrus but medial to that of the

[17] See also Reichert: Der Bau des menschl. Gehirns.
Leipzig 1861, part II, p. 77.
[18] On the anatomy of vertebrates. Vol. III, London
1868, p. 118.

foreleg and somewhat more to the rear. The facial nerve (see 8 of the figure) is innervated by the middle part of the suprasylvic gyrus. The place in question often exceeds 0.5 cm. in expansion and extends from the principal flexion above the sylvian fissure forward and backward.

We must add that we did not succeed in all the cases to set the cervical muscles in motion from the first-mentioned place. We have been able often enough to cause contraction of the muscles of the back, tail and abdomen from the parts lying between the designated points, but a circumscribed place, from which they could be stimulated separately, could not be determined with certainty. We also found the entire part of the convexity,[19] which lies posterior to the center of the facial nerve, to be absolutely nonexcitable by quite disproportionate intensities of current. Even when the shunt circuit was disconnected, therefore when a current of 10 daniells was in action, no spasms of muscles occurred.

The character of the spasms produced by stimulation of these motor centers differs according to the kind of stimulation. The stimulation by simple metallic closing of the chain current gives only a simple, rather fast-passing spasm. If, instead of the chain being closed in its metallic part, this is done by putting up the electrodes, then greater strengths of current are needed in order to obtain the same effect. Therefore here too the law of DuBois-Reymond applies. Metallic reversal always produces a ceteris paribus greater effect of stimulation than mere closing, but without the occurrence of two spasms (the second for the opening). However, in this kind of stimulation sometimes tetanus of the group of muscles concerned also appears, especially when the digital flexors are involved, although additional stimulating factors do not occur. When one of the electrodes has first acted, even only a short time, then the other one produces immediately at the same place a greater stimulating effect than it can before or afterwards.

While this agrees completely with what is known about the characteristics of peripheral nerves, we cannot, for good reason, omit to call attention to a different, moreover physiologically highly interesting stimulating factor. This is the absolutely constant predominance of the anode. In fact it seems as if within the minimum strengths of current only the anode incites spasms. Because the determination of this point is absolutely necessary for making the examination easier, we performed the following experiments which we often repeated.

1) With the ordinary distance between the electrodes, the place was sought from which spasms could be incited with the minimal strength of current, and in order to be entirely sure of that, we first performed repeated metallic closings. Then we used the current in open chain, without changing the place of the electrodes and closing them again. Now the spasms failed to appear. When we again opened, turned and closed, the stimulating effect was somewhat greater than in the first closings. This could be repeated as often as desired. If one or the other electrode left its place under repeated closings of the chain, this could be the cathode, without impairing the effect of stimulation. But the anode could not be shifted far from the point of stimulation, without either cessation of spasms, or spasms occurring in other groups of muscles.

2) The anode rested on the extension center, the cathode on the flexion center for the anterior extremity. Closing gave extension, reversal (in closed chain)—flexion, reversal—extension, reversal—flexion, and so forth. Therefore, each time the center corresponding to the anode was stimulated.

With regard to newer physiologic studies, it is tempting to attach to this fact some considerations concerning chemical processes in nerve activity. However, we prefer to abstain from that for the time being. The new facts which appeared in this study are so manifold, and their consequences extend in so many directions that it would be of little advantage to wander through these paths that require close investigation.

We must add here that in a somewhat longer closing of the chain, the more strongly stimulating effect of the change of the electrodes also expresses itself in the following manner. When we had produced a spasm while the anode lay on a center and the cathode lay on a spot which was indifferent to the strength of current used, and we left the chain closed for a somewhat longer time, then the closing of the reversed current sometimes incited, after previous opening, a single spasm, very seldom a repeated spasm. This means that, after a somewhat longer action of the anode, the central nerve substance reacted for a short time, even in minimal currents, also to the cathode. For several reasons one must use for this experiment only very weak currents, especially because stronger currents immediately destroy the substance by electrolysis.

In stimulation with tetanizing induction currents the effects of stimulation, depending on the kind, are not so constant. Frequently, tonic contractions of the masses of muscles concerned occur, which slacken in intensity only after a long time. Often there is an initial maximum contraction which is followed, after seconds-long duration of the current, by such a considerable diminution that the contraction could be regarded as completely expired if at the moment of the opening a

---

[19] We intentionally avoid the designation according to lobes, since in dogs neither a distinct formation of lobes exists nor anything similar corresponds to the human cerebral lobes based on location, finally, also because we do not yet know which parts of the dog can be regarded adequately as analogous to definite parts of man.

small movement in the sense of slackening contraction did not occur. These differences, as well as some phenomena which will be mentioned below, seem to be in causative connection with the individuality of the experimental animal—its greater or lesser excitability.

In continued use of stronger currents, symptoms of exhaustion occur—the necessity of stronger currents for obtaining the same effect, also complete absence of spasms. Very often, blood suffusions of the cortical substance take place. But more often one observes, even after weak currents, a series of symptoms, to which the opposite meaning must be given.

Eduard Weber[20] has already stated that after a current has been opened that tetanizes the spinal cord of a frog, secondary movements occur in all the muscles of the body. This fact seems to be entirely forgotten. At least we would assume that otherwise it would be used as an argument by the supporters of the excitability of the spinal cord.

Something very similar takes place after tetanization of the cerebral substance. After a stimulation of a few seconds, secondary movements occur in the dependent musculature, which show a clearly quivering character in the region of the facial nerve. The extremities show rather the picture of clonic spasmodic movements—differences which in any case depend on the different kind of muscular attachment. Even when the brain is at rest, these local spasmodic attacks can often repeat themselves. In isolated cases they also occur after insult of the cerebral substances with closings of the chain current. But as a rule, they are not observed after stimulation with these currents. In two of our experimental animals, well-characterized epileptic attacks were formed from these subsequent movements. The attack began on one side with spasms in the previously stimulated musculature, but later spread to all the muscles of the body, so that it developed to a complete extensor tetanus. The pupils widened to the maximum. One of the animals had two such attacks, the other had three. One could object and say that the dogs had been epileptic previously. But one of the dogs had been with the same master for 6 years, without having ever suffered from spasms. The background of the other dog remained unknown.

Now we shall mention the objections which could be raised against our experiments.

The first objection, which is always raised in electrical stimulation experiments by experts[21]

and nonexperts, is based on the current loops which can reach distant parts. If we disregard the question whether cortices or medullary substance of the cerebrum are excitable, this objection is easier to remove than any other. In the first place, the currents used by us for the demonstrative experiments were generally weak. And since the substance of the brain possesses a very great resistance, since other conducting parts were not in the vicinity, and finally since the distance between the electrodes was small, the density of the current, according to the laws of current distribution in nonprismatic conductors, could be only a minimal one at a very short distance from the inlets. This would sufficiently refute a priori the objection in question. We also have a long series of direct proofs for us. If the current loops reached the peripheral nerves first, then the nerves of the same side always lay closer, and they did not have the remotest reason to turn exclusively to the other side. Also the motor nerves of the eyes on the same side lay much closer to them than any other nerves that may come into question. The very mobile eye, which is so well balanced in labile equilibrium, forms, without requiring any preparation, the most excellent physiologic rheoscope; in minimal current loops it would also move much more easily than an anterior extremity, not to speak of the posterior extremities. But on the entire convexity, so far as it can be exposed, there is not a single place from which eye movement can be obtained even with stronger currents than the ones we ordinarily used. Hereby, also one part of the question would be disposed of, which caused one of us to institute these studies.

Finally, we wish to mention a fact of great physiologic and pathologic interest. It is the fact that, with fatal hemorrhage, the excitability of the brain decreases unusually fast and disappears almost entirely, even before death. Immediately after death it is completely extinguished even to the strongest currents, while muscles and nerves still react excellently. This seems to suggest that experiments about the excitability of the central organs should be instituted with undisturbed circulation.

In the second place, it could be assumed that not peripheral nerves or the spinal cord, about which the same thing can be said, but other cerebral regions than the large hemispheres could be hit by current loops. If this were the case, then the proof of electrical excitability of other cerebral regions would also be an important discovery. For at the present time it is generally asserted that most of them are inaccessible to direct stimulation. However, as it can be proved, even for electrical stimulation, that is not so. Those parts, which are said by a few investigators to possess direct excitability, are the posterior parts (cauda) of the corpus striatum, optic thalamus,

[20] R. Wagner's Handwörterb. d. Physiol. Vol. III, part II, p. 15.

[21] Moreover it should be interesting for one or another reader to note that among the many physicians to whom we showed our experiments, there were several specialists who were very competent in this respect, for example, Professors Nasse (Marburg) and Munk (Berlin).

cerebral peduncle, corpora quadrigemina, pons. If we exclude the corpus striatum, then all the other morphologic constituents of the brain just mentioned lie so much in the rear that in frontal sections they are only found if one, working posteriorly, arrives at the parts of the cerebrum that no longer react. The only exception is the corpus striatum, the cauda of which lies, however, in the nonexcitable zone.[22] Therefore, it could be possible that precisely the anterior or middle portion of this ganglion, the portion which is supposed to be nonexcitable, is excitable and is the place of origin for the effects of our stimulation. From the very beginning this appeared improbable because in equal strength of current the spasms ceased as soon as the electrodes changed their place by a few millimeters. For if straight lines are drawn through the two assumed admission points and a perpendicularly lying point drawn below their connecting line in the corpus striatum, an equilateral triangle is obtained whose equal sides would give off current paths of least resistance. Since the resistance of the two must be approximately the same, then ceteris paribus, the effect of stimulation should also be the same, which is not the case.

Not satisfied with these conclusive aprioristic evidences, we also tried to obtain direct proof. For this purpose we gave Carlsbad insect needles a dense insulating cover by immersing them repeatedly in a gutta-percha solution in chloroform. Only the tip and the head were kept conductive. When we introduced these needles into the rear part of the cerebrum, we obtained no trace of a spasm even with very much stronger currents, until the rheophores, which had penetrated several cm. deep, touched the cerebral peduncle. But then the animal received, with a lively jump, general agitation of the muscles. That was different when the anterior half of the brain was stimulated in the same manner. If it was to be assumed that current loops, penetrating up to the corpus striatum, incited the spasms which occurred by superficial stimulation, then the spasms should gradually become stronger with the penetration of the electrodes. However, this did not take place, but rather the spasms spread to other muscles and showed a different behavior which we shall not describe here in detail. Consequently, it can be assumed with certainty that neither the above-mentioned ganglion nor the structures composing the brain stem participated in the spasms stimulated from the convexity.

Another objection which could be raised and has been raised against all the previous successful experiments on stimulation of the central organs (spinal cord, brain stem) would be based on reflex occurrence of the contractions. This objection too can be eliminated by conclusive proofs.

Reflexes could be incited by the nerves of the dura and those of the pia mater, but we were protected by abundant exposition of the cerebral surface against stimulations of neighboring nerves of the cranial coverings. However, at one edge of the wound lay the partly detached temporal masses of muscles. These structures, which most probably had preserved their excitability, would have immediately revealed to us weak current loops. But sensitive fibers in the cerebrum itself have not yet been demonstrated or even assumed. Also, the complete insensibility of its substance does not give the slightest evidence for such an assumption.

As regards the dura, we have already stated above[23] that it already possesses a certain inherent sensitiveness in the physiologic state, but that this sensitiveness increases very rapidly after opening the skull. For this reason it is advisable to operate quickly, because otherwise the experimental animal, even if it is tied firmly, makes, by powerful jumps, the sparing of the cerebral substance very difficult during excision of this membrane. But if it is excised up to the edges of the bones, one is sufficiently protected against reflexes of its nerves. We assured ourselves of that in various manners. In the first place, in our stimulation experiments we incited crossed spasms, while reflexes always occur first on the same side (Pflueger). In the second place, the spasms ceased when the place was slightly changed but the distance from the remaining dura was the same. In the third place, they also ceased when we came closer to the dura, provided we did not find any motor centers. We did not even obtain any spasms, always under the last-mentioned provision, when the electrode lay close to the dura but still on the cerebral substance. However, if, in the fourth place, we touched the dura itself, there appeared in many cases, even if no current flowed through, but upon electrical stimulation, very lively reflex movements in an extremely characteristic form. But these movements looked quite different from the effects of our other stimulations. In the former, they always presented the aspect of fitness; extension of the head, contractions of the muscles of the spine, cries and moans even under morphine narcosis, seldom movements of the extremities. The picture of our experiments was quite different. Even non-narcotized animals lay motionless, indifferent, while we set in motion at one time an anterior extremity, at another time a posterior extremity by an electrical stimulus.

The pia cannot be reflected back in the same manner; on the contrary, it must be handled as carefully as possible. For the injury of a single one of its numerous swollen vessels overflows the field of operation with blood and can wreck the entire experiment, thus making the sacrifice of the animal useless. However, this does not hinder the

---

[22] We call nonexcitable, without prejudice, all those regions from which no spasms can be produced.

[23] In agreement with Longet and others.

proof of its being unessential for the occurrence of effects of our stimulation. Apart from all the reasons which we have already mentioned when we discussed the dura, the following is more than sufficient. Like Longet and others, we found the pia to be insensitive. We cut around it over a motor center, sparing the larger vessels, without any change of the effect of stimulation. We excised it at such a place—the spasms never failed to appear. We stuck insulated needles into the cerebral substance, and the muscles still twitched when we did that in the region of the motor sphere; they did not twitch under any of these conditions when we went beyond the posterior limit of this sphere. Moreover, it should be of interest to state here that neither morphine- nor ether-narcosis had an essential influence on the success of the experiments.

Finally, one may ask how it is that so many earlier investigators—among them the most brilliant ones—arrived at opposite results. To this we have only one answer: "The method creates the results." It is impossible that our predecessors had exposed the entire convexity, for in that case the spasms would have been elicited. The posterolateral wall of the dog's cranial vault, under which there are no motor parts, is recommendable, because of its formation, for placing the first trephine openings. Probably they began the operation here and neglected to break open anteriorly, under the erroneous opinion that the individual areas of the surface were equivalent. This was based upon the still widespread assumption that all the psychic functions were omnipresent in all the parts of the cerebral cortex. If they had thought of a localization of the mental functions, they would have regarded the apparent nonexcitability of individual parts of the substrate as something self-evident and would have examined all its parts. Perhaps none of the previous investigators had assumed that we could arouse ideas with our stimuli or could demonstrate something aroused on the vivisected animal.

This leads us to the discussion of a question which could be addressed to us, although without justification. Some people may ask us to explain the observations which exist in sufficient number about surgical injuries of the brain without disturbance of any function.[24] In the first place it is not our task to solve this apparent contradiction;

[24] One of us (Hitzig) has also observed such a case during his activity as head physician in the general military hospital in Berlin in the year 1866. A splinter of a shell had penetrated into the glabella of a soldier (Angelmeier) and had made there a triangular hole. From this hole, cerebral substance discharged itself continuously for at least 14 days. Finally the wound healed up by itself. This patient was not very ingenious; on the contrary, he seemed to be of inert intelligence. However, he did not present any gross motor or sensory disturbances.

for, before this duty becomes incumbent upon us, they must prove to us that the parts in question were injured or lost—a somewhat difficult undertaking. But neither we nor others know anything more accurate about other parts of the convexity, except perhaps what is known of the third frontal convolution, and this speaks precisely for us. As we have said before, the contradiction is only an apparent one; the parts of the cerebrum are not equivalent.

It also seems to us very appropriate to remind the reader of Griesinger's[25] following remark which fits this point very well:

"Some kinds of doubts were expressed about these observations. In almost all the cases only the intelligence was considered, while the disposition and the volition have remained entirely without consideration, and usually only the slightest demands were made on the intelligence, for example, the answering of simple medical questions, in order to declare it uninjured. In none of these observations was the intelligence tested in its entire scope, and in many of them, namely, in all hospital observations, a comparison of the mental condition after the illness or the loss of substance with the previous status was utterly impossible, etc."

As his matter requires, Griesinger looks only at the psychic condition. With regard to somatic functions we can ask, even with greater justification, exactly what he wants from the investigation of the psychic condition. Where are the studies on muscular characteristics or the qualities of the sense of touch, which would be more at the right place here than in other places where they—a scientific humbug—serve only to spray sand in the eyes of harmless readers! Some experiments, which will be mentioned in the following discussion, will show how well-founded this demand of ours is.

If we now look back at the results of our studies and ask ourselves what we have obtained through them in knowledge of the characteristics of the central organ, then it is our duty to distinguish between that which can rightly be concluded as certain, and that which has been made only probable.

In the first place, as a certain accomplishment we can mention the definitely proved fact—which can be reproduced at any moment—that structures of the central nervous system respond to one of our stimuli with a visible reaction. In principle, this alone would be of certain significance for physiology, since thereby the contradiction in the definition is removed, to which Fick rightly pointed recently and which refers to the beginning of this work.

Also confirmed is the fact that a considerable part of the nerve masses which compose the large

[25] Die Pathologie und Therapie der psychischen Krankheiten. 2. ed., Stuttgart 1861, p. 4.

hemispheres—it can be said almost one-half of them—is in direct connection with muscular movement, while another part apparently has nothing to do directly with it. Although this seemed very simple and self-evident, it was hardly clarified up to now. We refer for this purpose to what was said in regard to the historical synopsis. Whenever one spoke of such centers in the brain, even in most recent times, only basal parts— pons, thalami, etc. were mentioned,[26] and when those postmortem results were explained, the common expressions were carefully used. Only a few specialists in brain anatomy, among them especially Meynert, had expressed themselves, to be true in a different manner from Gall, in favor of a strict localization of the individual psychic faculties.

However, if we raise the question whether the effects of stimulation incited by us are produced by direct influence on those centers of the gray cortex in which the motor impulse of volition occurs, or whether one must think of stimulation of the medullary fibrillation, or whether a third thing is possible, then our answer must be much more reserved.

Even if we assume that it has been proved that the motor phenomena in question are incited by the ganglionic substance—and this is not the case—it would still not be proved in those motor phenomena which are liberated by internal occurrence, that precisely this part of the cortex supplies the substrate for the first externally directed link in the chain which begins with the first occurrence of a sensual impression, and whose preliminary end meets the expression of volition which appears as muscular movement.

It is rather not inconceivable, and it cannot be excluded by what we know in anatomy about the anastomosing structure of these parts, that the cerebral portion, which includes the birth place of the volition of movement, is just another one or perhaps a more manifold one, and that the regions called centers by us act only as mediators, collecting places in which similar but more suitable arrangements of muscular movements occur than in the gray substance of the spinal cord and the base of the brain. We shall soon see to what extent we have even uncovered a certain physiologic justification to allow a place for this point of view.

After we have granted, in this reservation, the widest scope to the purely psychologic possibilities—and we emphasize this expressly—we turn to the discussion of the question concerning the value of the gray and of the white substance for the occurrence of the effects of stimulation described by us. If the question is put in this form, then it should be partly possible now to answer it

satisfactorily. But if, instead of the more common concepts of gray and white substance, the words fibers and cells were compared, the possibility of a solution could not be perceived, for, since in the gray substance fibers and cells are inseparably mixed, an isolated examination of the individual morphologic constituents cannot be performed. Therefore, even if the direct proof of excitability were also produced for the gray substance, one could still object that, not the ganglion cells, but the interspersed nerve fibers of this substance provide the truly excitable part. At the present time the state of the question is that, by means of the above-mentioned experiments concerning the introduction of insulated needles, we have proved adequately the excitability of the medullary substance. Since the essential nervous constituents of the medullary substance—the nerve fibers— continue with the same anatomic characteristics into the cortical substance, there is no reason to assume an essential change of their physiologic characteristics before their anatomic continuity is interrupted by new structures. For this reason, the excitability of a part of the fibers, also of the cortex, can be rightly assumed. As said before, by the means available up to now it cannot be decided definitely whether the fibers alone or also the cells are excitable.

However, in an indirect manner a somewhat probable conclusion can be drawn concerning the function if not concerning the excitability of the cellular part of the cortex. In the description of our experiments we saw that, with a minimum strength of current, contractions of muscles occur only if the electrodes are in very specific places, and that they cease or they appear in other muscles when the electrodes deviate even only slightly from the aforementioned places. This behavior admits only two possibilities. Either the stimulus is picked up by the ganglion cells lying in the immediate vicinity of the electrodes and is converted by them into muscular movement, or precisely at these points excitable medullary fibers appear very near the surface, so that they are very favorably situated for stimulation. Since no other reason can be detected as to why the medullary fibers in question should mostly approach the ganglion cells precisely here, rather than go and meet their fate by penetrating into the others, it can be assumed that precisely those ganglion masses are intended for precisely those nerve fibers for the production of organic stimuli.

By the methods used up to now it cannot be decided whether a certain, ordinarily cooperating sum of these organic stimuli produces exactly the same motor manifestations as our electrical stimulus. For the simple theory of specific energies does not suffice here; we must develop a new viewpoint for the new facts found. We do not have here nerve fibers which run straight to the

---

[26] See for example, Griesinger in the place cited, page 4, and many other authors, but the same on page 23.

end organ, but rather fibers which emanate from the most central place of the cerebrum and can arrive there after they have passed a number of more and more peripherally situated stations, in each of which their liberated tensions are converted in a certain manner that is not exactly known, so that the result is what we call an appropriate movement. Of course, by a stimulus produced at any point of this path we can at the most show only what usually occurs in the more peripherally situated stretch and the more peripherally situated stations, while the functions of the central stations are not observed. Even this can be expressed only with a certain restriction since the stimulation of a larger sum of fibers is necessary for producing a certain motor modality, which fibers, however, do not lie together as comfortably in the central organs as in the trunk of a peripheral nerve. However, there is another way of solving the question according to the significance of the individual parts of the cortex; it is the extirpation of circumscribed and well known parts of it. We have also begun to embark upon this protracted road in the following manner.

After the soft parts of two dogs were reflected back, the skulls were opened by means of a crown trephine at the place where we presumed the center for the right anterior extremity to be. We chose the center for an extremity because possible motor phenomena should appear most distinctly in an extremity, and we did not choose the center for the posterior extremity because its position would possibly lead to the opening of the longitudinal sinus. Then the dura of the exposed place was removed; by electrical stimulation we ascertained that we had hit the desired place; so far as necessary, the pia was cut around and somewhat lifted from the cortical substance by means of a fine scalpel. In one case the removed piece was about as large as a small lentil, in the other case a little larger. Then the skin wound was united by means of button sutures. In the first case the animal had lost only a few drops of blood during the entire operation; in the other case the bleeding was not inconsiderable. The first case healed by first intention, the other case did not. But the two experimental animals presented symptoms which differed only in degree. The aspects of their disorder regarding motor disturbances were as equal as possible. This complete agreement of the results of the two experiments and their importance for all the observations which resulted from our other experiments cause us to mention them here, although we would like to collect additional similar experiences before any kind of publication is done. The necessity of giving this work a preliminary conclusion has prevented us from doing this up to now; moreover, it will be seen that a single successful experiment is sufficient for conclusions to be drawn by us ad hoc.

Both experimental animals showed immediately after operation, which occurred under morphine-narcosis, some general weakness which soon disappeared. But later the following was observed:

I. When running, the animals set the right front paw inappropriately more inward or more outward than the other one, and slid with this paw, never with the other, slightly outward, so that they fell to the ground. No movement disappeared entirely; however, the right leg was drawn up somewhat more weakly.

II. When standing, very similar phenomena. Besides, the front paw was placed on the dorsum instead of on the sole, without the dog being aware of it.

III. When sitting on the hind part, when both front paws rested on the ground, the right front leg slid gradually outward, until the dog lay entirely on the right side.

But under any circumstances the dog could immediately get up again. On the right front paw, the skin sensibility and the sensitivity to deep pressure showed no demonstrable abnormalities.

Most striking was the following experiment in the first dog[27] even after the wound had healed for a long time, after all the reactions had ceased, and it was on the 15th and even on the 28th day after the operation.

While the dog was standing, his right front paw was set on its anterior, upper edge so much inward and to the rear that it lay between the other three legs. If, by patting, the dog was prevented from moving away, the dog let the paw stay in this uncomfortable position for any length of time. But if he received any kind of motor impulse, he ran away, moving his sick leg almost as briskly as the other three. It was not possible to make the same experiment with the left leg, because the small animal always withdrew this limb and brought it into its previous comfortable position.

We also save here all the additional conclusions and observations, especially certain comparisons with human pathology, for another occasion, and regard the following only as essential for the present work. By extirpation of a part of what we call the center of the anterior extremity, the two experimental animals had lost only incompletely the ability to move the anterior extremity, and probably they lost no sensibility whatever. But they obviously had lost a partial consciousness of the conditions of this limb, the ability to form complete concepts about it; therefore, they suffered from a symptom which occurs in a very similar manner in a form of the disease group tabes, except that injury of a sensory conducting path surely did not exist here. In order to denote this condition better, one could perhaps express one-

[27] The second one is not mentioned here because, for experimental reasons, it was only three-legged.

self as follows: there still existed some motor conduction from the psyche to the muscle, while there was an interruption somewhere in the conduction from the muscle to the psyche. This interruption possibly concerned the end station of the hypothetical path for the muscular sense; but in any case it had its seat at the place of the center which was injured by us.

No matter how this was, it is certain that an injury of this center only alters, but does not remove, the voluntary movement of a limb which surely depends on the center, and that therefore other places and paths are also open to a motor impulse, in which this impulse can be born and hasten to the muscles of that leg, so that our reservation . . . was well founded. But it is also equally sure that such an injury, although small in comparison to the ablations of Flourens, Hertwig and others, produces very distinctly perceptible symptoms when the right spot is found;

and the symptoms are perceptible precisely on that limb whose muscles previously contracted upon electrical stimulation of the now destroyed masses.

From the above it becomes evident that in previous colossal mutilations of the brain either other parts were chosen, or the necessary attention was not paid to the finer functions of the motor mechanisms. It also results from the sum of all our experiments that by no means, as Flourens and most of the others after him believed, is the psyche a kind of total function of the entire cerebrum, whose expression can be removed as a whole but not in its individual parts by mechanical means, but that rather individual mental functions, probably all of them, contribute to the occurrence of the matter in circumscribed centers of the cerebral cortex.

Berlin, 28 April, 1870

Neurosurgical Classic—4

ARVEY CUSHING's interest in the pituitary gland resulted in more than 50 publications over a period of 30 years.[1-57] The title of one of these, "Is the pituitary gland essential to the maintenance of life?", indicates how little was known about this structure in 1909.[47] During the years that followed, Dr. Cushing played a significant role in the elucidation of pituitary function by closely examining clinical examples of pituitary malfunction. He established the surgical treatment of the pituitary adenomas and crystallized the concepts of hypo- and hyperpituitarism.[39,45,46,48]

Cushing's interest in patients with pituitary disorders was not limited to their scientific aspects.

"Cushing was always fascinated by the circus, particularly by the sideshows where he obtained histories of the giants, fat women, and midgets, and any other freak that might happen to be on display. In this way he made friends with many circus personalities and over the years managed to keep in touch with several well-known giants and midgets. Sir Arthur Keith, the distinguished curator of the Hunterian Museum, consented some years ago, on Cushing's insistence, to removing the top of the skull of the famous Irish giant whose skeleton had long been on display in the Museum, in order to ascertain the condition of the sella turcica where the pituitary body would have been. Sure enough, the sella was grossly enlarged and there was evidence that there had been a sizeable intracranial extension of the pituitary tumor.[39]

"But H. C. was as much interested in dwarfs as in giants, and many of his friends will remember that during the hot summer of 1929 after the family went to Little Boar's Head he surreptitiously filled the house with dwarfs on whom an attempt was being made to test the efficacy of some growth hormones recently purified by Herbert Evans. . . . "[39]

One of the circus patients " . . . was the subject of a letter which H.C. felt impelled to send to *Time* magazine after she had been made the object of ridicule in a previous issue. The letter, which *Time* published under the caption 'Skin Deep', ran thus:

"Sirs: . . . May I accordingly tell you something of the woman whose picture you published on p. 17 of *Time*, May 2, [1927] under the caption of 'Uglies'? This unfortunate woman who sits in the sideshow of Ringling Brothers 'between Fat Lady and Armless Wonder' and 'affects white lace hats, woolen mittens and high laced shoes' has a story which is far from mirth-provoking. Could it have been written up for you by O. Henry, it would have provoked tears rather than laughter. The facts are as follows: She is, as you say, a peasant of Kent and four times a mother. The father of these four children, a truck gardener, died some years ago and left her their sole support. She, previously a vigorous and good-looking young woman, has become the victim of a disease known as acromegaly. This cruel and deforming malady not only completely transforms the outward appearance of those whom it afflicts but is attended with great suffering and often with loss of vision.

"One of Mr. Ringling's agents prevailed upon her to travel with the circus and to pose as the 'ugliest woman in the world' as a means of livelihood. Mr. Ringling is kind to his people and she is well cared for. But she suffers from intolerable headaches, has become nearly blind, and permits herself to be laughed at and heckled by an unfeeling people in order to provide the wherewithal to educate her four children. Beauty is but skin deep. Being a physician, I do not like to feel that *Time* can be frivolous over the tragedies of disease."[39]

Because of Cushing's interest in chromophobe and acidophile adenomas of the anterior hypophysis, many patients with these tumors were referred to him. Of the 2023 patients with verified brain tumors seen in his clinic, 360 had pituitary adenomas.[26]

"Among his pituitary patients Cushing over the years had observed a special group with a condition which had been somewhat vaguely labelled 'polyglandular syndrome.' They were seldom subjected to operation because, unlike his other pituitary cases, they did not exhibit visual difficulty or signs of increased intracranial pressure; and since none had come to autopsy he had had no opportunity of definitely establishing the fact that their difficulties were of pituitary origin. . . . Until 1930 Cushing had never seen a basophilic tumor of the pituitary but he had often suspected that such might occur. . . .[39]

" . . . It is a matter of some interest that at the time of Cushing's original paper on basophilism no one of his own cases had yet come to autopsy. Three patients, however, who died after the paper was published all proved at autopsy to have basophilic adenomas."[39]

" . . . Cushing first described his deductions concerning the basophil tumors before the New York Neurological Society on 5 January 1932. He presented the same material again at the Harvard Medical Society on the 20th, and on 24 February he made it the subject of an Alpha Omega Alpha Lecture in New Haven. . . . These first three accounts of basophilism were merely curtain raisers, for his official presentation was given before the Johns Hopkins Medical Society on 29 February, and the full text appeared in the March number of the *Johns Hopkins Hospital Bulletin*."[39]

During the century prior to 1932, basophil adenomas had been described (as unimportant curiosities), experiments had shown that relationships existed between the pituitary gland and the adrenal cortex, and the clinical changes associated with adrenal cortical hyperfunction had been recognized.[49] Dr. Cushing's observations substantiated and correlated these findings.[25,27–29,38,39,52–54] Ideas about the underlying pathological lesions have changed since 1932, but because of the classical descriptions by Cushing, the clinical picture presented by these patients has become widely known as Cushing's syndrome.[49]

"For those who believe that the originality of most men reaches its peak before the age of forty and that it would be a good thing if most of us were chloroformed at sixty, it is a fact of some significance that one of Cushing's most original single contributions to clinical medicine was made in his sixty-third year as he was about to retire."[39]

References

1. BAILEY, P., and CUSHING, H. Studies in acromegaly. VII. The microscopical structure of the adenomas in acromegalic dyspituitarism (fugitive acromegaly). *Amer. J. Path.*, 1928, *4:* 545–564.
2. CROWE, S. J., CUSHING, H., and HOMANS, J. Effects of hypophyseal transplantation following total hypophysectomy in the canine. *Quart J. exp. Physiol.*, 1909, *2:* 389–400.
3. CROWE, S. J., CUSHING, H., and HOMANS, J. Experimental hypophysectomy. *Johns Hopk. Hosp. Bull.*, 1910, *21:* 127–169.
4. CUSHING, H. Sexual infantilism with optic atrophy in cases of tumor affecting the hypophysis cerebri. *J. nerv. ment. Dis.*, 1906, *33:* 704–716.
5. CUSHING, H. The hypophysis cerebri. Clinical aspects of hyperpituitarism and of hypopituitarism. *J. Amer. med. Ass.*, 1909, *53:* 249–255.
6. CUSHING, H. Partial hypophysectomy for acromegaly with remarks on the function of the hypophysis. *Ann. Surg.*, 1909, *50:* 1002–1017.
7. CUSHING, H. The functions of the pituitary body. *Amer. J. med. Sci.*, 1910, n.s. *139:* 473–484.
8. CUSHING, H. Dyspituitarism. *Harvey Lect.*, 1910–1911, 31–45.
9. CUSHING, H. The pituitary body and its disorders. Clinical states produced by disorders of the hypophysis cerebri. An amplification of the Harvey Lecture for December, 1910. *Philadelphia: J. B. Lippincott Co.*, 1912, x, 341 pp.
10. CUSHING, H. Concerning the symptomatic differentiation between disorders of the two lobes of the pituitary body: with notes on a syndrome accredited to hyperplasia of the anterior and secretory stasis or insufficiency of the posterior lobe. *Amer. J. med. Sci.*, 1913, *145:* 313–328.
11. CUSHING, H. Concerning diabetes insipidus and the polyurias of hypophysial origin. *Boston med. surg. J.*, 1913, *168:* 901–910.
12. CUSHING, H. Operative experiences with lesions of the pituitary body. *Trans. Amer. surg. Ass.*, 1913, *31:* 467–468.
13. CUSHING, H. The correlation of the organs of internal secretion and their disturbances. *Lancet*, 1913, *2:* 546–547.
14. CUSHING, H. Affections of the pituitary body. *Lancet.* 1913, *2:* 565.
15. CUSHING, H. Psychic disturbances associated with disorders of the ductless glands. *Amer. J. Insan.*, 1913, *69:* 965–990.
16. CUSHING, H. The perimetric deviations accompanying pituitary lesions (preliminary note). *J. nerv. ment. Dis.*, 1913, *40:* 793–794.
17. CUSHING, H. Surgical experiences with pituitary disorders. *J. Amer. med. Ass.*, 1914, *63:* 1515–1525.
18. CUSHING, H. Disorders of the pituitary gland. Retrospective and prophetic. *J. Amer. med. Ass.*, 1921, *76:* 1721–1726.
19. CUSHING, H. Les syndromes hypophysaires au point de vue chirurgical. *Rev. neurol.*, 1922, *38:* 779–808.
20. CUSHING, H. Prefatory note to: A consideration of the hypophysial adenomata. By N. M. Dott and P. Bailey. *Brit. J. Surg.*, 1925, *13:* 314–366 (see pp. 314–316).
21. CUSHING, H. The pituitary gland as now known. *Lancet*, 1925, *2:* 899–906.
22. CUSHING, H. Ductless glands (discussion). *Trans. Congr. Amer. Phys. Surg.*, 1925, *13:* 61–64.
23. CUSHING, H. Studies in intracranial physiology and surgery. The third circulation. The hypophysis. The gliomas. *London: Oxford Univ. Press*, 1926, xii, 146 pp.
24. CUSHING, H. Acromegaly from a surgical standpoint. *Brit. med. J.*, 1927, *2:* 1–9; 48–55.

25. CUSHING, H. The basophil adenomas of the pituitary body and their clinical manifestations (pituitary basophilism). *Johns Hopk. Hosp. Bull.*, 1932, *50:* 137–195.

26. CUSHING, H. Intracranial tumours. Notes upon a series of two thousand verified cases with surgical-mortality percentages pertaining thereto. *Springfield, Ill.: Charles C Thomas*, 1932, xii, 150 pp.

27. CUSHING, H. Further notes on pituitary basophilism. *J. Amer. med. Ass.*, 1932, *99:* 281–284.

28. CUSHING, H. Papers relating to the pituitary body, hypothalamus and parasympathetic nervous system. *Springfield, Ill.: Charles C Thomas*, 1932, vii, 234 pp.

29. CUSHING, H. "Dyspituitarism": twenty years later. With special consideration of the pituitary adenomas. *Arch. intern. Med.*, 1933, *51:* 487–557.

30. CUSHING, H. Posterior pituitary activity from an anatomical standpoint. *Amer. J. Path.*, 1933, *9:* 539–547.

31. CUSHING, H. Hyperactivation of the neurohypophysis as the pathological basis of eclampsia and other hypertensive states. *Amer. J. Path.*, 1934, *10:* 145–175.

32. CUSHING, H., and DAVIDOFF, L. M. The pathological findings in four autopsied cases of acromegaly with a discussion of their significance. *New York: Rockefeller Institute for Medical Research* (Monograph No. 22), 1927, 131 pp.

33. CUSHING, H., and DAVIDOFF, L. M. Studies in acromegaly. IV. The basal metabolism. *Arch. intern. Med.*, 1927, *39:* 673–697.

34. CUSHING, H., and GOETSCH, E. Concerning the secretion of the infundibular lobe of the pituitary body and its presence in the cerebrospinal fluid. *Amer. J. Physiol.*, 1910, *27:* 60–86.

35. CUSHING, H., and GOETSCH, E. Hibernation and the pituitary body. *Proc. Soc. Exp. Biol., N. Y.*, 1913, *11:* 25–26.

36. CUSHING, H., and GOETSCH, E. Hibernation and the pituitary body. *J. exp. Med.*, 1915, *22:* 25–47.

37. DAVIDOFF, L. M., and CUSHING, H. Studies in acromegaly. VI. The disturbances of carbohydrate metabolism. *Arch. intern. Med.*, 1927, *39:* 751–779.

38. EISENHARDT, L., and THOMPSON, K. W. A brief consideration of the present status of so-called pituitary basophilism. With a tabulation of verified cases. *Yale J. Biol. Med.*, 1939, *11:* 507–522.

39. FULTON, J. F. Harvey Cushing. A biography. *Springfield, Ill.: Charles C Thomas*, 1946, xii, 754 pp. (see pp. 299–304, 614–616, 658, 661 and 689).

40. FULTON, M. N., and CUSHING, H. The specific dynamic action of protein in patients with pituitary disease. *Arch. intern. Med.*, 1932, *50:* 649–667.

41. GOETSCH, E., and CUSHING, H. The pars anterior and its relation to the reproductive glands. *Proc. Soc. exp. Biol., N. Y.*, 1913, *11:* 26–27.

42. GOETSCH, E., CUSHING, H., and JACOBSON, C. Carbohydrate tolerance and the posterior lobe of the hypophysis cerebri. An experimental and clinical study. *Johns Hopk. Hosp. Bull.*, 1911, *22:* 165–190.

43. HARVEY CUSHING SOCIETY, A bibliography of the writings of Harvey Cushing. Prepared on the occasion of his seventieth birthday April 8, 1939 by the Harvey Cushing Society. *Springfield, Ill.: Charles C Thomas*, 1939, xv, 108 pp.

44. HENDERSON, W. R. The pituitary adenomata. A follow-up study of the surgical results in 338 cases (Dr. Harvey Cushing's series). *Brit. J. Surg.*, 1939, *26:* 811–921.

45. HORRAX, G. Some of Harvey Cushing's contributions to neurological surgery. *J. Neurosurg.*, 1944, *1:* 3–22.

46. JOHNSON, H. C. Surgery of the hypophysis. In: A history of neurological surgery. A. E. Walker, Ed. *Baltimore: Williams & Wilkins Co.*, 1951, xii, 583 pp. (see pp. 152–177).

47. REFORD, L. L., and CUSHING, H. Is the pituitary gland essential to the maintenance of life? *Johns Hopk. Hosp. Bull.*, 1909, *20:* 105–107.

48. SCARFF, J. E. Fifty years of neurosurgery, 1905–1955. *Int. Abstr. Surg.*, 1955, *101:* 417–513 (see pp. 439–442).

49. SOFFER, L. J., DORFMAN, R. I., and GABRILOVE, J. L. The human adrenal gland. *Philadelphia: Lea & Febiger*, 1961, 591 pp. (see pp. 350–366; 423–440).

50. TEEL, H. M., and CUSHING, H. The separate growth-promoting and gonad-stimulating hormones of the anterior hypophysis: an historical review. *Endokrinologie*, 1930, *6:* 401–420.

51. TEEL, H. M., and CUSHING, H. Studies in the physiological properties of the growth-promoting extracts of the anterior hypophysis. *Endocrinology*, 1930, *14:* 157–163.

52. THOMPSON, K. W., and CUSHING, H. Experimental pituitary basophilism. *Proc. roy. Soc.*, 1934, *115 B:* 88–100.

53. THOMPSON, K. W., and CUSHING, H. Inhibition of action of pituitary hormones by animal sera. *Proc. roy. Soc.*, 1937, *121 B:* 501–517.

54. THOMPSON, K. W., and EISENHARDT, L. Further consideration of the Cushing syndrome. *J. clin. Endocrin.*, 1943, *3:* 445–452.

55. WALKER, C. B., and CUSHING, H. Distortions of the visual fields in cases of brain tumor. (Fifth paper) Chiasmal lesions, with especial reference to homonymous hemianopsia with hypophyseal tumor. *Arch. Ophthal., N. Y.*, 1918, *47:* 119–145.

56. WEED, L. H., and CUSHING, H. Studies on cerebro-spinal fluid. VIII. The effect of pituitary extract upon its secretion (choroidorrhoea). *Amer. J. Physiol.*, 1915, *36:* 77–103.

57. WEED, L. H., CUSHING, H., and JACOBSON, C. Further studies on the rôle of the hypophysis in the metabolism of carbohydrates. The autonomic control of the pituitary gland. *Johns Hopk. Hosp. Bull.*, 1913, *24:* 40–52.

THE BASOPHIL ADENOMAS OF THE PITUITARY BODY AND THEIR CLINICAL MANIFESTATIONS (PITUITARY BASOPHILISM[1])*

HARVEY CUSHING, M.D.

Professor of Surgery, Harvard Medical School

Introduction. In a long since superseded monograph on the pituitary body and its disorders, published in 1912, a section was devoted to a group of cases which showed peculiar and sundry polyglandular syndromes. It was stated at the time that the term "polyglandular syndrome" implied nothing more than that secondary functional alterations occur in the ductless-gland series whenever the activity of one of the glands becomes primarily affected; and further, that the term, as employed, was restricted to those cases in which it was difficult to tell where the initial fault lay.

That a primary derangement of the pituitary gland, whether occurring spontaneously or experimentally induced, was particularly prone to cause widespread changes in other endocrine organs was appreciated even at that early day, and it was strongly suspected that this centrally placed and well protected structure in all probability represented the master-gland of the endocrine series. The multiglandular hyperplasias of acromegaly, so evident in the thyroid gland and adrenal cortex, were already known, and the no less striking atrophic alterations in these same glands brought about by the counter state of pituitary insufficiency were coming to be equally well recognized. But in spite of these hopeful signs, we were still groping blindly for an explanation of many other disorders, obviously of endocrine origin, like those associated with pineal, parathyroid or suprarenal tumors. Out of this obscurity, those seriously interested in the subject have, step by step, been feeling their way in spite of pitfalls and stumbling blocks innumerable.

The usual method of progression has been somewhat as follows. A peculiar clinical syndrome has first been described by someone with a clarity sufficient to make it easily recognizable by others. This syndrome in course of time has been found to be associated either with a destructive lesion or with a tumefaction primarily involving one or another of the organs in question. These tumefactions have proved in most cases to be of an adenomatous character and it was finally recognized (first in the case of the thyroid) that adenomata of this kind were functionally active structures that produced hypersecretory effects. It then gradually came to be realized that the tumor need not necessarily be bulky but, quite to the contrary, striking clinical effects might be produced by minute, symptomatically predictable adenomas. So *it is the degree of secretory activity of an adenoma*, which may be out of all proportion to its dimensions, *that evokes the recognizable symptom-complex in all hypersecretory states.*

The pituitary adenomas. The anterior-pituitary body, as distinct from the neuro-hypophysis, is a compact of cellular elements of three recognizable sorts, divided by histologists, on the basis of their staining reactions, into two principal types: (1) those having a non-granular cytoplasm, and (2) those with a cytoplasm which is distinctly granular. Cells of the former type are known as neutrophil (chromophobe) elements and of the latter—the granular type—as chromophil elements of which there are two sorts: (a) those whose granules show an affinity for acid dyes (acidophil cells) and (b) those with an affinity for basic dyes (basophil or cyanophil cells). Each of these three cellular types—chromophobe, acidophil and basophil—is capable of producing its own peculiar adenomatous formations.

Whether these three types of cells are fixed in character or whether they represent different stages in activity of the same original cell is a matter of dispute. The most recent advocate of the unitarian view is Remy Collin of Nancy who, purely on anatomical grounds, presents[2] a convincing argument to show (*cf.* Fig. 1) that the non-granular cell (*cellule principale:* mother-cell) represents the primitive stage of activity of an element which in the process of ripening acquires a granular cytoplasm that is primarily acidophilic (eosinophilic) but which may in turn become basophilic (cyanophilic). When the ripened granular cytoplasm comes to be discharged, little is left but the nucleus and membrane of the cell which may then either degenerate or, in a renewed cycle, once more pass through these same stages to be again discharged under proper stimulus.[3] But if this is actually what takes place,

[1] The subject matter of this paper was ventilated at the New York Academy of Medicine, January 5, 1932; at the Yale Medical School, February 24, 1932, and at the Johns Hopkins Hospital Medical Society, February 29, 1932.

* Reprinted from *Bulletin of The Johns Hopkins Hospital*, 1932, *50:* 137–195, with the kind permission of the Editors of the *Bulletin* and The Johns Hopkins Press.

[2] Collin, R., La neurocrinie hypophysaire. Etude histophysiologique du complexe tubéro-infundibulo-pituitaire. Paris, G. Doin et Cie., 1928, 102 pp.

[3] Nothing of precisely this same sort, to be sure, occurs in other glands of internal secretion; but this need not unduly disturb us, for the pituitary body, whether taken from a morphological or functional aspect, is a tissue of surprises. It is now recognized by histologists that secretory cells discharge in three different ways. They may merely extrude their accumulated granules

the fact that each of these varieties of cells is capable of forming adenomata whose elements appear to be of fixed rather than of a changing type is highly peculiar. What is more, one would naturally expect that adenomata composed of the non-granular mother-cells (*Hauptzellen: cellules principales*) would be more likely to show evidences of cell division than would adenomata composed of elements in the more advanced stages of secretory activity. But just the opposite occurs; the elements composing the common chromophobe adenomata rarely if ever show cell division, whereas those of a chromophil adenoma, whether acidophilic or basophilic, are frequently multinuclear (*cf.* Figs. 2b, 16, 23) and show numerous mitotic figures.[4]

Meanwhile, experimental pathology has provided us with some fairly definite facts concerning the function not only of the anterior pituitary considered as a whole, but, in turn, of its different cellular constituents. When its frequent association with a pituitary tumor came to be recognized, it was at first supposed that acromegaly was an expression of glandular deficiency and theoretically should be reproducible by experimental extirpation of the gland. This, however, in the majority of cases led to early death, at least of adult animals (chiefly dogs), whereas younger animals when hypophysectomized, though they might recover for long periods, ceased to grow and remained sexually infantile.

It had already been observed that tumors, grossly indistinguishable in situation and type from those associated with acromegaly, were of far greater frequency and provoked a syndrome, so far as its endocrinological manifestations were concerned, of a wholly different character. Individuals affected by these tumors when of adult age, instead of a tendency to overgrowth, showed on the contrary a tendency to become adipose, to

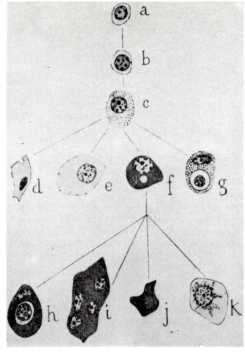

FIG. 1. Evolution of anterior-pituitary cell (Collin): (*a*) chief cell; (*b*) eosinophilic non-granular cell; (*c*) acidophilic granular cell; (*f* and *i*) typical basophilic forms; (*d* and *e*) degenerative eosinophilic cells; (*j* and *k*) degenerative basophilic cells; (*g* and *h*) endocytogenetic rebirth of chief cells.

lose their secondary sex-characters, and to become impotent, in company with recognizable atrophic changes in the sexual organs. When altogether comparable changes were seen occasionally to occur in animals (dogs) after incomplete experimental hypophysectomy, it became evident that the syndrome represented a deficiency state which was termed *hypo*pituitarism; and this furnished an added reason to assume—what had already been conjectured—that acromegaly almost certainly represented the counter state of *hyper*pituitarism.[5]

The final experimental proof of the correctness of this assumption was delayed until Evans and Long,[6] by daily parenteral injections of an alkaline anterior-lobe extract, succeeded in producing experimental overgrowth (gigantism) in the rat, an animal whose epiphyses do not close throughout

---

without particular change in form, as in gastric secretion; they may wholly disgorge their ripened cytoplasm, as in mammary secretion; or the entire cell may be cast off, as in sebaceous secretion—and this apparently is what takes place more particularly in the neurohypophysis from whose epithelial envelope (pars intermedia) degenerating cells are cast off which migrate through the pars nervosa where they become transformed into the hyaline bodies that presumably represent the active principle of this part of the gland.

[4] It would seem that the only possible way this question of fixity or changeableness of the elements composing pituitary adenomas could be conclusively answered would be by cultivating the cells of the different types to determine whether they breed true to their original form or whether their cytoplasm undergoes progressive alteration. Efforts in this direction have so far proved unconvincing owing largely to technical difficulties due to want of experience with the artificial growth of neoplastic tissues.

[5] Cushing, H.: The hypophysis cerebri: clinical aspects of hyperpituitarism and of hypopituitarism. J. Am. M. Ass., 1909, *53*, 249–255.

[6] Evans, H. M., and J. A. Long: The effect of the anterior lobe administered intraperitoneally upon growth, maturity, and oestrous cycle of the rat. Anat. Record, 1921, *21*, 62–63.

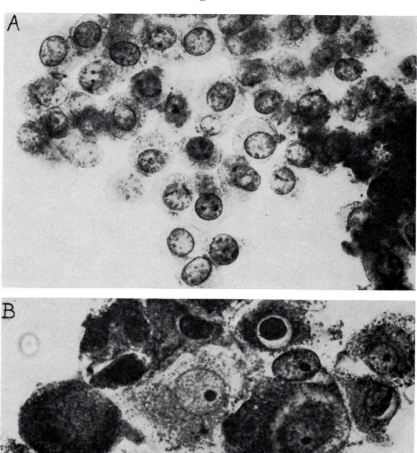

FIG. 2. Supravital preparation (Eisenhardt): (*A*) chromophobe adenoma (×850); (*B*) field from a chromophile adenoma (×850).

life; and subsequently in the dog, whose epiphyses like those of man normally do unite, Putnam, Benedict and Teel[7] produced a condition of overgrowth comparable in all respects to that characterizing acromegaly.

But this is only half the story. There was evidently a complicating element in these experiments. If only a single pituitary principle (hormone) had been involved in experimental hyper-

[7] Putnam, T. J., Benedict, E. B., and H. M. Teel: Studies in acromegaly. VIII. Experimental canine acromegaly produced by injection of anterior lobe pituitary extract. Arch. Surg., 1929, *18*, 1708–1736.

pituitarism of this kind, one might well enough have expected increased growth to go hand in hand with increased activation of the reproductive functions. But quite to the contrary, while the injections unmistakably served to promote growth, they at the same time checked the normal ovulatory cycle of the animals. In consequence of this observation, Dr. Evans was led to suspect the presence of dual glandular hormones and he came to believe, indeed, that they were in some peculiar way opposed in their action.

At another time and place a review has been given[8] of the steps leading to the disclosure that

the growth-provoking and sex-maturing principles—the former almost certainly elaborated by
the acidophil and the latter presumably[9] by the
basophil elements of the lobe—are chemically
separable hormones. Hence the former working
conception of hyperpituitarism *versus* hypopituitarism as an indication on the one hand of
secretory over-activity leading to acromegaly or
gigantism, and on the other hand of secretory
under-activity leading to a counterposed syndrome, wholly falls to the ground. Or, if not quite
so bad as this, it at least must be replaced by
hyperpituitary *versus* hypopituitary states due to
excessive or insufficient secretion not only of the
acidophil elements concerned with growth but
also of the basophil elements chiefly concerned,
presumably, with the ovulatory mechanism.[10]

In an attempt to interpret in terms of human
pathology the highly informing later-day disclosures of experimental biologists, we may properly
review, with necessary brevity, the development
of the idea that the adenomas which affect the
organs of internal secretion are not mere static
conglomerations of cells but represent lesions
possessing an incredible degree of physiological
activity, those which have most recently attracted
attention being the tiny adenomas of the parathyroid glandules and those of the pancreatic
islets.

The common tumors of the anterior pituitary—
first looked upon merely as a local expression of
acromegalic overgrowth, and subsequently as
sarcomas or "strumas" of the gland—were first
clearly differentiated by Benda in 1900 as vari

eties of adenoma; and we have slowly come to
understand with some degree of definiteness the
clinical pictures produced by those whose cells
possess a granular and acidophilic cytoplasm and
those with a non-granular or chromophobe cytoplasm. The former, even when so small that they
may easily escape postmortem detection, are productive of unmistakable acromegaly or gigantism
or a combination of the two. The more common
chromophobe adenomas, on the other hand,
usually attain a size sufficient to distort the
chiasm before they give appreciable clinical symptoms, and it is quite probable that the cells which
comprise them possess no secretory activity—
that is, produce no hormone. They nevertheless
cause their own peculiar constitutional disorder,
this being a deprivation syndrome[11] brought about
in all probability through compression of the
residual acidophil and basophil elements which no
longer are able to produce their peculiar secretory
product (Fig. 3).

This in general terms at least approximates the
truth. It must, however, be admitted that there
are certain borderline syndromes in which a primary wave of pathological overgrowth appears to
have been succeeded by a hypopituitary state—a
condition which for lack of a better term has been
called "fugitive acromegaly,"[12] the adenoma in
these states proving to be of a mixed cellular type.
Though the cells of these mixed adenomas are
predominantly chromophobe, a few of them show
a peripheral disposition of acidophil granules
suggesting the functional retrogression of previously mature acidophil elements; and since these
cells resemble the hypoacidophilic ("hypoeosinophilic") stage of development as described by
Collin, the observation might be construed as an
argument favoring his views. In other words, the
supposed functional immutability of the cells of an
anterior-pituitary adenoma may prove to be a
misconception; but this need not particularly concern us here.

Two examples of a third type of anterior-
pituitary adenoma, composed of basophil elements, were first described twenty years ago by
Erdheim,[13] the tiny lesions having been looked
upon as curiosities of morbid anatomy rather than
as findings of any conceivable clinical significance.
In one instance a small basophil adenoma, 1.5 mm.

---

[8] Teel, H. M., and H. Cushing: The separate growth-
promoting and gonad-stimulating hormones of the
anterior hypophysis: an historical review. Endokrinologie (Leipzig), 1930, vi, 401–420.

[9] The evidence of this is suggestive rather than conclusive. It is based on the facts: (1) that following castration, at least in the rat though not definitely in other
species, there is an increase in the basophil elements;
and (2) that the extracts of the pituitary glands of castrates of all species are more active than normal glands
in their gonad-stimulating properties. P. E. Smith
showed, moreover, that the central portion of the bovine anterior-pituitary which is particularly rich in
basophil elements has a more pronounced effect in
stimulating the thyroid to activity than the more eosinophilic cortical portion of the gland. The effect of these
injections on the adrenal cortex and the genital system
unfortunately was not noted.

[10] Time has shown that *hyper*pituitarism and *hypo*-
pituitarism are long words whose distinguishing syllable
is easily misread and misprinted. And now that it becomes necessary or advisable to recognize two hypersecretory states, the terms *pituitary acidophilism* and
pituitary basophilism are suggested as less unwieldy and
more easily interpreted than acidophilic hyperpituitarism (for acromegaly) and basophilic hyperpituitarism
(for the syndrome under discussion).

[11] *Cf.* Henderson, W. R.: Sexual dysfunction in adenomas of the pituitary body. Endocrinology, 1931, *15*,
111–127.

[12] Bailey, P., and H. Cushing: Studies in acromegaly.
VII. The microscopical structure of the adenomas in
acromegalic dyspituitarism (fugitive acromegaly). Am.
J. Path., 1928, *4*, 545–564.

[13] Erdheim, J.: Zur normalen und pathologischen
Histologie der Glandula thyreoidea, parathyreoidea
und Hypophysis. Beitr. f. path. Anat. u. Path., 1903,
33, 158–234.

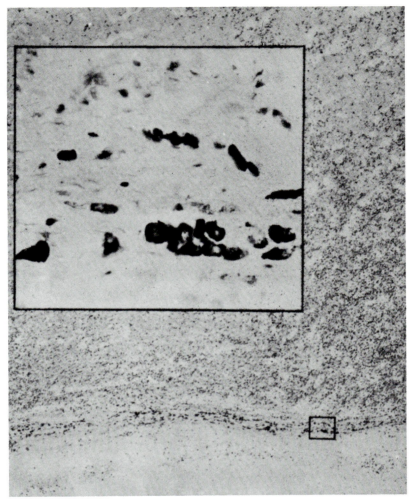

FIG. 3. Margin of large pituitary adenoma (×50) stained with ethyl violet-orange G for granules. Note peripheral rim of compressed granular cells shown in insert (×600).

in diameter, was found in a woman forty years of age supposedly the victim of Basedow's disease. The other example was found in a 43-year-old acromegalic whose relatively small pituitary body was chiefly occupied by a fair-sized eosinophil adenoma, the minute basophil adenoma measuring only 1 mm. in diameter having been regarded as an accessory finding.[14]

[14] It is quite conceivable that acidophil and basophil adenomata may not infrequently coexist in cases of acromegaly, but I know no other example than this in the literature. Such a coincidence might account for the differing syndromes shown by acromegalic patients some of whom exhibit disturbances which in the past we have been inclined to ascribe to the effects of secondary hyperplasia or adenoma-formation in the adrenal cortex.

PRESUMPTIVE EXAMPLES OF BASOPHIL
HYPERPITUITARISM

After this explanatory digression, let us return to a consideration of the peculiar polyglandular syndrome to which allusion was made in the introductory paragraph. The original example of the syndrome around which the present discussion hinges was described in my monograph (Case XLV, page 217) as having shown *a syndrome of painful obesity, hypertrichosis and amenorrhoea with overdevelopment of secondary sexual characteristics.* Whether these symptoms were chiefly attributable to disordered pituitary, adrenal, pineal or ovarian influences was uncertain.

Case 1. (J. H. H. Surgical No. 27140) Minnie G., an unmarried Russian Jewess, aged 23, referred by Dr.

Stetten of New York, was admitted to the Johns Hopkins Hospital on December 29, 1910.

Clinical history. One of a numerous and healthy family, though slight and undersized, she was well until 16 years of age, having escaped the customary children's ailments.

Her menses which started at the age of 14 were regular for two years and then suddenly ceased. She began to grow stout and in the two years prior to admission her weight had increased from 112 to 137 pounds. She suffered greatly from headaches, nausea and vomiting sometimes accompanying the more severe attacks. She complained also of aching pains in the eyes which latterly had become prominent, and there had been occasional periods of seeing double.

Other noteworthy symptoms were insomnia, tinnitus, extreme dryness of the skin, frequent sore throats, shortness of breath, palpitation, purpuric outbreaks, recurring nose-bleeds, and marked constipation accompanied by bleeding piles. A definite growth of hair had appeared on the face with thinning of hair on the scalp. She had become increasingly round-shouldered. Muscular weakness had become extreme and there was constant complaint of backache and epigastric pains.

Physical examination. This showed an undersized, kyphotic young woman 4 feet 9 inches in height (145 cm.), of most extraordinary appearance (Fig. 4). Her round face was dusky and cyanosed and there was an abnormal growth of hair, particularly noticeable on the sides of the forehead, upper lip and chin. The mucous membranes were of bright colour despite her history of frequent bleedings. Her abdominous body had the appearance of a full-term pregnancy. The breasts were hypertrophic and pendulous and there were pads of fat over the supra-clavicular and posterior cervical regions. The cyanotic appearance of the skin was particularly apparent over the body and lower extremities (Fig. 5) which were spotted by subcutaneous ecchymoses. Numerous purplish striae were present over the stretched skin of the lower abdomen and also over shoulders, breasts and hips; and a fine hirsuties was present over the back, hips and around the umbilicus. The skin which everywhere was rough and dry showed considerable pigmentation, particularly around the eyelids, groins, pubes and areolae of the breasts. The peculiar tense and painful adiposity affecting face, neck and trunk was in marked contrast to her comparatively spare extremities.

From a neurological aspect nothing was notable other than what at the time were taken to be signs of intracranial pressure: namely, headaches, slight exophthalmos, diplopia, puffiness of the eyelids and congestion of the optic discs [due, as would now appear, to deposition of intraorbital fat]. The cranial x-ray showed what for the day was regarded as a normal sella turcica. The epiphyseal lines (radial and phalangeal) were still roentgenologically visible. Not only did the skin bruise easily but spontaneous ecchymoses frequently appeared. Lumbar puncture, pricking of ear, etc., caused subcutaneous extravasations. Blood examination showed 5,300,000 erythrocytes and 12,000 leucocytes (polymorphonuclears 77 per cent), with a haemoglobin of 85 per cent. The systolic blood pressure was consistently high, averaging 185 mm. Hg.

There were no clear therapeutic indications and she

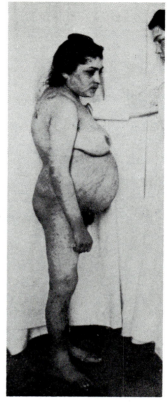

Fig. 4. Case 1. The original example (1902) of basophil (unverified) obesity.

was discharged. She reentered the hospital again in July 1911, at which time, owing to the assumption that her continued cephalalgia might be due to intracranial pressure, an oldtime subtemporal decompression was performed, a wet brain being disclosed without subsequent protrusion at the site of the bone defect. She also at this time complained so greatly of backache and pain in the left side that an exploration of the kidney and adrenal gland was under contemplation.

It was at this stage of the story that the case was first reported. Its most striking feature was the rapidly acquired adiposity of peculiar distribution in an amenorrhoeic young woman. At the time, Dercum's adiposis dolorosa (usually a menopausal disorder) Bartel's and Fröhlich's adiposogenital dystrophy (commonly associated with hypophysial-duct tumors) and the adipositas cerebralis of Aschner and Erdheim (due to hypothalamic lesions) were but vague terms; and the possible relation of the basophilic elements in the anterior pituitary to the reproductive functions was not even suspected.

In commenting on the case at the time, it was pointed out that a somewhat similar polyglandular syndrome had previously been recorded not only in association with pinealomas but with adenomatous or hyperplastic adrenal tumors. A chance remark that we might be on the way toward the recognition of the consequences of hyperadrenalism may possibly have inclined some of those, who soon reported similar cases, to believe that the source of the trouble in all probability lay in the adrenal gland. To this I shall return.

The case of Minnie G. further: Because of her continued complaints with an increase of weight up to 151 pounds, on Dr. Stetten's recommendation she again came under observation for a period of two months from May to July, 1913, at the Brigham Hospital in Boston.

Her symptoms and general condition at this time were found to be essentially unaltered. Though there was no protrusion at the site of the old decompression, the optic discs were still hyperaemic and congested with hazy margins, while the fields of vision were contracted and the acuity considerably reduced. Her blood-pressure fluctuated around 180/110, on one occasion reaching 210/140. She was still somewhat polycythemic, the erythrocytes slightly exceeding five million, the highest count having been 5,248,000 with a haemoglobin estimation of 105 per cent. Several differential blood counts were essentially within normal limits.

She was for a time studied by my medical colleague, Dr. Christian. On the basis of a defective excretion of phenolsulphonephthalein and the presence in the urine of a slight trace of albumin with occasional hyaline casts, he felt that a vascular type of nephritis was the probable cause of her hypertension. She was again discharged with no therapeutic recommendations.

On November 15, 1922, after an interval of nine years, she was for the second time admitted to the Brigham Hospital. It was then learned that her menses, after complete cessation for ten years, had late in 1913 again become irregularly re-established; also that in 1917 she had had an exploratory operation for a stone in the left kidney, but she was uncertain whether a calculus had actually been found.

The blood-pressure at this time averaged in the neighborhood of 160/95; the blood-count showed 5,240,000 erythrocytes; the basal metabolism was minus nine. Her general appearance was much as before, though she had lost some weight. The cranial roentgenograms taken at this time show [as subsequently reread] an unmistakable diffuse decalcification of the bones. Renal pyelograms were made, no trace of stone or other renal abnormality being disclosed. There was no evidence of advancing nephritis and on the whole she seemed at least no worse than in 1913. She accordingly was discharged once more without further light having been thrown on the nature of her disorder.

From correspondence it may be gathered that she at present (1932) is in reasonably good health though some of the stigmata of her malady still persist.

In the intervening years six other examples of the same or a highly similar disorder have been carefully studied at the Brigham Hospital. The patients were all comparatively young women who, in association with a more or less abrupt

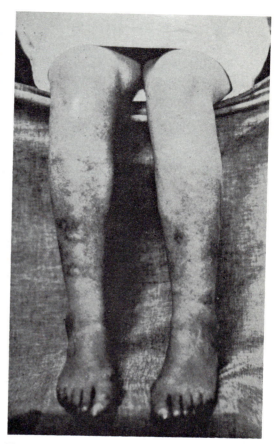

Fig. 5. Case 1. To show acrocyanosis with scars and ecchymoses of lower limbs.

amenorrhoea, had become rapidly obese with a peculiar tense and more or less painful adiposity chiefly affecting head, neck and trunk. They were all plethoric in appearance, all had become abnormally hirsute, all but one showed purplish cutaneous striae. Vascular hypertension with a high red blood count and haemoglobin percentage was usually present, and all complained of aches and pains and general enfeeblement. In some of the cases the acuteness of the condition appeared to subside, and only one, so far as known, succumbed to her malady.

Meanwhile, soon after the case of Minnie G. had been reported in 1912, descriptions of polyglandular syndromes closely resembling hers began to appear in the literature; and in a few instances, owing to the fatal outcome of the disorder, a systematic study of the organs was made possible. Such of these cases as have come to my attention may be given in the chronological order in which they appeared in print. The first of them was recorded in 1913 by Dr. H. G. Turney of London.[15]

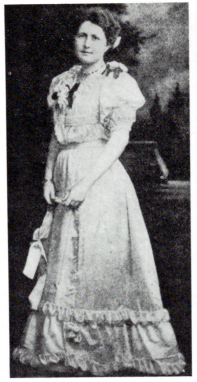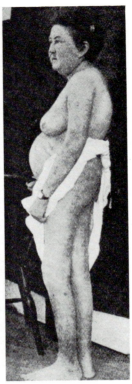

Figs. 6 AND 7. Dr. Turney's patient at the age of 20 and five years later (1913) at the height of the disorder.

Case 2. [Dr. Turney's patient.] *Amenorrhoea. Acute plethoric obesity with hypertrichosis. Spinal kyphosis from skeletal decalcification. Vascular hypertension. Polycythaemia. Duration 7 years. Autopsy.*

Miss A. O., a previously healthy and normal young woman, in 1907 when 20 years of age, suddenly ceased menstruating and began to grow obese. Three years later, she observed a tendency for her extremities to bruise easily. She gradually became increasingly round-shouldered (kyphotic) thereby losing two and a half inches (6.4 cm.) in height. Her chief complaints were of pain in the back.

The face was extremely fat and florid and the texture firm. The hair of the head was dry and somewhat scanty, as was the pubic and axillary hair, but there was a growth of fine short hair over the back and upper legs. Notable were the large pendulous mammae and the great obesity of the abdomen, which had the contour of a full-term pregnancy (*cf.* Figs. 6, 7).

The obesity of the trunk was in marked contrast to the somewhat thin extremities which below the knee were of a dark brownish color, interspersed with recent ecchymoses. The skin had a parchment-like texture. Numerous broad, red, atrophic striae were present over the abdomen and thorax. An apparent partial absorption of the posterior clinoid processes was shown by cranial roentgenograms. A glistening subretinal exudate was present in the right eye, probably from an absorbed haemorrhage. The systolic blood-pressure was high, varying between 200 and 185 mm. Hg. There had been a tendency to polycythemia, the erythrocytes on one occasion having been counted at eight million and on another at six million. The urine contained no albumin. Carbohydrate tolerance was normal.

The subsequent history of this patient was briefly given in a later article by Dr. Parkes Weber.[16] Several spontaneous fractures occurred from time to time, involving sternum, clavicle, and ribs. Multiple ulcers and subcutaneous abscesses developed, and in May 1914, seven years from the symptomatic onset of the disorder, death ended the story.

An *autopsy* was performed. The body was that of an hirsute woman with "abundant hair on the chin" and multiple subcutaneous abscesses and ulcers. There was found a chronic nephritis, an hypertrophic ventricle of the left heart, a fatty infiltrated liver, and *an enlarged left suprarenal gland* of "bulky cortex." The ovaries were small. The bones showed calcareous deficiency ("fibrous osteitis" and were so soft they could be easily cut with scissors. "Nothing abnormal was found in the *pituitary and thyroid glands*." [How thorough an examination of the former was made is not stated.]

---

[15] Turney, H. G.: Discussion on disease of the pituitary body. Proc. Roy. Soc. Med. (Sec. Neurol. and Ophth.), 1913 ,6, lxix–lxxviii.

[16] *Cf. infra.*, Brit. J. Dermat., 1926.

Dr. Turney at the time of his report, while the patient was still living, apparently favored a pituitary origin for the symptoms, but this opinion may have been modified by the post-mortem findings; Dr. Parkes Weber, on the other hand, in his subsequent discussion of the case appears to have regarded it as unquestionably due to a primary adrenal disorder. The next example of which I have knowledge was reported two years later (1915) by Dr. John Anderson of Glasgow.[17]

Case 3. [Dr. Anderson's patient.] *Amenorrhoea. Plethoric obesity. Hypertrichosis. Vascular hypertension. Asthenia. Duration 5 years. Autopsy: osteomalacia; adenoma of anterior pituitary and of adrenal cortex.*

A women, at the age of 23, in association with a menstrual irregularity which in two years was followed by total amenorrhoea, became increasingly obese, the adiposity sparing the limbs. The adipose areas were tender on palpation. She suffered much from headaches, pains in the chest and eyeballs, the eyes having become somewhat exophthalmic. She acquired a reddish complexion and facial hirsuties, developed a tendency to petechial haemorrhages and purpuric outbreaks on her arms and legs, the slightest contusion provoking ecchymoses. The systolic blood-pressure was 185 mm.; the red blood count approximated five million. Muscular weakness became extreme, and she finally died from increasing asthenia. The whole course of the malady was something over five years.

At the postmortem examination, arteriosclerosis with "chronic interstitial nephritis" was found. The ribs were brittle and easily fractured. The *ovaries* and uterus were senile in character; the *thyroid* was slightly enlarged; the *parathyroids* were normal, the *thymus* atrophic. In the medulla of one of the *suprarenal glands* which were "slightly enlarged" was a small pea-sized tumor, microscopically resembling the structure of the zona fasciculata. The *anterior pituitary* contained a small adenoma [type unrecorded] the size of a millet seed close to the pars intermedia. In the rest of the anterior lobe "the basophil cells were apparently increased at the expense of the eosinophil cells."

In his discussion of this case, Dr. Anderson expressed the belief that it was primarily a pituitary disorder, his interpretation being that it was an example of hypopituitarism [*sic*] with secondary hyperfunctioning of the suprarenal glands (hyperadrenalism) accounting for the development of the secondary male sexual characteristics. Needless to say, it was not well known at the time that true hypopituitary states are associated with atrophy rather than hyperplasia of the adrenal cortex, a similar dystrophy likewise affecting the thyroid and reproductive organs.

In 1919, another example of a syndrome which appears to be related to the disorder under discussion was reported by Dr. Reichmann[18] from the Medical Clinic of Jena. Apart from a swollen and plethoric face, the patient was not adipose but on the contrary was rather emaciated. She showed vascular hypertension with negative urine. There was bowing of the back and she had lost several centimetres in height. Because of the prominence of the eyes and fulness of the lids she was supposed to have Basedow's disease. This was excluded as was also cardio-renal hypertension; and under the belief that the condition was ascribable to a sympathico-adrenal disorder the left adrenal gland was surgically removed with a fatality a few days later from a generalized peritonitis. The autopsy showed a cardiac hypertrophy, hyperplastic arteriosclerosis, skeletal osteoporosis with spinal curvature, the bones being easily cut with a knife. The pituitary body, while macroscopically normal, was found on section to contain within a compressed mantle chiefly composed of basophilic elements a tumor "resembling a small-celled sarcoma." This was found to be an adenoma composed of chromophobe cells some of which contained eosinophilic [*sic*] granules. The thyroid was small; the remaining adrenal was hyperplastic; the ovaries fibrotic.

In his discussion of the case, the author, if correctly understood, was inclined to regard it as a form of acromegaly, the hyperpituitary changes being confined to the thickened and cyanotic face; the other symptoms were ascribed to a secondary adrenal origin.[19]

Chronologically the next fairly unmistakable case of which I have knowledge was described in Professor Zondek's monograph (1923) on the ductless glands[20] among other examples of so-called pluriglandular insufficiency.

Case 4. [Dr. Zondek's patient.] *Amenorrhoea. Acute adiposity. Facial hirsuties. Spinal kyphosis. Glycosuria. Duration 5 years. Autopsy: Skeletal osteoporosis; pituitary tumor (adenoma?).*

This concerned a 24-year-old Russian woman who had previously been normal in all respects and in good health. At the age of 19, amenorrhoea set in and she began rapidly to grow adipose, accumulations of fat being limited to the head and trunk, while the extremities remained thin (Figs. 8, 9). She began to lose the hair of her head, whereas on the cheeks and upper lip a somewhat definite beard began to appear; and as time

[17] Anderson, J.: A case of polyglandular syndrome with adrenal hypernephroma and adenoma in the pituitary gland—both of small size. Glasgow M. J., 1915, *83*, 178–192.

[18] Reichmann, V. Ueber ein ungewöhnliches Krankheitsbild bei Hypophysenadenom. Deutsch. Arch. f. klin. Med., 1919, *130*, 133–150.

[19] It may be assumed from the postmortem findings that this was a typical example of pituitary basophilism. The case has not been counted because of the absence of adiposity of the trunk which is so marked a feature of all the others. It suggests that the disorder may not necessarily be accompanied by abdominous obesity.

[20] Zondek, H.: Die Krankheiten der Endokrinen Drüsen. Berlin, Julius Springer, 1923, 287 pp.

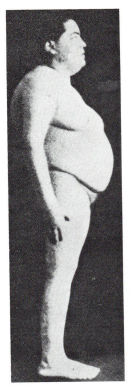 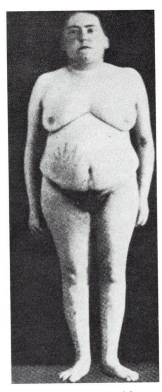

FIGS. 8 AND 9. Photographs of Dr. Zondek's case of pituitary tumor with osteomalacia (1923).

passed she became increasingly round-shouldered.

Glycosuria was found and the urine at one time showed as much as 3 per cent of sugar. The skin became pigmented, suggesting an adrenal disorder. The cutaneous dryness from lack of normal secretion strongly suggested myxoedema. Hence there were polyglandular disturbances which appeared to affect the function of the adrenals, thyroid, ovary and pancreas. She finally died of an intercurrent erysipelas.

An *autopsy* was performed. A marked osteoporosis of the skeleton was found, it being easily possible to cut the vertebral bodies with a knife, the spongy part of the bone having largely disappeared. There was follicular atresia of the ovaries, marked lipomatosis of the *pancreas*, an increase of colloid in the abnormally small *thyroid*, hypoplasia of the *thymus*, and capillary dilatation of the *parathyroid glandules*. [The adrenal glands are not mentioned and presumably would have been had they shown any change.]

The *pituitary body* showed no apparent abnormality until examined microscopically when it was found: "that the anterior lobe was enormously reduced and diminished mesially to a narrow ledge. As contrasted with this finding, the intermediary layer, as well as the posterior lobe, was rather more than normally developed. Between the gliomatous fibres of the posterior lobe, there were enlargements of the intermediary spaces, the exact nature of which, whether hydropical enlargements or myxomatous degenerations, could not be determined. In the vicinity of the diminished anterior lobe a tremendously developed fibrous tissue was encountered, into which the glandular elements of the anterior lobe gradually passed over. As to the kind of destroying process, involving particularly the anterior lobe, no definite decision was possible, this being the more difficult, as *there were nests of an adenomous-like structure enclosed in the masses of fibrous tissue.* The identity of these cells with the anterior-pituitary cells could not with certainty be determined, but Professor Benda, who saw the specimens, favored more the diagnosis of a tumor arising from the hypophysial duct."

This briefly reported case, in which some clinical details are unfortunately lacking, was, properly enough, regarded as one of pluriglandular nature, the most significant postmortem findings seemingly having been the lesion of somewhat obscure nature in the anterior pituitary. The adrenal glands at least we may assume to have shown no abnormality. Attention may be drawn to the fact that, as in the two preceding cases, the bones were described as being markedly softened and fragile, so much so indeed, that in his discussion of osteomalacia Zondek refers to this case (*loc. cit.*, p. 235) as illustrating one type of the disease.

In the following year, 1924, Drs. B. S. Oppenheimer and A. M. Fishberg of New York published a paper[21] in which the association of non-nephritic

[21] Oppenheimer, B. S., and A. M. Fishberg: The association of hypertension with suprarenal tumors. Arch. Int. Med., 1924, *34*, 631–644.

hypertension with suprarenal tumors was under discussion. Two illustrative cases were given. The first of them was that of a man said to have had an acromegalic appearance who was found after death to have had a tumor of the suprarenal cortex associated with cardiac hypertrophy. It is merely stated that the head and neck organs were negative, no specific mention being made of an histological examination of the pituitary body. It need scarcely be said that adenomas of the adrenal and cardiac hypertrophy are common in acromegaly. However, I have no wish to pick possible flaws in this highly interesting paper but rather to call attention to the authors' second case which bears a close resemblance to those under discussion. The essentials of the clinical history are as follows:

Case 5. [Patient of Drs. Oppenheimer and Fishberg.] *Plethoric obesity. Facial hirsuties. Cardiac hypertrophy. Vascular hypertension. Glycosuria. Cutaneous pigmentation and abscesses. Duration 5 years. Death without autopsy.*

S. G., an undersized child, 12 years of age, was admitted to the Montefiore Hospital complaining of weakness and adiposity. In her sixth year she suddenly began to put on flesh and became disproportionately adipose, gaining about 75 pounds (34 kg.). She was seen by many physicians and treated symptomatically with various glandular preparations. About a year prior to her admission the parents noticed a change in coloration of the skin and the patient developed a tendency to fall asleep. A routine urine examination revealed 4 per cent of sugar. Polyuria and nocturia developed about this time. At the age of 11, hair began to grow on the face, axilla and pubis. The patient had never menstruated.

Physical examination. An undersized child, appearing many years older than her actual age (Figs. 10–12). She was exceedingly obese and had a very red, plethoric facies. There was a well marked growth of hair on the chin and lower cheeks; pubic and axillary hair was abundant. The skin was dry and on the abdomen were pigmented striae. There were abscesses on the back and neck, a mycotic infection of the nails, and ulcers on the legs. There was no oedema whatever.

The heart was enlarged to the left. The sounds were of good quality, the second sound being accentuated over the aortic area. There were no murmurs. The blood pressure was 190 systolic, 130 diastolic.

The urine contained sugar but no acetone bodies. There was a heavy cloud of albumin but neither casts nor cellular elements were found. Phenolsulphonephthalein elimination, 45 per cent (after intravenous injection). The basal metabolic rate was normal. The blood showed 260 mg. of sugar per hundred cubic centimeters; erythrocytes, 4,500,000; white cells 11,800 with 78 per cent polymorphonuclears; haemoglobin, 90 per cent (Sahli). Roentgenologically the sella turcica was slightly larger than normal and showed bone absorption in the neighborhood.

The patient was placed on an anti-diabetic diet and digitalized. The urine rapidly became normal; the sugar and albumin disappeared completely. At one time signs

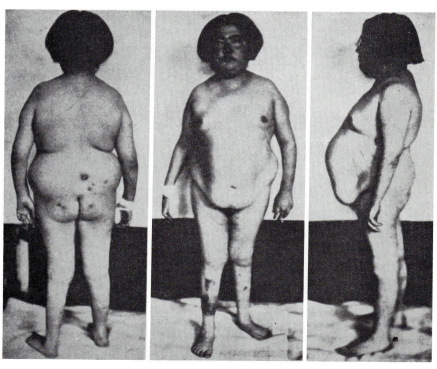

Figs. 10–12. Drs. Oppenheimer and Fishberg's patient with "adrenal hypertension" (1924).

and symptoms of broncho-pneumonia appeared but cleared up. The abscesses of the neck and back finally healed. At this juncture, the parents insisted on removing her from the hospital and she died three weeks later. Though no postmortem examination was obtained, the clinical picture, in the authors' words, "was so characteristic of suprarenal hyperplasia as to leave little doubt of the diagnosis."

It can be seen that the syndrome presented by this patient, though it was of preadolescent onset, bore a close resemblance to that of the others so far presented: *viz.*, a rapidly acquired adiposity sparing the extremities, a plethoric facies with pigmented abdominal striae, an exaggeration of the secondary sexual characters accompanied by a growth of hair on cheeks and chin, vascular hypertension, and glycosuria. Her precocious secondary sex-characters were unaccompanied by any signs of menstruation.

The close resemblance to the original case of Minnie G. shown by these last four patients, in their symptomatic history, in their physical appearance, and in their clinical findings, is unmistakable. They are examples unquestionably of a highly similar polyglandular disorder the interpretation of which to this point remains highly obscure in spite of the three postmortem examinations. A tendency to chronic nephritis with cardiac hypertrophy probably secondary to the hypertension was noted in Cases 2, 3 and 5. A peculiar softening of the bones was mentioned in all three autopsied cases. The adrenal glands showed a unilateral enlargement in Case 2, a pea-sized adenoma in Case 3, and are not mentioned in Case 4. The pituitary body was said to be normal in Case 2, to show a minute adenoma (type undesignated) in Case 3, and an "adenomatous-like structure" of undetermined nature in Case 4.

We now come to a particularly well recorded example of the disorder published in 1926 from which something more definite can be learned. I have taken the liberty of quoting fully from the author's vivid description[22] of the case.

Case 6. [Dr. Parkes Weber's case.] *Plethoric obesity. Amenorrhoea. Purpuric ecchymoses and cutaneous striae. Facial hirsuties. Exophthalmos. Vascular hypertension. Duration 4 years. Autopsy: cardiac hypertrophy; nephritis; pituitary adenoma (basophilic).*

"The patient, Mrs. E. B., aged 28 years, an Englishwoman, suffers from a 'coarse' plethoric-looking type of obesity, chronic purpura (Fig. 13), and large 'striae cutis distensae' ('striae atrophicae') of the trunk and limbs. The purpura recurs from time to time in the form of 'crops' of cutaneous petechiae and ecchymoses. Constriction of the veins of the arm at once produces ecchymoses. The 'striae' are of different dates and vary correspondingly in color, the newer ones being purplish, the older ones paler. The face is coarsely hyperaemic. The obesity is shown chiefly in the trunk, by the large fatty pendulous breasts and the corpulent projecting abdomen (Fig. 14).

"The limbs are not specially large, and the legs below the knees are relatively thin and have a striking appearance. They show transverse 'striae' (like the thighs do), and besides petechiae and ecchymoses there is a peculiar brownish discoloration, especially over the anterior surface, resulting probably from previous multiple haemorrhages. Moreover, a good deal of the skin in front of both legs has become shiny or parchment-like owing to some atrophic change. In spite of the obese appearance of her trunk, her body-weight is actually

[22] Parkes Weber, F.: Cutaneous striae, purpura, high blood-pressure, amenorrhoea and obesity, of the type sometimes connected with cortical tumours of the adrenal glands, occurring in the absence of any such tumour— with some remarks on the morphogenetic and hormonic effects of true hypernephromata of the adrenal cortex. Brit. J. Dermat., 1926, *38*, 1–19.

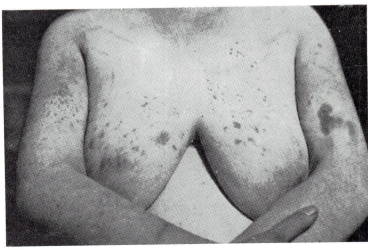

FIG. 13. Case 6. Dr. Parkes Weber's patient (1926) showing cutaneous hemorrhages and striae ascribed to adrenal hyperplasia.

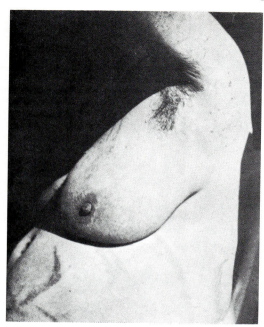

Fig. 14. Case 6. Left side of patient's trunk showing adiposity and purple striae of abdomen and mamma.

only 54 kgrm. [119 pounds], her height being 159 cm. [5 ft. 3 in.].

"The blood-pressure is high, the brachial systolic blood-pressure ranging from 205 to 230 mm. Hg.[23] The urine contains a little albumin, but is practically free from tube-casts. The administration of 100 grm. of sugar causes the appearance of a little sugar in the urine. The blood-sugar, when fasting, is within normal limits, but the curve after the administration of sugar by the mouth reaches its maximum height only after two hours. The blood-count shows nothing special, except-ing a moderate polymorphonuclear leucocytosis, pos-sibly connected with pyorrhoea alveolaris; the throm-bocytes are 180,000 to the c.mm. of blood. Ophthalmo-scopic examination (Dr. C. Markus, June 5th, 1925): In both eyes there is optic neuritis with white foci surrounding the optic discs; no haemorrhages; no macular changes. No tumour can be felt by abdominal palpation and no enlargement of the spleen or liver can be made out; by vaginal examination the uterus is like that of a nulli-para; there is no sign of any intra-thoracic disease. By roentgen-ray examination the *dorsum sellae turcicae* gives only an extremely faint shadow, but the pituitary fossa appears of normal size. There is slight bilateral exophthalmos. The basal meta-bolic rate is 20 per cent above the normal. . . . There is slight hairiness of the chin and upper lip. The Wasser-mann reaction is negative. . . .

"The *history* is that the patient was a twin, her fellow twin being born dead. Her father and mother are both living, aged 56 and 49 respectively, and the blood-

[23] On May 31st, when the brachial systolic blood-pressure was 220 mm. Hg., the brachial diastolic blood-pressure was 170 mm. Hg.

pressure of each of them is high. They have had eleven children, of whom only four are living. . . . She was married in December, 1922, and has never been preg-nant. Her menstrual periods ceased suddenly about September, 1921, but she had three slight periods again after her marriage. Since then (March, 1923) there has been complete amenorrhoea. About March 1922, she already began to get fatter, especially in the face and abdomen. But it is only since about March, 1923, *with the onset of permanent amenorrhoea*, that her chief symptoms have gradually developed: headaches, pains in her whole body, attacks of dyspnoea (accompanied by a sensation of suffocation), feelings of sickness (for which she sometimes induces vomiting by putting her finger in her mouth), frequent slight, epitaxis, the 'coarse' type of obesity already mentioned, the cutane-ous 'striae,' the purpura, the slight exophthalmos.

"The patient died on July 4th, 1925, in an attack clinically resembling acute pulmonary oedema. She had had a similar attack previously in the hospital, relieved apparently by blood-letting."

At the *postmortem examination:* There was no tumour in either *adrenal gland*, but the medullary substance was apparently rather in excess. The left ventricle of the heart was hypertrophied. There was slight chronic inter-stitial nephritis (slight renal sclerosis). In the anterior lobe of the *pituitary gland* was a minute adenoma con-sisting of basophil cells. There was no evidence of dis-ease in the *thyroid gland* or in the *ovaries;* the latter were said to have been rather small but histologically normal.

Microscopical examination "The *pituitary gland:* Its three parts can be easily distinguished. In the anterior part is a rounded nodule ($3 \times 4\frac{1}{2}$ mm. in the hardened sections) of basophil cells, in alveolar arrangement (with some minute calcareous spots), contained in a thin connective-tissue capsule; it is evidently a basophil adenoma. The remainder of the anterior part and the middle and posterior parts of the pituitary gland are of normal appearance. In the anterior lobe-spur of the pedicle of the pituitary gland there are many relatively large epithelial islands (Erdheim) [cf. Case 4]. This is remarkable, but must not be considered pathological. No special immigration of cells from the middle lobe into the posterior lobe can be made out."

Dr. Weber states in conclusion: "In my opinion it belongs to a group of cases characterized by complete amenorrhoea and by symptoms [given in the title of his paper] sometimes connected with cortical adrenal tumours, occurring in the absence of any such tumour. The main features cannot be explained by the small adenoma of the pituitary gland found at the post-mortem exami-nation."

In search of further information regarding this important case, Dr. Weber was written to and he obligingly forwarded the original paraffin block from which further sections of the tumor have been made. He also referred me to Professor Herbert M. Turnbull of the London Hospital who first recognized the nature of the lesion as a baso-phil adenoma and who kindly sent me the ac-companying photographs (Figs. 15, 16) from the single section in his possession.

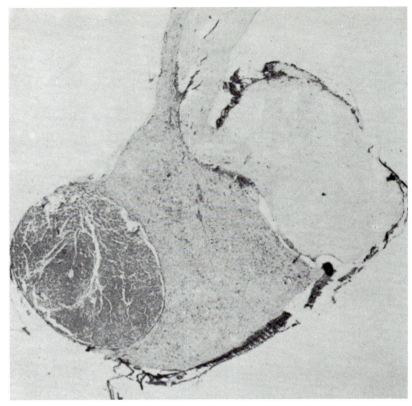

Fig. 15. Case 6. The anterior basophil adenoma (aniline blue-fuchsin, ×10). Kindness of Professor H. M. Turnbull.

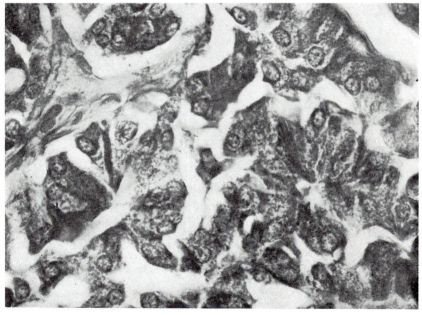

Fig. 16. Case 6. From the centre of the basophil adenoma to show the blue basophil granules in the often multinuclear cells (aniline blue-fuchsin, ×1020). Kindness of Professor Turnbull.

Much has been learned since 1926 concerning the influence of the pituitary body on the development and regulation of the genital system,[24] and Dr. Weber would have been more likely today than at that time to suspect the probable influence on his patient's syndrome of a pituitary adenoma which was then so easily explained away in favor of an adrenal influence even in the absence of any definite microscopical abnormality in these latter glands.

It was at about this time that it had become possible by crude chemical methods to separate the growth and sex hormones from bovine hypophyses and though Dott and Bailey in a study of the pituitary adenomas in the Brigham collection had stated in 1925[25] that basophil adenomata occur only in the form of minute intraglandular nodules that give rise to no known clinical manifestations, some of us soon began to suspect that this was probably a matter of not knowing what to look for.

This at least was the conclusion arrived at as the result of a survey of the then known facts regarding the dual anterior pituitary hormones which, chiefly for our own information, my junior co-worker, Dr. Harold Teel, and I shortly afterward came to put together.[26] The prepared mind was what enabled Dr. Teel during his house officership at the Lakeside Hospital in Cleveland for the first time to predict the presence of a basophil adenoma which, as will be told, was confirmed at autopsy.[27] The case history, which unfortunately is lacking in many details, may be briefly summarized as follows:

Case 7. [Dr. Teel's patient.] Obesity. Hypertrichosis. Menstrual irregularity. Meningitis. Autopsy: basophilic adenoma.

An exceedingly obese and abundantly hirsute young woman, 20 years of age, admitted to hospital in a comatose condition due to a meningococcal meningitis, was under clinical observation for only three days before she died.

Owing to her physical condition, a personal history was not obtainable, but it was learned that at the age of nine she had a continuous menstrual flow lasting four months. Subsequently, at the age of 14, she was said to have attained a normal adolescence, but her periods were subsequently most irregular. From the age of 15 she had grown exceedingly stout, the maximum weight

of 206 pounds (93.4 kg.) having been recorded seven months before her hospital admission. Because of excessive fatigability she had consulted a physician at about that time, when and he found she had a basal metabolic rate of +33, her enlarged thyroid was roentgenologically radiated. This is said to have caused little or no symptomatic improvement.

At *autopsy*, a suppurative meningococcic leptomeningitis was found to be the obvious cause of death. The *pituitary body* appeared to be of normal size, but suspecting from the patient's general appearance what might be found, Dr. Teel had the gland serially sectioned and a small though unmistakable basophil adenoma measuring 2.5 mm. in diameter was disclosed (Fig. 17). There was a persistent *thymus*, a slight enlargement of the *thyroid*, questionable enlargement of the pancreatic islets, and a definite enlargement (20 gm.) of the *suprarenals* with no histological change of structure, no definite secondary adenomata being present in any of these organs. The *ovaries* were enlarged apparently from increase in stroma; there was a single large corpus luteum with a small central haemorrhagic area and several smaller ones in various stages of organization. The only true neoplastic growth was the small anterior-pituitary adenoma to which the other endocrine changes were regarded as purely secondary.

THE SYNDROME AS IT OCCURS IN THE MALE

To this point, examples have been presented of this peculiar polyglandular syndrome as it occurs in women who seem to be more commonly victimized than do men. Why this should be so, if it is actually so, is not fully apparent. It is perhaps reasonable to assume that the combination of amenorrhoea, adiposity and heterosexual hirsuties may excite the attention of physicians and be recorded as a freakish disorder more often than would corresponding maladies in men.

However this may be, five cases of the same or a comparable disturbance, three of them with and two without autopsy, can be cited in the male. The first case, unfortunately unaccompanied by photographs of the patient, was briefly reported after careful study by Dr. E. D. Friedman of New York.[28] The essentials only need here be given.

Case 8. [Dr. Friedman's case.] Obesity. Hypertrichosis. Vascular hypertension. Glycosuria.

E. C., a student, 19 years of age, complained of obesity, hypertension and recurrent pains in the region of the spine for six months.

He was an undersized young man who at the age of ten in the course of two months had grown rapidly stout. Treatment with thyroid extract was without avail. His abdomen became pendulous and face ruddy. More recently he had been having shooting pains in the region of the spine, chest, and abdomen. He was thought to have "kidney trouble." There was shortness of breath, palpitation and tremor on exertion, dimness of vision and occasional headaches with impairment of memory. Nycturia was present; libido absent.

[24] *Cf.* Smith, P. E., and E. T. Engle: Am. J. Anat., 1927, *40*, 159–217. Also: Zondek, B., and S. Aschheim; Klin. Wchnschr., 1927, *6*, 248–252.

[25] Dott, N. M., and P. Bailey: Hypophysial adenomata. Brit. J. Surg., 1925, *13*, 314–366.

[26] Teel, H. M., and H. Cushing: The separate growth-promoting and gonad-stimulating hormones of the anterior hypophysis: an historical review. Endokrinologie (Leipzig), 1930, *6*, 401–420.

[27] Teel, H. M.: Basophilic adenoma of the hypophysis with associated pluriglandular syndrome. Arch. Neurol. & Psychiat., 1931, *26*, 593–599.

[28] Friedman, E. D. An unusual hypophyseal syndrome. N. York M. J., 1921, *114*, 113.

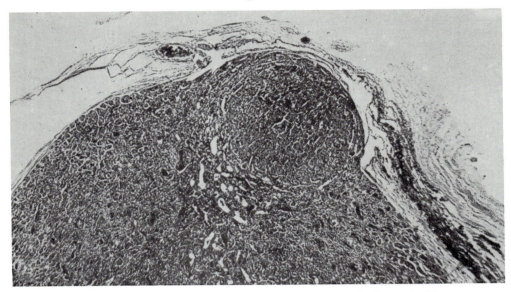

Fig. 17. The basophilic adenoma clinically predicted in Dr. Teel's case (1931).

Physical examination. The patient was round shouldered and short (136.5 cm.: 4 ft. 7 in.), obese (46.4 kgm.: 102 lbs.), with an erythematous face and a pendulous, distended abdomen. The mammae were well developed, the genitals small, and the fat distribution was of feminine type. There was an overgrowth of hair at the bridge of the nose and the body was covered with a fine lanugo. The heart was somewhat enlarged to the left. The skin, which was dry, showed ringworm in the axillae and pubes; erythema and telangiectasis of the face; and "striae distensae" on the abdomen and thighs.

Blood-pressure was 198/110 and there were two minute haemorrhages in the outer side of the left optic disc. The basal metabolic rate was −5 per cent. The urine showed glycosuria with a faint trace of albumin; the phenolsulphonephthalein excretion was diminished. The blood showed 95 per cent haemoglobin, 4,860,000 erythrocytes, 13,400 white cells of which 76 per cent were polynuclears. Chemical examination disclosed, in mgm. per cent, an excess of non-protein nitrogen (46.6); of cholesterin (308); and of sugar (240).

Roentgenograms: of the skull, showed markedly atrophic and thin bones of sella and sphenoid; of the hands, "a development of bones such as is usually seen in persons about 13 years of age." [Dr. Friedman informs me that the patient died of pneumonia in November of the year in which his report was made: there was no autopsy.]

It was recognized that this boy's syndrome had no relation to hyperpituitarism (acromegaly) nor to hypopituitarism (syndrome of Fröhlich). This condition nevertheless was thought to be of pituitary origin though the tendency to hypertrichosis and high cholesterin content of the blood suggested an involvement of the adrenals.

In the same year as the foregoing (1921) a highly suggestive example with a detailed post-

mortem examination was recorded by Dr. Hermann Mooser from the Pathological Institute of Zurich then under the direction of Professor Busse.[29] Though the protocol specifically states that the pituitary body was normal, the case so definitely fits into the polyglandular syndrome under consideration it cannot properly be neglected any more than can examples of acromegaly without gross changes in the pituitary body be excluded in a general consideration of acromegaly.

Case 9. [Dr. Mooser's case.] *Acute painful obesity sparing extremities. Cutaneous pigmentation. Spinal deformity from osteoporosis. Duration three years. Autopsy: osteomalacia with multiple fractures; cardiac hypertrophy; atheromatous vessels; contracted kidneys; acute pancreatic necrosis; testicular atrophy. Pituitary body large but said to be normal.*

Clinical history. The patient, aged 27 (born in 1890), the eldest of eleven children, one of them a pituitary [?] dwarf, was an unmarried merchant, a polylinguist, and fond of sport. Previously spare and of slight build (Fig. 18) at the age of 24, while in military service during the autumn of 1914, he began to grow so stout as scarcely to be recognizable. The adiposity was so rapidly acquired that broad striae atrophicae appeared over the trunk and extremities. The tension of the skin was such it gave the disagreeable feeling of being electrically stimulated. Ere long, he began having pain in his spine, which the military surgeon thought indicated a tuberculous spondylitis and he was sent to a sanitarium. There his disorder was diagnosed as adiposo-genital dystrophy of pituitary origin.

[29] Mooser, Hermann: Ein Fall von endogener Fettsucht mit hochgradiger Osteoporose. Ein Beitrag zur Pathologie der inneren Sekretion. Virch. Arch., 1921, *229*, 247–271.

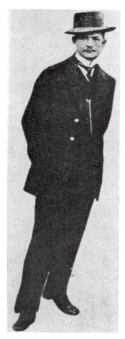

FIG. 18. Case 9. Dr. Mooser's patient in 1912, aged 22.

The adiposity, which was confined to face, neck and trunk (Fig. 19), progressively increased and the suffering from his tense skin which greatly disturbed his sleep became scarcely endurable. In the course of the next six months he became so weak he could scarcely hold a pencil or feed himself. He was given heliotherapy, which he bore badly, as it provoked alternating attacks of hyperaemia, cyanosis and sweating lasting from a few minutes to half an hour.

At first, there was little complaint of headache, but this for a time became more marked and later on again subsided. He was made sleepless by trembling of the body, noises in the ears, dreams and visions. He also complained of visual disturbances on moving his head. Ophthalmoscopic investigation, apart from a slight lessening of visual acuity, showed no abnormality. He had a marked polydipsia which obliged him to get up

three or four times at night. The genitalia became dystrophic. The urine examination showed during 1916–1917 a slight trace of albumin with a few hyaline casts and no sugar; amount was not recorded.

His height diminished from 165 cm. in 1914 to 158 cm. in 1917. The body circumference increased from 91 cm. in November 1915 to 96 cm. in January 1917, with a gain in weight from 52 to 63.9 kgm.

Roentgenological studies in 1916 showed that the contours of the sella turcica were scarcely visible, the bones porous. An examination a year later showed these conditions to be still more advanced. There was apparent destruction of the bodies of the mid-thoracic vertebrae associated with a gibbus which was diagnosed in 1915 as osteitis vertebralis; in 1916 as spondylitis tuberculosa; in 1917 recognized as part of a non-tuberculous generalized porosity or decalcification of the skeleton.

Following a brief period of asthmatic dyspnoea and haemoptysis, he died on November 27, 1917, three years from the onset of symptoms.

Postmortem examination.[30] The body was that of a man whose head, neck and body were exceedingly adipose in marked contrast to his relatively thin extremities. The abdomen was likened to a pillow, the circumference being 99 cm. at the level of the navel. The color of the skin was everywhere strikingly brown, the region of the pelvis being of a lighter color, presumably from the fact that during his periods of heliotherapy this region was protected by swimming tights. Radiating scars were present on inner surface of thigh and upper arm. The hairiness of the lower body was normal in distribution.

Head: The inner part of the calvarium showed sharply circumscribed red spots, the largest of which had a diameter of 5 to 3 cm. The cerebral vessels were markedly atheromatous. The sella turcica was not enlarged. The hypophysis measured 14 by 8 by 7 mm. The neurohypophysis was plainly evident. The organ was put immediately in formalin. The base of the sella turcica was of red but smooth bone. *Thorax:* Subcutaneous fat 3.5 cm. thick. The ribs were found to be greatly softened; the upper part of the sternum greatly thickened. The heart was enlarged; the aorta atheromatous; the

---

[30] Professor Busse's detailed protocol is herein greatly abbreviated.

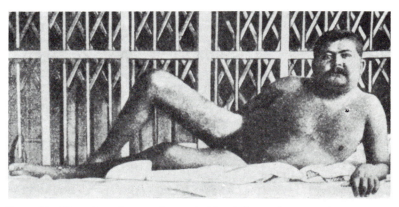

FIG. 19. Case 9. Dr. Mooser's patient, aged 27, at height of disease three years from onset.

thymus not to be identified in the abundant mediastinal fat. The thyroid gland was fibrotic, difficult to cut, and contained but little colloid.

Abdomen: Panniculus 4.5 cm. thick; omentum exceedingly large and fat; perirenal fat abundant. The *adrenal glands*, though buried in fat, were of average size and of normal appearance. In the *pancreas* was found an area of central necrosis. The *testes* were small.

The investigation, particularly of the bones, showed that the thickened sternum was due to the callus of a healing fracture; several ribs also showed old healed fractures. The manubrium was intensely red and soft, and contained great holes of soft marrow. The ribs were easily cut, as was true of the spinal column, part of which was removed. The greatly compressed bodies of the vertebrae, in places only 1 cm. thick, were so soft they could easily be cut with a knife.

The *gross pathological diagnosis:* lipomatosis; osteomalacia (seu rachitis tarda); multiple fractures of the ribs; vertebral collapse; hypertrophy of the cardiac ventricles; atheromatosis of aorta and of the cerebral vessels; encephalomalacia of the right occipital lobe; fibrino-purulent peritonitis; necrosis of the pancreas; hypoplasia of the thymus; granular atrophy of the kidneys.

The principal *histological findings* of note were those relating to the peculiar structure of the softened bones. The kidneys showed slight glomerular fibrosis; the cerebral vessels an endarteritis proliferans. No abnormality was found in the *adrenals, pineal* or *pituitary* glands.

The small [from a Swiss standpoint] *thyroid* showed an increase of intralobar connective tissue with small and atrophic intermedial follicles; the single *parathyroid* detected was closely attached to the capsule of the thyroid, measured 4 by 3 by 2 mm., and showed an increase of connective tissue. The *thymus* could scarcely be identified in the mediastinal fat. The *pancreatic islets* were relatively few and atrophic in the part of the gland that had escaped necrosis. The *testes* also showed fibrosis with atrophic changes, though some active spermatogenesis was still present.

The outstanding symptomatic features of this remarkable case were: (1) The suddenly acquired, and peculiarly disposed, painful obesity; (2) The softening of the bones affecting the entire skeleton but more particularly the vertebrae, leading to multiple fractures (*cf.* Case 2); (3) The ultimate enfeeblement with fatality at the expiration of three years. In view of the slightly contracted kidneys, the enlarged heart and the arteriovascular changes found after death, vascular hypertension was probably present during life. Plethora was not particularly emphasized nor purplish abdominal striae, but pigmentation of the skin was noted by the pathologist.

The author, in his analysis of the case, comes to the conclusion that the disorder represents a polyglandular deficiency, and ascribes the skeletal decalcification to sclerosis of the parathyroid glandules; the adiposity was taken to be chiefly thyroidal in origin though something was to be said in favour of a pancreatogenous insufficieny.

A possible pituitary origin was discussed only insofar as to point out the lack of resemblance of the syndrome to that of adiposo-genital dystrophy. Whether the gland was scrutinized for the possible presence of an adenoma is not apparent. The gross measurements were certainly in the upper limits of normal.

The next case, also with autopsy, figures in a report made from Professor Biedl's clinic in Prague in 1924 by Dr. William Raab[31] on the general topic of hypophysial and cerebral adiposity, or what is commonly called adiposo-genital dystrophy. The subject was approached largely from its roentgenological aspects, and it was a mere chance that in 1920 when preparing for my Lister Lecture[32] I happened to hit upon the fact in reading this paper that in one of the patients (Case 2) a basophil adenoma had been disclosed at autopsy. The photographs of the patient were so striking and bore such a close resemblance to the appearance of a patient at the time under observation in my own wards (*cf.* Case 11) that I felt little doubt but that they had been afflicted in all certainty with the same disorder. The translation of Dr. Raab's brief note of his case is as follows:

Case 10. [The Raab-Kraus case.] *Acute recent plethoric obesity, sparing extremities. Purplish striae. Backache with kyphotic spine. Death from infection. Autopsy: osteoporosis of skeleton; testicular atrophy; basophil adenoma of pituitary body.*

"Karel W., a man aged 31, showed gigantism of moderate degree (192 cm.), with very long extremities, externally well-developed genitalia and distribution of hair of normal masculine type. Patient complains of suffering from headaches for the past two weeks previous to his admission into the clinic and claims to have taken on 10 kgm. in weight during the same [sic] short period. This was confirmed by the family doctor.[33] The libido had always been rather low; he had been impotent for the past fortnight.

"There is a marked obesity of the face which appears, therefore, considerably disfigured when compared with former photographs (slit-eyes), and a marked adiposity of the abdomen (Figs. 20, 21). There is no adiposity of the long, slender extremities and of the nates. The abdomen is tremendously prominent and shows flame-shaped striae of dark-red color which are, in part, more than 2 cm. broad. The hips reveal the same feature. Weight 96 kgm. [211 pounds]. The X-ray plate shows a sella which, while not being excessively large, reveals

[31] Raab, W.: Klinische und röntgenologische Beiträge zur hypophysiären und zerebralen Fettsucht und genital Atrophie. (Case 2) Wien. Arch. f. inn. Med., 1924, 7, 443–530.
[32] Cushing, H.: Neurohypophysial mechanisms from a clinical standpoint. Lancet (Lond.), 1930, 2, 119–127; 175–184.
[33] In view of the postmortem findings of advanced testicular atrophy and decalcification of the skeleton, the disease presumably was of longer duration than this statement would indicate.

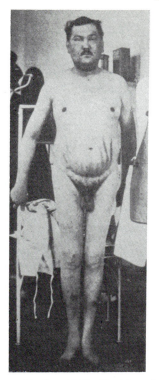 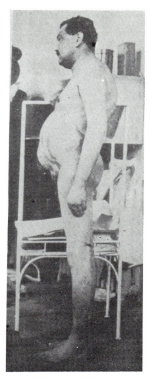

Figs. 20 and 21. Case 10. Dr. Raab's patient (1924) with verified basophilic adenoma.

nevertheless the characteristic deconfiguration produced by a process enlarging the intrasellar space. *Diagnosis:* tumor hypophyseos.

"The headaches improving and the weight remaining unchanged, the patient left the clinic, but returned in a few weeks, feverish and suffering from excessive pains in the lumbar vertebral column. Shortly afterwards he acquired a streptococcal phlegmon of the hand and died from acute sepsis in spite of generous incisions and amputation of his arm.

"The *autopsy* revealed an operculum sellae which was, as usual, concave; the pituitary body was scarcely enlarged; the posterior lobe was softened supposedly by postmortal changes. The pathologist emphatically denied the presence of a growth. Histologically, however, a small basophil adenoma was discovered which had almost entirely replaced the posterior lobe and showed central softening—a verification of the clinical diagnosis. An osteoporosis of extreme degree involving the vertebral column and the long bones accounted for the vertebral pain."

Further details of the postmortem examination of this case were given in a separate report in the same year (1924) by Professor E. J. Kraus[34] of Prague who has been kind enough to send me sections of the pituitary body (*cf.* appended Figs. 22, 23) for study, and whose personal description is translated as follows:

[34] Kraus, E. J.: Zur Pathogenese der Dystrophia adiposogenitalis. (Case 3) Med. Klinik, 1924, *20*, 1290–1292; 1328–1330.

"The *autopsy* reveals besides signs of a general septic infection a marked enlargement of the pituitary body which, however, does not protrude out of the pituitary fossa. There was, in addition to these findings, a definite osteoporosis of the vertebral column, sternum and ribs, there being a slight degree of kyphosis of the thoracic spine. There was a small diffuse colloid struma of the *thyroid*. The *testes* were strikingly small. The thickness of the fat layer was on the neck 1.3 cm., on the upper arm 2 cm., above the sternum 2 cm., on the abdomen 3.5 cm., and the upper leg 2 cm.

"The *morphological examination* of the endocrine organs reveals: *hypophysis* 0.93 gm. In the posterior lobe there is an infiltrating basophil adenoma, situated especially in its anterior two-thirds, having destroyed about two-thirds of the adjacent substance of the anterior lobe. In the non-affected third of the lobe there are several small cysts as big as hemp-granules. The tumor, almost in its entirety, is sharply demarcated, slightly compressing the adjacent glandular parenchyma, and infiltrating the neurohypophysis. Furthermore, the tumor sends a pointed process into the stalk of the pituitary body, thus replacing about the half of its cross-cut area. The numerous eosinophil cells on an average are somewhat smaller in size than normal. There are strikingly few ripe basophil cells. Many cells which have lost their granules (*Entgranulierte*) represent former basophil elements. There are many mother-cells (*Hauptzellen*), augmented apparently in relation to the diminished number of basophil cells. The pharyngeal-hypophysis could not be found in the many histological slides.

"The *pineal body* is of normal size and also histologi-

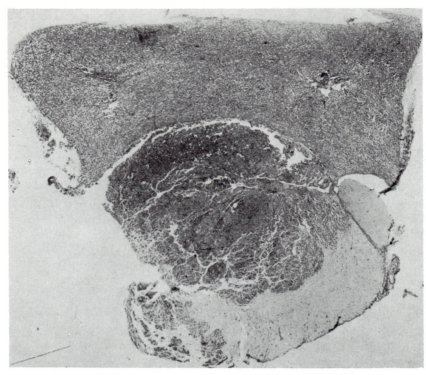

Fig. 22. Case 10. The basophilic adenoma from Dr. Raab's patient. Tumor lying between pars anterior above and pars nervosa below. (Hematoxlyin and eosin, ×9). Kindness of Professor Kraus.

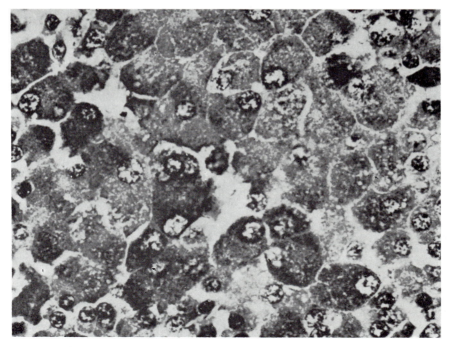

Fig. 23. Case 10. The adenoma of the Raab-Kraus case (hematoxylin and eosin×850) showing a cluster of basophilic cells, many of them multinuclear.

cally normal. The slightly enlarged *thyroid gland* contains much colloid, reveals enlarged vesicles, a partly cubic, partly flat epithelium, and a delicate interstitial tissue. Three *parathyroid glands* (weight together 9.16 gm.!) are strikingly infiltrated by fat tissue, and here and there occur rather large nests of oxyphil cells. The *pancreas* (weight 94 gm.) shows marked postmortal autolysis as do also the *adrenal glands*. The two *testes* (without the epididymes) weigh 18.3 gm. The canalicules of the testes have a delicate tunica propria. Spermatides, spermatoblasts and spermatozoa are wanting; only heads of spermotozoa are found in a very few canalicules. The epithelium for the most part shows four or five rows; the amount of lipoid is somewhat diminished. The interstitial cells are definitely diminished; the epididymes histologically normal."

Professor Kraus, if I understand him correctly, looked upon the hypophysial tumor as "an incidental finding" without relation to the clinical features shown by the patient, whereas Dr. Raab believed that the adenoma in some way influenced the secretory activities of the posterior lobe, the relation of which (pituitrin) to adiposity he has made the special object of study.[35] With neither of these views do I find myself in accord; and inasmuch as Professor Kraus not only was one of the first to describe basophilic adenomas,[36] but has since made other important contributions to the subject,[37] his seeming reluctance to correlate the adenoma with the clinical syndrome is the more surprising. This may be explained by the fact that only in later years, largely through the work of P. E. Smith and his collaborators, has the functional importance of these cells been pointed out. However this may be, I quite agree with Professor Kraus' opinion that the adiposal syndrome presented by this case was something wholly different from that seen in adiposo-genital dystrophy, which is a deprivation syndrome due usually to inactivation of the hypophysis by compression. The adipose disorder under consideration, on the contrary, is almost certainly due to a hyper-secretory influence of some kind, and since the adrenal glands, apart from their postmortal change, were supposedly normal in this case whereas an adenoma was found in the pituitary body, the latter would seem to be the most probable primary seat of the trouble.[38]

[35] Raab, W.: Das hormonal-nervöse Regulationssystem des Fettstoffwechsels. Ztschr. f. d. ges. exper. Med., 1926, *49*, 179–269.
[36] Kraus, E. J.: Die Beziehungen der Zellen des Vorderlappens des menschlichen Hypophyse zueinander unter normalen Verhältnissen und in Tumoren. Beitr. z. path. Anat. u. z. allg. Path., 1914, *58*, 159–210.
[37] Kraus, E. J.: Über die Bedeutung der basophilen Zellen des menschlichen Hirnanhangs auf Grund morphologischer Studien. Med. Klinik, 1928, *24*, 623, 662.
[38] Kraus has pointed out, particularly in relation to hypertension, that whenever there is an hyperplasia of the adrenal cortex an increased number of basophilic cells are found in the anterior pituitary, and the reverse

We may now turn to the next of the male patients whose syndrome bears so close similarity to the foregoing case that even without a postmortem examination it may safely be ascribed to a lesion of the same primary sort. Fortunately the somewhat meagre clinical record for the preceding case, in which many details are missing, can now be supplied:

Case 11. (P. B. B. H. Surgical No. 37076) *Rapidly acquired and painful adiposity, sparing limbs. Purplish striae. Vascular hypertension. Glycosuria with azoturia. Progressive weakness till bedfast. Clinical diagnosis: basophilic adenoma. Radiotherapeusis of pituitary gland. Marked improvement.*

E. G. F., a dentist 30 years of age, referred for therapeutic recommendations by Drs. R. T. Woodyatt and A. R. Colwell of Chicago, entered the Brigham Hospital August 11, 1930, with the principal complaints of painful obesity, loss of strength, irritability, polyuria and polyphagia.

Family and Personal history. The patient was one of twelve children of healthy parents, both living and well, none of this large family having had any known endocrinological disorders. He had been married for ten years and was the father of two children, the first of whom died following an instrumental delivery at birth, the second being a healthy girl one year of age. Until the past year the patient had always enjoyed excellent health. He was a tall man, standing over six feet, his normal average weight having been 160 pounds.

Present illness. This, he thinks, started five years before admission, when he began slowly to grow round-shouldered and stout. In the course of the next three years he gained 25 pounds and during the fourth year there was a more rapid gain of 35 pounds, his weight reaching 220 pounds (100 kgm.). He then began limiting his diet and finally succeeded in losing a few pounds, but under this régime he soon found himself without energy, easily fatigued, unable to concentrate his mind on his work, and fits of unnatural irritability alternated with periods of depression.

At this juncture he consulted a physician who restored some carbohydrates to his self-imposed dietary restrictions. He immediately felt better but his weight quickly increased, his abdomen became prominent, and for the first time he noticed a peculiar disposition of localized masses of fat on his face and neck. These fat deposits, which appeared in symmetrical regions over the head (cheeks, temples, orbital region, supramental and suprasternal regions, as well as over the cervico-dorsal spine), were at first soft, but tended to become increasingly firm and tense. They moreover were accompanied by most uncomfortable "drawing sensations," presumably from stretching of the cutaneous nerves. The tense skin over these swellings acquired a peculiar florid reddish-bronze color and showed telangiectases so altering his appearance that he was scarcely recognizable to his friends (cf. Figs. 27, 28).

At about this time (December 1929) he began to have an excessive thirst associated with a polyuria which was more marked at night when he would be obliged to void

is true—namely, an adrenal hypoplasia is accompanied by few basophils. He suggests that the "hypercholesterinämie" of hypertension may be the common basis or at least play an important rôle.

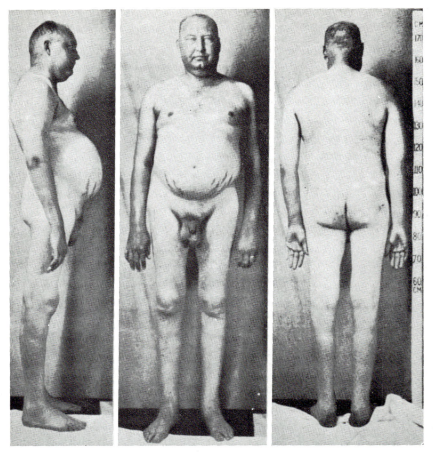

FIGS. 24–26. Case 11. To show the patient's abdominous configuration, thin extremities, plethoric face, kyphosis and striae (*cf.* Figs. 20, 21).

from four to six times. He experienced also susceptibility to fatigue, forgetfulness, restlessness, palpitation on slight exertion, swelling of the feet and ankles, generalized weakness, and impotence. A distinct loss of body hair was observed.

In January 1930, he was found to have a glycosuria and this led to his admission to the Presbyterian Hospital in Chicago where, by Drs. Woodyatt and Colwell, his condition was carefully investigated at various periods during the course of the next six months. They found, to make the story short:

(1) "A slight *leucocytosis* of from 10 to 18 thousand, with some preponderance of neutrophilic polymorphonuclear elements; erythrocytes in normal limits.

(2) "A variable *glycosuria* and hyperglycaemia, together with increased nitrogen excretion. On a diet with a daily glucose value of 201 grams, there was a daily excretion of 5.7 grams sugar (glucose) which was controlled by 50 units of insulin daily. This glycosuria was looked upon as a truly diabetic phenomenon, but it was accompanied by an unexpectedly great and wholly unrelated polydipsia and polyuria, the largest daily excretion observed having been 6720 cc. Attempts to modify this polyuria by pituitrin injections up to a dosage of 3 cc. in twelve hours were wholly ineffective.

(3) "*Azoturia.* On a diet containing 81 gm. of protein

daily (13 gm. nitrogen), there was a daily nitrogenous excretion of 20–24 gm. despite approximate caloric balance. This loss was later balanced by increasing the protein intake. Since then there has been a continuous excretion in the urine of 20 to 30 gm. daily.

(4) "*Blood chemistry:* urea N. 19.0; uric acid 3.8; creatinine 1.1; total N. P. N. 36.0; chlorides 466; calcium 7.1–8.9; cholesterol 147.5 (all values in mg. per 100 cc. blood); CO_2 77.7 vol. per cent. Wassermann reaction negative.

(5) "*Basal metabolic rate:* minus 10% to plus 1% on repeated readings.

(6) "A moderate degree of *vascular hypertension,* from 165/70 to 178/100, without evidences of arteriosclerotic change.

(7) "The administration of iodine was without effect. One of the *fat pads* on the front of the neck was removed for study and proved to be fatty tissue of customary pannicular type."

Finally, when a suspicious *enlargement of the pituitary fossa* was roentgenologically detected suggesting a possible pituitary or hypothalamic disorder, he was referred to the Brigham Hospital for an opinion.

Physical examination (on admission). This showed (Figs. 24–26) a tall (184.2 cm.), extremely abdominous, and somewhat round-shouldered man with patchy

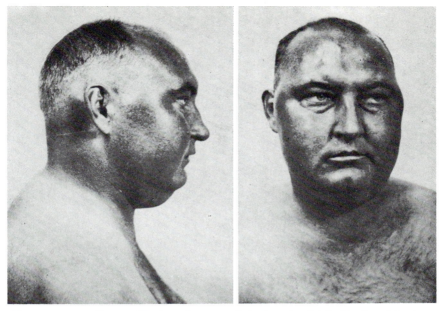

FIGS. 27 AND 28. Case 11. To show the tense, plethoric and painful adiposity of the face.

adiposity of the face, neck and trunk, and comparatively spare extremities (weight 86.8 kgm.). All his movements, such as those incidental to rising from a chair, were obviously made with great effort, as though his limbs were scarcely strong enough to support his huge body. His face was peculiarly florid and dusky, and on forehead, cheek bones, temples, and chin were deposits of fat which were tender to the touch and covered by tense, glistening skin (Figs. 27, 28). Similar accumulations of fat were present on the anterior aspect of the neck and over the cervico-thoracic region in the back.

Owing to the puffiness of his face and eyelids, the palpebral slits were narrow, the eyes being injected and somewhat prominent. Vessels of the fundus oculi were exceedingly tortuous and the edges of the discs were blurred, but there was no measurable swelling. The fields of vision were normal.

Wide purplish striae radiated from the groins over the abdomen and smaller striae were present over medial aspects of both thighs (Fig. 29). There was some pitting oedema about the ankles and some swelling of the hands, so that he was unable to remove a ring. He was partially bald and the hirsuties of the extremities and axillae was scanty, but there was abundant hair on the

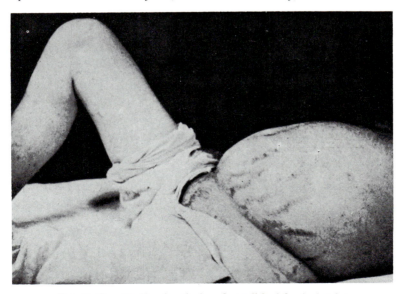

FIG. 29. Case 11. Showing the broad purplish abdominal striae

chest which was normal in deposition and texture. The skin of the axillae, groins and crotch was pigmented and scaly.

He was free from headache, but complained greatly of discomforts associated with the adiposity and also of variable pain in the back and shoulders. Roentgenograms were made of the entire skeleton, which in Dr. Sosman's opinion showed no evidence of decalcification. The pituitary fossa was not enlarged but the posterior clinoids appeared to show some absorption. No acromegalic changes were present. The spine and pelvis, so far as could be seen, were normal.

The blood examination, frequently repeated, averaged 4,600,000 red cells, 16,700 white cells, 85 per cent of them being polymorphonuclears. Haemoglobin was variously estimated at 90 to 100 per cent. The basal metabolic rate was −10 per cent; a specific-dynamic test with a 200 gm. steak-breakfast showed (possibly because of his nitrogen imbalance) a rise only to +4 per cent at the end of a four-hour period. The systolic blood-pressure was over 170 mm. of Hg., indicating a moderate vascular hypertension. There were no renal elements or albumin in the urine.

When admitted to hospital, he was still on the somewhat restricted diet which finally had been worked out by Dr. Woodyatt as most effective in caring not only for the diabetes but also for the increased nitrogen output. In order to balance this and to keep up the patient's strength, it had been found necessary to increase the protein in the diet from 200 to 475 grams. He was taking in addition 65 units of insulin daily, divided into two doses, 40 in the morning and 25 at night. This, however, had been found in Chicago, as it was found here, to be most variable in its effect. His polyphagia was most striking. He was hungry all the time, and even when allowed a full meal, of which he would partake greedily, he would feel ravenous again after an hour's interval.

Laboratory studies. During his long hospital sojourn of 71 days, his condition was investigated from every angle, both when under dietary restrictions and when free from them. Various authorities on diabetes and the blood, among them Dr. Reginald Fitz, Dr. W. P. Murphy, and Dr. E. P. Joslin, saw him in consultation but had no therapeutic suggestion to make. Under the supervision of one or another of them frequent detailed studies were made of the blood and during the entire period daily record was kept of the total protein, total nitrogen, total uric acid, and total sugar elimination in the urine, both diurnal and nocturnal.

Soon after his admission, a study of the fasting blood was made in Dr. Murphy's laboratory the morning after he had been on a wholly unrestricted diet for comparison with the findings after a period of dietary restriction, with the results shown in the subjoined table of blood studies.

During the 24 hours prior to the test on the morning of August 18th, the diet was estimated to contain 412 gm. carbohydrate, 188 gm. protein, and 256 gm. of fat with an approximate glucose value of 546 gm. The corresponding urinary output had been 5410 ccm. containing: 58.4 gms. sugar; 20.4 gms. total nitrogen (127.5 gms. total protein); and 855 mgm. uric acid.

During the 24-hour period preceding the August 22nd test, the diet contained 92 gm. carbohydrate, 178 gm. protein, and 177 gm. fat with a glucose value of 212

BLOOD STUDIES	AUGUST 18, 1930, DIET UNRESTRICTED	AUGUST 22, 1930, DIET RESTR CTED
Erythrocytes........	4,600,000	4,260,000
White cells.........	13,000	9,200
Haemoglobin.......	13.88 gm.	13.32 gm.
Cells..............	40.9%	36.6%
Plasma............	59.1%	63.4%
Individual cell volume.............	8.8×10⁻¹¹cc.	8.5×10⁻¹¹cc.
Blood iron.........	43.5 mgm. %	41.6 mgm. %
Blood sugar........	219 mgm. %	164 mgm. %
Non-protein nitrogen	36.8 mgm. %	45.8 mgm. %
Amino-acid nitrogen.............	17.0 mgm. %	6.8 mgm. %
Blood urea nitrogen	9.0 mgm. %	18.0 mgm. %
Creatinine.........	2.2 mgm. %	2.4 mgm. %
Uric acid.........	5.9 mgm. %	3.88 mgm. %
Whole-blood chlorides	255 mgm. (NaCl)	290 mgm. (NaCl)
Calcium...........	10.0 mgm. %	10.0 mgm. %
Cholesterol........	246 mgm. %	190.8 mgm. %
Total protein......	7.05 gm. %	6.94 gm. %
Albumin.........	3.98 gm. %	3.02 gm. %
Globulin.........	2.91 gm. %	3.53 gm. %
Fibrinogen........	0.16 gm. %	0.39 gm. %

gms. The corresponding urinary output had been 4550 ccm., containing: 15.5 gm. sugar; 36.4 gm. total nitrogen (227.5 gm. total protein); and 1595 mgm. uric acid.

During the month of August, also, acting on the assumption that a basophil adenoma might conceivably show a sex-maturing substance in the urine similar to that present during pregnancy, a series of observations was made by Mr. D. W. Gaiser to test this point. The urine was highly toxic for immature rats but the survivors showed no change in ovaries or seminal vesicles at the end of 120 hours. Similar tests on immature mice were equally without result.

On September 12, 1930, during a period when he was again on a restricted diet without insulin [he showed on this particular day a fasting blood sugar 0.214, with the elimination of 4300 cc. of urine containing 24.4 grm. sugar, 183 grm. total protein, 29.2 grm. total nitrogen, and 1495 mgm. total uric acid], an estimation in Dr. Joslin's laboratory was made of his plasma lipids (the patient's brother and an insulinized case of diabetes of nine years' duration serving as controls), with the following results:

Plasma lipids

	CHOLES-TEROL	TOTAL FATTY ACIDS	LECITHIN	TOTAL LIPINS
	mgm. per 100 cc.	mgm. per 100 cc.	mgm. per 100 cc.	mgm. per 100 cc.
Normal average......	230	390	210	680
The patient, E. G. F..	326	575	344	901
Controls:				
Patient's brother...	189	259	230	448
A 9-year diabetic...	391	286	330	667

Though the patient's fatty acids and total lipins were considerably in excess of the controls, they were regarded as "approximating those seen in cases of mild or moderate diabetes in the days before the introduction of insulin."[39]

[39] Attention may be drawn to two recently published papers by Anselmino and Hoffman (Klin. Wchnschr., 26 Dec. 1931, pp. 2380–86) in which the presence in the anterior pituitary of what is called a metabolizing (*Stoffwechsel*) hormone is claimed. This appears to be related to but is separable from the gonad-stimulating hormone. Its injections increase the acetone-body content in the blood by accelerating fat combustion.

As weeks passed, he became increasingly more feeble, was reluctant to get out of bed, and appeared rapidly to be going downhill, the progressive loss of strength causing him great concern. Not only did he suffer from pain in his hips and shoulders but from such extreme sensitiveness of his face he could not bear the pressure of a pillow against it. It was very difficult to make him comfortable in bed, recourse being finally had to an air mattress. He ceased to take an interest in his surroundings; became so feeble he was unable even to turn in bed; and he finally acquired a carbuncular infection at the lower end of his spine which began rapidly to spread. Knowing that other patients with this syndrome had died either from or with ulcerative cutaneous infections (*cf.* Case 10), it was feared that his end was near.

From the outset, he had been pleading for an exploratory operation which was considered impracticable, but in view of the growing conviction that his trouble must be due to a basophil adenoma, which might conceivably be amenable to radiation, he was given, between October 14th and 17th, four x-ray treatments. During their course, he felt particularly miserable, but by the 19th his downward progression for the preceding month was unmistakably checked. The improvement in his general condition was so striking it must have been something more than coincidence. He felt stronger, began to show an interest in his surroundings, to make efforts to move himself about, was conscious of a diminution in thirst, and of lessening in his discomforts. The carbunclar infection of the lower spine began to show improvement, and though he was unable as yet to get out of bed, he at this juncture (October 21, 1930) insisted on being taken home. There he continued rapidly to improve and the infected area on his back and hip soon healed.

According to his frequent letters he continued to complain of the backaches and of the painful sensations in the tense, adipose areas; and on March 6, 1931, he reported a further gain in weight up to 235 pounds. But on the whole, he made steady progress and by July 1931, was able to walk a half-mile or more at a time without over-fatigue. In October 1931, he stated that the "tumorous growths" of his head had nearly disappeared, and two months later he wrote from Florida, where he had gone for the winter, stating that he was still improving and no longer showed sugar on an ordinary diet, even without insulin.

The sudden improvement following radiation of the patient's pituitary body was looked upon as something more than mere coincidence. As will be pointed out in the next section, the average duration of life of the fatal cases had been in the neighborhood of five years and all the patients succumbed to progressive enfeeblement associated in most of the cases with terminal infections, a happening which in this particular instance there was every reason to anticipate when recourse was finally had to radiotherapeusis.

The exhaustive laboratory studies of the blood and urine gave no information of value though attention may be called to the consistently high nonprotein nitrogen percentages and to the high

cholesterol reading, on a single occasion, of 246 mgm. per cent. In this connection it is interesting that Professor Kraus, after the painstaking enumeration of the number and condition of the basophilic elements in the anterior pituitary in various pathological states, expresses the conclusion in a recent paper (*loc. cit.*, 1928) that a definite relationship exists between the number of these cells, those of the adrenal, the blood-pressure and cholesterin metabolism.

Another matter to which attention may be called is the fact that the patient's diabetes, like that complicating cases of acromegaly, was far more difficult to regulate and control by insulin than is the diabetes primarily of pancreatic origin. What, if anything, this may have to do with the known counter-effect of posterior lobe extract (pituitrin) on the action of insulin needs further ventilation.

Another unmistakable example of this same disorder, recently reported by Dr. Wieth-Pedersen from the Rigshospital of Copenhagen, has been called to my attention by a Danish student in our Medical School. The author gives a detailed report[40] of two cases both of which showed marked striae distensae cutis to which factor attention is particularly drawn. One of the patients had a malignant adrenal tumor with metastases, the other a pituitary tumor associated with adrenal hyperplasia, the syndrome in both having been ascribed to the adrenal factor.

The first case was that of a woman, 158 cm. in height, with headaches, puffy skin (without hypertrichosis), dimness of vision, increase of 16 kg. in weight, with reddish-blue striae distensae, hypertension 245/150, cardiac enlargement and polydipsia. She died a year after the onset of symptoms. An adrenal tumor 12 by 6 cm. with metastases was found at autopsy. The pituitary body was said to be normal but was not examined microscopically. An abbreviated report of the second case follows:

Case 12. [Dr. Wieth-Pedersen's patient.] *Delayed adolescence. Plethoric adiposity with striae. Albuminuria. Hyperglycaemia. Glycosuria. Vascular hypertension. Cardiac hypertrophy. Duration 4 years. Autopsy: pituitary adenoma (type unverified); adrenal hyperplasia.*

Clinical history. A young man, 24 years of age, entered the hospital May 6, 1930, and died there three months later. He had always been well but his puberty was delayed until the age of 20 when he began to grow abdominous and the color of his face and hands became bluish red. He had polyphagia, polydipsia, and polyuria. He perspired freely when at work. He needed to shave only twice weekly. There was no headache or dizziness. His vision had become impaired in later years and he

[40] Wieth-Pedersen, G.: Et Tilfaelde af Binyretumor og et af Hypofysetumor med Binyrehyperplasi, begge med Striae distensae cutis. Hospitalstidende, 1931, *74*, 1231–1244.

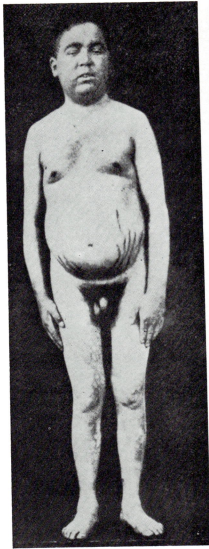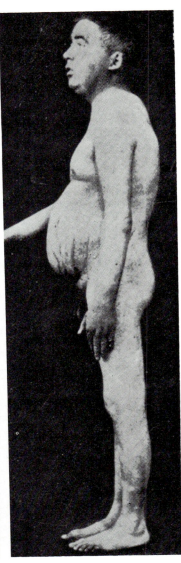

FIGS. 30 AND 31. Case 12. Photographs of Dr. Wieth-Pedersen's patient with pituitary adenoma of unrecorded type.

had lost some weight under treatment during the nine months prior to admission.

Physical examination. The appearance was that of a man older than his age. He was of slight stature. Height 161.5 cm. (5 ft. 3 in.); weight 61.3 kg. (135 lbs.). There was quite marked adiposity, localized around abdomen, thorax and face, the extremities not being affected. No dyspnoea while resting. The teeth were carious. The thyroid gland was covered by a cushion of fat, but not enlarged. No peripheral adenitis. No cardiac enlargement was detected. There were numerous pigmented naevi on the chest.

On both sides of the abdomen were reddish striae distensae, 1 cm. in width and 5 to 6 cm. in length; otherwise nothing abnormal. The external genitalia were not hypoplastic. The face and hands showed a

deep red-blue color. There was cyanosis of the lower legs with spots of light brownish pigmentation which contrasted with the varices which were present. At the time of the examination there was a four days' growth of beard which amounted to 2 mm. at the most. The hair on the head, eyebrows, axillae and pubis was normal.

The urine contained sugar and albumin with a few hyaline casts. Blood-pressure 190/170: haemoglobin 93 per cent (Sahli). Wassermann negative. The cranial roentgenograms showed no abnormality; the sella was normal (10 by 12 mm.) with no evidence of a destructive process. The epiphyseal lines in both knees and wrists were open, corresponding with 16 to 17 years of age. No signs of atherosclerosis.

The basal metabolic rate was approximately normal.

Renal function was unimpaired. The eyes were normal, except for a polar cataract visible in both of them. Blood urea [non-protein nitrogen ?] 44 mgm.%; fasting blood sugar, highest estimate 263 mgm.%. No ketonuria observed. Only on days of fasting was it possible to make the patient sugar-free; even on an anti-diabetic diet with greatly reduced calories the urine still showed sugar. Insulin was not used.

Course of disease. There was considerable variation from day to day, not only in the hypertension, but in the albuminuria and in the percentage of sugar in the blood. The patient complained of headache, of pains in the ears, and became dull and sleepy. On one occasion, he had subjective dimness of sight, marked dizziness, and vomited, the blood-pressure registering 185/120 with a rapid pulse. The abdominal striae grew more pronounced and finally reached all the way up to the axillae on both sides. Ecchymoses occurred from time to time on the legs and arms; his left hand became oedematous. On August 1st, the patient became dyspnoeic and cyanotic and died that evening.

Autopsy: August 2nd. The extremities were lean compared with the trunk. There were striae distensae on the abdomen, running longitudinally to thorax and even to axillae. The skin was without oedema, apart from that on the left forearm and back of hand. The growth of the hair was natural, except the beard, which was scanty. Broncho-pneumonia was found, also marked hypertrophy of the left ventricle and atheroma of the aorta and common iliacs. The mesentery was exceedingly fat. The kidneys were slightly granular.

The *thyroid gland* was small (each lobe measuring 3 by 1.3 cm.) and firm. The *right adrenal* was normal, but the left was hyperplastic, weighing 27 grams; the tissue on fresh section appeared normal, but the medullary portion was oedematous and of a brownish-green color. The *pituitary gland*, on removal of the brain, was found to be replaced by a soft tumor-like growth of reddish color, which measured 3 by 2 by 2.5 cm. The brain itself was oedematous, the ventricles moderately dilated.

Microscopical examination. The *thyroid gland* showed changes like those found in a colloid struma, the epithelial lining of the follicles being low cuboidal, with no proliferation and no increase of connective tissue. The *pancreas* showed slight increase of connective tissue, with an unusual number of islets. The *left adrenal gland* had a normal structure without oedematous cell proliferation. Toward its centre, there was some oedema and congestion of the vessels without cell degeneration. The hyperplasia was evenly distributed between cortex and marrow, the two structures being indefinitely contrasted with indistinct arrangement of cell columns. The *kidneys* showed no definite change, though casts were found in the tubules.

Hypophysis: "The tumor tissue consists of a coarse network of rather delicate connective tissue, often containing thin-walled, wide, congested vessels. Although there are postmortem changes, one is of the impression that the network of connective tissues with its branches all throughout has been covered by cells of epithelial nature. These cells are polygonal, at times somewhat extended, and containing a nucleus of varying sizes and shape with a dark nucleolus. Quite often there are seen large plump complexes of nuclei, a few mitoses. These cells form, as a rule, a quite dense layer and line

irregularly-shaped vacuoles which are filled with granular material consisting of necrotic and degenerative cells. Thus, the tumor tissue appears papillomatous in structure. The connective tissue, which is increased in amount in the periphery of the tumor, is also infiltrated with tumor cells. There is no evidence of sarcoma. The endothelium of the vessels appears normal."

Pathological diagnosis: Tumor of the hypophysis. Hyperplasia of the suprarenal glands, of the thyroid and of the pancreas. Hypertrophy of the left heart. Chronic granular nephritis. Compression of the left optic nerve. Hydrocephalus internus. Oedema of pia and arachnoid. Dilation of sella turcica. Atheromatosis of mitral valve and aorta. Oedema of face and back of hand. Striae distensae cutis. Pigmentation and ecchymoses of the skin.

In his interesting discussion of the two cases, the author naturally ascribed the polyglandular disorder in the first of them to the adrenal tumor. In the second case, he laid chief emphasis (as did Dr. Parkes Weber in Case 6) upon the unilateral adrenal hyperplasia. He however ascribed the delayed puberty, retarded ossification and the adiposity to a pituitary effect as an example of dystrophia adiposo-genitalis [sic].

COLLATION OF SYMPTOMATIC AND PATHOLOGICAL DATA

The twelve patients whose case histories have been presented, as will have been noted, were all relatively *young adults.* Their *average age* at the onset of the malady, so far as can be estimated (Case 10 being eliminated for want of information) has been 18 years; the youngest was six (Case 5) and the oldest 25 (Case 11).

In *stature,* the female patients all appear to have been definitely undersized. Where heights were given, the tallest (Case 6) was 159 cm. (5 ft. 3 in.), the shortest (Case 1), 145 cm. (4 ft. 9 in.). Two of the male patients, on the other hand, were tall: Case 9, 192 cm. (6 ft. 1½ in.); Case 11, 184.2 cm. (6 ft. ½ in.).

The *average duration* of the disease from onset to death in the cases where definitely stated (Case 10 again eliminated) has been slightly over five years, the extremes being three (Case 9) and seven [?] years (Case 8).

The following features are characteristic of all cases: (1) A rapidly acquired, peculiarly disposed and usually painful *adiposity* (in one instance representing a 40 per cent gain in weight) confined to face, neck and trunk, the extremities being spared; (2) A tendency to become round-shouldered (kyphotic) even to the point of measurable loss of height (*cf.* Cases 2 and 9) associated with lumbo-spinal pains; (3) A sexual dystrophy shown by early *amenorrhoea* in the females and ultimate functional *impotence* in the males; (4) An alteration in normal hirsuties shown by a tendency to *hypertrichosis* of face and trunk in all the females as well as the preadolescent males (Cases

8 and 12) and possibly the reverse in the adult males; (5) A dusky or plethoric appearance of the skin with *purplish lineae atrophicae;* (6) *Vascular hypertension*, present in all cases except Cases 4, 7 and 9 where no mention was made of blood-pressure; it varied from the highest recorded in Case 6 of 230/170 to the lowest in Case 11 of 178/100; (7) A tendency to *erythraemia*, a count exceeding five million having been present in five of the nine cases in which blood counts were recorded; (8) Variable *backaches, abdominal pains, fatigability* and ultimate extreme *weakness.*

Other features less consistently recorded have been as follows: *Acrocyanosis (e.g.,* Cases 1, 12); *Purpura-like ecchymoses*, whether from bruising or occurring spontaneously (Cases 1, 2, 3, 6, 12); *Aching pains in the eyes*, associated with slight exophthalmos (Cases 1, 3, 6, 11), with transient diplopia (Case 1), with suggestive papilloedema (Cases 1, 6, 11), with dimness of vision (Cases 8, 9, 12), with subretinal exudate (Case 2) and retinal haemorrhage (Case 8); Extreme *dryness of skin (e.g.,* Cases 1, 2, 4, 6, 8), with pigmentation *(e.g.,* Cases, 1, 4, 6, 11, 12); *Polyphagia,* poly-dipsia and polyuria *(e.g.,* Cases 11, 12); *Oedema of the lower extremities* was noted in several cases and in Case 12, of the hand; A *susceptibility to pulmonary infections* (Cases 5, 6, 8, 9, 12); *Albuminuria* of slight degree with occasional casts was found in six patients (Cases 1, 5, 6, 8, 9, 12); A *sense of suffocation* and difficulty in swallowing were occasionally noted (Cases 1, 6); *Insomnia* was a not uncommon complaint; An increase of non-protein nitrogen and of cholesterin in the blood was recorded in the only patients (Cases 8, 11 and possibly 12) in which it was estimated; A *poly-morphonuclear leucocytosis* was noted in Cases 1, 5, 6, 8, 11.

Secondary endocrine disturbances conceivably affecting the *adrenal glands* were suggested not only by the hypertension, by the pigmentation (particularly noted in Cases 1, 4, 9, 12) but by the terminal extreme weakness; on the part of the *pancreatic islets*, by the glycosuria (Cases 4, 5, 8, 11, 12); conceivably on the part of the *thyroid gland*, by the increased metabolic rate (Cases 6, 7), though this was once recorded as low (Case 11) and in most cases was not noted; of the *para-thyroid glandules*, possibly by the osteoporosis from decalcification, either roentgenologically apparent (Case 1) or demonstrated at autopsy, and to which the marked upper thoracic kyphosis *(e.g.,* Cases 1, 2, 4, 9, 10, 11) and the spontaneous fractures (Cases 2, 9) are attributable. There was no increase of blood calcium in Case 10; in no instance was calcium elimination estimated.

Postmortem findings. The malady appears to leave the patients with a definite *susceptibility to infections.* Death in the nine fatal cases, eight of which came to postmortem examination, was

ascribable to, or associated with, multiple cutaneous abscesses and ulcers (Cases 2, 5), intercurrent erysipelas (Case 4), acute pulmonary complications (Cases, 5, 6, 12), intercurrent meningitis (Case 7), a streptococcal phlegmon (Case 10), pancreatic necrosis (Case 9). *Chronic nephritis* of mild degree was found, in the absence of any definite clinical signs, in Cases 2, 3, 6, 9 and 12; *hypertrophy of the cardiac ventricle* in Cases 2, 6, 9 and 12; and vascular atherosclerosis was noted in Cases 3, 9, 12. An *osteoporosis of the skeleton* most marked in the spine was specifically described in six (Cases 2, 3, 4, 6, 9, 10) of the eight autopsies, Cases 7 and 12 being the exceptions and in these it may have escaped notice.

The ductless glands. A *basophilic adenoma of pituitary body* was found in Cases 6, 7 and 10; undifferentiated adenoma in Cases 3 and 12; what was described as an adenomatous-like structure in a fibrosed area of the anterior pituitary was noted in Case 4; and in Cases 2 and 9, the gland was said to be "normal." The *thyroid* was described as slightly enlarged (colloidal) in Cases 3, 7, 10, 12; as small in Case 4; as fibrotic in Case 9. The *parathyroids* were described as normal in Case 3; to have shown capillary dilatation in Case 4; to be fibrotic in Case 9; and infiltrated with fat in Case 10. The *suprarenal glands* in Cases 2 and 6 showed a cortical hyperplasia; in Case 3, a small adenoma; while in Cases 4, 7, 9 and 10, no abnormality was noted. The *ovaries* and uterus were said to be senile in Case 3; in Case 4 to show atresia; in Case 6, to be small but normal; and in Case 7, to show hypertrophy with signs of increased functional activity. The *testes* in Cases 9 and 10 showed atrophy of the spermatogenous epithelium.

DISCUSSION AND RECAPITULATION

In ascribing this obscure polyglandular syndrome to a pituitary rather than to an adrenal source, I am aware that much might be said in favour of the latter seat of origin. Indeed, it was my original belief in the case of Minnie G. that her malady was in all probability associated with an adrenal tumor. What light the contemporary literature served to shed on the subject was strongly in favour of such an interpretation, containing, as it did, numerous examples of precocious sexual development in children or of the masculinization of women who were found to have large suprarenal tumors. A striking example was that reported in 1911 by Launois, Pinard and Gallais[41] of a bearded and amenorrhoeic woman who showed plethoric adiposity with an abundance of purplish lineae over the trunk. A supra-

[41] Launois, P.-E., M. Pinard, et A. Gallais: Syndrome adiposo-génital avec hypertrichose, troubles nerveux et mentaux d'origine surrénale. Gaz. d. hôp., 1911, *84*, 649–654.

renal tumor of cortical type with metastases to liver and lungs was found at autopsy in association with what was said to be a normal pituitary body, though the sella turcica was said to have measured 18 mm. in its largest diameter which, to say the least, is at the upper limit of normal for her age, this being 14.4 mm. according to Erdheim and Stumme's measurements.

About this same time, twenty years ago, I had the opportunity in London to see with Dr. Gordon Holmes a striking example of masculinization or heterosexual virilism in a woman from whom an adrenal tumor was subsequently removed by Sir Percy Sargent with prompt restoration of the patient's original normal feminine appearance and reactions.[42] This woman had a lean, mannish habitus quite unlike the highly plethoric and adipose individuals herein depicted, and the case may possibly have unduly coloured my impressions of hyperadrenalism of which, to be sure, several differing types have been described. Primary adrenal tumors, therefore, may cause striking constitutional transformations, but there nevertheless is justification in again emphasizing the fact that all known primary pituitary disorders inevitably cause marked secondary changes in the adrenal cortex, a pathological observation which is amply supported by what occurs after experimental pituitary dwarfism or gigantism. And if the acidophilic adenomas of acromegaly inevitably cause hyperplasia not infrequently associated with actual adenomata of the adrenal cortex,[43] it is reasonable to assume that basophilic adenomas may well enough do the same.

An excess or deficiency of anterior-pituitary hormones, in other words, secondarily affects the function of the adrenal cortex with established certainty, whereas nothing comparable to this occurs in the reverse direction. Hence, if further study should prove that adrenal tumors in the absence of any demonstrable change in the pituitary body may cause a polyglandular syndrome in many respects similar to that under discussion, it may well enough be assumed that, when the same features characterize the syndrome of a basophilic adenoma, they in all probability are secondarily ascribable to a hypersecretory influence of adrenal cortex even in the absence of any histologically appreciable abnormality as exemplified by the Parkes Weber and by the Raab-Kraus cases cited above.[44]

The disorders under discussion in all probability are much more common than would appear from the present assembly of twelve examples which with four exceptions have been restricted to cases in which a postmortem examination has been held. Acromegaly was once looked upon as a rare disease, and in its extreme form may still be so considered. However, one encounters on every hand persons with unmistakable traces of pituitary acidophilism (acromegalic overgrowth) so mild in its effects medical advice has not been sought; and the same is probably true of persons affected by transitory or mild degrees of pituitary basophilism.

I am quite aware that in ascribing the disorder to the basophilic elements, even were their association with maturation and the ovulatory mechanism established beyond peradventure, many questions arise which are at present unanswerable. For example: (1) If the sex-maturing principle, which during pregnancy appears to spill over into the urine, is excreted by the basophilic cells, should it not be found (cf. Case 11) in the urine of patients with basophilic adenomas if the polyglandular disorder under consideration is actually due to the hypersecretory effect of such a lesion?[45] (2) Whereas premature sexual maturity appears to characterize the disorder in children of either sex, why, in adult women, should amenorrhoea occur together with an apparent reversal of the secondary characters of sex? (3) If in this syndrome we are actually dealing with an oversecretion of the gonad-stimulating factor, why should atretic ovaries be found in the females instead of over-follicularized or over-luteinized ("mulberry") ovaries such as occur in immature or adult female rats after repeated injections with extracts containing one or the other gonad-stimulating factors?[46] (4) If the polyglandular features of the disorder are partly due, as premised, to a secondary hyperplasia of adrenal cortex, why has this not been observed in rats after injection with the gonad-stimulating extracts whereas it is a striking effect of injecting growth-promoting extracts?[47] An answer to these and other questions

---

[42] Holmes, G.: A case of virilism associated with a suprarenal tumour: recovery after its removal. Quart. J. Med., 1924–25, *18*, 143–152.

[43] Cushing, H., and L. M. Davidoff: The pathological findings in four autopsied cases of acromegaly with a discussion of their significance. Monogr. Rockefeller Inst. M. Research, No. 22, 1927, p. 109.

[44] Smith and Engle, as may be recalled, found that pituitary transplants in the immature female rat produced precocious sexual maturity even after bilateral adrenalectomy. Loc. cit., 1927.

[45] The hypophysial hyperplasia which occurs in pregnancy, described by Erdheim and Stumme (1909), is composed of modified chief cells which are non-granular. One would assume that this means the cells are not advancing to secretory maturity. The source of the gonad-stimulating substance in the urine, unless it is provided by the placenta (cf. Collip), is therefore not clear.

[46] Cf. Fevold, H. L., F. L. Hisaw, and S. L. Leonard: The gonad-stimulating and the luteinizing hormones of the anterior lobe of the hypophysis. Am. J. Physiol., 1931, *97*, 291–301.

[47] Cf. Smith and Engle, 1927, loc. cit.

will doubtless in time be forthcoming.

A *chronological recapitulation* of the facts that have chiefly served to throw light on this subject during the past twenty years are as follows: (1) Primary anterior-pituitary disorders are commonly produced by adenomas; (2) Adenomas of the endocrine series are as a whole functionally active lesions; (3) Even minute adenomatous tumors of parathyroid glandules and pancreatic islets may lead to serious constitutional derangements of hypersecretory type; (4) Pituitary adenomas are of three principal varieties—neutrophil, acidophil and basophil, no constitutional disorder heretofore having been definitely ascribed to the last; (5) There is experimental evidence to suggest that the basophilic elements of the anterior pituitary secrete the sex-maturing hormone; and finally, (6) A polyglandular syndrome hitherto supposed to be of cortico-adrenal origin characterized in its full-blown state by acute plethoric adiposity, by genital dystrophy, by osteoporosis, by vascular hypertension, and so on, has been found at autopsy in six out of eight instances to be associated with a pituitary adenoma which in the three most carefully studied cases (Cases 6, 7, 10) has been definitely shown to be composed of basophilic elements, the lesion in one instance (Case 7) having been clinically predicted before its postmortal verification.[48]

[48] Since Erdheim and Stumme's classical paper (Über die Schwangerschaftsveränderung der Hypophyse. [III. Adenome der Hypophyse.] Ziegler's Beitr., 1909, *46*, 1–132), no one appears to have made a systematic search for the presence of adenomata in supposedly normal pituitary glands. These authors found adenomas in approximately one out of ten of the glands that were serially sectioned.

Conclusions. Of all subjects that engage the attention of the profession at the present day, that of endocrinology particularly lends itself to the temptation of impressionistic speculation. During the past ten years, innumerable syndromes of so-called polyglandular type, some of them bearing a certain resemblance to that under consideration, have often been described in print. Examples of "diabetes in bearded women," of rapidly acquired obesity, of hypertension, of masculinization in the female and of sexual precocity in children of either sex, often associated with hyperplasias or tumors of one sort or another of the suprarenal glands, have been so many and varied as to baffle analysis.

Some of these syndromes have unquestionably been due to cortico-adrenal tumors and in not a few instances, indeed, such a tumor has been removed at operation with definite amelioration of symptoms. What is more, in similar states suprarenal tumors have been found after death in the absence of any recognizable abnormality in the pituitary body, though all too often the protocol refers to the examination of this structure either in the briefest terms or not at all.

While there is every reason to concede, therefore, that a disorder of somewhat similar aspect may occur in association with pineal, with gonadal, or with adrenal tumors, the fact, that the peculiar polyglandular syndrome, which pains have been taken herein conservatively to describe, may accompany a basophil adenoma in the absence of any apparent alteration in the adrenal cortex other than a possible secondary hyperplasia, will give pathologists reason in the future more carefully to scrutinize the anterior-pituitary for lesions of similar composition.

Neurosurgical Classics—5 and 6

T HE nineteenth century French surgeon, Pierre Paul Broca, is remembered today for his accomplishments in two fields. As an anthropologist he made valuable studies of human skulls, and he founded the Société d'Anthropologie and the *Revue d'Anthropologie*.[5,10–13] As a neuropathologist he made his most significant contributions when he reported the pathological lesions in two cases of "aphemia."[6–9] These and subsequent reports played a major role in establishing the concept of cerebral localization which was an important prerequisite to modern neurological surgery.[16,20,27–29,30]

During the first half of the nineteenth century, the brain was thought to act as a whole, with no localization of its functions.[1,4,14,15,18,19,26,30,31] Franz Joseph Gall, however, held the opposite view.[21,25] He " . . . placed the faculty of memory for words in the frontal lobes of the brain because of his observation that his schoolmates with prodigious memories had rather prominent eyes, presumably due to the overgrowth of the inferior aspect of the frontal lobes. Gall buttressed this observation from his study of a patient with a fencing foil wound in the frontal lobe of the brain with attendant speech disturbance. Unfortunately, Gall's name is linked closely with the pseudoscience of phrenology which was strongly advocated by Spurzheim, an early associate of Gall . . . "[20]

"Bouillaud, a French physician, in 1825 reiterated the view of Gall and produced autopsy material to substantiate the idea that, 'the principal lawgiver of speech is to be found in the anterior lobes of the brain.'[3] Bouillaud, who later became a popular professor of medicine, repeatedly defended his view in prolonged discussions at medical gatherings. On one occasion, he offered a reward of 500 francs to anyone who could produce a brain from a patient with a significant lesion of the frontal lobes who did not have a disturbance of speech. About this time, Velpeau reported a brain tumor involving both frontal lobes in a patient who not only had no speech difficulty but was actually loquacious. Whether he had the temerity to claim the reward is not known . . . "[20]

Further advances in understanding disturbances of speech were made in 1861. " . . . In February 1861, before the recently formed Société d'Anthropologie, Gratiolet,[17] who had previously exhibited a primitive Mexican skull, discussed the significance of the volume of the brain. Auburtin,[2] the pupil and son-in-law of Bouillaud, opposed the view that the total volume of the brain gave an exact measurement of intelligence, and opposed Gratiolet's view that the functions of all parts of the brain were the same. Broca,[6] who was Secretary of the Society, joined in the debate."[4]

"The discussion aroused so much interest that it was continued at subsequent meetings. Auburtin reported a case in which haemorrhage into both frontal lobes caused no symptoms beyond loss of speech, and another in which pressure with a spatula upon the exposed frontal lobe caused immediate interruption of speech. He localized in the frontal lobes 'the faculty of co-ordinating the movements peculiar to language' . . . "[4]

On April 11, 1861, a patient named Leborgne ("Tan") was admitted to the surgical service of the Bicêtre, a hospital in Paris for chronic diseases, under Broca's care. Apart from his acute illness, a diffuse phlegmon of the right lower extremity, the patient had an interesting neurological disorder that had begun with aphasia 21 years previously. Because of the discussions at the Société d'Anthropologie, Broca asked Auburtin to see "Tan" in consultation. "Tan" died on April 17, 1861, and at a meeting of the Société d'Anthropologie on the following day, Broca described the findings present at autopsy.[6] Significantly, Broca did not section the brain but left it intact for the anatomical museum.[6,7]

"Broca concluded from the history, clinical examination, and pathological studies of his patient that the loss of speech was a consequence of a lesion in one of the frontal lobes, probably in the third convolution. Broca referred to this loss of speech as aphemia (from a = not + phēmē = voice). He extended his observations by asserting that if speech function resided in a specific area, other mental faculties are probably situated in circumscribed loci in the cerebral hemispheres. Thus, Broca unwittingly became one of the champions of discrete localization of function within the brain."[20]

A few months later a similar case came under Broca's care.[8,19] The patient had been admitted to the Bicêtre eight years previously, at the age of 76, because of senile debility. In April, 1860 he had suddenly become unconscious, and although he had partially recovered, he remained aphasic. In October, 1861 the patient fractured his left femur in a fall, and was transferred to the surgical service. There he died twelve days later. At autopsy a lesion was found in the second and third left frontal convolutions, and Broca's ideas about cerebral localization were reinforced.

"This started a controversy so heated that Head,[19] who extensively reported the writings on the subject at that time, said it became a political issue. The older Conservatives, still frightened by the impact of phrenology, held the holistic view that the specific functions could not be localized. The younger Republicans and Liberals quickly espoused the view put forward by Broca."[20]

"Hughlings Jackson . . . opposed Broca's concepts at a medical meeting where Broca made a later report now further strengthened by more autopsy material. Broca's finding seemed so incontrovertible that he was deemed the winner of the discussion.[16]

Another detractor was the eminent French clinician, Trousseau, who not only attacked Broca's hypothesis of localization but also made carping criticism of the term aphemia, that Broca had employed. Trousseau, in consultation with a Greek physician, pointed out that aphemia meant 'infamy' in later Greek usage and substituted the term aphasia."[20]

"Over 40 years after 'Tan's' death, his brain was re-examined by Pierre Marie. Marie, one of the most celebrated French neurologists, succeeded to the post of neurology at the Bicêtre in 1897. There he did a careful study of the previously undissected brain of 'Tan.' In a series of provocative papers,[22-24] the first of which was pointedly entitled 'The Third Frontal Convolution Does not Play Any Special Role in the Function of Language,' he attempted to demolish the views put forth by Broca. Marie demonstrated that the lesion reported in 'Tan' was much more widespread than Broca reported. The frontal areas were destroyed as previously described, but there was also extensive damage in the temporal and parietal areas . . . "[20]

"To emphasize the dubious nature of Broca's concept of localization and to overlook his contribution establishing the left hemisphere as the dominant half of the brain would be unjust. A few years after the examination of his famous patient and fortified by other autopsy findings, he suggested that the left cerebral hemisphere had a unique role in the formation of speech. Even the honor of establishing this doctrine was contested. Marc Dax in a communication to the Academy of Medicine in 1864 stated that his father, Marc Dax senior, had suggested this nearly 30 years before in 1836. Broca was naturally piqued by this usurpation of priority and could find no mention of this report in the literature. However, Dax actually produced the manuscript and republished it.[14] Nonetheless, the honor must remain with Broca, who brought this important observation to the general attention of the medical world."[20]

Reproduced below are translations of

Broca's reports of his first two cases of aphasia, which represent a major milestone in the development of modern neurological surgery.

References

1. Ask-Upmark, E. Swedenborg as a pioneer in cerebral localization. *J. Amer. med. Ass.*, 1963, *183*: 805–806.
2. Auburtin. Reprise de la discussion sur la forme et le volume du cerveau. *Bull. Soc. anthrop. Paris*, 1861, *2*: 209–220.
3. Bouillaud, J. Recherches cliniques propres à démontrer que la perte de la parole correspond à la lésion des lobules antérieurs du cerveau, et à confirmer l'opinion de M. Gall, sur le siège l'organe du langage articulé. *Arch. gén. Méd.*, 1825, *8*: 25–45.
4. Brain, [R.] Speech disorders. Aphasia, apraxia and agnosia. *London: Butterworth & Co., Ltd.*, 1961, 184 pp. (see pp. 30–53).
5. Broca, P. Sur le volume et la forme du cerveau suivant les individus et suivant les races. *Bull. Soc. anthrop. Paris*, 1861, *2*: 139–204.
6. Broca, P. Perte de la parole, ramollissement chronique et destruction partielle du lobe antérieur gauche du cerveau. *Bull. Soc. anthrop. Paris*, 1861, *2*: 235–238.
7. Broca, P. Remarques sur le siège de la faculté du langage articulé, suivies d'une observation d'aphémie (perte de la parole). *Bull. Soc. anat. Paris*, 1861, s. 2, *6*: 330–357.
8. Broca, P. Nouvelle observation d'aphémie produite par une lésion de la moitié postérieure des deuxième et troisième circonvolutions frontales. *Bull. Soc. anat. Paris*, 1861, s.2, *6*: 398–407.
9. Broca, P. Sur le siège de la faculté du langage articulé. *Bull. Soc. anthrop. Paris*, 1865, *6*: 377–393.
10. Broca, P. Mémoires d'anthropologie. *Paris: C. Reinwald*, 1871–1888, 5 vols. (see *5*: 1–161).
11. Broca, P. Instructions craniologiques et craniométriques de la Société d'anthropologie de Paris. *Paris: G. Masson*, 1875, vii, 203 pp.
12. Broca, P. Sur la trépanation du crâne et les amulettes crâniennes à l'époque néolithique. *Paris: E. Leroux*, 1877, 74 pp.
13. Broca, P. Instructions générales pour les recherches anthropologiques à faire sur le vivant. *Paris: G. Masson*, 1879, 2nd ed., xii, 289 pp.
14. Critchley, M. The study of language-disorder: past, present, and future. In: *The centennial lectures cemmemorating the one hundredth anniversary of E. R. Squibb & Sons.* J. T. Culbertson, Ed. New York: G. P. Putnam's Sons, 1959, x, 292 pp. (see pp. 269–292).
15. Gibson, W. C. Pioneers in localization of function in the brain. *J. Amer. med. Ass.*, 1962, *180*: 944–951.
16. Goldstein, K. Pierre Paul Broca (1824–1880). In: *The founders of neurology.* W. Haymaker, Ed. Springfield, Ill.: Charles C Thomas, 1953, xxvii, 479 pp. (see pp. 259–263).
17. Gratiolet. Sur la forme et la cavité crânienne d'un Totonaque, avec réflexions sur la signification du volume de l'encéphale. *Bull. Soc. anthrop. Paris*, 1861, *2*: 66–71.
18. Head, H. Aphasia: an historical review. *Brain*, 1921, *43*: 390–411.
19. Head, H. Aphasia and kindred disorders of speech. *Cambridge, England: University Press*, 1926, 2 vols. (see *1*: 1–141).
20. Joynt, R. J. Centenary of patient "Tan." His contribution to the problem of aphasia. *Arch. intern. Med.*, 1961, *108*: 953–956.
21. Magoun, H. W. Development of ideas relating the mind and brain. In: *The centennial lectures commemorating the one hundredth anniversary of E. R. Squibb & Sons.* J. T. Culbertson, Ed. New York: G. P. Putnam's Sons, 1959 x, 292 pp. (see pp. 247–267).
22. Marie, P. Revision de la question de l'aphasie: la troisième circonvolution frontale gauche ne joue aucun rôle spécial dans la fonction du langage. *Sem. méd.*, *Paris*, 1906, *26*: 241–247.
23. Marie, P. Revision de la question de l'aphasie: que faut-il penser des aphasies sous-corticales (aphasies pures)? *Sem méd., Paris*, 1906, *26*: 493–500.
24. Marie, P. Revision de la question de l'aphasie: l'aphasie de 1861 à 1866; essai de critique historique sur la genèse de la doctrine de Broca. *Sem. méd., Paris*, 1906, *26*: 565–571.
25. Riegel, R. E. Early phrenology in the United States. *Med. Life*, 1930, *37*: 361–376.
26. Riese, W. The early history of aphasia. *Bull. Hist. Med.*, 1947, *21*: 322–334.
27. Schiller, F. Leborgne—in memoriam. *Med. Hist.* 1963, *7*: 79–81.
28. Stookey, B. Jean-Baptiste Bouillaud and Ernest Auburtin. Early studies on cerebral localization and the speech center. *J. Amer. med. Ass.*, 1963, *184*: 1024–1029.
29. Thorwald, J. The triumph of surgery. R. Winston and C. Winston, Transl. *New York: Pantheon Books, Inc.*, 1960, xi, 454 pp. (see pp. 7–12).
30. Walker, A. E. The development of the concept of cerebral localization in the nineteenth century. *Bull. Hist. Med.*, 1957, *31*: 99–121.
31. Wilkins, R. H. Neurosurgical classic—XII. *J. Neurosurg.*, 1963, *20*: 904–916.

Loss of speech, chronic softening and partial destruction of the left anterior lobe of the brain*

by paul broca

Paul Broca, on the occasion of this report, presents the brain of a man, aged fifty-one, who died in his department of the hospital at Bicêtre and who had lost the use of speech twenty-one years ago. Before the specimen is deposited in the Dupuytren Museum and before the complete observation is published in the *Bulletin de la Société anatomique*, we shall present a short summary here because the brain is quite similar to those of which Mr. Auburtin spoke at the last meeting.

* Translation of: Perte de la parole, ramollissement chronique et destruction partielle du lobe antérieur gauche du cerveau, by Paul Broca. *Bulletins de la Société d'Anthropologie*, 1861, *2*: 235–238. Printed with the kind permission of Masson & Cie, Paris, France.

When the patient was admitted to Bicêtre twenty-one years ago, he had lost, shortly before that, the use of speech. He could pronounce only a single syllable, which he ordinarily repeated twice in succession. Whatever the question might be that was addressed to him, he always answered *tan, tan* while adding quite varied expressive gestures. That is why all over the hospital he was known only by the name of *Tan*.

At the time of his admission, *Tan* was perfectly healthy and intelligent. At the end of ten years he commenced to lose the movement of his right arm. Then the paralysis reached the lower limb of the same side so that after six to seven years he continually stayed in bed. After some time it was noticed that his sight was failing. Finally, those who were close to him noted that his intelligence deteriorated a great deal in the final years.

On April 12, 1861, he was brought into the surgical department of the hospital for a vast, diffuse, gangrenous phlegmon, which was present in the entire length of the right lower extremity (of the paralyzed side) from the instep to the buttock. It was then that Dr. Broca saw him for the first time. The study of this poor man who could not speak and who, being paralyzed in the right hand, could not write, indeed presented some difficulty. It was ascertained, however, that the general sensibility was everywhere preserved, that the left arm and leg obeyed the will, that the muscles of the face and of the tongue were not at all paralyzed, and that the movements of the latter organ were perfectly free.

The state of the intelligence could not be determined exactly, but there was proof that *Tan* understood almost all that was said to him. Being able to show his ideas or his desires only by the movements of his left hand, he often made incomprehensible gestures. Numerical responses were those which he made best, by opening or closing his fingers. Without making a mistake he indicated the time of a watch down to the seconds. He knew how to say exactly how many years he had been at Bicêtre, etc. Nevertheless, various questions for which a man of ordinary intelligence would have found the means to answer by gesture remained without intelligible response. At other times the response was clear, but did not refer to the question. Hence, there is no doubt that the intelligence of the patient had undergone profound injury, but he certainly preserved more of it than he needed in order to speak.

The patient died April 17, 1861. At autopsy the dura mater was found thickened and vascularized, its inner surface covered with a thick layer of pseudo-membrane, and the pia mater was thickened, opaque and adherent to the anterior lobes, especially to the left lobe. The frontal lobe of the left hemisphere had softened over the greatest part of its extent; the convolutions of the orbital lobule, although atrophied, had preserved their form; most of the other frontal convolutions were entirely destroyed. There resulted from this destruction of cerebral substance a large cavity, capable of accommodating a hen's egg and filled with serous fluid. The softening reached the ascending gyrus of the parietal lobe posteriorly, the marginal gyrus of the temporosphenoidal lobe inferiorly, and finally, in the depths, the lobe of the insula and the extraventricular nucleus of the corpus striatum. It is to the lesion of this latter organ that the paralysis of the movement of the two limbs of the *right* side should be attributed, but it is enough to glance at the report to recognize that the principal center and initial site of the softening was the middle part of the frontal lobe of the left hemisphere. It was there that the most extensive lesions, the most advanced, and the oldest were found. The softening then spread slowly into the surrounding parts, and it can be considered as certain that there had been a very long period during which the affection occupied only the convolutions of the frontal lobe. This period probably corresponds to the eleven years that preceded the paralysis of the right arm, during which the patient, having preserved all his intelligence, had lost only his speech.

Therefore, everything points to the fact that, in the present case, the lesion of the frontal lobe was the cause of the loss of speech.

NEW OBSERVATION OF APHEMIA PRODUCED BY A LESION OF THE POSTERIOR HALF OF THE SECOND AND THIRD FRONTAL CONVOLUTIONS*

by Paul Broca

In the first observation of aphemia which I communicated to the Society some months ago I described a rather complicated cerebral lesion, a progressive softening which had successively destroyed three frontal convolutions, the lobe of the insula, the extraventricular nucleus of the corpus striatum, and finally the upper marginal convolution of the temporosphenoidal lobe. Knowing that at the start of the illness and for a long period of ten years the patient had lost only the faculty of articulating words, while preserving entirely intact all his other intellectual faculties, sensory and motor, I have been led to think that the loss of speech had been the consequence of a lesion rather circumscribed at first and that the central

* Translation of: Nouvelle observation d'aphémie produite par une lésion de la moitié postérieure des deuxième et troisième circonvolutions frontales, by Paul Broca. *Bulletin et Mémoires de la Société Anatomique de Paris*, 1861, s.2, 6: 398–407.

organ of articulated speech was probably that in which this lesion had begun. To discover this organ among all those which were injured at the time of death I looked for the point at which the alteration appeared the oldest, and I found that in all probability the softening must have started in the third frontal convolution, perhaps also the second.

I did not overlook the fact, however, that the oldness of the injury and the extent of its ravages rendered this determination somewhat uncertain. I have, therefore, let some doubts hover over my conclusions. The new fact that I am presenting today to the Society will permit me to be more affirmative. The aphemia had begun abruptly a year and a half before death. The lesion which I found at autopsy was perfectly circumscribed and existed precisely, without the least difference, at the point where I had assumed that the lesion must have begun in my first patient.

Observation. Lelong, the person named, aged 84, an old laborer, was brought to the infirmary of the hospital at Bicêtre, the surgical department, Saint-Prosper ward, October 27, 1861, to be treated for a fracture of the neck of the left femur.

This man had been admitted to the hospital eight years before because of senile debility. At that time he had no paralysis; he had kept all his senses, all his intelligence. However, his limbs, weakened by the progress of age, refused to work; and his hand, which had become trembling, could no longer write. Furthermore, he never again knew how to write.

In April 1860, during the Easter holiday while descending stairs, he suddenly collapsed. He recovered in time to prevent hurting himself, but he appeared to have lost consciousness. He was taken to the infirmary, the medical service, and was treated for cerebral apoplexy.

He was able to walk within a few days. He never showed the least appearance of paralysis of his limbs. However, his daughter, from whom I have this information, thought that he had a paralyzed tongue. The fact is that at the moment of his accident he had suddenly and definitely lost the ability to speak. He no longer pronounced certain words that are articulated with difficulty. His gait was somewhat uncertain, but he did not limp. His intelligence had undergone no appreciable damage. He understood all that was said to him, and his short vocabulary, attended by a mimical expression, permitted him to be understood, in turn, by persons who habitually lived with him.

This state was maintained without change up to October 27, 1861. On that day, while getting up from bed, he lost his balance, fell on his left hip, and broke the neck of the femur. I pass over in silence all that is relative to this fracture.

The paralysis of the tongue, of which we had

been told, did not exist. This organ was quite mobile, it deviated not at all and showed the same thickness on the right and on the left. The act of swallowing was done well, his sight and hearing were preserved, and his limbs obeyed his will with the exception of the fractured limb, and when sitting up he was again as strong as another of his age. Emission of urine and fecal matter was regular. Finally, general sensibility persisted without alteration, and the patient suffered much from his fracture, which was complicated by a rather severe contusion.

To questions addressed to him, this man responded only by signs accompanied by one or two syllables articulated abruptly with a certain effort. His syllables had meaning, they were French words, namely: *yes, no, three* (trois mispronounced tois), and *always*. There was a fifth word that he pronounced only when he was asked his name; he then answered *Lelo* for *Lelong*, which was his true name.

The first three words of his vocabulary each corresponded to a definite idea. To affirm or approve, he said, *yes*. To express the opposite idea, he said, *no*. The word *three* expressed all numbers, all numerical concepts. Finally, whenever none of the preceding three words was applicable, Lelong used the word *always*, which, consequently, had no fixed meaning.

I asked him if he knew how to write. He answered, *yes*. I asked him if he would. He said *No*. I said, "Try!" He tried but he could no longer succeed in directing the pen.

The applications which he made of the word *three* are rather curious and should be indicated with some details. This word was always accompanied by a sign made with the fingers because our patient, knowing that his tongue betrayed his thought, therefore rectified by gesture this involuntary error. For greater clarity I shall take the liberty to report here some of his responses.

"How many years have you been at Bicêtre?" —*Three*, and he raised eight fingers.

"Have you any children?"—*Yes.*

"How many?"—*Three*, and he lifted four fingers.

"How many sons?"—*Three*, and he lifted two fingers.

"How many girls?"—*Three*, and he lifted two fingers.

That was all perfectly accurate.

"Do you know how to read the time?"—*Yes.*

"What time is it?"—*Three*, and he lifted ten fingers. (It was ten o'clock.)

"What age are you?" We expected to see him open both hands eight times and then make an added four fingers, because we knew that he was eighty-four years old. Instead of that, he made only two gestures while saying, *three*, and I believed for a moment that he had lost the concept of numbers greater than ten. However, the intern, Mr. Bernadet, made a remark that immediately revealed to us that this man knew his age very well and that he counted perfectly. With the first gesture he had raised eight fingers, with the second he had raised four. That undoubtedly meant eight tens and four units. The thing merited being verified. I repeated the question, and he made exactly the same signs accompanied by the word *three*. And when he saw that we had this time understood his language, he added, *yes*, with an affirmative sign of his head.

He had some very expressive gestures which permitted him to make very intelligible responses. Thus, he let us know his occupation before we had instructed him on this point. "What trade did you follow before entering Bicêtre?"—*Always*, and at saying this he made the gesture with his hands of a man who takes a shovel, drives it into the soil, lifts it, and then hurls a shovelful of soil.— "Then are you a laborer?"—*Yes*, with an affirmative sign of his head. He was actually a laborer.

His answers deceived us only once. When we asked him how long ago he had lost his speech, he answered, *three*, while lifting eight fingers. Perhaps he confused the date of his apoplexy with that of his entry into Bicêtre. Perhaps also he wished to say eight months, which was still inaccurate. We thought at that time, according to the supervisor's report, that this mishap dated back three years. It was only after his death that his elder daughter, while giving us confirmation of his other responses, informed us that he had lost his speech in April, 1860, eighteen months before his death. I then asked myself if the gesture *eight* had not been preceded by a gesture *one* which might have passed unperceived. This interpretation today appears to me very likely. However, even though this was the one and only time the patient made a mistake or had not known how to express himself, we know enough about him to assert: 1) that he understood all that was said to him; 2) that he employed with discernment the four words of his vocabulary; 3) that he was healthy in mind; 4) that he knew the written numbering and at least the value of the first two orders of units; 5) that he had lost neither his general ability for language nor the voluntary motility of the muscles of phonation and articulation, and that he had consequently lost only the *faculty of articulated language*.

He was, therefore, stricken with *aphemia*, but this aphemia differed in several respects from that which I had studied in my first patient. The latter had only one invariable response to all questions. It was the monosyllable "*tan*," always repeated twice, and this word was not even a French word. This was not the last remains of his native tongue. This was a chance sound entirely devoid of meaning. It can be said, on the contrary, that Lelong had a vocabulary. In addition to his family name (*Lelo*), four words, French words, had survived the wreckage, and he used them with every possible meaning, while giving to three of them definite preferences. Hence, these were two varieties of aphemia, perfectly distinct from one another. It is true, one might assume, that in the long run, through the progress of his disease, Lelong would have descended to the level of the other patient. There was, however, one embarrassing circumstance. It is that, in the latter, the aphemia had been, from the start, as complete as it was twenty-one years later at the time of his death. The cerebral softening, while spreading, had altered or abolished the functions and the various organs, having destroyed at first only one small part of the frontal convolutions. The disease had terminated by hollowing out an area in the anterior lobe, with a vast loss of substance, and the intelligence of the patient had at the same time undergone a noticeable deterioration, and, nevertheless, whereas all the other functional disturbances had been increasing, the sole symptom of the aphemia had constantly remained the same. It was, therefore, permissible to ask whether Tan's aphemia and that of Lelong were of the same nature. There were both negative and affirmative explanations. Consequently, I hesitated to admit that the site of the lesion must be the same in the second case as in the first, and I awaited, without making any pronouncement on the matter, the results of the autopsy. Indeed the patient had lost strength rapidly. Some eschars at the sacrum occurred unexpectedly and he died on November 8, 1861, only twelve days after his fall.

Autopsy. The thoracic and abdominal viscera revealed nothing remarkable. It is not necessary to speak here of the fracture of the neck of the femur. I shall speak only of the brain.

All the sutures had ossified. The walls of the cranium were somewhat thickened, but were no harder than usual. The bones were healthy, as well as the dura mater which was not thickened. There was a rather large amount of serous fluid in the arachnoid cavity; the pia mater was neither thickened nor congested.

The entire encephalon with its membranes weighed 1136 grams at removal from the cranium, a lower-than-average figure and almost equal to the minimum for the encephalon of *adult* individuals of the *male sex* and *healthy* mind. Among the weights known up to the present this minimum has been 1133 grams. However, it is known that in the aged the average weight of the encephalon diminishes in a marked manner. It will be seen later, furthermore, that one of the hemispheres had undergone a rather pronounced atrophy. These two considerations combined had contributed to make the weight of the encephalon of our patient go well below the average.

When the brain was placed on the table, at first glance a surface lesion was seen which occupied the left frontal lobe immediately below the anterior end of the fissure of Sylvius. At this level the surface of the hemisphere was appreciably sunken, and the depressed pia mater permitted seeing through the transparency a collection of serous fluid, which occupied at the surface an expanse very nearly equal to that of a one-franc piece. This lesion was incomparably more circumscribed than that which existed in Tan's brain. However, in comparing the two areas, it was determined that the center of the lesion was identically the same in both cases.

Before lifting up the pia mater, I separated the cerebellum, the pineal body, and the medulla oblongata, which together weighed 142 grams; then I divided the so-called brain along the median line and weighed the two hemispheres separately. The right weighed 514 grams, the left only 480 grams. The latter, which was the center of the disease, was hence 34 grams lower than the healthy hemisphere. The comparative weight was repeated after ablation of the pia mater and draining of the serous fluid from the lateral ventricles. The right hemisphere at that time weighed 487 grams, the left 455, the difference being 32 grams instead of 34. That indicated that the center of the left frontal lobe contained about 2 grams of serous fluid. It was seen that the left hemisphere underwent a considerably greater reduction in weight than might have been expected from the small extent of the lesion of the frontal lobe. Despite that, the consistency of the cerebral substance was exactly the same on both sides. It was very firm, more so than the brain of the aged ordinarily is. The surface of the right and left convolutions showed the most normal color; there was no difficulty in removing the pia mater.

The right hemisphere was perfectly healthy in all parts, as was also the cerebellum, the medulla oblongata, and the pineal body. There were appreciable lesions only on the left hemisphere.

In this hemisphere the optic layer, the fornix, the corpus callosum, the taenia pontis, the corpus striatum, the occipital and parietal lobes, the lobe of the insula, and the orbital convolutions that form the lower layer of the frontal lobe were normal. It seemed to me, however, that at the union of the anterior end of the ventricular nucleus of the corpus striatum with the medullary substance of the frontal lobe the consistency of the cerebral tissue was slightly reduced; but, this lesion, if it was one, was entirely independent of the principal lesion, from which it was separated by a considerable thickness of healthy tissue. It is the latter lesion that I am going to describe now.

The collection of serous fluid located under the pia mater, the site of which has been indicated above, occupied a cavity hollowed out in the substance of the convolutions. At this level the third frontal convolution, which runs along the upper edge of the fissure of Sylvius, as is known, was completely cut across and had undergone throughout its entire depth a loss of substance, the extent of which appeared to be about 15 millimeters. Our cavity was, therefore, continuous outward with the fissure of Sylvius at the level of the lobe of the insula. On the inside it encroached on the second frontal convolution, which was very deeply notched, but the innermost layer of which was spared to a depth of 2 millimeters. It was this thin tongue which alone maintained the continuity of the second frontal convolution. The first was perfectly healthy. The transverse or posterior frontal convolution which forms the boundary in front of the fissure of Rolando was likewise healthy. Finally, the two diseased convolutions, in their anterior two-thirds, showed complete integrity. Consequently, it could be asserted that in our patient the aphemia had been the result of a deep lesion, but a very clearly circumscribed one, of the second and third frontal convolutions in one part of their posterior third.

It is certain that this lesion was not a softening. The cerebral tissue was so far from being softened near the walls of the lesion that still today, although the portion has been examined and handled several times, the thin tongue which maintains the continuity of the second frontal convolution has preserved its solidity. That seems to me also to indicate that the cerebral tissue in the immediate vicinity of the lesion was more resistant than in the normal state.

On the other hand, on the walls of the central point some small spots were seen of a yellowish-orange color which appeared of hematic origin, and microscopic examination, made by my intern Mr. Piedvache, showed that there were crystals of heme at this level. Hence it was a case of an *old apoplectic center*, and there was no doubt that our patient had lost his speech suddenly in an attack of apoplexy eighteen months before his death.

This observation offers very remarkable analogies with that of my first patient, and it was much more revealing, since the disease here was perfectly limited. In the first case there could be some doubt about the initial site of the lesion. It was only by a reasoned analysis of the anatomical disorders that one was led to recognize that the aphemia had been the result of the softening of the two external frontal convolutions. In my second patient, on the contrary, this determination was evident. There had been no symptom other than the aphemia, no other lesion than that of the two convolutions mentioned above, and it was incontestable that in this man the disease which had affected these two convolutions had been the direct cause of the aphemia.

In both cases the second frontal convolution was much less deeply altered than the third. It may be concluded from this that the latter had been, in all probability, the principal site of the initial lesion. Two facts are too few when it is a matter of solving one of the most obscure and most controversial questions of cerebral physiology. I cannot, however, keep from saying, until there is more information, that the integrity of the third frontal convolution (and perhaps of the second) appears indispensable for articulated speech.

In my preceding report I expressed the thought that if the doctrine of the particular localizations was one day recognized as accurate, this was probably not at the points in the more or less clearly limited areas corresponding to the points determined from the vault of the cranium, that one could localize the various cerebral faculties. In other words, I thought that if ever there were a science of phrenology, this was the phrenology of the convolutions, and not the phrenology of the bumps. I therefore shall not conceal the fact that I felt astonishment neighboring on stupefaction when I found that in my second patient the lesion occupied *strictly* the same site as in the first. These were not only the same convolutions that were diseased; they were in exactly the same point, immediately behind their middle third, namely the lobe of the insula, and precisely on the same side (left side). The initial site of the disease, consequently, corresponded in the two cases *to the same point of the wall of the cranium.*

I do not hide from myself that the partisans of the phrenology of bumps might bring together from these two facts an argument favorable to their system. However, without daring to make a pronouncement again, and without attaching too much importance to the too few detailed observations, which have preceded mine, I cannot doubt that in several of the facts published aphemia has been seen to follow lesions which occupied principally (if not exclusively) the anterior half of the frontal lobes. These facts, perfectly compatible with the hypothesis of the localizations by convolutions, appeared very difficult to reconcile with the principle of the localizations by districts or, if one wishes, by compartments corresponding to invariable points of the cranial box. I am, therefore, disposed to attribute to pure coincidence the absolute identity of the site of the lesions in my two patients.

As for the well-manifested difference that exists between the two varieties of aphemia that I have described in my two observations, a difference that I was tempted to attribute, before the second autopsy, to a difference in site, I now suppose that it depended on the nature of the lesions. In my first patient it was a case of progressive softening, a lesion which was never clearly limited. The second was only a very limited apoplectic center. It is, for that reason, probable that, in the first case, the diseased convolution was, from the start, altered to a more considerable extent. Thus, it can be understood, up to a certain point, why the aphemia was more complete and more serious in the first man than it was in the one the observation of whom I have just reported.

Neurosurgical Classic—7

APPROXIMATELY fifty years ago Dr. Walter E. Dandy converted a personal disappointment into a major advancement in the understanding of a common neurological disorder—hydrocephalus.[2] Following his graduation from the Johns Hopkins Medical School in 1910, Dandy worked for a year with Dr. Harvey Cushing in the Hunterian Laboratory of Experimental Medicine. He then spent 1911–1912 as Cushing's clinical assistant, and was invited to accompany Cushing the following year to the newly built Peter Bent Brigham Hospital in Boston. Because of clashes of personality between the two men, the offer was withdrawn. By that time, however, Dr. William S. Halsted had filled all of the positions on his surgical house staff for 1912–1913, and Walter Dandy was left without an appointment. Through the kindness of the director of the hospital (Dr. Halsted was on vacation), Dandy was given a room and was allowed to work in the Hunterian Laboratory. There Dandy and Kenneth D. Blackfan, instructor in pediatrics, performed their basic studies of hydrocephalus and the circulation of the cerebrospinal fluid which were to revolutionize medical thought in these areas.[19–22]

Until that time there had been no adequate theories advanced to explain the circulation of the cerebrospinal fluid or the development of hydrocephalus. Furthermore, there were still no satisfactory methods of treating hydrocephalus. Although this condition was known to the ancients, the only operative treatment developed prior to the nineteenth century was ventricular puncture. Then open ventricular drainage to the surface of the head was proposed in 1881, and later was carried out by a number of surgeons. During the following three decades a great variety of other operations were also devised for the treatment of hydrocephalus. Ventricular fluid was shunted into the subcutaneous or subarachnoid spaces, into the venous system, or into the peritoneal cavity. The choroid plexuses were destroyed or removed, and operations were developed for the drainage of the spinal subarachnoid fluid into the peritoneal or retroperitoneal spaces. However, the results of these ingenious operations were very discouraging.[1,23,25,28,31,32]

Then Dandy and Blackfan began their important investigations.[19–22]

"Dandy was able, in the dog, to produce dilatation of the lateral and third ventricles by obstructing the aqueduct of Sylvius, to produce distention of one lateral ventricle by obstructing its foramen of Monro and to prevent the latter by previous removal of its choroid plexus. By separating the Pacchionian granulations from the great venous sinuses both over the vertex and at the base of the dog's brain, he demonstrated that hydrocephalus did not result, and, therefore, that cerebrospinal fluid absorption did not occur in that manner (as was widely believed) but rather, directly into the blood vessels in the subarachnoid spaces.

"In the autopsy room an obstruction either at the aqueduct of Sylvius or at the foramina of Luschka and Magendie or along the basilar cisterns was demonstrated in every case of 'idiopathic' hydrocephalus. This disorder was thus reclassified, upon a solid basis of anatomical and physiological study and of clinical observation, into communicating and non-communicating types. . . . "[1]

These studies, and the operations that Dandy devised as a result of them (third ventriculostomy, choroid plexectomy, and catheter drainage of the third ventricle through the aqueduct of Sylvius) were of basic importance to the development of successful shunting procedures for hydrocephalus.[26,27,29,31–38] Throughout his life Dandy continued to contribute to the understanding of hydrocephalus,[1–25,30] and his last published work was on this subject.[17,24]

References

1. CAMPBELL, E.   Walter E. Dandy—surgeon, 1886–1946. J. Neurosurg., 1951, 8: 249–262.

2. CROWE, S. J. Halsted of Johns Hopkins. The man and his men. *Springfield, Ill.: Charles C Thomas,* 1957, ix, 247 pp. (see pp. 86–88).

3. CUSHING, H. Studies in intracranial physiology & surgery. The third circulation. The hypophysis. The gliomas. *London: Oxford Univ. Press,* 1926, xii, 146 pp. (see pp. 1–51).

4. DANDY, W. E. Exhibition of a case of internal hydrocephalus. *Johns Hopk. Hosp. Bull.,* 1918, *29:* 153–154.

5. DANDY, W. E. Extirpation of the choroid plexus of the lateral ventricles in communicating hydrocephalus. *Ann. Surg.,* 1918, *68:* 569–579.

6. DANDY, W. E. Experimental hydrocephalus. *Ann. Surg.,* 1919, *70:* 129–142.

7. DANDY, W. E. The diagnosis and treatment of hydrocephalus resulting from strictures of the aqueduct of Sylvius. *Surg. Gynec. Obstet.,* 1920, *31:* 340–358.

8. DANDY, W. E. Hydrocephalus in chondrodystrophy. *Johns Hopk. Hosp. Bull.,* 1921, *32:* 5–10.

9. DANDY, W. E. The diagnosis and treatment of hydrocephalus due to occlusions of the foramina of Magendie and Luschka. *Surg. Gynec. Obstet.,* 1921, *32:* 112–124.

10. DANDY, W. E. The cause of so-called idiopathic hydrocephalus. *Johns Hopk. Hosp. Bull.,* 1921, *32:* 67–75.

11. DANDY, W. E. Cerebral ventriculoscopy. *Johns Hopk. Hosp. Bull.,* 1922, *33:* 189.

12. DANDY, W. E. An operative procedure for hydrocephalus. *Johns Hopk. Hosp. Bull.,* 1922, *33:* 189–190.

13. DANDY, W. E. Intracranial tumors and abscesses causing communicating hydrocephalus. *Ann. Surg.,* 1925, *82:* 199–207.

14. DANDY, W. E. Where is cerebrospinal fluid absorbed? *J. Amer. med. Ass.,* 1929, *92:* 2012–2014.

15. DANDY, W. E. Surgery of the brain. In: *Lewis' practice of surgery.* Hagerstown, Md.: W. F. Prior Co., Inc., 1932, *12:* 671+17 pp. (see pp. 213–243).

16. DANDY, W. E. The operative treatment of communicating hydrocephalus. *Ann. Surg.,* 1938, *108:* 194–202.

17. DANDY, W. E. Diagnosis and treatment of strictures of the aqueduct of Sylvius (causing hydrocephalus). *Arch. Surg., Chicago,* 1945, *51:* 1–14.

18. [DANDY, W. E.] Selected writings of Walter E. Dandy. Compiled by C. E. Troland and F. J. Otenasek. *Springfield, Ill.: Charles C Thomas,* 1957, vii, 789 pp.

19. DANDY, W. E., and BLACKFAN, K. D. An experimental and clinical study of internal hydrocephalus. *J. Amer. med. Ass.,* 1913, *61:* 2216–2217.

20. DANDY, W. E., and BLACKFAN, K. D. Internal hydrocephalus. An experimental, clinical and pathological study. *Amer. J. Dis. Child.,* 1914, *8:* 406–482.

21. DANDY, W. E., and BLACKFAN, K. D. Hydrocephalus internus. Eine experimentelle, klinische und pathologische Untersuchung. *Beitr. klin. Chir.,* 1914, *93:* 392–486.

22. DANDY, W. E., and BLACKFAN, K. D. Internal hydrocephalus. Second paper. *Amer. J. Dis. Child.,* 1917, *14:* 424–443.

23. DAVIDOFF, L. M. Treatment of hydrocephalus. Historical review and description of a new method. *Arch. Surg., Chicago,* 1929, *18:* 1737–1762.

24. FAIRMAN, D. Evolution of neurosurgery through Walter E. Dandy's work. *Surgery,* 1946, *19:* 581–604.

25. FISHER, R. G. Surgery of the congenital anomalies. In: *A history of neurological surgery.* A. E. Walker, Ed. Baltimore: Williams & Wilkins Co., 1951, xii, 583 pp. (see pp. 334–361).

26. NULSEN, F. E., and SPITZ, E. B. Treatment of hydrocephalus by direct shunt from ventricle to jugular vein. *Surg. Forum,* 1952, *2:* 399–403.

27. PUDENZ, R. H., RUSSELL, F. E., HURD, A. H., and SHELDEN, C. H. Ventriculo-auriculostomy. A technique for shunting cerebrospinal fluid into the right auricle. Preliminary report. *J. Neurosurg.,* 1957, *14:* 171–179.

28. RIECHERT, T., and UMBACH, W. Die operative Behandlung des Hydrocephalus. *Olivecrona u. Tönnis Handb. Neurochir.,* 1960, *4,* pt. 1: 599–672.

29. ROBERTSON, J. T., SCHICK, R. W., MORGAN, F., and MATSON, D. D. Accurate placement of ventriculoatrial shunt for hydrocephalus under electrocardiographic control. *J. Neurosurg.,* 1961, *18:* 255–257.

30. SACHS, E. The history and development of neurological surgery. *New York: P. B. Hoeber, Inc.,* 1952, 158 pp. (see pp. 90–92).

31. SCARFF, J. E. Fifty years of neurosurgery, 1905–1955. *Int. Abstr. Surg.,* 1955, *101:* 417–513 (see pp. 445–455).

32. SCARFF, J. E. Treatment of hydrocephalus: an historical and critical review of methods and results. *J. Neurol. Neurosurg. Psychiat.,* 1963, *26:* 1–26.

33. TORKILDSEN, A. A new palliative operation in cases of inoperable occlusion of the Sylvian aqueduct. *Acta chir. scand.,* 1939, *82:* 117–124.

34. TORKILDSEN, A. A new palliative operation in cases of inoperable occlusion of the Sylvian aqueduct. *Acta psychiat., Kbh.,* 1939, *14:* 221.

35. TORKILDSEN, A. Ventriculo-cisternostomy. A postoperative study. *Acta chir. scand.,* 1941, *85:* 254–260.

36. TORKILDSEN, A. Ventriculocisternostomy. A palliative operation in different types of non-communicating hydrocephalus. *Oslo: J. G. Tanum Forlag,* 1947, 240 pp.

37. TORKILDSEN, A. Should extirpation be attempted in cases of neoplasm in or near the third ventricle of the brain? Experiences with a palliative method. *J. Neurosurg.,* 1948, *5:* 249–275.

38. TORKILDSEN, A. A follow-up study 14 to 20 years after ventriculocisternostomy. *Acta psychiat., Kbh.,* 1960, *35:* 113–121.

INTERNAL HYDROCEPHALUS

An Experimental, Clinical and Pathological Study*†

WALTER E. DANDY, M.D.
and
KENNETH D. BLACKFAN, M.D.
BALTIMORE

Part 1.—Experimental Studies

1. INTRODUCTION

The term "hydrocephalus" is merely a symptomatic designation for an idiopathic disease. The subdivisions into acute and chronic, internal and external, congenital and acquired, are made according to no one standard, but according to several—pathological, clinical and embryological. Such subdivisions do not clarify the pathogenesis, but serve to obscure it. Chronic internal hydrocephalus, whether congenital or acquired, is the most important and frequent form encountered.

Internal hydrocephalus is characterized by a progressive accumulation of cerebrospinal fluid in the ventricles, causing their dilatation and a consequent cortical atrophy and, when possible, enlargement of the head. The disease is usually fatal; spontaneous recovery, however, does occur in a small percentage of cases.

Numerous forms of treatment have been suggested and tried, but, as the number of methods indicates, they have been almost uniformly unsuccessful. The etiology being so obscure, any treatment is necessarily empirical and consequently unsatisfactory. Successful therapy must depend on the identification and the treatment of the cause of the disease.

It is evident that internal hydrocephalus is due to an abnormality either in the formation or in the absorption of cerebrospinal fluid or possibly in both. Our studies—experimental and clinical—have been concerned with the development, the pathology and the diagnosis of internal hydrocephalus.

2. HISTORICAL

Reference to hydrocephalus is made by the earliest medical writers. Hippocrates is credited with suggesting surgical treatment by trephining the anterior part of the skull. He evidently thought that the accumulation of fluid was extracerebral.

Galen was the first to give special consideration to this disease, which played a conspicuous part in his theory of the "animal spirit." Galen was really advanced in his knowledge of the anatomy of the ventricles of the brain. He thought they were in free communication with one another and that they formed a closed system. He knew of the aqueduct of Sylvius and of the foramina of Monro. Galen, however, believed that the soul or "animal spirit" was contained in the ventricles and that here it underwent a process of purification; the purified products were supposed to pass into the pores of the brain and the waste products found their way through the pituitary body and were discharged into the nose as "pituita." He considered hydrocephalus due to some defect in this process of elaboration of the "animal spirit."

The teachings of Galen were accepted without question until Vesalius, in 1543, denied the existence of the "animal spirit." Following Vesalius a succession of distinguished anatomists have been interested in the study of hydrocephalus. Among them have been Willis, Sylvius, Rhazes, Celsus, Petit, Pacchionis, Brunner, Littré, Morgagni, Cotugno, Monro, Haller, Robert Whytt, and in the nineteenth century Magendie, John Hilton, Luschka and Key and Retzius.

Many theories regarding the content of the ventricles have been considered since the overthrow of Galen's theory of the "animal spirit." It has at various periods been regarded as water, air, vacuum, vapor, until finally it was proved to be a fluid. Verduc, about 1700, insisted that fluid was never present in the normal ventricles, and this agitation led to Haller's vapor theory. Haller had the advantage of a correct knowledge of the circulation of the blood and supposed the vapor to be exhaled by the arteries and inhaled by the veins.

* Received for publication April 27, 1914.

From the Departments of Surgery and Pediatrics of the Johns Hopkins University and Hospital. A preliminary communication of this study appeared in the Journal of the American Medical Association, 1913, lxi, 2216.

† Reprinted from the *American Journal of Diseases of Children*, 1914, *8:* 406–482, with the kind permission of the American Medical Association.

Cotugno (1770) first proved the existence of the subarachnoid space and in addition found fluid in this space in living fishes and turtles, but was unable to demonstrate fluid in dogs because the spinal cord so closely filled the dural envelope. Though he was the real discoverer of the existence of cerebrospinal fluid in the living animal, his findings were not accepted because of the firm belief in Haller's vapor theory. At this time all fluid was explained on the basis of some pathological process or as a postmortem condensation of the vapor.

Galen's teaching that the pituitary body was the portal of exit of the ventricular contents was held by many until the end of the eighteenth century. Haller denied this function to the pituitary body, but Petit (1718) and even Monro (1793) supposed that hydrocephalus was due to sclerosis of the pituitary body, which effectually closed the channels of exit from the ventricles.

Monro (1793), after whom the foramen of Monro is named, was also interested in the study of hydrocephalus. The presence of a foramen (the foramen of Magendie), leading from the fourth ventricle to the subarachnoid space as claimed by Haller and Cotugno, was denied by many, including Monro. He said:

> The bottom of the fourth ventricle has no such communication with the cavity of the spinal marrow as Dr. Haller supposed, being completely shut off by its choroid plexus and pia mater. As further proof that the four ventricles communicate with each other and that they do not communicate with the cavity of the spinal marrow, I have observed in the bodies of every one of fifteen children who died from internal hydrocephalus that all the ventricles were distended; that on cutting into one of the lateral ventricles, all the ventricles were emptied, that in these cases, the passages above described were greatly enlarged, and that in none of them was water contained in the cavity of the spinal marrow or between its pia and the dura mater.

So near to the cause of hydrocephalus, in his zeal to prove a closed foramen, Monro, unfortunately, mistook it for the normal condition and left the discovery of the communication between the ventricles and the subarachnoid space to Magendie.

Without doubt, Magendie's contribution is the most important that has been made to the subject of hydrocephalus. He demonstrated by experiments on animals (1) that fluid normally fills the ventricles and the subarachnoid space; (2) that free communication exists between the ventricles and the subarachnoid space by means of a foramen which now bears his name; (3) that the central and spinal subarachnoid cavities form a single freely communicating space, and (4) that the aqueduct of Sylvius or the foramen of Magendie was obstructed in several cases of hydrocephalus.

Magendie, however, did not understand why hydrocephalus should result from an obstruction, for he thought the pia secreted the cerebrospinal fluid. He was led to believe that in some way the fluid could readily make its way upward through these membranous obstructions, but for some reason which he did not understand, its return was impeded and accumulation in the ventricles resulted.

The existence of cerebrospinal fluid has since been admitted, but the other observations of Magendie have been opposed. The controversy over Magendie's various claims and the views of more recent workers will be considered later.

3. INTERNAL HYDROCEPHALUS EXPERIMENTALLY PRODUCED

Flexner has noted that internal hydrocephalus sometimes follows the injection of the meningococcus into the subarachnoid space of monkeys. With this exception, we have been able to find no instance of hydrocephalus experimentally produced. The more common pathological processes producing internal hydrocephalus are usually so large (tumors) or so diffuse (inflammations) that it has been difficult to determine their exact part in the production of this disease. It is obvious that if hydrocephalus can be produced by experimental means, it will be possible to obtain definite information regarding its cause.

We conducted two series of experiments. In one, the aqueduct of Sylvius was occluded and in the other, the vein of Galen or the straight sinus or both were ligated. In each series the experiment was such that the function of either the aqueduct or of the vein was not disturbed.

I. EFFECT OF OCCLUSION OF THE AQUEDUCT OF SYLVIUS

In this series of experiments, in which an obstructing body was placed in the aqueduct of Sylvius, an internal hydrocephalus invariably resulted. It should be emphasized that the obstructing body was so placed *in* the aqueduct that the topographical relations were undisturbed and the lumen of the vein of Galen unaffected. The resulting hydrocephalus was therefore due solely to the mechanical occlusion of this channel. It is preferable to use a small obstructing body and depend on the formation of adhesions gradually to produce total occlusion. When this is done, practically no postoperative irritative effects result. A small pledget of cotton proved most efficient as the obstructing body.

These experiments were performed most successfully on dogs. Cats and monkeys were tried, but without success. When carefully done, the operative mortality in dogs was negligible. The animals at the time of operation were from 2 to 6 months of age. At this age the sutures of the skull are united so that the resulting hydrocephalus causes cerebral atrophy rather than enlargement of the head. Cerebral atrophy and cephalic enlargement are merely different expressions of the same underlying cause—increased intracranial pressure. Until the sutures are united, enlargement of the head is permitted by diastasis; after union the ventricular dilatation can be compensated only by cerebral atrophy and to a lesser degree by the displacement of external fluid and the absorption of bone.

The obstruction was placed in the aqueduct of Sylvius through a subcerebellar route as follows: Under ether anesthesia and strict surgical precautions, a bilateral, suboccipital decompression was made through a posterior median incision. The defects in the bone and dura were made as large as possible to facilitate the subsequent procedure. The pia-arachnoid binding the cerebellum and the medulla was carefully cut on each side of the midline and an opening made corresponding to the foramen of Magendie, which is absent in the dog. The cerebellum and the roof of the fourth ventricle were raised by a small retractor. Through the artificial opening in the roof of the fourth ventricle a small pledget of cotton on the end of a graduated carrier was passed along the floor of the fourth ventricle into the aque-

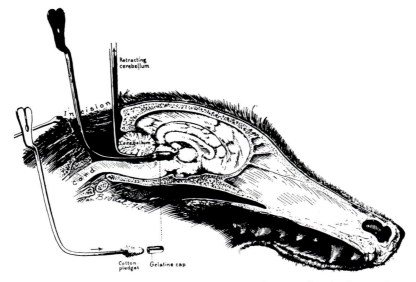

Fig. 1.—Midsagittal section of a dog's head to illustrate the method of procedure in the experimental production of internal hydrocephalus. The obstruction is placed in the aqueduct of Sylvius by the subcerebellar route.

duct of Sylvius (Fig. 1). The pledget of cotton was deposited by withdrawal of the carrier. A refinement of technic, though of doubtful benefit, consisted in enclosing the cotton in a gelatin capsule immersed in liquid petrolatum. The cerebrospinal fluid dissolves the capsule surrounding the cotton (Fig. 2). The introduction of the cotton was rendered easier when it was enclosed. This, however, was not essential and was of questionable value, as adhesions form less readily about the cotton.

With care, an accurate deposition of the obstructing body can be obtained. The anterior tip of the fourth ventricle can be determined from the reading on the graduated carrier. Often additional evidence was afforded by resistance to the carrier's progress. It is very easy to deviate slightly and force the instrument into the mesencephalon, naturally with destructive results on account of the immediate proximity of the pyramidal tracts and the nuclei of the upper cranial nerves.

The recovery following operation was uneventful. Frequently a slight spasticity, disturbance of equilibrium and weakness of the extraocular muscles persisted for several days following the operation, but all soon disappeared. Vomiting and lethargy, general pressure signs were evident from the time of operation and these were the principal manifestations of internal hydrocephalus. Doubtless a bilateral choked disk would have been present and given the best evidence of the onset and progress of the intracranial pressure. Unfortunately, however, the eye-grounds were not examined. The animals were painlessly killed from three to eight weeks after operation. They were in good condition at the end of this time.

The citation of one experiment may be taken as representative of the entire group. Ether anesthesia was used in all experiments.

EXPERIMENT 1.—Jan. 9, 1911. Mongrel puppy, aged about 3 months; weight, 4½ pounds.

Operation.—A small piece of unencapsulated cotton was passed into the aqueduct of Sylvius by the subcerebellar route described above—no operative complications.

Postoperative History.—January 11: Marked loss of equilibrium with tendency to fall backward. Slight dissociation of ocular movements; slight spasticity but no paralyses; frequent vomiting; marked lethargy. January 17: General condition good. Equilibrium normal. Walks around slowly but no tendency to playfulness; spasticity has disappeared, ocular movements normal, vomiting persists. January 28: Lies curled up in the cage most of time; takes no interest in surroundings. Sluggishly responds to stimuli; tendency to stupor. Ocular movements normal; vomiting more frequent. Losing weight. February 9: *Killed by ether thirty days after operation.*

Pathological Note.—During the removal of the calvarium the forceps punctured a greatly thinned cortex and entered a large, distended lateral ventricle. The intraventricular pressure was so great that cerebrospinal fluid spurted a distance of three feet. The accompanying photograph (Fig. 2 *b*) shows the obstruction in the aqueduct of Sylvius well organized and apparently impermeable. The third and lateral ventricles were greatly dilated and the

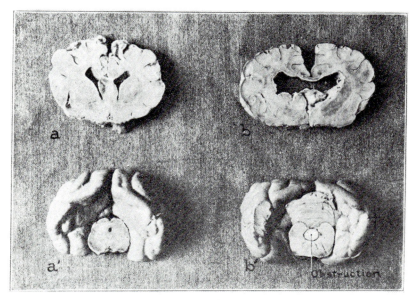

Fig. 2.—*a*, Cross-section of a normal brain of a dog at the level of the optic chiasm; *a'*, cross-section of the normal mid-brain of a dog to show the size of the aqueduct of Sylvius; *b*, cross-section of brain showing an experimental internal hydrocephalus of one month's duration; note the complete atrophy of the septum lucidum and fusion of the ventricles; *b'*, cross-section of the mid-brain of same animal showing the obstruction which had been placed in the aqueduct of Sylvius.

thickness of the cortex was correspondingly diminished. Only an occasional shred of septum lucidum remained. The vein of Galen was normal.

II. OCCLUSION OF THE AQUEDUCT OF SYLVIUS FOLLOWED BY EXTIRPATION OF THE CHOROID PLEXUSES OF BOTH LATERAL VENTRICLES

Though we removed the choroid plexus from one or both lateral ventricles in a series of experiments, the bilateral removal was followed by the insertion of an obstruction in the aqueduct of Sylvius in only one experiment. The object of this experiment was to see if extirpation of the choroid plexus modified the development of the internal hydrocephalus. The operative procedure was as follows: A bilateral, subtemporal decompression was made. On each side the dura was opened and a transcortical incision was carried into the lateral ventricle at the junction of the body and the descending horn. By dilating the cerebral opening with a nasal dilator, a good exposure of the entire lateral ventricle was obtained and the choroid plexus almost completely extirpated. Despite the great vascularity of the choroid plexus, bleeding was slight and was readily controlled by cotton pledgets.

At the same operation a suboccipital decompression was performed and an obstruction passed along the subcerebellar or transventricular route and deposited in the aqueduct of Sylvius. The choroid plexus of the third ventricle and probably remnants of the choroid plexus of the lateral ventricles still remained in front of the obstruction. Prevention of fluid accumulation was possible only to a modified degree. There was lethargy and occasional vomiting.

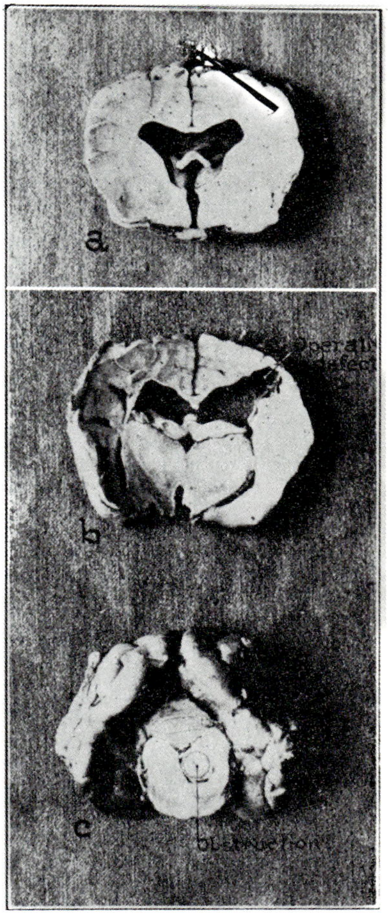

Fig. 3.—Cross-section of a brain of a dog showing an internal hydrocephalus of five weeks' duration which resulted from obstructing the aqueduct of Sylvius. The choroid plexuses of the two lateral ventricles were simultaneously extirpated: *a*, at level of optic chiasm; note atrophy of septum lucidum and dilated lateral ventricles; *b*, to show the operative defect in the cortex; the dilated ventricles are closed only by the meninges; the remains of the septum lucidum are still evident; *c*, midbrain showing the obstruction in the aqueduct of Sylvius.

Thirty-five days after the first operation, the suboccipital wound was reopened and found in perfect condition. The cerebellum was herniated through the osseous defect made at the previous operation. This showed an increased intracranial pressure. A fine pair of forceps was passed along the floor of the fourth ventricle and the obstructing body readily located and grasped. It was firmly in position; there was beginning organization, and some force was required to dislodge it. On its release there was a gush of cerebrospinal fluid. An internal hydrocephalus had resulted from the occlusion placed in the aqueduct of Sylvius thirty-five days previously, *in spite of the almost complete bilateral extirpation of the choroid plexuses of the lateral ventricles.*

The obstructing body was replaced at once in the aqueduct, the animal killed and the brain hardened *in situ* with formaldehyde solution. Subsequent examination showed a completely occluded aqueduct. The pia had healed, covering the operative wound in the cortex. The hydrocephalus was distinctly modified, being much less than a hydrocephalus of the same duration, in which the choroid plexuses had not been removed. The difference is well shown by comparing the ventricles (Fig. 3) in this specimen with the ventricles in Figure 2. The obstruction in each was of practically the same duration, and in both the occlusion of the aqueduct was complete. The contrast is less striking, however, than it should be, because the brain of the former animal (Fig. 3) was hardened *in situ* and the ventricles more nearly resembled their actual size, whereas the brain in the latter (Fig. 2) was hardened after removal, and the opening of the ventricles, before fixation, resulted in considerable shrinkage. The inference is to be made that the extirpation of the choroid plexuses modifies the degree of the internal hydrocephalus.

The preceding experiments prove that *an internal hydrocephalus results from a simple mechanical occlusion of the aqueduct of Sylvius. From this it is apparent that cerebrospinal fluid forms in the ventricles, at least more rapidly than it is removed, and that the aqueduct of Sylvius is necessary for its escape.*

III. LIGATION OF THE VENA GALENA MAGNA AND THE SINUS RECTUS

That internal hydrocephalus may be due to an obstruction of the great vein of Galen or of the straight sinus has been suggested. In most of the pathological specimens used to support this theory, tumors have been present in the corpora quadrigemina, the pineal gland, the cerebellum or in this immediate neighborhood, and compression of the aqueduct of Sylvius in all probability has also resulted. The most conclusive clinical proof is given in a few recorded instances of a thrombosis of the great vein of Galen or straight sinus. Newman (1882) reported a case of hydrocephalus in which a small thrombus was present in the vena Galena magna at its junction with the sinus rectus. Browning also presented a case with a small thrombus in the sinus rectus.

Internal hydrocephalus resulting from venous obstruction is dependent on the venous collateral circulation. A good description of the venous collateral circulation of the veins of Galen is given in Poirier and Charpy's "Anatomy," 1901, iii, 60. This work is based largely on that of Browning, Hedon and Trolard. The internal cerebral system of veins, of which the great vein of Galen is the trunk, is largely independent of the external venous system. It is not, however, a completely closed system. Collateral circulation is definitely established with the external system by the basilar, superior cerebellar, internal occipital, temporal, posterior corpus callosal and several smaller tributaries of the vena Galena magna. This is demonstrated by the fact that colored solutions injected into the straight sinus pass to the external system by these channels. Poirier and Charpy, however, minimize the importance of this collateral circulation and think it is insufficient to prevent internal hydrocephalus when the vein of Galen is obstructed. They further state that the small veins of Galen which drain practically the whole interior of the brain have almost no collateral circulation.

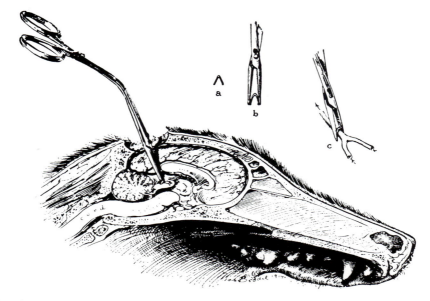

Fig. 4.—Drawing to indicate method of ligating the vena Galena magna. The silver clip is similar to that devised by Dr. Cushing. *a* shows the silver clip; *b*, in position in the clip holder, and *c*, its application on the vein.

To determine the importance of venous obstruction in the production of internal hydrocephalus, we occluded the vein of Galen or the straight sinus or both in ten dogs. To do this a trephine opening was made just above the external occipital protuberance a little to either side of the midline. This opening was then enlarged with rongeur forceps. The dura was opened, reflected over the superior longitudinal sinus and the occipital lobe separated from the falx cerebri. The straight sinus in the tentorium cerebelli (osseum) was traced downward to the vena Galena magna which is situated directly under the splenium of the corpus callosum. By careful blunt dissection the vein of Galen was isolated to permit the application of one or more silver clips (Fig. 4). These clips are similar to those designed by Dr. Cushing and act as most effective ligatures in wounds of such depth that ligation is impossible.

In the ten dogs in which a ligation was thus accomplished, only one developed an internal hydrocephalus. In the other animals there was no evidence of ventricular enlargement.

Following the operation there was invariably an immediate recovery; in none were there any signs to indicate that the dogs were abnormal. All were as active and playful as the control animals. The animals were under observation from one to eight months, and one gave birth to a litter of healthy puppies six months after the operation.

The single instance in which hydrocephalus resulted is of importance. The clip was placed just at the origin of the vena Galena magna, much lower than in any of the other experiments, thus barring the principal tributaries mentioned above from participation in the collateral circulation; the stasis resulting is no doubt similar to that in ascites which results from an obstruction to the vena cava, where the

Fig. 5.—Internal hydrocephalus of three and one-half months' duration, produced by ligation of the vena Galena magna near its origin: *a*, dilated lateral ventricles, with atrophy of septum lucidum; *b* to show the resultant dilated aqueduct of Sylvius; compare with normal Figure 2, *a'*.

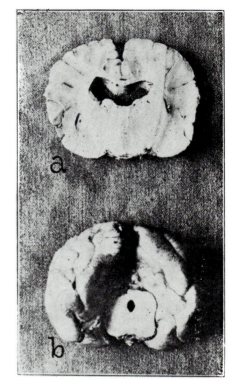

collateral circulation is insufficient to take over the additional work. The hydrocephalus was of three and one-half months' standing. The septum lucidum was largely destroyed, only shreds remaining. The ventricular dilatation was considerably less than in the dog in which the aqueduct of Sylvius was obstructed for thirty-five days and the choroid plexus of both lateral ventricles extirpated. The aqueduct of Sylvius was also larger than normal, showing the effects of its participation in the transmission of the increased ventricular fluid (Fig. 5).

In those dogs in which hydrocephalus did not develop, the clip was placed higher on the vein of Galen and nearer its junction with the sinus rectus. When the clip was so placed, or when the straight sinus alone was ligated, there was no evidence of fluid stasis and the ventricles remained normal in size, showing that below this point there was sufficient venous collateral circulation to prevent the formation of hydrocephalus.

It is therefore evident that a low obstruction of the vena Galena magna may result in the production of an internal hydrocephalus, but that a high ligation has no such effect.

4. THE FORMATION OF CEREBROSPINAL FLUID

I. THE EXISTENCE OF CEREBROSPINAL FLUID

Since the introduction of lumbar puncture by Quincke (1891), the existence of cerebrospinal fluid can be demonstrated at any time. That fluid rapidly reforms after withdrawal either from the ventricles or the subarachnoid space can also be demonstrated. Following ventricular puncture in hydrocephalus or after lumbar puncture in cerebral tumor with a postoperative cerebral hernia, the rapidity of the formation of fluid can be estimated. In either case the tension prior to the puncture is reestablished within a few hours, showing that the fluid removed by puncture has reformed during this time. The rapidity of formation can be observed in the rare condition known as rhinorrhea, in which the cerebrospinal fluid discharge may be 200 c.c. or even more in twenty-four hours.

The problem of the formation of cerebrospinal fluid concerns both the place and the manner of its formation.

II. THE PLACE OF FORMATION OF CEREBROSPINAL FLUID

Magendie thought cerebrospinal fluid was formed from the pia, saying:

The pia is almost exclusively a tissue of blood-vessels, and resembling very closely the pulmonary parenchyma, offers the most favorable conditions for a secretion, prompt and considerable. Everything, therefore, leads us to suppose the pia to be the secretory organ of the cerebrospinal fluid.

Magendie tried some injection experiments which tended to confirm this opinion, though he realized the necessity of further proof of a more direct character. He also realized the difficulty of harmonizing this view with his anatomical observations in hydrocephalus.

Lewandowsky was of the opinion that cerebrospinal fluid was a brain product and that only a small part of it could be ascribed to transudation from the choroid plexuses. Spina concurred with this view, but thought the cerebrospinal fluid was a product of transudation not only of the capillaries in the brain, but also in the pia mater. Schmorl noted serological differences in the cerebrospinal fluid of the ventricles and the subarachnoid space and concluded that fluid was formed both in the ventricles and in the pia. He further asserted that no communication existed between the ventricles and the subarachnoid space. Kafka, in a series of eighteen cases, was unable to verify these differences in serological (mainly Wassermann) tests.

The experiments concerning the production of internal hydrocephalus show that fluid forms in the ventricles. This is substantiated in hydrocephalus, in which there is obstruction to the outlets from the ventricles. The experiment in which a modified grade of hydrocephalus followed the total occlusion of the aqueduct of Sylvius and the bilateral extirpation of the major part of the choroid plexuses of the lateral ventricles is evidence of a direct character that the choroid plexuses, as has been suggested, are the organs from which this fluid is produced.

We do not maintain, however, that all cerebrospinal fluid is formed in the ventricles or from the choroid plexuses. Since transudation is partly responsible for this fluid formation, it is possible that fluid might be formed externally in the subarachnoid space, as has been suggested by Schmorl. Evidence for the extracerebral formation of cerebrospinal fluid is found in internal hydrocephalus, in which the foramina of Luschka and Magendie are occluded and all the choroid plexuses are enclosed in the ventricles. In such conditions though cerebrospinal fluid may be obtained by lumbar puncture it is always very small in amount and reforms very slowly. In Case 4, Group 1 (N.M.), never more than 3 c.c. were obtained, and frequently lumbar puncture yielded no fluid. In Case 5 of Group 1 (M.R.), all the choroid plexuses were enclosed in the cerebral ventricles and the clinical and pathological observations showed an absence of communication between the ventricles and the subarachnoid space. By lumbar puncture, however, 5 c.c. of spinal fluid could be obtained. The ventricular and spinal fluids differed but little in composition. The amount of reducing substance (Fehling) was equal in the two. Hexamethylenamin, given by mouth, appeared in each in the same minute quantity, and the cell-count of the two fluids was the same. The choroid plexuses of this patient could obviously play no *direct* part in the formation of the fluid in the subarachnoid space. This fluid, small in amount, which reformed only after several hours, could be derived from one of two sources, either as a transudate from the pial vessels or as a transudate through the thin wall of the dilated fourth ventricle.

In Case 7, Group 1 (M.N.) the spinal and ventricular fluids were of similar composition, and an absence of communication between the ventricles and the subarachnoid space was clinically demonstrated. Twelve hours after a ventricular injection of phenolsulphonephthalein a minute trace of this color was present in the spinal fluid.

Since phenolsulphonephthalein, when present in concentration in the blood, does not appear in the cerebrospinal fluid, it is probable that the trace in the spinal fluid of this patient also was derived by transudation from the ventricles. The foregoing data are, however, insufficient to permit us to assert that the spinal fluid is formed in such a manner.

Although the choroid plexuses were known to Herophilus of Alexandria, Galen gave them the name by which they are known at the present day. Various functions have been ascribed to these structures. Willis (1664) thought they were blood-filters; Varoli, that they sucked up the ventricular fluid; Riolanus noted their exceptional vascularity and called them *rete morabile;* Nuck (1696) first believed them to be glands, a view which was soon received with favor, though various fanciful suggestions regarding them have been expressed since. Ruysch (1700) modified this general glandular conception to that of a cerebrospinal fluid-forming gland. Purkinje (1836) noted the epithelial character of their lining cells, but did not draw any conclusions concerning their function. Special attention was attracted to the secretory nature of this epithelium by Faivre (1854) and Luschka (1855).

Even at the present day there is no agreement of opinion as to the manner of production of cerebrospinal fluid.

One group favors the view that cerebrospinal fluid, like other body fluids, is produced by simple filtration through an animal membrane and that their differences depend on osmotic pressure between the capillaries and the serous spaces. This view is supported by Leonard Hill, Starling and Mestrezat. Another group, influenced by Heidenhain, chiefly, explains the formation of fluids on the basis of a cellular activity, or an active rather than a passive formation. In favor of this view are Galeotti, Cappelletti, Cavazzani, Studnicka, Goldmann, Schläpfer, Kingsbury, Mott and others.

1. The Manner of Formation, Based on the Composition of Cerebrospinal Fluid

Schmidt (1850) was the first to demonstrate differences between the composition of the cerebrospinal fluid and other serous fluids and between the blood-plasma and the cerebrospinal fluid. On this basis he suggested a secretory process of formation for cerebrospinal fluid. That which principally differentiates this fluid from other body fluids is its very low solid content and consequently its low protein content. The total solids are about one-seventh or one-eighth and the protein content about one three-hundredths of the blood-plasma content. This difference is most marked between the cerebrospinal fluid and the blood-plasma, but also obtains between the cerebrospinal fluid and the pericardial, peritoneal and other serous fluids. The specific gravity of the cerebrospinal fluid is 1.003, as compared to 1.028 for the blood-plasma. It is difficult, indeed, to understand how differences of osmotic pressure alone, acting on a common fluid medium and through the same vascular endothelium, could produce such differences as exist in the chemical composition of the various fluids.

As further evidence of the secretory theory of formation, it has been pointed out that the composition of cerebrospinal fluid resembles saliva more closely than it does the other serous fluids; while the salt content of saliva is somewhat higher, the water, total solids, protein content and specific gravity in cerebrospinal fluid are very similar. For some time a reducing body—pyrocatechin of Halliburton—was regarded as specific for cerebrospinal fluid. Halliburton has since shown this reducing substance to be glucose. Nawratzki confirmed the presence of sugar and estimated that it was present in about the same amount as in the blood. Cavazzani noted a minimum alkalinity of the cerebrospinal fluid as contrasted to the blood. He also declared that he had found a diastatic ferment, but Panzer and Lewandowsky were not able to confirm this finding. Kafka noted a lipolytic ferment. Other differences of a specific character have been reported, but most have been disputed, so that they are not now available as evidence of secretory activity.

Against the secretory theory of formation of cerebrospinal fluid is the mineral content of cerebrospinal fluid. Halliburton, Schmidt and Nawratzki determined that it was essentially the same as that of the parent blood-plasma and the other serous fluids. Simple filtration would seem to explain best this similarity of salt content.

2. The Manner of Formation Based on the Anatomy and Histology of the Choroid Plexus

The choroid plexuses are unique specialized structures, placed in every ventricle. That they are endowed with an exceptional blood-supply and covered by cells of a special character would seem to indicate that they are structures with a special function.

The elaborate blood-supply might well appear to indicate a filter-bed, while the specialized epithelium would indicate a gland. It would seem that there could be little doubt, from an anatomical point of view alone, that by one or both of these methods cerebrospinal fluid is supplied to the ventricles from the choroid plexuses. As noted above, Faivre and Luschka first emphasized the character of the epithelium and from analogy insisted on its secretory character. Their views have since been strengthened by the histological observations of Petit and Girard, Meek, Galeotti, Schläpfer, Goldmann, Immamura, Voshimura, Hworostuchin, Francini and others. The choroidal epithelial cells are large, cubical and often columnar, with a granular cytoplasm and basal nuclei. The cells are similar in appearance to gland cells, and such a histological picture is hardly conceivable without a secretory activity.

In addition to the general glandular appearance, granules, presumably of a secretory character, have been observed, both post-mortem and by intra-vitam staining methods. Galeotti (1897) first noted basophil and acidophil granules. These findings were substantiated by Bibergeil and Levaditi, Francini, Schläpfer and Goldmann, principally by the use of intra-vitam staining methods. Hworostuchin observed mitochondria, which he thought indicated the secretory activity of the plexuses. In addition, he noted the presence of nerves in the choroid plexus.

3. The Manner of Formation Based on the Action of Drugs on the Rate of Production of Cerebrospinal Fluid

It has been suggested that cerebrospinal fluid is formed by the secretory activity of the epithelium of the choroid plexus, because after the administration of drugs which stimulate glandular secretion there is supposed to be an increased production of cerebrospinal fluid and the cells show a histological change similar to the discharged appearance of the cells of the salivary glands. Petit and Girard, and Meek observed a swollen appearance of the choroid epithelium, a peripheral cytoplasmic clear zone and often cellular rupture following the administration of pilocarpin; Cappelletti, Cavazzani and Petit and Girard obtained after the injection of pilocarpin an increased flow of cerebrospinal fluid from a subarachnoid fistula and compared this with the effect on the salivary glands. They also noted an increase following ether, amyl nitrite and a diminished flow following atropin and hyoscyamin. Sicard was unable to confirm this. Dixon and Halliburton recently considered this subject in detail. They found only a slight increase of cerebrospinal fluid following injection of pilocarpin, atropin, amyl nitrite and various salts; and a definite increase following ether, chloral hydrate, chloroform, choroid plexus extract and brain extract.

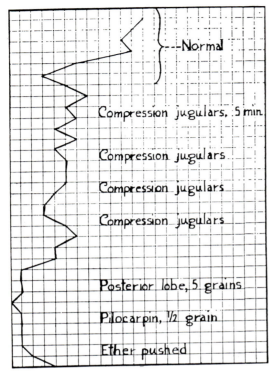

Fig. 6.—Curves representing actual flow of cerebro-spinal fluid from subarachnoid fistula, as influenced by drugs and mechanical factors. The base line represents time, each division being a five-minute interval. The vertical line represents the actual number of drops in each five-minute interval. The drugs used are entered during the progress of the curves.

FIGURE 6 A.

In order that conclusions of value may be drawn from experiments of this nature, several precautions are necessary. The anesthetic must be constant and the animal must be sufficiently anesthetized to insure perfect quiet throughout the experiment. Vapor anesthetics cause great variations in the rate of flow of the fluid, and change of respiration produces similar results. To minimize these influences we used chlorbutanol, administered by stomach-tube; with this drug a very even anesthesia was secured. Rather than insert a cannula at random into the subarachnoid space, we exposed and trephined the atlas, and opened the dura by a stellate incision. Into the trephine opening in the atlas a special fitting cannula was inserted. The animal was then placed in a sling in such a manner that the cannula was at the most dependent part, and the fluid from both the head and the spinal canal ran into this as into a funnel. By this technic, bloody fluid was not obtained, and fluid did not accumulate as occurs when a needle is inserted through the dura. Clogging of the cannula does not occur and the experiments may be continued for several hours. To insure a steady outflow of cerebrospinal fluid we waited from fifteen to twenty minutes, or until the accumulated fluid had escaped. Drops were counted over arbitrary periods of five minutes. The results of these observations are represented in the accompanying charts (Fig. 6).

The most striking and uniform result obtained in these experiments followed the temporary compression of the jugular veins. Except in one instance there was always a marked and instantaneous increase of cerebrospinal fluid following jugular compression. We believe this can be explained only by an increased production of fluid. It is conceivable that it might be due to displacement of fluid by the cerebral congestion. If this were so, a retarded flow would be expected after the restoration of the equilibrium in the blood-vessels, but in each instance the previous level of fluid escape was reestablished. Moreover, the same results were obtained following jugular compressions frequently repeated at short intervals. When pressure on the jugular veins was maintained for a longer period of time, the increased flow did not continue, but gradually returned to normal. This was due, no doubt, to rapid establishment of collateral venous circulation.

Since general cerebral venous stasis (jugular compression) results in increased cerebrospinal fluid formation, the place of formation of this fluid is probably from the vessels on the surface of the brain as well as in the ventricles. Owing to the efficient collateral on the surface of the brain, the formation of the fluid there is but transient, whereas in obstruction to the vein of Galen (low ligation and poor collateral) the increased production in the ventricles is continuous.

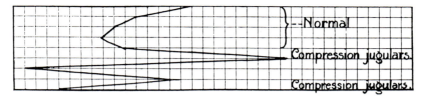

Figure 6 B.

In a number of experiments ether caused an increased production of fluid. It is probable that this increase is also due to venous stasis. The effect is not continuous, but occurs regularly with each application of ether. Amyl nitrite caused no such increase of fluid. The effect of pilocarpin on the increase of fluid production is slight, but always positive. When compared to the secretion which results from the stimulation of the salivary glands, however, it is practically negligible. An animal when given pilocarpin will drown in its own salivary secretion, but the cerebrospinal fluid outflow increases only a few drops. We hesitate to make any positive deductions of glandular activity on such small though fairly constant results. Though no mechanical factors which might cause congestion and thereby filtration were noted during these experiments, this possibility must be borne in mind.

Repeated intravenous injections of freshly prepared aqueous extracts of choroid plexus and of posterior lobe of the pituitary body of the ox or sheep failed to produce an increased rate of flow of cerebrospinal fluid. This is contrary to the results of Dixon and Halliburton. They obtained a definite increase after the injection of extract of choroid plexus.

Following the experiments with pilocarpin the choroid plexuses were removed for microscopic examination. We were unable to find definite histological alteration in the structure of the gland. Frequently, ruptured cells were observed, but these are often seen in the normal choroid plexus. From a purely

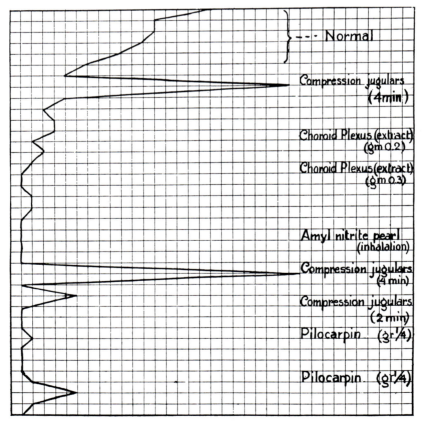

Figure 6 C.

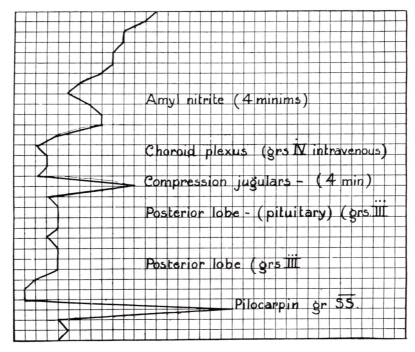

Figure 6 D.

objective point of view, it was impossible to tell from the choroid plexus whether or not a previous injection of pilocarpin had been made.

4. The Manner of Formation Based on the Impermeability of the Choroid Plexus

One of the strongest arguments in favor of the secretory theory of cerebrospinal fluid formation is the difficulty with which foreign substances pass from the blood to the cerebrospinal fluid. Were it entirely a simple mechanical process of filtration, it is difficult to understand why simple substances should not readily pass through into the cerebrospinal fluid. It has been observed frequently that when very large doses of potassium iodid are administered, none passes into the cerebrospinal fluid. It has also been noted that in obstructive jaundice, bile pigments cannot be demonstrated in the cerebrospinal fluid. It is evident that a mechanism which can prevent the passage of certain substances into the cerebrospinal fluid must play a very important rôle in the prevention of the hematogenous transmission of infections

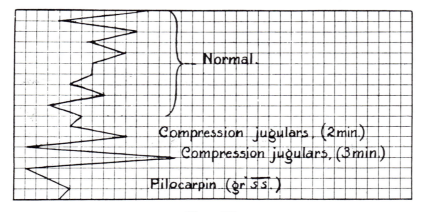

Figure 6 E.

to the central nervous system, and, for the same reason, when affections of the central nervous system exist, they are correspondingly refractory to remedies conveyed by the blood.

Such an impermeability to the cerebrospinal fluid has been shown to exist for numerous substances. Sicard was unable to obtain methylene-blue or potassium iodid in the cerebrospinal fluid when large doses were given subcutaneously, intravenously or by mouth. Rotky was unable to detect iodids, bromids, salicylates, mercury or bile pigments. These observations have been extended to include serological investigations. Widal and Sicard could not demonstrate agglutinins or immune bodies in the cerebrospinal fluid in typhoid fever. The behavior of the Wassermann reaction in the cerebrospinal fluid of hereditary syphilis without involvement of the central nervous system gives further evidence of the impermeability of the choroid plexus to foreign substances. In the majority of patients[1] whom we examined, the reaction was positive in the blood, but in no instance was there a positive reaction in the cerebrospinal fluid.

This impermeability, however, is not absolute; traces of many substances have been found in the cerebrospinal fluid. In certain diseases affecting the central nervous system there is a permeability. Sicard, Rotky, Capka and Mott showed this in meningitis, diabetes and uremia. Achard and Ribot observed traces of potassium iodid, Lewin and Bernard traces of salicylates, and Sicard traces of mer-

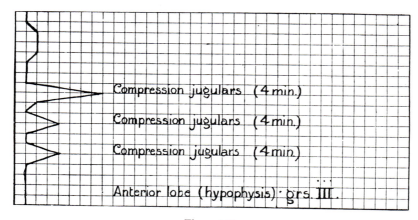

Figure 6 F.

cury in chronic mercurial poisoning, Olmer and Tian, Castaigne and others noted bile pigments in jaundice. Crowe noted hexamethylenamin, Rotky uranin and Lewandowsky strychnin. Zaloziecki observed immune bodies and agglutinins in typhoid fever, and thought that their quantity was dependent on the albumin content of the cerebrospinal fluid and the high concentration of immune bodies in the blood. We determined the presence or absence in the cerebrospinal fluid, of various substances after ingestion, and intravenous and subcutaneous administration. These observations were made on animals and in patients from the hospital wards. The results are given in Table 1.

These results confirm those of many previous investigators. Of the various substances used, only hexamethylenamin and sodium salicylate were detected in the cerebrospinal fluid. The test for these substances is very delicate, and this may explain their detection in the cerebrospinal fluid. It is worthy of note that in dogs sodium salicylate and hexamethylenamin were obtained, in traces, in the vitreous humor. In several of the animal tests the aqueous humor was examined and the findings were almost identical with those of the cerebrospinal fluid.

It is striking that in spite of the actual flooding of the blood with colored solutions, such as phenolsulphonephthalein, indigocarmin, trypan blue and bile pigments, not even traces are present in the cerebrospinal fluid. In our experiments the animals were deeply colored following intra-vitam staining with trypan blue, and even the choroid plexuses were deeply stained, but the cerebrospinal fluid remained colorless—an observation frequently made by Goldmann. Indigocarmin *was found in both the peritoneal and the pericardial fluids,* but *not* in the cerebrospinal fluid or in the aqueous humor.

From these observations it would appear certain that the passage of substances into the normal cerebrospinal fluid is very difficult, and that when it occurs they appear only in faint traces. It is also apparent that there is greater difficulty in the passage of substances into the cerebrospinal fluid than into the

1. These were patients from the Pediatric Clinic and the observations have not been published.

TABLE 1.—EXPERIMENTS TO DETERMINE THE PRESENCE OR ABSENCE OF VARIOUS
SUBSTANCES IN THE CEREBROSPINAL FLUID AFTER ORAL, INTRAVENOUS AND
SUBCUTANEOUS ADMINISTRATION

I. ANIMAL TESTS

Substance used	Amount	How given	Time of test after administration	Test in C.S.F.*	Other fluids
Methylene blue	30 c.c.	Intravenous	45 min.	−	Aqueous humor negative.
Indigocarmin	60 c.c.	Intravenous	30 min.	−	Peritoneal and pericardial positive; aqueous humor negative.
Phenolsulphonephthalein	100 mg.	Subcutaneous	90 min.	−	Pericardial and aqueous humor negative.
Potassium iodid	30 gr.	Subcutaneous	60 min.	−	
Potassium iodid	60 gr.	Mouth	4 hrs.	−	None in aqueous humor.
Potassium iodid	50 gr.	Intravenous	30 min.	−	Pericardial fluid negative.
Strychnin	$\frac{1}{4}$ gr.	Subcutaneous	15 min.		
Morphin	$\frac{1}{2}$ gr.	Subcutaneous	30 min.		
Trypan blue	1 gm.	Intravenous	60 min.	−	
Hexamethylamin	45 gr.	Mouth	60 min.	+	Pericardial pleural fluids and aqueous humor positive.

II. CLINICAL TESTS

Substance used	Amount	How given	Time of test after administration	Test in C.S.F.*	Other fluids
Hexamethylamin	10 gr.	Mouth	2 hrs.	+	
Bile pigments	Obstruction 2 months	—	2 mos.	−	
Bile pigments	Catarrhal jaundice 3 weeks	—	3 wks.	−	
Bile pigments	Obstruction 3 weeks	—	3 wks.	+	
Sodium salicylate	30 gr.	Mouth	60 min.	+	
Potassium iodid	40 gr.	Mouth	40 min.	−	

* In this column +means positive and −negative.

other serous fluids. It seems difficult to attribute this fact to mechanical inhibition alone, but rather to a selective or discriminating cellular activity.[2]

IV. SUMMARY OF THE FORMATION OF CEREBROSPINAL FLUID

It can be definitely stated that cerebrospinal fluid forms in the ventricles. From evidence partly direct, but more largely indirect, there can be but little doubt that the choroid plexuses (possibly including the ependyma) produce this fluid. Whether this formation is alone by secretory or mechanical means or by both is impossible to say absolutely from the evidence at hand. Certainly fluid is readily and rapidly formed by the induction of venous stasis, and when the collateral circulation is insufficient (as the small veins of Galen and the beginning of the large vein of Galen), the increased production may be continuous and hydrocephalus result. How far the normal differences of intravascular pressure cause transudation or production of cerebrospinal fluid cannot, however, be inferred by the production of artificial pressures. The similarity of the saline content of the blood and cerebrospinal fluid would seem to be undoubted evidence that filtration must be partially responsible for this fluid production.

2. Ducrot makes an interesting observation which, if substantiated, is indicative of therapeutic possibilities. He asserts that injections of methyl violet are followed by the appearance of the contents of the blood-plasma in the cerebrospinal fluid and in the proportions found in the blood. In jaundice, bile also readily passes into the cerebrospinal fluid following methyl violet injection. His explanation is that methyl violet paralyzes the secretory choroidal epithelium and the result is a temporarily inactive membrane. Filtration is then inhibited. This he also uses as proof of the secretory formation of cerebrospinal fluid. After several hours the effects of this drug wear away and the normal action of the choroid plexus is again restored.

On the other hand, the histological character of the choroid plexus epithelium, the radical difference in the chemical composition of the cerebrospinal fluid in comparison to the blood and other serous fluids and the protection of the cerebrospinal fluid from substances in the blood (impermeability) necessitate the assumption of a cellular or secretory activity. It therefore seems most probable that cerebrospinal fluid is formed both by filtration and by secretion.

5. ABSORPTION OF CEREBROSPINAL FLUID

The maintenance of a proper amount of cerebrospinal fluid in the ventricles and the subarachnoid space requires that there shall be an absorption equal to the formation. The first proof of an active circulation of cerebrospinal fluid was obtained by the experiments of Magendie. He demonstrated, after draining the subarachnoid space of as much fluid as possible, that there was such an active reformation that an equal amount of fluid could be again obtained on the following day or even sooner. He also demonstrated an active absorption of colored solutions when they were injected into the subarachnoid space and noted their presence in the jugular veins and in the urine.

Long before this absolute evidence, an active discharge of the ventricular content, whether fluid, vapor or animal spirits, had been presumed. As previously mentioned, Galen believed that the discharge of the material resulting from the purification of his animal spirits took place through the infundibulum and cribriform plate into the nose, where it was recognized as "pituita." Though Galen's theories of the animal spirits were attacked by Vesalius (1543) and later overthrown, his view that the infundibulum was the portal of exit for the ventricular content was accepted by many even until the time of Magendie (1825).

I. HISTORY

Lymphatics in the dura were described by Mascagni about 1775. Meckel (1777) supported this observation and referred to them as "vasa resortentia lymphatica." Arnold (1838) asserted the presence of lymphatics in the pia-arachnoid membranes and ascribed absorption of the cerebrospinal fluid to them. His (1850) and von Recklinghausen (1863) agreed with this observation and also noted the presence of perivascular lymphatics.

Böhm (1869) asserted the existence of a unique, independent system of valveless lymphatics which directly connected the subarachnoid space with the pial vessels, forming in reality an accessory system to the blood-vessels. He maintained that there were large stomata which allowed free access to these vessels from the subarachnoid space. During congestion these vessels filled with blood, but despite the unguarded openings the blood did not pass into the cerebrospinal fluid. Milk and granular substances injected into the subarachnoid space, however, passed readily over into the veins through these stomata and the intermediary system of lymphatics. These stomata, demonstrable by silver nitrate staining, were similar to the diaphragmatic stomata, advocated only a short time before by von Recklinghausen.

Key and Retzius (1875) attributed the absorption of cerebrospinal fluid to the pacchionian granulations. During the injection of colored solutions under pressure into the subarachnoid space, they were able to observe such solutions passing through the pacchionian bodies into the longitudinal sinus.

II. METHODS OF TECHNIC

Though many investigations have been conducted to determine the method of exit of the cerebrospinal fluid, the results have been variable and inconclusive. They have been inconclusive chiefly because the experimenters have used artificial pressures, or the injections have been made post mortem. In all experiments here submitted the conditions have been as near normal as possible; no pressure was used, and the animals were alive (ether anesthesia). The results of the experiments represent as nearly as can be determined the natural processes of absorption.

The principal method used in solving this problem was by substituting inert colored fluids for an equal amount of cerebrospinal fluid and then determining the quantitative output of these substances in the urine. The substance must necessarily be one that is readily absorbed and quickly eliminated by the kidney.

We tried indigocarmin, methylene-blue and phenolsulphonephthalein. Methylene-blue and indigocarmin were of little value in these experiments, so almost sole reliance was placed on phenolsulphonephthalein. Methylene-blue was but slowly excreted and appeared in the urine as a leuko-body, which rendered its quantitative estimation uncertain. Indigocarmin appeared more rapidly in the urine, but its color was affected by urinary pigments to such an extent that even an approximate quantitative value could not be estimated. Phenolsulphonephthalein met all requirements. The question of the excretion of phenolsulphonephthalein by the kidney has been investigated thoroughly by Rowntree and Geraghty, who introduced it as a test of the renal function. By virtue of its stability, its inert character, its rapid, uniform and almost complete elimination by the kidney, its easy and accurate quantitative estimation, phenolsulphonephthalein is well adapted for this study. It has been used recently by Dandy and Rowntree in the estimation of absorption of fluids from the pleural and peritoneal cavities.

On account of the difficulty and uncertainty of performing lumbar punctures on dogs, owing to the great length of the cord, we obtained the cerebrospinal fluid from the cisterna magna. After exposing the occipito-atlantal membrane it was possible to puncture the transparent arachnoid membrane and siphon off the desired amount of fluid. The fluid was replaced by an equal amount of phenolsulphonephthalein solution at body temperature. One c.c. (6 mg.) of phenolsulphonephthalein was chosen as the amount for injection in these experiments. In each instance the time of the appearance of the substance in the urine and the quantitative output in the urine over periods of one and two hours were determined. The quantity excreted in the urine was determined by colorimetric readings in Rowntree and Geraghty's modification of the Autenrieth-Königsberger colorimeter.

It should be emphasized that these percentages should not be taken as absolute, for the total amount of phenolsulphonephthalein injected cannot be recovered in the urine. In the peritoneal and pleural cavities one can recover from 80 to 90 per cent, but, for some reason which is not evident, only 60 to 90 per cent can be recovered after injection into the subarachnoid space. The results are sufficiently accurate for all practical purposes. The accompanying figures represent the percentage recovered of the amount injected.

TABLE 2.—Phenolsulphonephthalein Excretion in Experiment 2.

Hours After Injection	Time	Output of Phenolsulphonephthalein Per Cent
1	11:07 a.m.	16.6
2	12:07 a.m.	17.8
3	1:07 p.m.	13.6
4	2:07 p.m.	7.2
5	3:07 p.m.	4.5
6	4:07 p.m.	2.2
7	5:07 p.m.	1.3
8	6:07 p.m.	.3
9	7:07 p.m.	+
	Total amount excreted in 9 hours	63.5

III. THE RATE OF ABSORPTION OF CEREBROSPINAL FLUID IN DOGS

The following experiment is characteristic of the series:

EXPERIMENT 2.—May 26, 1911. Female dog, weight, 14½ pounds. One c.c. (or 6 mg.) of phenolsulphonephthalein substituted for 1 c.c. of cerebrospinal fluid (ether anesthesia). Time of injection, 10:02 a. m. Time of first appearance in urine, 10:07 a. m., five minutes. The hourly output is given in Table 2.

Five days later another injection on the same animal gave identical results.

We can conclude that there is an active circulation of cerebrospinal fluid. For a period of from three to four hours the absorption is fairly regular and after this time progressively diminishes. This diminution is in all probablity due to the dilution by the fluid which is being constantly formed. It may be said that the cerebrospinal fluid is completely absorbed and renewed at least every four or six hours, or at least from four to six times every twenty-four hours. Experiments in which methylene-blue and indigo-carmin were used were similar in time of appearance and disappearance, though a quantitative value could not be obtained.

The quantitative results of absorption from the human subarachnoid space are similar to these results in animals.

IV. DOES ABSORPTION OF CEREBROSPINAL FLUID TAKE PLACE INTO THE BLOOD OR INTO THE LYMPH?

There are two ways by which absorption of cerebrospinal fluid could occur—the blood and the lymph. Mott, who is the strongest exponent of the theory of lymphatic absorption, thinks perivascular lymphatics perform this function. The prevalent view, however, is that, with the possible exception of lymphatic connections along the olfactory and optic nerves, the central nervous system, including the meninges, is destitute of lymphatics. The present conception of the lymphatic system is that it is everywhere closed by endothelial cells, and that all its branches converge either to the thoracic or to the right lymphatic duct. Except for the work of Key and Retzius, who believe that the filling of the lymphatics occurs along the nerve sheaths, we know of no evidence of lymphatic absorption. Their experimental injections, however, were made under high pressure and were performed post mortem. Evidence of this character is open to the most severe criticism. Normally the cerebrospinal fluid does not pass along the sheaths of the nerves with exception of the olfactory and optic nerves.

Hill showed that when a colored solution was injected into the subarachnoid space it appeared in the urine in from ten to twenty minutes, but that the cervical lymph-glands were only slightly tinged after one or two hours. He concluded that absorption was directly into the blood.

We performed a series of experiments to determine the manner of absorption of cerebrospinal fluid. A cannula was placed in the thoracic duct and phenolsulphonephthalein was substituted for cerebrospinal fluid. The total lymph was collected, and the output of phenolsulphonephthalein in the urine was estimated.

EXPERIMENT 3.—April 18, 1911. Thoracic duct fistula. Ether anesthesia. The substitution of 1 c.c. (6 mg.) phenolsulphonephthalein for 1 c.c. cerebrospinal fluid (through the occipito-atlantal membrane). Catheterization of bladder.

Time of injection, 12:03 p. m.; first appearance in urine, 12:09—six minutes; first appearance in lymph, 1:45—one hour, thirty-six minutes.

Excretion of phenolsulphonephthalein in urine: First hour, 1:09 p. m.—9.5 per cent; second hour, 2:09—12.2 per cent.

TABLE 3.—Results in Experiment 4

Time	Blood Examination	Lymph Examination
3:32 p.m.	0	0
3:33 p.m.	+	0
3:36 p.m.	+	0
3:58 p.m.	+	0
4:15 p.m.	+	0
Animal killed with ether.		

From this experiment it is evident that the cerebrospinal fluid is excreted in the urine long before it appears in the lymph, and that in two hours over 21 per cent (even with an anesthetic) is excreted in the urine, while only a bare trace is present in the lymph. Presumably absorption took place directly into the blood. Proof of this is supplied by experiments, of which the following is an example:

EXPERIMENT 4.—April 30, 1913. Thoracic duct fistula. Chlorbutanol anesthesia. *Specimens of blood* taken from the carotid artery. Substitution 1 c.c. (30 mg.) phenolsulphonephthalein for 1 c.c. cerebrospinal fluid, through the occipito-atlantal membrane.

Time of injection, 3:30 p. m. The results are given in Table 3.

Absorption took place directly into the blood and was very rapid. The dye was detected in specimens of arterial blood in three minutes, whereas there was no trace in the lymph after forty-five minutes. In one experiment of a similar nature a trace was found in the lymph in eighteen minutes after injection. In no case was there more than a trace even at the end of two hours—a striking contrast to the content in the blood and urine. The trace of color in the lymph appearing after a considerable interval might readily be derived from the blood.

It may be objected that absorption had taken place through the tributaries of the right lymphatic duct. For this reason the following experiment was performed:

EXPERIMENT 5.—May 10, 1911. Ether anesthesia. Thoracic duct fistula; dorsal laminectomy, the spinal cord and dura ligated at level of fifth dorsal vertebra. As a further precaution a second ligation was made 2 cm. above the first. Injection of 1 c.c. (30 mg.) phenolsulphonephthalein into the subarachnoid space of the segment distal to both ligations. Time of injection, 2:06 p. m.

Blood examination 2:12 p. m., +; 2:20 p. m., +.
Lymph examination, 2:12 p. m., 0; 2:20 p. m., 0.
Animal killed with anesthetic.

It is therefore evident from these experiments that the lymphatics play no part in the absorption of the cerebrospinal fluid, but that absorption takes place directly into the blood.

V. ABSORPTION IS A DIFFUSE PROCESS INVOLVING THE ENTIRE SUBARACHNOID SPACE

The preceding experiment shows that absorption takes place also from the spinal subarachnoid space. When phenolsulphonephthalein is injected into the cisterna magna it is, as will be shown subsequently, distributed to all parts of the cerebral and spinal subarachnoid space in a very short time. It is believed by some that absorption is limited to the superior longitudinal and the other venous sinuses, and that the remaining cerebral and spinal vessels take no part in this absorption. In order to determine the part of the spinal subarachnoid space in the absorption of cerebrospinal fluid, experiments like the following were done:

EXPERIMENT 6.—June 2, 1911. Dorsal laminectomy; chlorbutanol anesthesia; ligation of dura and cord at the level of the fourth thoracic vertebra. A second ligature was placed 2.5 cm. above the first, to prevent absolutely the direct transmission of fluid from the lower segment into the cranial subarachnoid space. Fluid withdrawn from distal spinal segment and substitution of 1 c.c. (12 mg.) phenolsulphonephthalein. Animal killed with anesthesia.

Time of injection, 12:47 p. m.; time of appearance in urine, 12:53 p. m.—six minutes; 18.2 per cent was excreted the first hour and 10.4 per cent the second hour.

EXPERIMENT 7.—Similar to Experiment 6. June 8, 1911.

Time of injection, 2:32 p. m.; time of appearance in urine, 2:38 p. m.—six minutes; 15.1 per cent was excreted the first hour and 13.2 per cent the second hour.

Animal killed with anesthesia.

It will be seen that there is a very high absorption from the spinal subarachnoid space; in fact, the amount of phenolsulphonephthalein excreted is nearly as much as from the entire subarachnoid space. There is, however, with such experiments an increase in pressure which cannot be prevented. The spinal subarachnoid space in the dog contains comparatively little fluid, so closely do the arachnoid and dura envelop the spinal cord. For this reason it is impossible accurately to substitute the amount of fluid which is withdrawn. The injection is consequently under tension, which must alter the rate of absorption and probably accounts for the rapid excretion. This permits the deduction that an active and rapid absorption takes place from the spinal subarachnoid space. Absorption is, therefore, a diffuse process. It takes place from the entire subarachnoid space and is not restricted to any particular portion of this space. Our results, therefore, show that the absorption of cerebrospinal fluid is directly into the capillary network of the entire subarachnoid space.

VI. THE EVIDENCE AGAINST THE ABSORPTION BY MEANS OF STOMATA

The principal exponents of the theory of stomata as a means for the absorption of cerebrospinal fluid are Böhm, Adamkiewicz, Reiner and Schnitzler. The strongest argument in favor of stomata is that granules have been observed to pass from the subarachnoid space into the veins. This can readily be shown in embryos, and with much greater difficulty in adults; but as mentioned above, and as shown by Mall, this is entirely dependent on pressure and the consequent tearing or rupturing of delicate tissues.

Stomata in the subarachnoid space were originally suggested by Böhm (1869), but his observations lack confirmation. Stomata in lymphatics of the central tendon of the diaphragm, as described by von Recklinghausen, have been proved to be artefacts. That there are stomata in blood-vessels is even more difficult to believe. If there were stomata in the blood-vessels in the subarachnoid space one would expect to find bloody cerebrospinal fluid as the result of venous congestion. The absence of blood cannot be explained by valves, as these have never been demonstrated.

In our experiments, India ink and lampblack *granules in suspension were substituted for an equal amount of cerebrospinal* fluid, and the animals used were kept under anesthesia for varying periods of time. Even after two or three hours there was no evident egress of granules. Specimens of blood from superior longitudinal sinus were examined microscopically at frequent intervals for granules, but with uniformly negative results. At the end of one, two or three hours there was a perfectly uniform distribution of granules throughout the entire cerebral and spinal subarachnoid space. There was no evidence of an accumulation in any particular locality. A number of the animals were frozen, and subsequently placed in formaldehyde solution; the sinuses were later opened, examined by sections and the blood in the sinuses also examined. Granules were present in the pacchionian granulations and along the walls of the longitudinal and other sinuses, but there was no suggestion of any passage into the lumen of the sinus. In each case the granules were separated by the arachnoid membrane and a layer of dura.

The blood in the sinuses was also free from granules. That granules of this size never pass out of the subarachnoid space is not maintained. In all probability there is an elimination by some vital activity, but evidently not by a free transit through preformed openings.

Further evidence of the absence of stomata is offered by a number of experiments in which pressure was used. If granules are injected into the subarachnoid space of adult dogs under a pressure of 100 mm. of mercury or less there is no passage of the granules into the venous sinuses. These high pressures kill the animal. The longitudinal and lateral sinuses can then be exposed for their entire distance, but even after the lapse of an hour or even longer granules are not found in the sinuses. The pacchionian granulations are full of granules, but there is no passage through their walls. It is evident, therefore, that with the animals' own processes of absorption during life and even with highly artificial pressures after death, no evidence can be obtained of a passage of granules, by way of stomata, either into the sinuses or into any other part of the vascular system.

It has been shown in the foregoing experiments that absorption is by a general or diffuse process involving the capillaries in the entire subarachnoid space. Since the absorption from the spinal subarachnoid is *at least proportionally as great* as from the entire subarachnoid space, it is not necessary to attempt to explain the absorption of cerebrospinal fluid by means of stomata along the cerebral venous sinuses.

VII. THE EVIDENCE AGAINST THE ABSORPTION OF CEREBROSPINAL FLUID BY THE PACCHIONIAN GRANULATIONS

The theory that the pacchionian granulations play a part in the absorption of cerebrospinal fluid is due to the work of Key and Retzius. This view has received much support. The pacchionian granulations are really arachnoid diverticula which project into the lumen of the sinuses and into the bones of the vault of the skull. They are lined by a layer of arachnoid with a superimposed layer of dura, which is a far greater mechanical impediment to the passage of fluid than the simple endothelium lining of the capillaries in the pia arachnoid. The pacchionian granulations, moreover, are not present at birth or are developed so poorly as to escape notice. They increase in size and number with age and with intracranial pressure. It is asserted that in many animals they are absent.

Any evidence of the passage of fluid through the pacchionian granulations during life would be very difficult, if not impossible to obtain. Consequently, all proof is dependent on post-mortem injections. In such a condition it is possible to force fluid through the pacchionian granulations into the sinuses with very high pressure. Under a still higher pressure it is even possible to force water from the subarachnoid space into the nasal cavity.

The best evidence against the absorption of cerebrospinal fluid through the pacchionian granulations is the general character of the absorption from the subarachnoid space.

VIII. COMPARISON OF ABSORPTION OF CEREBROSPINAL, PERITONEAL AND PLEURAL FLUIDS

The absorption of fluids from the peritoneal and pleural cavities has been studied by Dandy and Rowntree. They showed that absorption of fluids from these spaces was a diffuse process, and was not dependent on the posture assumed. It was also demonstrated that absorption was directly into the blood and that lymphatics played no part. The absorption from these cavities is much more rapid than from the subarachnoid space. A comparison between the absorption of fluid from the pleural and peritoneal cavities with that from the subarachnoid space is shown in the accompanying chart. The time of first appearance of phenolsulphonephthalein in the urine was practically the same in all. The output from the pleural and the peritoneal cavities was more rapid than that from the subarachnoid space (Fig. 7).

IX. ABSORPTION FROM THE VENTRICLES

In order to complete the discussion of the absorption of cerebrospinal fluid it is necessary to consider briefly here some of the clinical observations, the details of which are given in a subsequent part of this article. In seven cases of hydrocephalus the communication between the ventricles and the subarachnoid space was found to be totally obstructed. An excellent opportunity to estimate absorption from the ventricles was thus allowed. When phenolsulphonephthalein was introduced into the ventricles of these patients its first appearance in the urine was greatly delayed (thirty or forty minutes or longer) and never was there an elimination of more than 1 per cent during the two hours following the first appearance in the urine. This was irrespective of the dilatation of the ventricles or the quality of fluid present.[3]

The excretion of phenolsulphonephthalein after such an injection continued ten days and even longer. The dye was present in the ventricles also for the same length of time. It is evident, therefore, that practically *no absorption takes place from the ventricles.*

6. COMMUNICATION BETWEEN THE VENTRICLES AND THE SUBARACHNOID SPACE

The preceding experiments show that fluid forms in the ventricles and that it is absorbed from the entire subarachnoid space. It is evident that the normal balance between the production and the absorption of cerebrospinal fluid depends on an adequate communication between the place of formation and the place of absorption, namely, between the ventricles and the subarachnoid space.

Six foramina of communication between the ventricles and the subarachnoid space have been de-

---

3. That tension of the intraventricular fluid has no effect on the absorption from the ventricles is shown by the fact that before and after the removal of 90 c.c. of ventricular fluid in Case 4, N. M., Group 1, the absorption was exactly the same (0.25 per cent in two hours).

scribed. The foramen or canal of Bichat was first described (1819) as a median opening accompanying the vena Galena magna and affording communication between the third ventricle and the subarachnoid space. Soon afterward, Bichat added a foramen at the tip of each lateral ventricle—the lateral foramina of Bichat. Magendie, Luschka, and Key and Retzius proved these three foramina to be artefacts, as they were evident only after pressure was used. Mierzejewsky and Merkel (1872) again asserted the existence of a foramen from the tip of each lateral ventricle. Though regarded by most anatomists as artefacts, they are still believed by many to exist.

Though a communicating foramen at the fourth ventricle was suspected by Cotugno and others, its existence was first demonstrated by Magendie in 1825. Renault (1829) proved that no such foramen existed in the horse and that hydrocephalus in this animal did not result from its absence. Magendie confirmed the findings of Renault, though he continued to maintain the importance of this foramen in man. Krause (1843) maintained that all the ventricles, including the fourth, were sealed by pia, and that the foramen of Magendie was an artefact produced either by pressure or by dissection. Todd

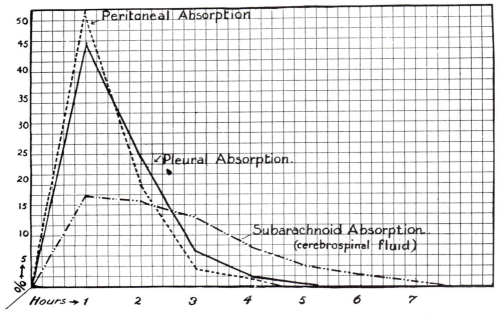

Fig. 7.—Curves to compare the total excretion of peritoneal, pleural and cerebrospinal fluids. The base line represents time divided into one-hour intervals. The vertical line represents absorption (percentage of excretion) of phenolsulphonephthalein in the urine.

(1847) and Reichert (1861) expressed similar views. Virchow (1854) strongly opposed the theory of the existence of the foramina and of any communication between the ventricles and the subarachnoid space or between the cerebral and the spinal subarachnoid spaces. "There is no direct communication between the subarachnoid spaces, either between each other or with the cavities of the brain, and the fluid contained in them cannot thus simply rise or fall."[4] The weight of his teachings was sufficient to retard greatly the acceptance of Magendie's views.

The existence of the foramen of Magendie was, however, supported by capable anatomists. Luschka (1854) verified the absence of this foramen in the horse and thought that the absence of hydrocephalus was explained by the lateral foramina which he described. These foramina are present in all animals and are larger in those in which there is no central foramen. He unquestionably substantiated the existence of the central foramen and named it in honor of Magendie. Key and Retzius (1875) confirmed the findings of Magendie and Luschka in every particular.

Retzius in 1896 examined one hundred brains and found the foramen of Magendie absent in two and the foramina of Luschka absent in three. This was confirmed by Hess and Cruveilhier. Cannieu (1898), however, after numerous injections and histological studies, concluded that the evidence in favor of

4. "Die subarachnoidealen Räume stehen in keiner offenen Verbindung, weder unter sich, noch mit den Hirnhöhlen, und die in ihnen enthaltene Flüssigkeit könne daher nicht einfach in ihnen auf- oder absteigen."

communication could be explained by artefacts and that the ventricles formed a closed system everywhere lined by ependyma. Testut also believed this. Schmorl expressed a similar view after noting serological differences between the fluid in the ventricles and the subarachnoid space. He believed that this
not only denoted a double origin of cerebrospinal fluid, but that the absence of the foramina of Magendie and Luschka was to be deduced therefrom.

We do not think that observations of a similar character can throw any additional light on this subject. The experiments which follow prove the existence and the function of these foramina between the
ventricles and the subarachnoid space.

I. THE DEMONSTRATION OF FUNCTIONAL COMMUNICATION

When phenolsulphonephthalein is introduced into the ventricles, it appears in the spinal fluid in from
one to seven minutes. In these cases there was no increased tension of the ventricular fluid and no pressure was used. The results can therefore be attributed only to the normal means of regulating the distribution of fluids. The time of appearance of the dye in the spinal fluid may occasionally be delayed in
cases of hydrocephalus even when there is free communication (Case 3).

When phenolsulphonephthalein is substituted for an equal amount of *spinal fluid* and introduced
into the spinal subarachnoid space, the dye is soon found *in the ventricles*. These observations demonstrate that an open communication exists between the ventricles and the subarachnoid space in both
directions. They also demonstrate that fluid readily passes upward into the ventricles even against the

TABLE 4.—TIME OF APPEARANCE OF PHENOLSULPHONEPHTHALEIN IN THE SUBARACHNOID
SPACE FOLLOWING ITS INTRODUCTION INTO THE VENTRICLES

Case 1	2 minutes
Case 2	7 minutes
Case 3	13 minutes
	20 minutes
Case 4	1 minute

stream of cerebrospinal fluid from the ventricles. Such results render untenable the theory, usually
credited to Key and Retzius and recently advocated by Propping, that valves, though not demonstrable, exist at these openings. The passage of fluids from the subarachnoid space into the ventricles is of
the greatest importance in its bearing on intraspinal anesthesia and the treatment of diseases of the
central nervous system by intraspinal injections.

II. THE LOCATION OF THE COMMUNICATION

If an obstruction exists either at the aqueduct of Sylvius or at the basal foramina of Magendie and
Luschka, phenolsulphonephthalein, after introduction into the ventricles, does not appear in the spinal
fluid. This was the case in seven patients, and the obstruction was found in four on whom post-mortem
examination was held.

This proves that there are no openings between the third and lateral ventricles and the subarachnoid
space, or in other words, that the foramina of Bichat and Mierzejewsky (or the lateral foramina of
Bichat) do not exist. The aqueduct of Sylvius is the only channel for the escape of fluid from the third
and lateral ventricles. The openings between the ventricles and the subarachnoid space must therefore
be posterior to the aqueduct of Sylvius and must lead from the fourth ventricle. These openings are the
foramina of Magendie and Luschka.

7. THE DISTRIBUTION OF GRANULES IN THE SUBARACHNOID SPACE

Those who favor the theory of absorption of cerebrospinal fluid by means of stomata or by specialized
structures along the longitudinal or other sinuses have assumed the presence of an intra-arachnoidal
current to carry the cerebrospinal fluid to these structures. This is very similar to the assumption that
an intraperitoneal current carries the fluids to the central tendon of the diaphragm. We have been unable to find any evidence to support such an assertion either in the peritoneal cavity (Dandy and Rowntree) or in the subarachnoid space.

To determine the presence or absence of a current in the subarachnoid space, we substituted for the
cerebrospinal fluid (withdrawn through the occipito-atlantal membrane) an equal amount of a suspension of lampblack granules. The animal was kept under anesthesia from one to two hours, and at the end
of this time was killed and frozen to avoid distribution of the granules after death. Subsequent examina-

tion showed a most uniform distribution of granules throughout both the cerebral and spinal subarachnoid space. In so far as could be determined there was absolutely no evidence of any accumulation along the sinuses or in any other locality. With the exception of four parts of cranial nerves, there were no granules along the nerve sheaths. Granules were present in the olfactory nerves to their termination, the optic nerves to the fundus, the trigeminus over the gasserian ganglion and the auditory nerve to the internal auditory meatus. This distribution represents the normal limits of the distribution of the cerebrospinal fluid. If pressure is used, and only then, the other cranial and spinal nerves may be injected for varying distances.

The even and quite rapid distribution of granules throughout the cerebrospinal fluid is more readily explained by the pulsation in the central nervous system.

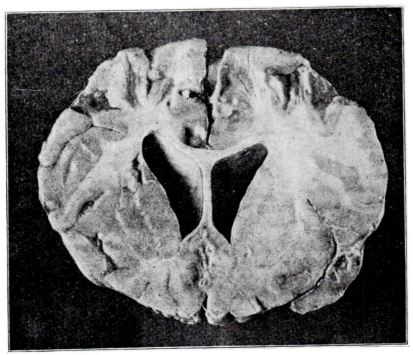

FIG. 8—Brain, cross-section of a normal child of 1 year; included as a standard for comparison with specimens of internal hydrocephalus which follow.

Part 2.—Clinical and Pathological Studies

In the following observations we determined the amount of absorption from the ventricles, the amount of absorption from the subarachnoid space and whether or not there was free communication between the ventricles and the subarachnoid space. Phenolsulphonephthalein[5] was used in these studies. After the introduction of a phenolsulphonephthalein solution into the ventricles and, at a subsequent test, into the subarachnoid space, the time of its first appearance in the urine was determined and the amount which was excreted in the urine for a two-hour period was estimated. The patency or occlusion of the communication was determined by the presence or absence in the spinal fluid of the phenolsulphonephthalein after its introduction into the ventricles.

5. It should be emphasized that the ordinary solution of phenolsulphonephthalein is made up with alkali; this is sufficient to prevent its use in the central nervous system. We used a neutral solution which, when diluted with cerebrospinal fluid, caused no symptoms whatever referable to the central nervous system. For ventricular use, 1 c.c. (6 mg.) of phenolsulphonephthalein was diluted with 3 c.c. of cerebrospinal fluid and for spinal subarachnoid use 1 c.c. (6 mg.) of phenolsulphonephthalein was diluted with 2 c.c. of cerebrospinal fluid.

8. ABSORPTION FROM THE VENTRICLES AND THE SUBARACHNOID SPACE WHEN HYDROCEPHALUS DOES NOT EXIST

In a number of patients in whom a ventricular or lumbar puncture was indicated for diagnosis, phenolsulphonephthalein was substituted for the cerebrospinal fluid removed. From these results a normal standard of absorption from the ventricles and the subarachnoid space and the average time of normal communication between them were obtained.

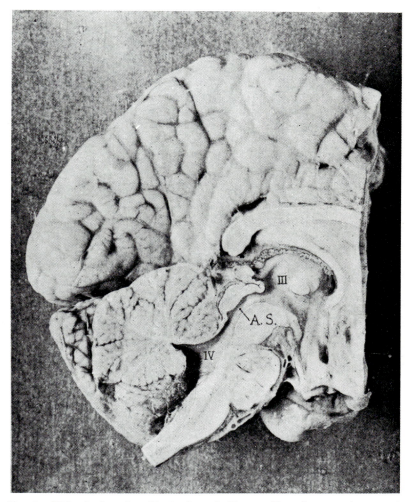

Fig. 9.—Midsagittal section of brain shown in Figure 8. Note the patent foramen of Magendie and the aqueduct of Sylvius.

It was found that after introduction into the ventricles, phenolsulphonephthalein appeared in the urine *in from ten to twelve minutes, and that during two hours from 12 to 20 per cent was excreted.* When introduced into the subarachnoid space it appeared in the urine in *from six to eight minutes, and from 35 to 60 per cent was excreted in two hours.* Phenolsulphonephthalein passed rapidly from the ventricles to the subarachnoid space, and appeared in the spinal fluid in from *one to three minutes.*

Pathological studies have shown that in some cases of hydrocephalus the communication between the ventricles and the subarachnoid space is open and that in others it is closed. It is obvious that a different operative procedure is indicated in these different types of cases. The inability to decide which type is present is undoubtedly one reason why the results of operation have been so unsatisfactory. We have endeavored to determine the presence or absence of the communication in hydrocephalus by the use of phenolsulphonephthalein after having demonstrated on animals that the method was harmless. In all cases permission for applying the tests was obtained from the parents.

9. STUDIES OF THE ABSORPTION FROM THE VENTRICLES AND THE SUBARACHNOID SPACE IN PATIENTS WITH INTERNAL HYDROCEPHALUS

It was possible to divide the cases which we studied into two groups. The introduction of phenolsulphonephthalein into the ventricles and a later examination for this substance in the spinal fluid will determine either by its absence that the communicating foramina are occluded (Group 1) or by its presence that they are patent (Group 2).

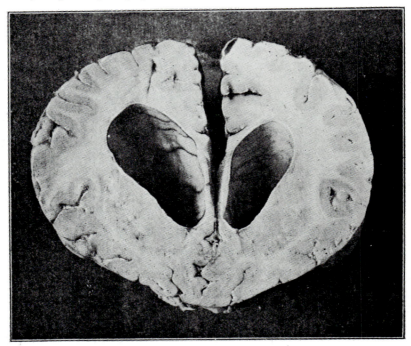

Fig. 10.—Cross-section of brain, showing moderately dilated lateral ventricles, in acute internal hydrocephalus (Case 1, Group 1, P. G.) due to occlusion of the foramina of Magendie and Luschka by a tuberculous exudate. There was no absorption from the ventricles.

GROUP 1.—INTERNAL HYDROCEPHALUS WITH OBSTRUCTION TO THE
CHANNELS OF EXIT FROM THE VENTRICLES

Case 1.—P. G., aged 7 months. Diagnosis: General miliary tuberculosis, tuberculous meningitis; internal hydrocephalus secondary to meningitis; meningocele.

Clinical Note.—Family History: Two other children living and well. No family history of hydrocephalus.

Past History: Full term, normal delivery. The patient was born with a meningocele. Dentition began at 3 months. Sat up at fourth month. No acute illness. No apparent disturbance from meningocele.

Present Illness: The patient had a severe cough and fever and had been very drowsy for a week.

Physical Examination: The patient was a well-nourished infant lying in a state of coma. In the sacral region was a large meningocele. Compression of the tumor caused bulging of the anterior fontanel. Von Pirquet test, positive.

Spinal Fluid from Meningocele: Clear fluid, 112 cells per cubic millimeter; tubercle bacilli present.

Tests.—1. There was no evidence of communication between the ventricles and the spinal subarachnoid space in forty-five minutes. 2. After ventricular introduction phenolsulphonephthalein did not appear in the urine for forty-five minutes. *In two hours only 0.75 per cent was excreted.* It was being excreted seventy hours later. 3. The absorption from the spinal subarachnoid space was rapid. Phenolsulphonephthalein first appeared in the urine six minutes after its introduction into the ventricles, and *62 per cent was excreted in the first two hours.*

Death from tuberculous meningitis.

Pathological Findings.—General miliary tuberculosis; tuberculous meningitis; myelomeningocele; internal hydrocephalus. The brain was normal in size. There was a plastic exudate over both parietal lobes, along the falx cerebri and the sylvian arteries, and scattered over the cerebral cortex were numerous tubercles. The base of the brain was covered with a thick exudate which extended from the optic chiasm posteriorly over the inferior surface of the pons and medulla, and the lower surface of both cerebellar hemispheres. The cisterna magna was filled with exudate. *The foramina of Magendie and foramina of Luschka were completely occluded by this exudate* (Figs. 10 and 11). On section, the ventricles were moderately dilated. A sagittal section continued through the midline showed the foramen of Monro to be moderately dilated, and the aqueduct of Sylvius patent. The fourth ventricle was about normal in size, and was partly filled with tuberculous exudate. This exudate, in addition to forming an external covering, firmly bound the medulla and the cerebellum together, thus doubly sealing the foramina of exit. It was also continuous with that which extended over the surface of the cerebellum and the base of the brain. Many tubercles were scattered over the ependyma of the third and of the lateral ventricles. The choroid plexus appeared normal except for tubercles demonstrated histologically. The pineal gland was very small, measuring about 2 mm. in diameter. The vein of Galen was patent.

    The spinal cord and its meninges did not appear abnormal, except for a few miliary tubercles; no exudate was present. *Meningocele:* The sac measured 8 by 7 cm. It projected through a median defect in the first and second sacral vertebrae and was firmly attached to the bodies of these vertebrae by a small pedicle 1.5 cm. in length. The cord ended at the upper part of the meningocele; the filum terminale and a few branches of the cauda crossed the cavity of the meningocele and became embedded in a cicatrix on the dorsal wall. The sac of the meningocele was directly continuous with the subarachnoid space.

    CASE 2.—A. H., aged 6 months. Diagnosis: Internal hydrocephalus, myelomeningocele (ruptured).

    Clinical Note.—Past History and Present Illness: Only child, full term, normal delivery. At birth the mother noticed a "swelling" the size of an apple over the lower part of the spine (meningocele), and the head appeared to be

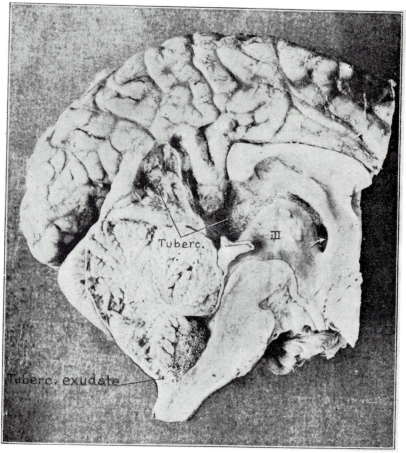

FIG. 11.—Midsagittal section of brain in Case 1. Observe the exudate which completely fills the space between the medulla and cerebellum and binds them together. This completely blocked the foramina of Magendie and Luschka. The aqueduct of Sylvius is patent.

larger than normal. The baby had never moved her legs. The head and the swelling on the back had steadily increased in size. Three days before admission the meningocele ruptured, after which there was a discharge of slightly blood-tinged fluid with consequent diminution in the size and in the tension of the sac.

Physical Examination: The patient was a fairly well-nourished infant with a moderate degree of hydrocephalus. The head measured 40 cm. in circumference. The anterior and posterior fontanels and the sutures were widely open. There was a downward dislocation of the eyes and a nystagmus in all directions. The neck was rigid and the arms slightly spastic. The lower extremities were flaccid and atrophied; the reflexes were absent. A collapsed meningocele sac was present in the lower lumbar and sacral region. From the ruptured medullovascular area a turbid, slightly blood-tinged fluid exuded.

Tests.—1. There was no evidence of communication between the ventricles and the spinal subarachnoid space *in two hours.* 2. *Forty minutes* after ventricular introduction of phenolsulphonephthalein it had not appeared in the urine. *In two hours only 1 per cent was excreted* in the urine.

Death occurred as a result of the rupture of the meningocele sac.

Pathological Findings.—The brain was enlarged. The sulci were shallow and the convolutions flattened. The meninges appeared normal, the foramina of Luschka and Magendie were patent. The lateral and third ventricles

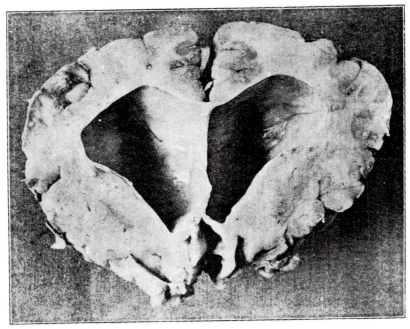

Fig. 12.—Cross-section of brain to show greatly distended lateral ventricles in case of internal hydrocephalus (Case 2, Group 1, A. H.) due to complete occlusion of the aqueduct of Sylvius.

were greatly and uniformly dilated, the relative and absolute size of which are shown in the photographs (Figs. 12 and 13). The fourth ventrical was flattened to a mere slit.

The aqueduct of Sylvius was completely obliterated. There was a small blind pouch at the position where the aqueduct should begin from the third ventricle, but beyond this there was no gross evidence of its presence. Cross-sections of the midbrain examined microscopically showed two independent, small spaces with a lining of ependymal cells. In one there was a small lumen and in the other the walls were in apposition. They undoubtedly represented remains of the aqueduct of Sylvius (Fig. 14). Microscopically there was a gliosis which had replaced the aqueduct of Sylvius. The corpora quadrigemina were very large but symmetrical.

The vena Galena magna was normal in size and the lumen was patent. The pineal gland was small. The choroid plexuses of the lateral ventricles were normal.

The meningocele sac measured 10 by 7 by 6 cm. It protruded through a defect in all the lumbar and the first sacral vertebrae and was attached by a broad base to these vertebrae. Its cavity was directly continuous with the subarachnoid space of the spinal cord. A series of from six to seven nerve roots rising from the cord at the line of attachment to the vertebrae ran transversely, on each side, through the cavity to the walls of the sac.

The spinal canal and subarachnoid space were otherwise normal.

Remarks.—The absence of communication was shown by the tests. This was substantiated by finding only microscopic remnants of the aqueduct of Sylvius. The dilatation of the third and lateral ventricles ahead of the obstruction and the collapsed fourth ventricle behind the obstruction were evidences of the influence of an obstruction in the aqueduct.

CASE 3.—N. P., aged 6 weeks. Diagnosis: Internal hydrocephalus.

Clinical Note.—Family History: Two other children aged 2 years and 4 years living and well. No history of syphilis or hydrocephalus.

Past History and Present Illness: Full term, normal delivery. At birth it was noticed that the child's head was large. When 2 weeks old she had general convulsions which lasted two or three days. Three weeks before death she had convulsions lasting over a period of three or four days. The head had grown progressively larger.

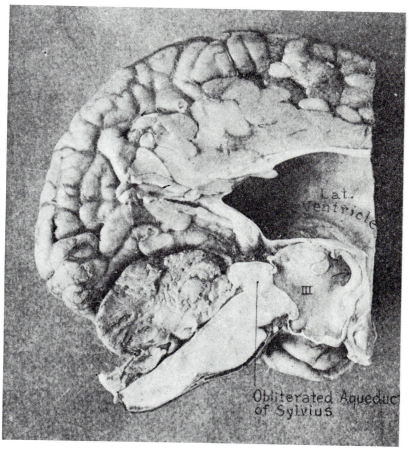

FIG. 13.—Midsagittal section of brain in Case 2 to show complete absence of the aqueduct of Sylvius and its replacement by neuroglia. Note the greatly dilated third and lateral ventricles anterior to the obstruction and the flattened slit-like fourth ventricle posterior to the obstruction. The septum lucidum is almost completely atrophied.

Physical Examination: The patient was an emaciated infant with hydrocephalus. The head measured 50.5 cm. in circumference. There was separation of nearly all of the cranial bones. There was displacement of the eyes downward and a nystagmus in all directions.

Tests.—1. There was *no evidence of communication* between the ventricles and the subarachnoid space *in twenty minutes.* 2. After ventricular introduction phenolsulphonephthalein did not appear in the urine in forty-five minutes. *During two hours only 1 per cent was excreted.*

Death from internal hydrocephalus.

Pathological Findings.—The cortex in places was only a millimeter in thickness and the brain collapsed into a shapeless mass when it ruptured. Sulci were present only over the temporal lobes; the remaining cortex was smooth. The size of the ventricles was almost equal to that of the calvarium. The foramina of Monro were from five to six times the normal size. There was complete atrophy of the septum lucidum. The fourth ventricle and the basal foramina of Luschka and Magendie were normal; the meninges were normal; the cerebellum was greatly flattened anteroposteriorly, as the result of the pressure of fluid in the lateral ventricles.

There was no aqueduct of Sylvius (Fig. 15). No trace of the aqueduct of Sylvius could be found in the gross or in sections when examined under the microscope, nor was there any evidence of epithelial remains as in the previous specimen. The choroid plexus was small but otherwise appeared normal. The vein of Galen was unobstructed. The pineal body was small. The spinal cord and the meninges, cerebral and spinal, were normal.

CASE 4.—N. M., aged 24 months. Diagnosis: Internal hydrocephalus.

Clinical Note.—Family History: Three other children living and well. No history of hydrocephalus or syphilis.

Past History and Present Illness: Full term, normal delivery. The patient's head was "large and round" at birth, but until he was 4½ months old it was not considered abnormal in size. He never held up his head, sat up or walked. Dentition began at the twelfth month. The patient had had no illness suggestive of meningitis. A puncture of the corpus callosum was performed when the patient was 1 year old. The head continued to increase in size.

Physical Examination: The patient was a well-nourished child, with a very large head, which measured 54 cm. in circumference. The anterior fontanel was 10 by 9 cm. in diameter; it was tense and bulging. The sutures were widely separated. There was ocular displacement downward, an internal strabismus of the left eye and a nystagmus in all

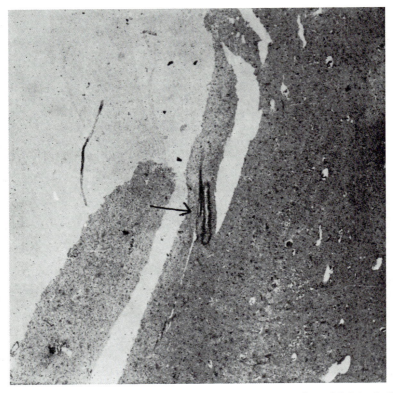

FIG. 14—Photomicrograph to show a microscopic remnant of the aqueduct of Sylvius in Case 2.

directions. The eye-grounds showed optic atrophy. There was a slight spasticity of the arms and legs. The reflexes were exaggerated and there was an ankle clonus. The head increased 11 cm. in seven months. The child's condition otherwise remained the same except for a partial weakness of both arms and legs.

Blood: Wassermann reaction, negative.

Ventricular Fluid: Clear. Noguchi globulin reaction negative, 6 cells per cubic centimeter.

Tests.—1. There was no evidence of communication between the ventricles and the subarachnoid space in two days. 2. After ventricular introduction phenolsulphonephthalein did not appear in the urine for forty minutes. *In two hours only 0.6 per cent was excreted. Phenolsulphonephthalein was being excreted after eleven days.* One month later, similar results were obtained. Phenolsulphonephthalein appeared in the urine in thirty-five minutes and 0.5 per cent was excreted in two hours. It was being excreted after eleven days. 3. After subarachnoid introduction, phenolsulphonephthalein appeared in the urine *in six minutes, and 35 per cent was excreted in two hours.* After twenty hours there was no trace of phenolsulphonephthalein in the urine. 4. The kidney function was normal; 45 per cent was excreted in two hours.

Remarks.—The results in this case were very similar to the one preceding: there was practically no absorption from the ventricle, and the appearance time of phenolsulphonephthalein in the urine was greatly delayed. In marked contrast were the results obtained from the subarachnoid space. It was evident that there was no communication between the ventricles and the subarachnoid space. The duration of excretion over eleven days in two separate experiments demonstrated the slow rate of absorption from the ventricles.

There could be no doubt that an obstruction existed either at the aqueduct of Sylvius or the basal foramina of Luschka and Magendie. We were never able to obtain more than 3 c.c. of cerebrospinal fluid by lumbar puncture. From the fact that so little spinal fluid could be obtained, we were inclined to infer that the obstruction was located at the basal foramina.

The patient is living.

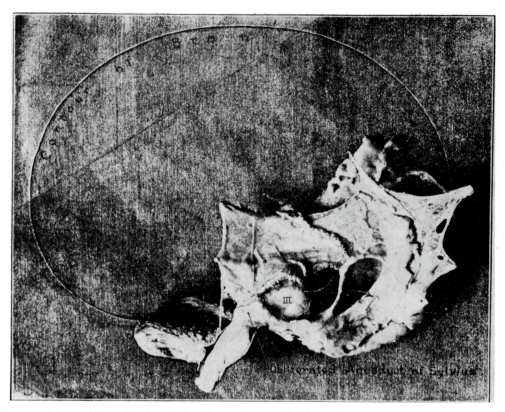

Fig. 15.—Advanced internal hydrocephalus (Case 3, Group 1, N. P.) caused by a completely occluded aqueduct of Sylvius. The cortex is a mere shell and could not be retained in its proper form. Note the exceedingly large foramen of Monro and the fringes of choroid plexus. Note the small fourth ventricle behind the occluded aqueduct of Sylvius, in marked contrast to the huge ventricles in front of this obstruction. The cerebellum is greatly flattened from the pressure of the distended lateral ventricles.

Case 5.—M. R., aged 13 months. Diagnosis: Internal hydrocephalus.

Clinical Note.—Family History: Mother and father living and well. The patient was a third child; a brother aged 5 years and a sister aged 3 living and well. No history of syphilis; no history of hydrocephalus.

Past History and Present Illness: The child was born at full term; instrumental delivery. The patient was well until 4 months old. Then she had a severe illness, which lasted one month. The body was rigid; there was marked opisthotonus and many convulsions of a general character; during this time the patient had a high fever. The mother noticed an enlargement of the head three weeks after the onset of this illness. The following four months, the increase in the size of the head was rapid. After that it grew larger but not so rapidly.

Examination: The patient was a well-nourished child. The head measured 55.5 cm. in circumference. The fontanels were open. The sutures were widely separated. There was marked downward displacement of the eyes, so that the pupils were almost entirely hidden behind the lower lids. A lateral and vertical nystagmus was present. There was a low grade (1 to 2 diopters) bilateral choked disk. Von Pirquet test, negative.

Spinal Fluid: Clear, six cells per cubic centimeter; Wassermann, negative. Reducing substance (Fehling's), present.

Ventricular Fluid: Five c.c. clear fluid, two cells per cubic millimeter; Wassermann, negative; reducing substance (Fehling's), present.

Tests.—1. There was *no evidence of communication between the ventricles and the subarachnoid space in one and one-half hours.* 2. After ventricular introduction, phenolsulphonephthalein did not appear in the urine for twenty minutes. *Only 0.9 per cent was excreted in two hours.* 3. After subarachnoid introduction, phenolsulphonephthalein appeared in the urine in eight minutes; *25 per cent was excreted in two hours.*

Patient died two months later of hydrocephalus.

Pathological Findings.—The brain was hardened *in situ* with formaldehyde solution. When removing the brain, an unusual accumulation of fluid filling the entire posterior cranial fossa was encountered. This could be likened to an encapsulated cyst. The walls were thin, transparent and in many places adherent to the dura. While freeing the

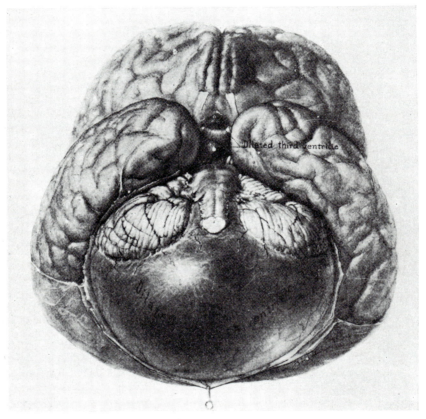

FIG. 16.—Ventral view of the brain in Case 5, Group 1, M. R. The foramina of Magendie and Luschka are absent and the fourth ventricle is distended into a huge cyst completely filling the posterior cranial fossa. The lateral lobes of the cerebellum are separated and crowded to either side. Note also the distended third ventricle.

lateral portions of the cyst, it was punctured and the brain collapsed. The cyst was a greatly dilated fourth ventricle, and the roof of the ventricle formed its walls (Fig. 16). Its size was limited only by the limitations of the posterior fossa. The cyst wall was adherent to the spinal cord and the lateral lobes of the cerebellum, making an impermeable membrane and preventing communication between the ventricles and the subarachnoid space. The lateral lobes of the cerebellum were separated 4 cm. and between them stretched this impermeable membrane. The aqueduct of Sylvius was considerably dilated. The septum lucidum was atrophied; the third and lateral ventricles and the foramina of Monro were greatly dilated. Their relative size is best shown in the accompanying drawings[6] (Figs. 17 and 18).

The pia arachnoid was everywhere fused with the "cyst wall" of the fourth ventricle; this membrane was greatly thickened over the base of the brain. The usual transparent bridge of the pia arachnoid between the inferior surface of the pons and the optic chiasm was so opaque that the underlying brain was invisible; this opaque thickened membrane was also continuous over and adherent to the floor of the third ventricle. It also completely covered and was

6. We wish to express our thanks to Mr. Max Brödel for the accompanying drawings and for his assistance in the preparation of many of the figures.

adherent to the optic chiasm. Over the entire base of the brain this thickening of the meninges was very apparent; over the surface of the cerebral lobes it was less apparent.

The vein of Galen and the straight sinus were normal; the choroid plexuses appeared to be normal. The choroid plexus of the fourth ventricle was entirely within the cyst. The pineal gland was small. The spinal cord was not obtained for examination.

Remarks.—In this case also an absence of communication was demonstrated by the phenolsulphonephthalein test. This was confirmed by the post-mortem findings. There was practically no absorption from the ventricles and a rather high though subnormal absorption from the subarachnoid space. The partial obliteration by adhesions of the subarachnoid space over these areas mentioned no doubt explains the diminished absorption from this space.

Case 6.—F. W., aged 6 months. Diagnosis: Internal hydrocephalus. Meningocele and syringomyelocele.

Clinical Note.—Family History: The patient was the youngest of four children. The other three were well. There was no evidence of syphilis. No history of hydrocephalus.

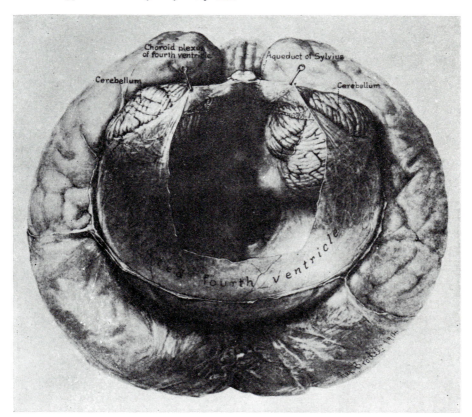

Fig. 17.—View of dilated fourth ventricle in Case 5 with window removed. Note the extent of the "cyst," the separation of the cerebellar hemispheres and the patent aqueduct of Sylvius.

Past History: Full term, difficult delivery, owing to large head, without instruments. Weight at birth, 10 pounds.

Present Illness: The mother noticed that the head was abnormally large at birth. There was also present a large "swelling" over the middle of the lower back. The circumference of the head and the swelling over the back gradually increased in size.

Examination: The patient was a well-nourished infant whose head measured 51 cm. in circumference. There was diastasis of the cranial bones. The anterior and posterior fontanels were widely open and tense. A large meningocele protruded from a spina bifida of the lower lumbar and all the sacral vertebrae. There was complete paralysis of the lower extremities. The head grew 5 cm. in one month.

Spinal Fluid: Clear, 3 cells per cubic millimeter. Noguchi globulin reaction negative. Reducing substance present (Fehling's).

Ventricular Fluid: Clear, 2 cells per cubic millimeter. Noguchi globulin reaction negative. Reducing substance present (Fehling's).

Tests.—1. There was very slight evidence of communication between the ventricles and the subarachnoid space in four and one-half hours. *A faint* trace of phenolsulphonephthalein was then present. 2. After ventricular introduction, phenolsulphonephthalein did not appear in the urine for sixteen minutes. *Two per cent was excreted in two hours.* The head increased in size and at a test after two months there *was only 1 per cent excreted in two hours.* Phenolsulphonephthalein appeared in the urine in twenty-five minutes. At this time there was no evidence of communication between the ventricles and the subarachnoid space after three hours. 3. After subarachnoid introduction, phenolsulphonephthalein appeared in the urine in twelve minutes, and *10 per cent was excreted in two hours.* 4. The kidney function was normal.

The patient died of hydrocephalus.

Pathological Findings.—The dura was firmly adherent to the cerebellum by fibrous bands, which had to be torn before the brain could be removed. These adhesions were present throughout the posterior fossa and extended almost

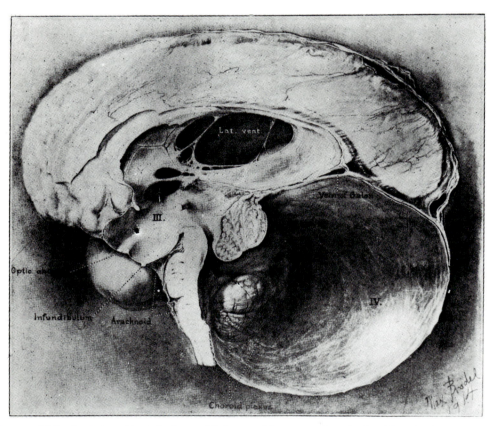

Fig. 18.—Midsagittal view of brain in Case 5. All the ventricles communicate freely with each other. There are no foramina of Magendie and Luschka. The choroid plexus is included in the "cyst." Note the patent and enlarged foramen of Monro (arrow) and aqueduct of Sylvius. The large openings in the septum lucidum show the effects of the intraventricular pressure.

the entire distance of the spinal canal, binding the spinal cord to the dura. The cerebellum was also firmly bound to the medulla by adhesions which occluded the foramina of exit from the fourth ventricle (Figs. 19 and 20).

The cerebral cortex was so thin that in places it was translucent. This was especially true over the temporal lobes. Here no convolutions were evident, the surface being entirely smooth. The convolutions were elsewhere flattened and the sulci shallow. Viewed from below the floor of the third ventricle appeared as a film. The third and lateral ventricles and the foramina of Monro were greatly dilated; only shreds of the septum lucidum remained. The aqueduct of Sylvius was about normal in size and everywhere patent. The fourth ventricle was compressed. The first portion of the central canal of the cord was dilated, but this soon became obliterated so that throughout its entire length there was no connection with the syringomyelocele. When the ventricles were filled, the fluid readily passed out of the central canal but not through the foramina of Luschka and Magendie. These were entirely occluded.

The corpora quadrigemina were very large. The pineal gland was small. The choroid plexus appeared normal in the gross. Microscopically the choroidal epithelium was flattened and the vascular spaces somewhat dilated.

Syringomyelocele and Meningocele: Two separate, non-communicating cavities were contained within the cutaneous covering. The sac protruded through a defect in the third, fourth and fifth lumbar and all the sacral vertebrae.

The walls of the sac were fused in part. The meningocele was in communication with the subarachnoid space and contained clear fluid. The syringomyelocele was connected for a short distance with the central canal of the cord. This cavity contained turbid straw-colored fluid. The central canal of the cord was obliterated between the syringomyelocele and the medulla. At those points, the canal was greatly dilated. There was no communication between the cerebral ventricles and the syringomyelocele.

Remarks.—This case is unusual in that at first a very slight communication existed between the ventricles and the subarachnoid space. One month later and shortly before death there was no evident communication in three hours, and absorption following ventricular injection had diminished to 1 per cent. The time of appearance in the urine increased to twenty-five minutes.

The subarachnoid absorption was low (10 per cent). An old inflammatory process was present obliterating all the basal foramina and tightly binding the cerebellum to the medulla. This accounts for the small size of the fourth ven-

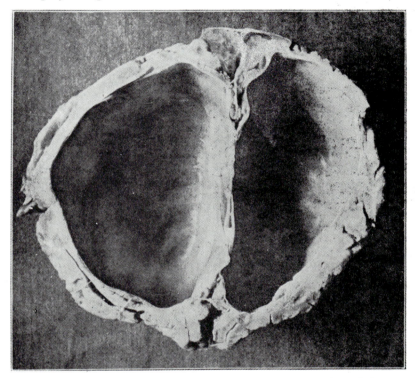

Fig. 19.—A very advanced internal hydrocephalus (Case 6, Group 1, F. W.) due to inflammatory adhesions at the base, which occluded the foramina of Magendie and Luschka.

tricle, which was unusual as the aqueduct was patent and the third and lateral ventricles were greatly dilated. On account of the strong adhesions, enlargement of the fourth ventricle was prevented. The hydrocephalus resulted from adhesions blocking the foramina of exit and preventing the cerebrospinal fluid from reaching the subarachnoid space. It must have occurred during intra-uterine life as the hydrocephalus was present at birth. Whether or not the adhesions from the inflammatory process which obliterated the cisterna were responsible for the low subarachnoid absorption can only be conjectured. This case may readily be regarded as a transitional type between those with total occlusion and those with communication (Group 2).

Case 7.—M. N., aged 5 months. Diagnosis: Internal hydrocephalus.

Clinical Note.—Past History: The patient was born at full term after a difficult instrumental delivery. The head was not noticed to be abnormally large at birth. Paralysis of the left side of the face was observed two weeks after birth. The baby had never moved his head in a normal manner, but the parents did not attribute this to any other cause than general weakness. The head had been increasing in size for about one month.

Physical Examination: The patient was a fairly well-nourished infant with moderate hydrocephalus. The circumference of the head was 47.5 cm. There was downward dislocation of the eyes and a nystagmus in all directions. The eye-grounds showed a marked choking of the disks, the swelling being about 3 diopters in each fundus. The left side of the face was completely paralyzed. The extremities were normal and the reflexes at the knee active. The Wassermann reaction of the blood and spinal fluid was negative.

Ventricular Fluid: Clear, 9 cells per cubic millimeter. Globulin test, negative. Fehling's test positive.

Spinal Fluid: Clear, 5 cells per cubic millimeter. Globulin test, negative. Fehling's test positive.

TABLE 5.—SUMMARY OF GROUP 1, INTERNAL HYDROCEPHALUS WITH OBSTRUCTION

Name and No.	Patient's Illness	Absorption after Ventricular Introduction		Absorption after Spinal Introduction		Communication, Ventricle and Subarachnoid space	Duration of Excretion		Etiology	Postmortem Findings
		Time of appearance Minutes	Two-hour absorption Per cent	Time of appearance Minutes	Two-hour absorption Per cent	Time of appearance	Ventricle	Spinal canal		
1. P. G.	Tuberculous meningitis; internal hydrocephalus	45	0.75	6	62	None in 45 min.	3% excreted in 12 hrs. Three days later the concentration of 'phthalein in the urine was undiminished	Less than 12 hrs.	Tuberculous meningitis. Meningocele present since birth	Exudate over base of brain occluding the foramina of exit.
2. A. H.	Internal hydrocephalus	40	1	……	……	None in 2 hrs.	……	……	Congenital; myelomeningocele also present	Occlusion of aqueduct of Sylvius.
3. N. P.	Internal hydrocephalus	45	1	0	0	None in 20 min.	……	……	Congenital	Total absence of aqueduct of Sylvius. Living.
4. N. M.	Internal hydrocephalus	40, 35	0.50, 0.50	6	35	None in 2 days	11 days. 11 days. 6.1% first 24 hours. 7.5% second 24 hours. 5.7% third 24 hours.	21 hrs.	Congenital	Living.
5. M. R.	Internal hydrocephalus	40, 20	0.50, 0.9	8	25	None in 1½ hrs.	……	……	Meningitis at 4 mos. Previously normal	Absence of foramina of Luschka and Magendie. Fourth ventricle a large cyst. Marked thickening of pia arachnoid.
6. F. W.	Internal hydrocephalus	16, 25	2, 1	12	10	Trace in less than 4½ hrs. None in second observation 3 hours	7 days	48 hrs.	Congenital; no history of meningitis, meningocele and syringomyelocele	Chronic inflammatory process; adhesions at base occluding foramina of exit.
7. M. N.	Internal hydrocephalus	30	1.5	0	35	None in 30 min. faint trace in 14 hours	……	……	Congenital	Living.

Tests.—1. There was no evidence of communication between the ventricles and the subarachnoid space in thirty minutes. 2. After ventricular introduction, phenolsulphonephthalein did not appear in the urine for thirty minutes. Only *1.5 per cent was excreted in two hours.* 3. After subarachnoid introduction, *35 per cent phenolsulphonephthalein was excreted in two hours.*

Remarks.—From the results of the foregoing observations we know that there was an obstruction to the outflow of cerebrospinal fluid from the ventricles into the subarachnoid space. The excretion of phenolsulphonephthalein from the subarachnoid space (35 per cent) was normal.

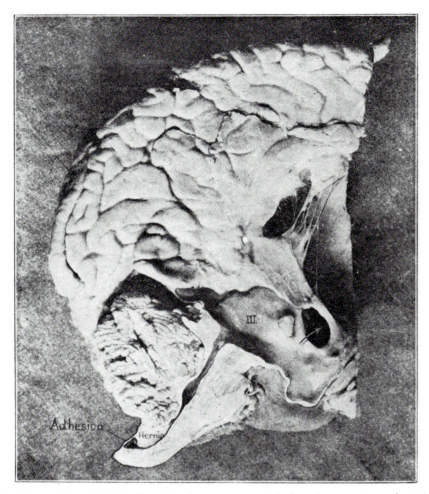

Fig. 20.—Cross-section of brain in Case 6, to show extreme ventricular enlargement, aqueduct of Sylvius patent. Dilatation of the fourth ventricle was prevented by adhesions between the dura and the cerebellum.

SUMMARY OF GROUP 1

The essential feature of this type of internal hydrocephalus is the absence of communication between the ventricles and the subarachnoid space. This lack of communication was demonstrated clinically in seven patients. It was confirmed at necropsy in five. In one (Case 1, P. G.) a thick tuberculous exudate covered the base of the brain and tightly sealed the communicating foramina. In two (Case 5, M. R., and Case 6, F. W.) the basal foramina were occluded by adhesions resulting from an old meningitic process; in the former, the illness occurred four months after birth, and in the latter it was evidently prenatal. In two there was complete occlusion of the aqueduct of Sylvius. In one of these (Case 2, A. H.) epithelial remnants of the aqueduct were demonstrated microscopically; in the other (Case 3, N. P.) no

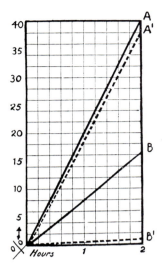

Fig. 21.—Curves comparing the normal absorption from the ventricles and the subarachnoid space with the absorption in internal hydrocephalus of the obstructive type. The base line represents a two-hour interval and the vertical line the percentage of absorption (excretion of phenolsulphonephthalein) during that time. The heavy lines represent the normal absorption and the dotted lines the absorption in hydrocephalus. *A*, normal subarachnoid absorption; *A'*, absorption from subarachnoid space of case of obstructive hydrocephalus; *B*, normal absorption of fluid placed in the ventricles; *B'*, absorption from ventricles in obstructive hydrocephalus.

trace of the aqueduct was present. In both the region of the aqueduct was occupied by neuroglia tissue. The sixth and seventh patients are living (Case 4, N. M., and Case 7, M. N.). In these seven patients the absorption from the ventricle was less than 1 per cent in six. In the one in whom the absorption was as high as 2 per cent, there was probably a minute communication between the ventricles and the subarachnoid space. At a subsequent examination the absorption in this case was less (1 per cent), and there was proof of the obliteration of the foramina. The absorption from the ventricles is independent of the size of the ventricles or the amount of the contained cerebrospinal fluid. In Case 1 (P. G.) the ventricles were only moderately dilated and the absorption was not greater than in the most distended ventricles. The excretion of phenolsulphonephthalein in the urine is prolonged in this group (from the normal period of several hours, to ten days). The time of appearance of the dye in the urine is greatly delayed also (from thirty to fifty minutes).

In marked contrast to the negligible ventricular absorption was the high subarachnoid absorption in all except the two postmeningitic cases (Cases 5 and 6). The appearance time in the urine and the duration of excretion following subarachnoid injections were normal.

This type of internal hydrocephalus results because the cerebrospinal fluid cannot escape from its place of origin in the ventricles, where the absorption is negligible, to the subarachnoid space, where the absorption normally occurs, because the channels of communication are occluded (Fig. 21).

GROUP 2.—INTERNAL HYDROCEPHALUS WITH FREE COMMUNICATION BETWEEN THE
VENTRICLES AND THE SUBARACHNOID SPACE

Case 8.—R. G., aged 1½ years. Diagnosis: Internal hydrocephalus.

Clinical Note.—Family History: Three other children living and well. No history of syphilis or hydrocephalus.

Past History: Full term. Weight at birth, 12 pounds. Spontaneous delivery. Patient held up head at the fourth month, sat up at the sixth month. Dentition began at the seventh month. He appeared a normal baby in every respect until 7 months of age.

Present Illness: When 7 months of age, he became ill with high fever, vomiting, great irritability and muscular rigidity. This condition lasted for three days and during the following two weeks he had an irregular fever. The appetite was poor and he lost in weight. After this illness the patient was unable to hold up his head. One month later it was noticed that the head was larger than normal and that the eyes were pushed downward. For the next three months, the head continued to increase rapidly in size.

Examination: The patient was a well-developed and well-nourished infant. The head measured 52 cm. in circumference. He was unable to raise his head. The child saw and heard and recognized the members of his family. The forehead was prominent and the occiput flattened. The anterior fontanel was widely open and the sutures separated. The eyes were displaced downward and there was weakness of both external recti. The eye-grounds were normal. The reflexes were active and equal; a bilateral ankle clonus was present.

Spinal Fluid: Clear, 6 cells per cubic millimeter. Noguchi globulin test, negative.

Ventricular Fluid: Clear, 6 cells per cubic millimeter. Noguchi globulin test, negative.

Tests.—1. There was communication between the ventricles and the subarachnoid space. Phenolsulphonephthalein was demonstrated in the spinal fluid *two minutes* after ventricular introduction. The test was repeated after one month and phenolsulphonephthalein appeared in the spinal fluid in one minute. 2. After ventricular introduction phenolsulphonephthalein appeared in the urine in thirty minutes and *2 per cent was excreted in two hours*. One month later, the test was repeated and phenolsulphonephthalein appeared in the urine in twenty minutes and 2.3 per cent was excreted in two hours. 3. After subarachnoid introduction, *11 per cent of phenolsulphonephthalein was excreted in two hours*. At the second test, phenolsulphonephthalein appeared in the urine in thirteen minutes and 7 per cent was excreted in two hours.

Remarks.—From the history it seemed very definite that an attack of meningitis was the ethiological factor responsible for the development of the internal hydrocephalus. From the rapid passage of fluid from the ventricles to the subarachnoid space it was evident that free communication existed. The absorption from the subarachnoid space was much diminished, from 7 to 11 per cent of phenolsulphonephthalein, as opposed to the normal of 35 per cent or over. The appearance of the dye in the urine following its introduction into the ventricles and into the subarachnoid space was also much delayed. The kidney function test was normal.

CASE 9.—M. R., aged 11 months. Diagnosis: Cerebrospinal meningitis with secondary internal hydrocephalus. *Clinical Note.*—Family History: No history of syphilis or hydrocephalus.

Past History: Only child, full term, normal delivery; breast fed. Dentition began at fourth month. Sat up at eight months. Always well until present illness.

Present Illness: This began suddenly three days before admission to the outpatient department (March 31, 1913) with high fever, drowsiness, vomiting and extreme irritability. She had had one convulsion. Temperature 101.6 F.

The following note was made: "An irritable colored girl, aged 11 months, appears very sick. She is well-nourished and well-developed. There is slight cervical rigidity. The sudden onset, drowsiness, fever, vomiting, convulsion and rigidity of the neck suggest meningitis." Lumbar puncture was not allowed and hospital treatment was refused by the parents. The first two weeks after the onset the baby was very sick. About April 12 she was unconscious for five days. Two weeks later (April 26, 1913) she vomited and began to have twitching movements of the face and extremities.

On admission to the hospital (May 2, 1913) the child, greatly emaciated, was in a stupor from which it was difficult to arouse her. The head measured 45 cm. in circumference, the anterior fontanel was small. The pupils reacted slowly to light. Vision was evidently impaired. There was rigidity of the extremities, exaggerated reflexes and ankle clonus. Temperature, 102 F. Leukocytes, 14,400. Von Pirquet test, negative.

Spinal Fluid: Twenty c.c. turbid fluid. Noguchi globulin reaction, positive; culture showed no growth. Smear: Many pus cells, no organisms.

Thirteen c.c. of antimeningitic serum were injected. The patient was removed from the hospital by her parents after twenty-four hours. The child was brought to the dispensary seven weeks later (June 25, 1913) because she could not see. On examination in the ward, July 5, 1913, the patient was poorly nourished, apparently blind, and very sensitive to sounds. The head was retracted and the neck rigid and there was spasticity of the extremities. The head measured 45 cm. in circumference. The pupils were unequal and reacted only slightly to light. There was no choking of the disks. There was a vertical and lateral nystagmus. Kernig's sign was positive. The reflexes were exaggerated and a bilateral ankle clonus was present. Temperature, 98.6 F. Leukocytes, 12,000. Wassermann reaction, negative.

Spinal Fluid: Clear, 10 c.c. Forty-two cells per cubic millimeter; Noguchi globulin reaction, positive; cultures negative; tubercle bacilli not found.

Ventricular Fluid: Clear fluid, 12 cells per cubic millimeter; Noguchi globulin reaction, positive.

The child was taken home after a few days, having made no improvement.

Tests.—1. There was communication between the ventricles and the subarachnoid spaces. Phenolsulphonephthalein appeared in the spinal subarachnoid space *seven minutes* after being introduced into the ventricle. 2. After ventricular introduction, phenolsulphonephthalein appeared in the urine in thirteen minutes and *6.5 per cent was excreted in two hours*. Later (two and one-half months) a second test was made and phenolsulphonephthalein appeared in the urine in twenty minutes and only *0.5 per cent was excreted*. 3. After subarachnoid introduction, phenolsulphonephthalein appeared in the urine in eight minutes and *14 per cent was excreted in two hours*. Two days later this test was repeated and 9.5 per cent of phenolsulphonephthalein was excreted in two hours. It was being excreted in the urine after seventy-two hours. 4. The kidney function was normal.

Remarks.—The child was seen at the onset of an attack of epidemic cerebrospinal meningitis. A month afterward she was brought to the hospital because of beginning blindness. The absorption after ventricular injection was low (about 50 per cent of the normal). The patient was admitted to the hospital two months after the onset, totally blind, and hydrocephalus was evident. There was very marked diminution in absorption, only 0.5 per cent after ventricular injection and 9.5 per cent and 15 per cent from the subarachnoid space. Free communication existed between the ventricles and the subarachnoid space.

CASE 10.—H. N., aged 8 months. Diagnosis: Internal hydrocephalus.[7]

Clinical Note.—Family History: No other cases of hydrocephalus in the family.

Examination: The child was well-nourished. The head measured 51 cm. in circumference. The anterior fontanel measured 10 by 8 cm.; it was tense and slightly bulging. There was a bilateral choked disk. The knee-reflexes were exaggerated though equal. Two and one-half weeks after the first admission the patient's head had increased 2 cm. in size. During another interval of eighteen days the head increased 0.9 cm. in circumference. At this time lumbar punc-

---

7. The phenolsulphonephthalein tests in this case demonstrated a communicating type of hydrocephalus. Repeated lumbar punctures were made for their therapeutic effect. The process has remained stationary for three months and the child is apparently cured.

ture was repeatedly done and fluid withdrawn for its therapeutic effect. Following this mode of treatment the child became able to hold up its head and the increase in size became less rapid. The Wassermann test was negative for the blood and the ventricular and spinal fluids. Von Pirquet test, negative.

Ventricular Fluid: Clear, 6 cells per cubic millimeter. Noguchi globulin test, negative.

Spinal Fluid: Clear, 6 cells per cubic millimeter. Noguchi globulin test, negative.

Tests.—1. Communication was demonstrated between the ventricles and the subarachnoid space. Phenolsulphonephthalein appeared in the spinal fluid *twenty minutes* after its introduction into the ventricle. 2. Phenolsulphonephthalein appeared in the urine twenty-five minutes after its introduction into the ventricles *and 4.4 per cent was excreted in two hours.* Two weeks later, the absorption was 4 per cent. 3. The absorption from the subarachnoid space *was 10 per cent during a two-hour period.* The same result was obtained two weeks later. 4. The kidney function test was normal.

Remarks.—Except for the brief illness shortly after birth there was nothing to suggest a cause for the hydrocephalus. We were unable to obtain any information either from the mother or the attending physician to warrant a diagnosis of meningitis. The clinical tests showed that there was a delayed absorption from the subarachnoid space. The time of appearance in the spinal canal following the ventricular injection was much longer than in either of the two preceding cases of this group. That there was adequate communication, however, was shown by the relatively high concentration of phenolsulphonephthalein in the spinal fluid two and one-half hours after the ventricular injection.

CASE 11.—J. C., aged 16 months. Diagnosis: Internal hydrocephalus.

Clinical Note.—Only child. Parents, healthy; instrumental and prolonged labor (thirty-one hours). A cephalhematoma developed soon after birth and disappeared in five weeks. The primary respirations were difficult to establish. No convulsions. The enlargement of head was not noticed at birth. The head appeared large when he was 3 months of age and thereafter steadily increased in size. In six weeks it increased 2 inches, and in two weeks $\frac{3}{4}$ inch. January, 1913, the head measured 55.5 cm.; September, 69.5 cm., and November, 1913, 72.5 cm. The child never had fever or convulsions or any illness suggesting meningitis.

Examination: The head was large and measured 72 cm. in circumference. The reflexes were exaggerated. The Wassermann reaction of the spinal fluid and blood was negative.

By lumbar puncture from 40 to 75 c.c. of clear fluid were obtained. Six cells per cubic millimeter. Globulin test, negative. Fehling's, slight reduction.

Tests.—1. There was communication between the ventricles and subarachnoid space. Phenolsulphonephthalein appeared in the spinal fluid in less than one minute after its introduction in the ventricle. 2. The absorption following the introduction of phenolsulphonephthalein in the ventricles was 4 per cent in two hours and the time of appearance in the urine was forty minutes.

Remarks. A subarachnoid test was not obtained. It was evident, however, from the rapid appearance of phenolsulphonephthalein in the subarachnoid space that communication was adequate.

SUMMARY OF CASES IN GROUP 2

In this type of hydrocephalus the communication between the ventricles and the subarachnoid space is patent, thus differing from Type 1, in which there is no communication between the ventricles and the subarachnoid space. Following intraventricular introduction of phenolsulphonephthalein, the dye appears almost immediately (from one to seven minutes) in the spinal fluid. In one case of this group on two separate occasions the time of appearance in the spinal fluid was delayed to fifteen and twenty minutes. We were unable to determine the reason for this delay. Communication in this type of hydrocephalus is further proved by the rapid appearance in the ventricular fluid of phenolsulphonephthalein after being introduced into the subarachnoid space.

The absorption from the subarachnoid space of these patients is greatly diminished (about 10 per cent in two hours). There is a corresponding increase in the time of first appearance of phenolsulphonephthalein in the urine and in the time required for its total excretion from the subarachnoid space. *The diminished subarachnoid absorption is the factor responsible for the production of the internal hydrocephalus* (Fig. 22).

The absorption after ventricular injection was also very low (about 4 per cent), but distinctly higher than in Group 1. *Since it has been shown that there is practically no absorption from the ventricles, the absorption following ventricular injection in normal cases or in cases of internal hydrocephalus of the communicating type must be due to absorption from the subarachnoid space after the fluid* has passed through the foramina of exit from the ventricles.

We have had no pathological examination on patients with hydrocephalus of this type demonstrated by these clinical tests. It is very likely that the diminished absorption from the subarachnoid space is due to adhesions which diminish the size of the subarachnoid space. Adhesions anterior to the foramina of Luschka, by causing obliteration of the cisterna magna, would prevent the passage of fluid into the general cerebral subarachnoid space as effectually as if the aqueduct of Sylvius were obliterated. The two groups would then be essentially similar, differing only in the fact that the spinal subarachnoid space participated in absorption in the communicating type. When there are adhesions at the base of the brain they are frequently present also between the cord and the meninges.

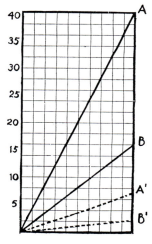

Fig. 22.—Curve comparing the normal ventricular and subarachnoid absorption with the absorption in internal hydrocephalus of the communicating type. The base line represents a two-hour period and the vertical line represents the absorption (percentage of phenolsulphonephthalein excreted) during this time. The heavy lines represent the normal absorption and the dotted lines the absorption in hydrocephalus. A, normal subarachnoid absorption; A', absorption from subarachnoid space in communicating hydrocephalus; B, normal absorption of fluid placed in the ventricles; B', absorption of fluid placed in ventricles of communicating hydrocephalus.

We have had the opportunity of examining the specimen from a patient who had hydrocephalus of this variety. There was a congenital internal hydrocephalus evidently the result of an intra-uterine meningitis. Dense adhesions were found along the cord and the base of the brain obliterating the cisterna magna. The foramen of Magendie was sealed by adhesions, but the foramina of Luschka were patent and greatly dilated. There was no cisterna for the reception of fluid.

How much alteration in the meninges alone, without adhesions, interferes with absorption, cannot be stated. It seems to us probable that the major part if not all of the disturbance is due to the limitation of the subarachnoid space.

That there is another type of hydrocephalus intermediate been Group 1 and Group 2 appears probable. There must be cases in which the obstruction to the outflow of fluid from the ventricles is not complete but partial, and in which the subarachnoid absorption is either normal or diminished. With such a combination a hydrocephalus must also result. Indeed, Case 6 (Group 1, F.W.) probably belongs to this intermediate group. That there was a slight communication was shown by the trace of phenolsulphonephthalein in the spinal fluid after ventricular introduction. The subarachnoid absorption was greatly diminished and corresponded in amount with the absorption found in the cases of Group 2. The slightly higher absorption, 2 per cent after ventricular introduction, is probably also to be explained by a partial communication. At a later observation a complete obstruction was found and the ventricular absorption was much less.

10. CLINICAL DIFFERENCES BETWEEN THE COMMUNICATING AND OBSTRUCTIVE TYPES OF INTERNAL HYDROCEPHALUS

There is no way by which a differentiation can be made between the obstructive and the communicating types of internal hydrocephalus except by the actual determination of the presence or the absence of communication between the ventricles and the subarachnoid space. While the increase in size of the head appears usually to be slower in many cases in which there is communication, there are other cases in which the increase is very rapid.

It is sometimes possible to tell by the large amount of fluid removed by lumbar puncture that the case is of the communicating type. This can be, however, only when the internal hydrocephalus is advanced in degree. When there is obstruction either at the aqueduct of Sylvius or at the foramina of Luschka and Magendie, 25 c.c. or more of fluid can frequently be obtained by lumbar puncture and the erroneous conclusion might be reached that the fluid was withdrawn from the ventricles. Differences in the cell count and in serological tests, between the spinal and ventricular fluids, are usually too slight to be of any value.

The only satisfactory method of differentiating these two groups is by the phenolsulphonephthalein test as described above.

11. THE RELATION OF OBSTRUCTION TO INTERNAL HYDROCEPHALUS

That obstruction may be responsible for internal hydrocephalus was first demonstrated by Magendie. John Hilton accepted Magendie's views and thought that probably every case was so produced. In his excellent lectures on "Rest and Pain," drawings are given to show the obstruction which he found quite constantly. Quincke, Bourneville and Noir, Spiller, Browning, Schlapp and Géré, Neurath and numerous other writers reported cases showing various types of occlusion which were held responsible for the internal hydrocephalus. Obstructions have been observed at the foramina of Monro producing a unilateral hydrocephalus, at the aqueduct of Sylvius producing dilatation of the third and lateral ventricles, and at the foramina of Luschka and Magendie producing enlargement of all the ventricles. The obstructions have been due to inflammations, tumors and congenital defects. Obstructions have also been noted in animals, especially in the horse, cow, dog and cat (Fig. 23). Dexler studied many cases of hydrocephalus, known as *Dummkoller*, in the horse, and found quite constantly an occlusion of the foramina of Luschka. It will be recalled that the foramen of Magendie does not exist in the horse.

In our series of seven patients in whom an obstruction was determined by the phenolsulphonephthalein test, necropsies were obtained in five, and in each of these the presence of an obstruction was demonstrated. Moreover, an obstruction experimentally placed in the aqueduct of Sylvius causes an internal hydrocephalus. Internal hydrocephalus is produced because the fluid forms in the ventricles and cannot escape to the subarachnoid space where it is absorbed. In this respect there is a close analogy between the ventricles of the brain and the renal pelvis. Just as hydronephrosis results from obstruction along the course of the ureter, so a hydrocephalus results from an occlusion of the channels of exit from the ventricles. In neither the pelvis of the kidney nor the ventricles of the brain is there sufficient absorption to overcome the effects of occlusion.

12. THE RELATION OF MENINGITIS TO INTERNAL HYDROCEPHALUS

In two specimens (Group 1) it was shown after the pathological examination that adhesions occluding the communicating foramina were responsible for the hydrocephalus. These were undoubtedly the result of a previous meningitis. In Group 2, two patients gave a definite history of meningitis, immediately preceding the onset of the internal hydrocephalus. Case 9 (M.R.) of Group 2 was seen during an attack of epidemic meningitis and during the subsequent development of the hydrocephalus. Case 8 (R.G.), Group 2, gave a typical history of meningitis. Before this illness the child was perfectly well and afterward he was not able to hold up his head and his head had enlarged.

Case 6 of Group 1 was an example of congenital hydrocephalus with a meningocele. Post-mortem examination, however, revealed the evidences of a marked basilar meningitis with occlusion of the foramina of Luschka and Magendie. There is, therefore, clinical and pathological evidence that meningitis is frequently the etiological factor in the production of internal hydrocephalus of both the obstructive and the communicating types, and there is every reason to believe that it occurs both before and after birth.

That meningitis is an important factor in the production of this disease has been clinically recognized at least since the beginning of the nineteenth century. Alexander Monro (1827) observed that hydrocephalus apparently of postnatal origin was frequently preceded by a severe illness, which was not then recognized as meningitis. Greater attention was directed to this disease as an etiological factor by Trousseau (1857), Foerster (1863), Ziemssen and Hess (1874). Joslin, Koplik, Gildesheim, Barlow and Lees, and Göppert recently called attention to the importance of this disease as a cause of internal hydrocephalus.

The pathological changes reported by various observers have not been uniform. Barlow and Lees, Hildesheim, and Bettencourt and Franca believe that the process always occluded the foramina of Magendie and Luschka. Barlow and Lees observed only two cases in a large series in which no occlusion was found and thought the hydrocephalus in these cases was due to an overproduction of fluid. Göppert, from post-mortem examination of twenty-three cases, classified the anatomical findings under three types: (1) total occlusion, four cases; (2) foramen of Magendie closed, but the foramina of Luschka large, six cases; (3) all the foramina patent, thirteen cases. Göppert's determination of the patency or occlusion of these openings was made by granular injections into the ventricles post mortem. The results of most observers have been based on inspection of the base of the brain, from which it is impossible to determine the condition of the foramina with certainty.

Why an internal hydrocephalus should result with patent foramina has never been demonstrated. We are unable to give the pathological basis for hydrocephalus of the communicating type owing to the fact that all of our patients are living; but the evidence here presented gives an explanation for the production of this type of hydrocephalus.

13. THE RELATION OF VENOUS STASIS TO INTERNAL HYDROCEPHALUS

Venous stasis due to obstruction of the small or the large veins of Galen is undoubtedly the cause of a small percentage of the cases of internal hydrocephalus. Experimental proof of this has been given. Internal hydrocephalus resulting from thrombosis by these veins has also been reported. Although such a cause of hydrocephalus is infrequent, it should always be looked for post mortem. It is also possible

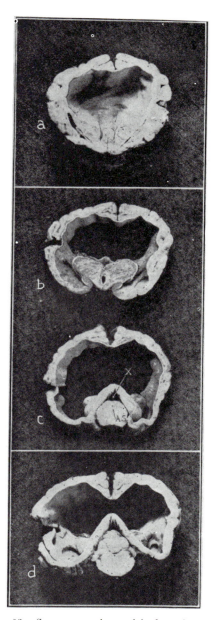

Fig. 23.—Spontaneous internal hydrocephalus in a dog found by Dr. A. P. Jones. The aqueduct of Sylvius (*A. S.*) is completely occluded. The lateral ventricles form a single cavity owing to the absorption of the septum lucidum. A free communication is present between the third ventricle and the subdural space at *X*, but the hydrocephalus is not modified owing to the poor absorption from the subdural space. Note the small fourth ventricle posterior to the obstruction.

TABLE 6.—SUMMARY OF GROUP 2, INTERNAL HYDROCEPHALUS WITHOUT OBSTRUCTION*

Case	Illness	Absorption after Ventricular Introduction		Absorption after Spinal Introduction		Communication between Ventricular and Subarachnoid space	Duration of excretion after		Kidney function 2 hours Per cent	Etiology
		Time of appearance Minutes	Two-hour absorption Per cent	Time of appearance Minutes	Two-hour absorption Per cent	Time of Appearance in Spinal Canal following Ventricular Introduction—Minutes	Ventricular introduction	Spinal introduction		
8. R. G.	Internal hydrocephalus	30	2	Not obt.	11	1	Longer than 2 days	0	44	Definite history of meningitis. Hydrocephalus followed immediately.
9. M. R.	Internal hydrocephalus following epidemic meningitis. Two months later	20 13–15	2.3 6.5	13	7	2 ?—	....	More than 24 hrs.	40 (1st hr.)	Followed meningitis.
10. H. N.	Internal hydrocephalus	20 25	0.5 4.4	8 Not obt. Not obt.	14 9.5 10	2 20	....	....	45	Hydrocephalus noted 6 weeks after birth. May have resulted from illness 3 days after birth.
11. J. C.	Internal hydrocephalus	About 25 30	4 4	Not obt. 0	10 0	13 1	0	0	Not tested.	

* No post-mortem examination in any case.

that tumors in the region of the midbrain might exert sufficient pressure to obstruct either the aqueduct or the veins of Galen. We are inclined to regard venous stasis as being of relative minor importance in the production of hydrocephalus.

Certainly in very young children tumors are uncommon, and the obstructive process is usually insufficient to produce a simultaneous involvement of the veins. In adults, among whom tumors are more common, it may play a more frequent but always a subsidiary rôle, because the aqueduct of Sylvius will usually also be occluded.

14. THE POSSIBILITY OF OTHER CAUSES OF INTERNAL HYDROCEPHALUS

Almost every conceivable cause, direct and indirect, has been suggested as being responsible for hydrocephalus. Alcohol, rickets, trauma, tuberculosis, syphilis, heredity, psychic disturbance during pregnancy, lack of resistance of the brain tissue, osteogenetic defects of the skull and many other less likely possibilities have been suggested. Syphilis is undoubtedly responsible for a certain number of cases, but to cause hydrocephalus, syphilis must produce a lesion which involves the cerebrospinal spaces and cause a diminished absorption of cerebrospinal fluid either by occlusion of the foramina or by an affection of the meninges. In not one of our cases was there any evidence by serological test that syphilis was the etiological factor. Elsner thought syphilis responsible in three cases out of eighteen, and Hadenfeldt in 10 per cent of his cases. It is very unlikely that as systemic diseases without localized manifestations syphilis, tuberculosis, rickets and alcoholism have any etiological bearing on the production of internal hydrocephalus.

There was no familial or hereditary history of hydrocephalus in our cases. Göhlis reports an instance of a woman who gave birth to six still-born, hydrocephalic children.

The production of hydrocephalus by trauma is very difficult to prove. We have seen one case (not here recorded) in which the father, who was a physician, insisted that the onset of the disease dated from a severe fall. Various congenital anomalies have been associated with hydrocephalus, such as hydrothorax, absence of kidney, cleft palate, bicornuate uterus, etc. The occurrence of internal hydrocephalus with spina bifida has been frequently noted. There were three such instances present in our series of cases.

Lack of resistance of cerebral tissue and imperfect development of the skull, though frequently suggested as causes of hydrocephalus, have been mentioned merely as possibilities. The cerebral atrophy and non-union of the sutures of the skull are undoubtedly secondary manifestations of the intracranial pressure.

15. INTERNAL HYDROCEPHALUS FOLLOWING THE REMOVAL OF A MENINGOCELE

Internal hydrocephalus following the extirpation of a meningocele has been frequently reported, but the cause for its development has never been satisfactorily explained. Muscatello, who has reported a series of cases of this character, attributed the hydrocephalus to an operative infection. His reason for doing this was based on the frequency with which ulceration of the meningocele was observed.

From our observations on the general character of absorption of fluid from the subarachnoid space, it is most likely that the hydrocephalus results from a diminution in the absorption of the cerebrospinal fluid. This diminished absorption takes place because a large part of the absorbing surface is removed at the time of the operation.

Before removing a meningocele, it is important to determine the absorption from the subarachnoid space in order to determine whether or not it is sufficient. If absorption is below the normal, operation in the light of our present knowledge would be contra-indicated.

16. SUGGESTIONS AS TO THE TREATMENT OF INTERNAL HYDROCEPHALUS

We have shown that there are two types of internal hydrocephalus differing physiologically and anatomically, and it is obvious that an entirely different therapy is necessary for each variety. In the treatment it is important to know which type of hydrocephalus is present—the obstructive or the communicating. This can be determined by the phenolsulphonephthalein test.

In the obstructive type of internal hydrocephalus, the treatment should be directed toward removal of the obstruction. If this is at the foramina of Magendie and Luschka, as in Cases 5 and 6 of Group 1, the obstruction without doubt could be relieved. If the occlusion is located at the aqueduct of Sylvius, as in Cases 2 and 3 of Group 1, the problem of making an opening is obviously more difficult, perhaps impossible. It would also be necessary, before undertaking such an operation, to determine the amount of absorption from the subarachnoid space. If there is a low subarachnoid absorption as in Case 6 of Group 1, it is probable that the relief of the obstruction would merely transform an internal hydrocephalus of the obstructive type into one of the communicating type.

In the communicating type, the internal hydrocephalus is the result of diminished absorption from the subarachnoid space. In one case the post-mortem findings indicated that adhesions from an old inflammation produced obliteration of the cisterna magna and prevented the cerebral subarachnoid space from participation in the absorption. At present, the rational treatment in this type of hydrocephalus would be to drain the fluid into other tissues where there is adequate absorption.

17. SUMMARY AND CONCLUSIONS

An internal hydrocephalus was experimentally produced in dogs by placing an obstruction in the aqueduct of Sylvius.

It is therefore evident that the cerebrospinal fluid is formed in the ventricles faster than it can be absorbed, and that the aqueduct of Sylvius is essential for its escape.

An internal hydrocephalus resulted from placing an obstruction in the aqueduct of Sylvius in spite of the extirpation of the choroid plexus of both lateral ventricles. This procedure apparently modifies the grade of the internal hydrocephalus.

An internal hydrocephalus may also result from an experimental ligation of the vena Galena magna near its origin; when the ligature is more distally placed or when the sinus rectus alone is ligated, an internal hydrocephalus does not result, owing to the efficient venous collateral circulation.

Cerebrospinal fluid is derived mainly from the choroid plexuses, probably both by filtration and by secretion.

An increase of cerebrospinal fluid is caused by general venous congestion as demonstrated by temporary jugular compression. This increase of fluid ceases when the congestion is relieved by the collateral circulation.

Drugs and glandular extracts produce but slight change in the rapidity of formation of cerebrospinal fluid. Pilocarpin produced a slight increase.

There is a definite impermeability of the fluid-forming structures. Of the various substances in solution in the blood, only traces of a few find their way into the cerebrospinal fluid. The cerebrospinal fluid is more strongly protected from substances in the blood than the peritoneal, pleural and pericardial fluids.

There is a rapid and constant formation and absorption of cerebrospinal fluid. A new supply is formed and absorbed at least every four to six hours.

The lymphatics play a negligible part in the absorption of cerebrospinal fluid.

Cerebrospinal fluid is absorbed directly into the blood. Absorption is from the entire subarachnoid space. It is a diffuse process and does not take place through specialized structures such as the pacchionian granulations or through stomata opening into the venous sinuses. That stomata do not exist is demonstrated by the fact that granules do not readily pass from the subarachnoid space into the blood.

There is practically no absorption from the ventricles.

The maintenance of an equilibrium between the formation and the absorption of cerebrospinal fluid necessitates a communication between the ventricles and the subarachnoid space.

Communication is solely by the foramina of Magendie and Luschka.

After the introduction of phenolsulphonephthalein into the subarachnoid space it soon appears in the lateral ventricles. There are therefore no valves at these openings.

If an obstruction exists at the aqueduct of Sylvius, phenolsulphonephthalein does not appear in the spinal fluid. The so-called foramina of Mierzejewsky and Bichat therefore do not exist.

Granules placed in the subarachnoid space, without pressure, are soon uniformly distributed throughout the entire spinal and cerebral subarachnoid space. There is no evidence of a current to the region of the venous sinuses. Granules pass along the olfactory and optic nerves, over the gasserian ganglion of the trigeminal nerve and a short distance along the auditory nerves, but not along the remaining cranial and spinal nerves.

Internal hydrocephalus can be divided into two anatomically different types, depending on the patency or occlusion of communication between the ventricles and the subarachnoid space.

In seven patients with internal hydrocephalus lack of communication was demonstrated clinically. In each of these seven cases there was practically no absorption from the ventricles, while the subarachnoid absorption was high. The internal hydrocephalus, therefore, resulted because the passage of fluid from the ventricles into the subarachnoid space was prevented.

Four cases of internal hydrocephalus in which there was communication between the ventricles and the subarachnoid space were studied. In these cases there was a low subarachnoid absorption. Meningitis was the cause of the hydrocephalus in two patients with the obstructive type and two with the communicating type of hydrocephalus.

The probable cause of internal hydrocephalus following the excision of a meningocele is the limitation of absorbing surface and consequent diminution in the absorption of cerebrospinal fluid.

Surgical treatment differs according to the variety of internal hydrocephalus. *In the obstructive type* the obstruction must be removed. *In the communicating type* it is necessary to increase the area for the absorption of fluid.

BIBLIOGRAPHY

Achard, C., and Ribot, A.: Passage de l'iodure de potassium dans liquide céphalo-rachidien normal, Compt. rend. Soc. de biol., Paris, 1909, lxvi, 916.

Adamkiewicz: Ueber den Sagen "Hirndruck," die Bewegung der Cerebrospinalflüssigkeit im Schädel und den "Druck im Gehirn," Neurol. Centralbl., 1897, xvi, 434.

Adamkiewicz: Sitz. d. k. Akad. d. Wissensch., Wien, 1883, lxxxviii, 11, 311.

Alexandroff, S.: Ueber fötalen Hydrocephalus auf Grund der Falle der Königlichen Charité, Inaug. Diss., Berlin, 1901.

d'Astros: Les hydrocéphalie, Paris, 1898.

Axhausen: Zur Kenntnis der Meningitis serosa acuta, Berl. klin. Wchnschr., 1909, xlvi, 244.

Ballance, Charles A.: Some Experiences in Intracranial Surgery, Tr. Am. Surg. Assn., 1906, xxiv, 160.

Bárány, R.: Ein operativ geheilter Fall von otitischem Kleinhirnabscez der rechten Hemisphäre, Wien. med. Wchnschr., 1911, lxi, 523.

Barlow and Lees: On Hydrocephalus, Allbutt's System of Medicine, vii.

Bartels, P.: Das Lymphgefässsystem, von Bardeleben's Handbuch der Anatomie des Menschen, Jena, 1909.

Baxter: Chronic Hydrocephalus with Meningocele, Med. Times and Gaz., March, 1882, i, 239.

Biedl, A.: Innere Sekretion, Berlin, 1913.

Bibergeil et Levaditi: Quoted by Francini.

Birch-Hirschfeld: Lehrbuch der path. Anat., 1894, ii, 277.

Blumenthal: Ueber Cerebrospinalflüssigkeit, Ergeb. d. Physiol., i, Abt. 1, 285.

Böhm: Experimentelle Studien über die Dura mater des Menschen und der Säugethiere, Virchows Arch. f. path. Anat., 1869, xlvii, 218.

Bonhoeffer, K.: Der erworbene Hydrocephalus, Lewandowsky's Handbuch der Neurologie, Spezielle Neurologie II, iii, 729.

Bonhoeffer, Obduktionsbefund bei iodiopath. Hydrocephalus, Jahresb. d. schles. Gesellsch. f. vaterl. Kult., 1908; Zwei Kranke mit akut entwickeltem Hydrocephalus, Allg. med. Central. Ztg., 1908.

Bourneville: Des quelques formes de l'hydrocéphalie. Recherches sur l'épilepsie, l'hystérie, l'idiotie et l'hydrocéphalie, Compt. rend. pour l'année, 1883.

Bourneville and Noir: Hydrocéphale, Progrès méd., 1900, xii, 17.

Bramwell, B.: On the Localization of Intracranial Tumors, Brain, 1889, xxii, 1.

Broca: Des exstirpations de spina bifida, Revue d'orthop., 1895, vi, 38.

Browning, W.: Veins of the Brain, Brooklyn, 1884.

Bruno, Cramer und Ziehen: Handbuch der Nervenkrankheiten im Kindesalter, 1913, p. 876.

Bettencourt and França: Ztschr. f. Hyg. und Infectionskrankh., 1904, xlvi.

Cannieu: Recherches sur la voute du quatrième ventricule des vertèbres, Bibliog. Anat., 1898, vi, 159.

Cappelletti, L.: L'écoulement du liquide cérébro-spinale par la fistula céphalorachidienne en conditiones normales et sous l'influence de quelques médicaments, Arch. ital. de biol., 1901, xxxvi, 299.

Cavazzani: Contributo alla fisiologie del liquido cerebrospinale, Centralbl. f. Physiol., 1901, xv, 216.

Claiso, P., and Levi, C.: Etude histologique d'un cas d'hydrocéphalie interne, Bull. Soc. med. de Paris, 1897, lxxii, 264.

Crowe, S. J.: On the Excretion of Hexamethylenamin (Urotropin) in the Cerebrospinal Fluid and Its Therapeutic Value, Johns Hopkins Hosp. Bull., 1909, xx, 102.

Cushing, H.: Physiologische und anatomische Beobachtungen über den intracraniellen Kreislauf, etc., Mitt. a. d. Grenzgeb. d. Med. u. Chir., 1902, ix, 773.

Cushing, H.: Keen's Surgery, 1911, iii.

Cushing, H., and Sladen, F. J.: Obstructive Hydrocephalus Following Cerebrospinal Meningitis, with Intraventricular Injection of Antimeningitis Serum (Flexner), Jour. Exper. Med., 1908, x, 548.

Dandy, W. E., and Rowntree, L. G.: Peritoneale und pleurale Resorption in ihren Beziehungen zu der Lagerungsbehandlung, Beit. zur klin. Chir., 1913, lxxxvii, 539.

Dexler, H.: Beiträge zur Pathogenese und pathologischen Anatomie der Hydrocephalus internus des Pferdes, Neurol. Centralbl., 1899, xviii, 924.

Dietzfelbringer, H.: Beitrag zur Lehre von Hydrocephalus, Inaug. Dissert., Erlangen, 1907.

Dixon, W. E., and Halliburton, W. D.: The Cerebrospinal Fluid. 1. Secretion of the Fluid, Jour. Physiol., 1913, xlvii, 341.

Dixon, W. E., and Halliburton, W. D.: The Rapidity of Absorption of Drugs Introduced into the Cerebrospinal Fluid, Jour. Physiol., 1912, xliv, Proc. Physiol. Soc., p. vii.

Dixon, W. E., and Halliburton, W. D.: The Action of Choroid Plexuses on the Secretion of the Cerebrospinal Fluid, Jour. Physiol., 1910, xl, Proc. Physiol. Soc., p. xxx.

Dochez, A. R.: Proteolytic Enzymes and Antienzymes of Normal and Pathological Cerebrospinal Fluids, Jour. Exper. Med., 1909, xi, 718.

Ducrot, R., and Gautrelet, J.: Présence des pigments biliaires dans le liquide céphalo-rachidien après suppression physiologique des plexus choroïdes. Les plexus choroïdes jouents le rôle de véritables glandes sécrétants le liquide céphalo-rachidien, Compt. rend Soc. de biol., 1905, lvii, 161.

Ducrot, R., and Gautrelet, J.: Présence des pigments normaux sérum sanguin dans le liquide céphalo-rachidien après suppression physiologiques des plexus choroïdes, Compt. rend. Soc. de biol., 1905, lvii, 289.

Engel: Ueber die Sekretionserscheinungen in den Zellen der Plexus choroidei des Menschen, Arch. f. Zellforsch., 1909, ii.

Faivre, E.: Recherches sur la structure du conarium et des plexus choroïdes chez l'homme et chez les animaux, Compt. rend. l'Acad. d. sc., 1854, xxxiv, 424.

Faivre, E.: Etude sur le conarium et les plexus choroïdes de l'homme et des animaux, Ann. d. sc. nat. Par., 1857, vii, 52; Gaz. méd. de Paris, 1854, No. 36.

Falkenheim and Naunyn: Ueber Hirndruck, Arch. f. exper. Path. u. Pharmakol., 1887, xxii, 261.

Findlay, J. W.: The Choroid Plexuses of the Lateral Ventricles of the Brain, Their Histology, Normal and Pathological (in Relation Especially to Insanity), Brain, 1897, xxii, 161.

Finkelnburg: Zur Differentialdiagnose zwischen Kleinhirntumoren und chronischem Hydrocephalus, Deutsch. Ztschr. f. Nervenh., 1905, xxix, 135. Beitrag zur Anwendung der Hirnpunktion bei chronischem Hydrocephalus, München. med. Wchnschr., 1910, lvii, 1871.

Flexner, S.: Experimental Cerebrospinal Meningitis in Monkeys, Jour. Exper. Med., 1907, ix, 142.

Foerster: Handbuch der speciellen pathologischen Anatomie, Jena, 1863, p. 598.

Foster, N. B.: Sugar in the Cerebrospinal Fluid of Diabetes: A Preliminary Report, Boston Med. and Surg. Jour., 1905, cliii, 441.

Francini, M.: Sur la structure et la function des plexus choroidieus, Arch. ital. de biol., 1907, xlviii, 352.

Fuchs: Ueber Beobachtungen an Sekret- und Flimmerzellen, Anat. Hefte, Abt. I, 1904, xxv, 503.

Fuchs: Die Veränderungen der Dura mater bei endocraniellen Drucksteigerungen, Arb. a. d. neurolog. Inst. a. d. Wien. Univ., 1903, x; Idiopathischen Hydrocephalus internus, ibid., 1904, xi, 62.

Galeotti: Studio morfologico e citalogico della volta del diencefalo in alcuni vertebrati, Riv. di patol. nerv., 1897, ii, 481.

Geigel, R.: Die Rolle des Liquor cerebralis bei der Circulation im Schädel, Arch. f. d. ges. Physiol., 1905, cix, 337.

Gerhartz, H.: Oppenheimer's Handbuch der Biochemie des Menschen und der Tiere, Jena, 1909.

Göppert, F.: Zur Kenntnis der Meningitis cerebrospinalis epidemica mit besonderer Berücksichtigung des Kindesalters, Klin. Jahrb., 1906, xv, 523.

Goldmann, E. E.: Vitalfärbung am Zentralnervensystem; Beiträge zur Physio-pathologie des Plexus choroideus und der Hirnhäute, Berlin, 1913.

Gowers: Diseases of the Nervous System, Philadelphia, 1892.

Gurlt: Ueber thierische Missgeburten. Ein Beitrag zur pathologischen Anatomie und Entwickelungsgeschichte, iv, Berlin, 1877.

Hadenfeldt: Ueber die Häufigkeit des chronischen Hydrocephalus in Kindesalter, Kiel, 1898.

Halben: Hydrocephalus internus idiopath., etc., Deutsch. med. Wchnschr., 1909, p. 438.

Halliburton, W. D.: Cerebrospinal Fluid. Jour. Physiol., 1889, x, 232.

Hart: St. Bartholomew's Hosp. Rep., London, 1876.

Hedon: Circulation veineuse de l'encéphale. Thèse de Bordeaux, 1888.

Heile: Zur Behandlung des Hydrocephalus, Deutsch. med. Wchnschr., 1908, p. 1468.

Henle, A.: Beitrag zur Pathologie und Therapie des Hydrocephalus, Mitt. a. d. Grenzgeb. d. Med. u. Chir., 1896, i, 264.

Herrick, F. C.: An Experimental Study into the Cause of the Increased Portal Pressure in Cirrhosis, Jour. Exper. Med., 1907, ix, 93.

Hess: Das Foramen Magendie, Morph. Jahrbuch., 1885, x, 578.

Heubner: Eulenberg's Encyclopädie.

Heuser, C. H.: The Development of the Cerebral Ventricles in the Pig, Am. Jour. Anat., 1913, xv, 215.

Hill, L.: The Physiology and Pathology of the Cerebral Circulation, London, 1896; Allbutt's System of Medicine, 1899, vii, 239.

Hilton: Rest and Pain, New York, 1879.

Horsley, J. S.: Surgical Treatment of Congenital Hydrocephalus, Jour. Am. Med. Assn., 1906, xlvii, 1.

Hworostuchin: Zur Frage über den Bau des Plexus Choroideus, Arch. f. mikr. Anat., 1911, lxxvii, 232.

Iscovesco, H.: Etude sur les constituants colloïdes des humeurs de l'organisme., Jour. de physiol. et pathol. gén., 1907, ix, 793; Le liquide céphalo-rachidien normal, Compt. rend. Soc. de biol., 1907, lxii, 181.

Joslin, E. P.: Internal Hydrocephalus Following Cerebrospinal Meningitis, Am. Jour. Med. Sc., 1900, cxx, 444.

Kafka: Die Cerebrospinalflüssigkeit, Ztschr. f. d. ges Neurol. u. Psychiat., 1912, vi, 321.

Kalischer, S.: Der angeborens Hydrocephalus, Lewandowsky's Handbuch der Neurologie, Spezielle Neurologie II, iii, 714.

Keen: Drainage der Hirnventrikel, Mercrédi méd., 1890; Surgery of the Lateral Ventricles of the Brain, Verhandl. d. x. internat. med. congr., Berlin, iii, Chirurgie, 1891.

Kestner, P.: Hydrocephalus und Hypoplasie der Nebennieren, Centralbl. f. allg. Path. u. path. Anat., 1907, xviii, 433.

Key, A., and Retzius, G.: Studien in der Anatomie des Nervensystems und des Bindesgewebes, Stockholm, 1875.

Knox, J. H. M., and Sladen, F. J.: Hydrocephalus of Meningococcus Origin, with a Summary of Recent Cases of Meningitis Treated by Antimeningococcus Serum, Arch. Pediat., 1908, xxv, 761.

Kochel, R.: Ueber Thrombose der Hirnsinus bei Chlorose, Deutsch. Arch. f. klin. Med., 1894, lii, 557.

Koplik: Hydrocephalus Complicating Epidemic Cerebrospinal Meningitis, Am. Jour. Med. Sc., 1907, xxxiii, 547.

Kramer: The Circulation of the Cerebrospinal Fluid and Its Bearing on the Pathogenesis of Poliomyelitis Disease, New York Med. Jour., 1912, xcv, 532.

Krause: Subcutane Dauerdrainage der Hirnventrikel bei Hydrocephalus, Berl. klin. Wchnschr., 1908, No. 29.

Lagriffaul, A., Roger H., and Mestrezat, W.: Le liquide céphalorachidien dans la fièvre de Malta, Compt. rend Soc. de biol., 1910, lxviii, 358.

Laquerie, J. Clémenceau de la: Glycometrie der Cerebrospinalflüssigkeit, Thèse de Paris, 1905.

Laworn, D.: Brit. Med. Jour., 1893, i, 1322.

Lazarus-Barlow, U. S.: Contribution to the Study of Lymph Formation, with Especial Reference to the Parts Played by Osmosis and Filtration, Jour. Physiol., 1896, xix, 418.

Leber: Der gegenwärtige Stand unserer Kenntnisse von Flüssigkeitswechsel des Auges, Ergebn. d. Anat. u. Entwcklgsgesch. Wiesb., 1894, iv, 144.

Lehmann: Chemistry of the Cerebrospinal Fluid, Handbuch der physiologische Chemie, 1854, p. 137.

Lewandowsky, M.: Zur Lehre von der Cerebrospinalflüssigkeit, Ztschr. f. klin. Med., 1900, xl, 480; Neurol. Centralbl., 1901, p. 447.

Luschka, H.: Die Adergeflechte des menschlichen Gehirns, Berlin, 1855.

Luschka, H.: Zur Lehre von der Secretionzelle, Arch. f. physiol. Heilkunde, 1854, xiii, 1.

Macewen: Pyogenic Infectious Diseases of the Brain, Spinal Cord, etc., Glasgow, 1893.

Mackenzie, S.: The Diagnosis of Tumors of the Cerebellum, Lancet, London, 1880, i, 559.

Magendie, F.: Recherches physiologiques et cliniques sur le liquide céphalorachidien ou cérébro-spinal, Paris, 1842

Mall, F. P.: On the Development of the Blood-Vessels of the Brain in the Human Embryo, Am. Jour. Anat., 1905, iv, 1.

Marc, See: Sur la communication des cavités ventriculares de l'encéphale, Rev. mens. de Chir., 1878–1879.

McClure, R. D.: Hydrocephalus Treated by Drainage into a Vein of the Neck, Johns Hopkins Hosp. Bull., 1909, xx, 110.

McGuillaio: La circulation de la lymphe dans le moelle épinière, Revue neurol., 1899, No. 23.

Meek, W. J.: A Study of the Choroid Plexus, Jour. Comp. Neurol. und Psychol., 1907, xvii, No. 3.

Merkel: Topographische Anatomie, 1907, i, 79.

Merkel, Gottlieb: Sechs Fälle von protrahirter Meningitis cerebrospinalis epidemica nebst einigen Worten über die mögliche Enstehungsweise des Hydrocephalus in solchen Fällen, Arch. f. klin. Med., 1866, i, 519.

Mestrezat, W.: Le liquide céphalo-rachidien normal et pathologique, Jour. de physiol. et de path. gén., 1912, xiv, 504.

Milian: Le liquide céphalo-rachidien, Paris, 1904.

Monro: On the Brain, the Eye and the Ear, Edinburgh, 1793.

Monro, A.: Observations on the Structure and Function of the Venous System, Edinburgh, 1783.

Morgagni: De Sedibus et Causis Morborum, Epist. anat. med., xii.

Mott, F. W.: Cerebrospinal Fluid, Lancet, London, 1910; Brit. Med. Jour., 1904, ii, 1554.

Mott, F. W., and Barratt, J. O. W.: Three Cases of Tumor of the Third Ventricle, Arch. Neurol., i, 434.

Muscatello, G.: Ueber die Diagnose der Spina Bifida und über die postoperativ Hydrocephalus, Arch. f. klin. Chir., 1902, lxviii, 267.

Muscatello, G.: Ueber einen nicht gewöhnlichen Fall von Cephalocele und die post-operativ Hydrocephalus, Arch. f. klin. Chir., 1902, lxviii, 248.

Nawratzki, E.: Zur Kenntniss der Cerebrospinalflüssigkeit, Ztschr. f. physiol. Chem., 1897, xxiii, 532.

Neumann, H.: Ein Fall von geheiltem Wasserkopf, Deutsch. med. Wchnschr., 1891, iii, 39.

Neurath: Demonstration of a Case of Internal Hydrocephalus, Neurol. Centralbl., 1896, xv, 87.

Olmer, D., and Tian, A.: Perméabilité des méninges normales au salicylates de lithium, Compt. rend. Soc. de biol., 1909, lxvi, 894.

Orton: A Pathological Study of a Case of Hydrocephalus, Am. Jour. Insan., lxv, 229.

Osterwald, K.: Beitrag zur Diagnose des Cysticercus Ventriculi Quarti, Neurol. Centralbl., March 16, 1906.

Oules, M.: Sur un cas d'hydrocéphalie chez un chien, Toulouse méd., 1909, 2 ser., xi, 250.

Panzer, T.: Zur Kenntniss der Cerebrospinalflüssigkeit, Wien klin. Wchnschr., 1899, p. 805.

Parkin, A.: Operative Treatment of Hydrocephalus, Lancet, London, 1893, ii, 21, 1244.

Petit, T., and Girard, J.: Sur la function sécréatoire et la morphologie de plexus choroïdes, Arch. d'Anat. Micro., 1902–1903, v, 213.

Poirier and Charpy: Traité d'anatomie humaine, 1901, iii, 152.

Power, D'Arcy: The Results of a Year's Experience in the Surgical Treatment of Hydrocephalus in Children, Internat. Clin., ser. 5, 1895, iii, 254.

Propping: Die Mechanik des Liquor cerebrospinalis und ihre Anwendung auf die Lumbal-Anästhesia, Mitt. a. d. Grenzgeb. d. Med. u. Chir., 1909, xix, 441.

Purkinje: Ueber Flimmerbewegungen in Gehirn, Müller's Archiv, 1836.

Quincke: Zur Pathologie der Meningen, Deutsch. Ztschr. f. Nervenh., 1909, xxxvi; 1910, xl.

Quincke: Die Lumbalpunktion des Hydrocephalus, Berl. klin. Wchnschr., 1891, xxxviii.

Recklinghausen: Recherches su le spina bifida, Arch. f. path. Anat. und Physiol., 1886, cv.

Von Recklinghausen: Pathologie des Kreislaufs.

Regnault, F.: Forme du crâne dans l'hydrocéphalie chez les animaux, Bull. et Mém. Soc. Anat. de Paris, 1901, lxxvi, 460.

Rehn: Ueber Rückenmarksanästhesie, Mitt. a. d. Grenzgeb. d. Med. u. Chir., 1909, xix, 806.

Von Reichmann: Zur Physiologie und Pathologie des Liquor cerebrospinalis, Deutsch. Ztschr. f. Nervenh., xlii.

Reiner, M., and Schnitzler, J.: Fragments aus der experimentelle Pathologie, Wien, 1894; abst. Neurolog. Centralbl., 1895, p. 19.

Retzius: Das Menschenhirn, 1896, p. 38.

Rosenblatt, L.: Der congenitale Hydrocephalus und seine Beziehung zur Geburt (Giessen), Inaug. Dissert., Wiesbaden, 1898.

Rotky: Untersuchungen über die Durchlössigkeit der Meningen für chemische Stoffe, Ztschr. f. klin. Med.,1912, lxxv, 494.

Roubinovitsch, J., and Paillard, J.: La pression du liquide céphalo-rachidien dans diverses maladies mentales, Compt. rend Soc. de biol., 1910, lxviii, 582.

Rous, F. P.: Clinical Studies of the Cerebrospinal Fluid, Am. Jour. Med. Sc., 1907, cxxxiii, 567.

Rowntree, L. G., and Geraghty, J. T.: An Experimental and Clinical Study of the Functional Activity of the Kidneys by Means of Phenolsulphonephthalein, Jour. Pharmacol. and Exper. Therap., 1909–1910, i, 576.

Ruffer, M. Armand: Chronic Hydrocephalus, Brain, 1890, xiii, 117.

Schlöpfer, V.: Ueber den Bau und die Funktion der Epithelzellen des Plexus choroideus in Beziehung zur Granuladehre und mit besondere Berücksichtigung der vitalen Färbungsmethoden, Beitr. z. path. Anat. u. z. allg. Path., Suppl. VII, p. 101.

Schmorl: Liquor cerebrospinalis und Ventrikelflüssigkeit, Verhandl. d. deutsch. pathol. Gesellsch., Erlangen, 1910.

Schultze: Die Krankheiten der Hirnhäute und die Hydrocephalie, Nothnagel's Spec. Path. u. Therapie, 1901, ix.

Sicard, A.: Les injections sous-arachnoidiennes et le liquide céphalorachidien, Thèse de Paris, 1899.

Spiller, W. G.: Internal Hydrocephalus, Jour. Am. Med. Assn., 1907, xliii, 1225.

Spiller, W. G.: Two Cases of Partial Internal Hydrocephalus from Closure of the Interventricular Passage, Am. Jour. Med. Sc., 1902, cxxiv, 44.

Spina, A.: Untersuchungen über die Resorption des Liquors bei normalen und Erhalten intercraniellen Druck, Neurolog. Centralbl., xx, 224; Arch. f. d. ges. Physiol., lxxxiii, 120, 415.

Starling, E. H.: Fluids of the Body, Chicago, 1909.

Storch, K.: Ungewöhnlich hoher Grad der Hydrocephalie mit consecutiver Missbildung des Schädels, der Augen und der Nase beim Kalb, Oesterr. Monatschr. f. Tierh., Wien, 1891, xv, 197.

Studnicka, F. K.: Untersuchungen über den Bau des Ependyma der nervösen Centralorgane, Anat. Hefte, 1900, xv, 303.

Stursberg: Ein Beitrag zur Kenntniss der Cerebrospinalflüssigkeit, Deutsch. Ztschr. f. Nervenh., 1911, xlii, 325.

Sutton: The Lateral Recesses of the Fourth Ventricle; Their Relation to Certain Cysts and Tumors of the Cerebellum and to Occipital Meningocele, Brain, 1887, ix, 352.

Thomson, St. Clair: The Cerebrospinal Fluid, Lancet, London, 1899, i, 577.

Toison and Lenoble: Note sur la structure et la composition du liquide céphalo-rachidien, Compt. rend. Soc. de biol., 1891, p. 373.

Tourneux and Martin: Contribution à l'histoire du spina bifida, Jour. d. l'Anat., 1881, xvii, 283.

Trolard: Les lacunes veineuses de la dure mère, Jour. l'anat. et physiol., 1892, xxviii, 28.

Virchow, H.: Ein Fall von angeborenem Hydrocephalus internus, Fest-Schr., Albert v. Kölliker, Leipz., 1887.

Virchow: Handbuch der speziellen Pathologie und Therapie, Erlangen, 1851, i, 112; Die krankhaften Geschwülste, Berlin, 1863, vol. i.

Walter, F. K.: Studien über den Liquor cerebrospinalis, Monatschr. f. Psychiat. u. Neurol., xxviii, Erganzungs., p. 80.

Weber, L. W.: Ueber erworbenen Hydrocephalus, Arch. f. Psychiat., vol. xli.

Westenhoeffer: Pathologisch-anatomische Ergebnisse der oberschlesischen Genickstarreepidemie von 1905, Klin. Jahrb., Berl., 1906, xv, 657.

Whytt, R.: Observations on the Dropsy in the Brain, Edinburgh, 1768.

Zalociecki: Zur Frage der Permeabilität der Meningen insbesondere Immunstoffen gegenüber, Deutsch. Ztschr. f. Nervenh., 1913, xlvi, 195.

Ziemssen: Handbuch. d. acuten Infectionskrankh., Part 2, 1874, p. 683.

Ziemssen and Hess: Klinische Beobachtungen über Meningitis cerebrospinalis epidemica, Arch. f. klin. Med., 1866, i, 72, 346.

Ziemssen: Ueber den diagnostischen und therapeutische Wert der Punktion des Wirbelkanalis, Verhandl. d. cong. f. innere Med., 1893, xii.

Neurosurgical Classic—8

ONE of the most interesting stories in the history of neurosurgery concerns the disagreement between David Ferrier and Friedrich Goltz at the 1881 International Medical Congress in London.[12,13,19,21—24,29,31,37] Their encounter was important because its outcome provided a vital stimulus to successful cerebral surgery.[2,3,26,27,33,34,38] Of incidental interest is the fact that, because of his presentation at the Congress, Ferrier was later forced to appear at the Bow Street Police Court to answer charges made by the Victoria Street Society for the Protection of Animals from Vivisection.[4—7,25,31]

Despite the fact that by 1881 the foundations of cerebral localization had been laid by Broca, Fritsch, Hitzig, Jackson, and others, there were still a considerable number of qualified persons who believed that the cerebrum acted as a whole.[30,35,36] Professor Goltz of Strassburg, a respected pioneer in the newly expanded field of neurophysiology, was their leader.[1,16—20] In experiments with dogs, Goltz had removed almost the entire cerebral cortex bilaterally without finding much change in their motor and sensory functions. He brought one of these dogs to London to provide demonstrable proof that discrete cerebral functional centers did not exist. Professor Ferrier, on the other hand, had just completed extensive experiments on primates which led to opposite conclusions.[8—11,13—15,28,32] The stage was therefore set for the "Discussion of Localization of the Vital Functions in the Cerebral Cortex" held in the hall of the Royal Institute on Thursday, August 4.

Goltz began with an address in German in which he challenged concepts basic to the hypothesis of cerebral localization.

" . . .'When as the result of a stimulus we observe a group of muscles twitching, say of the foot, we cannot say that the stimulus to a given nerve or system produced the reaction. Reactions of foot muscles can be produced by stimuli applied to the motor nerves, the spinal cord, the brain, or certain sensory nerves. Hence, the fact that stimulus of a section of the nervous system causes reactions in foot muscles does not necessarily lead to definite conclusions about the functional significance of the stimulated organ. I cannot know whether the origin of the stimulus was a motor or a sensory channel, or whether a central organ was directly stimulated. The problems are increased in experiments with the cerebrum because we do not even know the extent to which electric currents applied in depth to the brain are responsible for the results.'

"There was, he declared, only one reliable method of proving whether or not motor and sensory centers existed: removal of those parts of the brain which supposedly represented functional centers. If the part of the brain which according to Professor Ferrier governed the movements of a foot were removed from a living creature, the foot ought subsequently to be paralyzed. If the foot were not paralyzed, every thinking person must regard it as proof positive that the so-called center for that particular movement did not exist. If one removed the part of the cerebral cortex which according to Professor Ferrier's claims should govern hearing, deafness should ensue. If deafness did not ensue, the alleged center for hearing did not exist.

"Fritsch and Hitzig, Professor Goltz continued, had already perceived the flaws of the method of stimulus and had attempted a few experiments with extirpation. But only a few experiments. As he would undertake to prove, such meager experimentation was wholly insufficient. Moreover, initial disturbances of the motor faculties or the senses after removal of parts of the cortex did not signify. If the experimental animals were kept alive for a considerable period of time, such disturbances or temporary paralyses disappeared completely or very largely. That alone proved that the old concept of the brain's functioning as a whole, so that any part of it could at all times take over for any other part, came closer to the truth than the theory of functional centers. He, Goltz, had for the first time developed the method of extirpation in a manner hitherto untried, and had kept numerous animals alive long enough to

119

be able to draw valid conclusions. He would now outline the results of his work.

" . . . 'In a large number of experiments . . . I made it my task to excise the largest possible parts of the cerebral cortex and to keep the animal alive and under observation as long as possible. In order to avoid hemorrhage, I extirpated the brain matter by washing away whole areas with a jet of water at high pressure.'

" . . . Employing this simple 'rinsing' method, Goltz went on, he had determined that dogs were only temporarily paralyzed, or disturbed in their sight, hearing, and sense of smell, by removal of large parts of the brain. They soon regained complete mobility and full sensory perception. These experiments refuted the theory of localization and proved that Flourens's old hypothesis had been the correct one all along. At most Flourens had overestimated the speed with which restitution of motor and sensory abilities took place. Flourens had, however, been mistaken in regard to a single point. He had assumed that a small remnant of brain would suffice to assume both the physical and mental functions of all the rest of the cerebrum. This was true of the physical but not of the mental functions. This error of Flourens's, however, in no way accrued to the support of the localization theory of Ferrier and his followers. They had confined themselves to studies of muscular and sensory functions and had failed to observe that every sizable operation upon both hemispheres of the brain led to more or less severe disturbances of mental ability. Ferrier alone had spoken of such disturbances. But he had also assigned a particular site to intelligence, namely the frontal lobe of the brain, and declared that mental disturbances followed only if this lobe were injured. Experiment proved, however, that every extensive injury to the brain produced mental derangement.

"In order to establish these results, here briefly summarized, upon a firm scientific basis, Goltz continued, he had discarded the water-jet method and developed an entirely new procedure which enabled him to extirpate precisely determined parts of the brain. 'I employed Whit's mechanical drill, which enables one to impart rapid rotation to small instruments. For the most part I used a kind of helical saw. By means of such an instrument it is comparatively easy to remove portions of the brain of any desired size. . . . In the cases of some dogs I undertook two, three, and four or more operations, and observed the degenerative symptoms with utmost care.'

"He described how he had trepanned the skulls of his dogs at various planes, removed the bone and the parts of the brain lying beneath, especially those areas which according to Ferrier constituted motor and sensory centers. . . . 'A dog,'

Goltz said . . . 'which was deprived of both frontal lobes of the cerebrum—one, that is, which according to Ferrier had lost its psychomotor centers—can move all its limbs, its lower jaw, tongue, tail, eyes, and ears. In short, it shows no evidence of muscular or sensory deficiencies.'

"Goltz opened a suitcase which lay on the lectern and took from it an obviously damaged skull of a dog, and a tiny preserved remnant of brain. 'This dog,' he declared, 'whose skull and brain I have here, survived four major operations, and was not killed until a full year had passed after the last operation. The dog was completely idiotic, making no response to men or animals. All his sense perceptions were severely impaired. But he was neither deaf nor blind, had lost neither the sense of smell nor of taste. Not a muscle of his body was paralyzed, not a spot on his hide robbed of sensation. This animal's brain weighs only fourteen grams. The brain of a healthy dog of the same age, size, and breed weighs ninety grams. Clearly, nothing was left in this brain of Ferrier's motor or sensory centers.'

" . . . 'To demonstrate the truth of my claims,' Goltz continued . . . 'I have brought with me from Strassburg a dog from whose brain I have removed, in the course of five operations between November 15, 1880, and May 25, 1881, the cortex from both parietal and occipital lobes. . . . You will be able to recognize the enormous extent of cerebral extirpation by the peculiar deformation of the head. If you run your fingers along the edges of the large gaps in the bony structure you will realize even more clearly how extensive the operations were which the animal has survived.' . . . He would use this dog to show, he continued, that one did not paralyze any muscle by destruction of any segment of the cerebral cortex, or permanently stamp out any of the sensory functions. He undertook to prove beyond the shadow of a doubt that Ferrier's theory was, as he had stated, completely wrong."[31]

Ferrier's reply to this challenge is reproduced below.[13] Its effect was not entirely manifested until that afternoon, when the assemblage visited Professor Gerald Yeo's laboratory at King's College to see the animals mentioned by Goltz and Ferrier. Goltz presented his dog first.

" . . . 'This dog . . . has travelled with me from Strassburg to London. As I indicated to you in my talk this morning, the animal has been deprived of by far the greater part of the cortical substance of both parietal lobes and both occipital lobes. A series of five operations were needed to produce this enormous cerebral extirpation. . . . The deformation of the animal's head is quite obvious. You can easily thrust several fingers into the huge gaps in the bony structure.'

"Goltz went on to say that the dog would prove the claims he had made that morning. He made the animal run, jump out of its cage, and move its head. Then he picked up a whip and snapped it. 'Go on, get out, go away!' he ordered, and drew attention to the cringing movement which indicated that the animal heard. He demonstrated that the dog could also see. He described his observation that the dog not only avoided large obstacles with facility, but would retreat from splashes of light on the floor caused by sun streaming in through the window. 'Observing this,' he continued, 'I devised the following experiment. I had a kind of flag sewed, consisting of a brilliantly white, broad strip of linen framed by two black stripes. If this flag is laid on the floor, the dog avoids stepping on the white area. I have brought the flag with me and will endeavor to repeat the experiment here.'

" . . . Goltz . . . spread out the cloth. The dog hesitated, then walked around the flag in a cautious arc. Goltz removed the cloth, and the dog at once stepped upon the place it had covered. 'That the actions of this dog are determined by visual impressions,' Goltz continued, 'is furthermore proved by the changes in his behavior as soon as he is blindfolded. I have brought a hood which I shall draw over his head. Now not a ray of light can reach his eyes. You will see that the animal which a few moments ago easily avoided all obstacles will now repeatedly run into things. Observe how he tries to pull the hood off, using both forepaws.'

"Goltz then went on to demonstrate, using a pincers at various points in the dog's skin, that all parts of the surface of his skin and the mucous membranes as well were sensitive to pain. 'At the institute we had a small, lively, extremely playful puppy,' he declared. The bold little creature insisted on playing with the experimental subject, and had frequently bitten him. The dog now before us had in every case shown sensitivity to pain.

"Goltz demonstrated the dog's sense of smell by asking Professor Donders of Holland to blow some smoke from his cigar into the animal's nose. The dog turned its head away. Goltz admitted, however, that its sense of smell was evidently not so keen as that of a sound dog.

" . . . He proceeded to demonstrate that the dog had suffered loss of intelligence, and of nothing else, by placing the animal in a low, square pen which he had likewise brought from Strassburg. The dog could easily have jumped over the small wire fence. But although it was lured from outside, it ran around the inside of the fence and was unable to hit upon the idea of jumping over. It wagged its tail innocently when Goltz threatened it with his fist. A cat was brought from the college animal laboratory and held toward the dog. The dog showed no sign of hostility or fear, despite the cat's furious spitting; in fact, it attempted to lick the cat's paws."[31]

Goltz then declared:

" . . . 'I hope that I have convinced you that none of this animal's sensory functions have been destroyed. It can see, hear, smell, feel. It does, however, display remarkable deviations from normal in its reactions to sense impressions. Its actions are so aimless, and at times so contrary to intelligent behavior, that we must deny it all capacity for reflection and pronounce it a canine imbecile.' This, he continued, provided proof that the theory of localization was flatly wrong. . . . As announced, he concluded, the dog would shortly be killed by chloroforming and the brain exposed for all to see that the cerebrum had been almost completely extirpated."[31]

"Prof. Ferrier, London, then called attention to the condition of two of the monkeys which he had alluded to in his remarks at the morning meeting. The first was the monkey which had the motor area of the left hemisphere extensively destroyed seven months previously. The animal was in every other respect normal, except as to the movements of the right arm and leg. The condition of these was recognized as bearing the closest resemblance to hemiplegia of some duration in man—M. Charcot remarking, 'It is a patient!' The movements of the leg were seen to be greatly impaired, and the arm quite powerless, being maintained flexed at the elbow, the thumb bent on the palm, and the fingers semi-flexed. The animal took pieces of food offered it with its left hand, and neither in its struggles to get free, nor on any occasion whatever, did it show any volitional action with the right hand or arm.

"The second monkey exhibited was the one which had had the region of the superior temporosphenoidal convolution destroyed in both hemispheres ten weeks previously. The animal was seen to be active and vigorous without the slightest sign of motor paralysis in any part of the body. Its vision was evidently perfect, the animal snatching eagerly at pieces of food offered it. That it was deaf, however, was demonstrated most clearly. While the two monkeys were on the floor together before the audience, Dr. Ferrier snapped a percussion cap in their immediate proximity, whereupon the hemiplegic monkey started with the most lively signs of surprise, whereas the other exhibited not the slightest indication whatever of hearing. This experiment was repeated several times with the same result. The animal was admitted to be perfectly deaf, and no other deficiency could be detected."[13]

Professor Yeo summarized the demonstration of the animals with the following remarks:

"I should not presume, at this late hour, to make any remarks upon this subject, however interesting it be to me, were it not that I may lay claim to being in some measure a skilled witness in the matter. And I believe the interpretation of the behaviour of such animals as these requires a special training and experience in order to arrive at correct conclusions. Although I have watched the surgical questions involved in my operations on the brain with more special interest than any other consideration, I have never for a moment lost sight of the physiological deductions to be arrived at after the recovery of the animals. I have naturally, therefore, become very familiar, from almost daily observation with the peculiarities and changes in the animal's conduct, which have followed the injuries of the brain.

"Besides the fact of my having done all the operations and watched accurately the clinical history of the cases afterwards, thus learning how to interpret the various symptoms, I think my opinion about these animals is made worthy of record, by the fact that I have no personal bias concerning the question of localization, as I have no original view to put forward.

"I commenced this series of experiments with distinct misgivings as to the existence of local cortical centres, in Ferrier's sense, so that I may say I was rather prejudiced against, than in favour of, his views.

"The first point that strikes me is that these very remarkable negative results obtained by my friend, Professor Goltz, in the case of dogs, cannot be said to be an adequate argument against the positive results arrived at in our experiments upon monkeys; while, on the other hand, our positive results seem to curtail in an absolute manner the very extensive generalizations Professor Goltz wishes to draw from his experiments.

"First, let us consider the condition of this remarkable dog.

"Is he really deficient in intellectual power, and does he show no signs of persistent local incapacity?

"It is said that, though his sight be perfect, he is unable to reason concerning his visual impressions, because he can make his way about, but avoids a patch of black on the floor, as if it were a solid object, and is unmoved by threats of the fist or whip. He sniffs about as if he could smell perfectly, but yet he is said to have eaten substances that no intelligent dog would eat. He can

hear, but will not respond to a whistle or call as an ordinary intelligent dog. He moves about in an eccentric and silly manner, and, though he is said to have perfect power over the movements of his muscles, he will not leave the box in which he has been confined, nor will he jump out of a shallow frame.

"Now, while recognizing all these remarkable facts, so ably demonstrated by my friend Professor Goltz, I must say I think them capable of a very different interpretation.

"I remark that, as he runs about, the dog frequently has to halt suddenly before an object, as if he had only just seen it; and, further, he often strikes the right side of his head, as if he could not see so well on that side. From this I am inclined to believe that his field of vision is in some way restricted, or his sight deficient. This fact would also sufficiently well explain his avoiding the black patch on the floor. His want of fear of the whip or the threats of his master's fist shaken before his face may depend simply upon the fact that he is quite familiar with these manoeuvres, and experience has taught him that they are not followed by any unpleasant consequences. That he can reason accurately concerning his imperfect visual impressions, I think, is clearly shown by the manner in which he recognizes his friends by sight. If he ate dog's flesh he certainly must have had impaired senses of taste and smell: now, however, he sniffs about in a most systematic manner, and since he arrived in London he certainly has shown a considerable degree of discrimination about his food, and in three or four days has learned to recognize the person who gives him his meals.

"As to his getting out of the box, I must confess I can't recognize any want of desire to get out, or want of intellect on that point: in fact, he seems extremely anxious to jump out and looks appealingly for help, as if unable to accomplish the leap himself, and as if he were at the same time confident from experience that timely help would come. That he does not leave the frame I believe to be simply a matter of education: not that he has ever been systematically taught to remain there, but he recognizes an unconsciously expressed wish on the part of his master that he should remain; and, after repeated demonstrations, he has acquired this habit, so he seldom thinks of moving when placed in the frame.

"Does he show any signs of ordinary intelligence? Certainly there is no lack of spontaneous voluntary movements. He constantly runs about with joyous carelessness, like a dog who had been confined for some time. He shows distinct signs of appreciating pleasure and pain, and likes to be caressed and petted, just as any other dog, and, except in appearance and gait, shows no want of intellectual power. He doubtless has a silly look, which is much contributed to by the shortness of the hair on his head when compared with the rest of his body, and by the fact that his sense of sight is impaired. His gait is unnatural and awkward, not from want of intellectual power, but, as I believe, because he has distinct loss of power over his hind legs. The individual muscles may be quite strong, he may be able to stand perfectly, and the less complex acts of co-ordination may be skilfully executed; but, when called upon to perform some sudden or considerable movement requiring complex co-ordination and extensive efforts, the general voluntary co-operation necessary is quite wanting. This is seen in his attempts to turn suddenly, to run quickly, or to spring, when his hind legs slip about in a weak meaningless manner, and practically come from under him. In fact, he may be said to have paresis, best seen in his hind limbs; or, in other words, he behaves like a dog with part of his so-called motor centres removed. The paresis is, no doubt, wonderfully slight for an animal who has had all these centres destroyed, and his considerable motive power is to me most strange. Besides expressing how much I have learned from my learned friend Professor Goltz, I candidly admit that, should the entire of the so-called motor centres prove to be destroyed in this case, he has succeeded in completely changing my views on the question of cerebral localization.

"The general behaviour of the dog, together with the difficulties I have experienced in exposing and completely removing certain parts of the cerebral cortex of other animals, makes me rather sceptical as to the exact extent of the lesion. One often thinks one has destroyed much more than really turns out to be the case at the autopsy. It may seem extremely bold on my part, but I cannot refrain from expressing my conviction that much of this dog's cerebral cortex will be found intact. Professor Goltz admits that all the anterior lobes and the extremities of the occipital lobes have not been removed. This latter omission would quite explain his vision, such as it is. I feel sure that much grey matter is also left untouched in the immediate neighbourhood of the longitudinal fissure and on the lateral aspects of the hemispheres. In short, I regard the animal as intensely interesting, as showing how great a portion of many centres can be taken away without the complete annihilation of any of their functions, and further as demonstrating how very extensively such an animal may be deprived of his income of impressions without becoming a perfect idiot by deprivation.

"Now let us criticise the monkeys. We have seen only two of many that have been operated upon by the same method and with the same localization of result. Those who have experience of

the aseptic method of operation will excuse my presumption in saying that I think absolute localization of the cortical lesion has not been arrived at with at all the same exactness in any set of experiments undertaken without its aid. In these cases there is no sign of any local or constitutional disturbance. The wounds heal in ten days, the scalp adhering to the injured brain surface and the membranes in the immediate neighbourhood remaining to all appearances perfectly normal.

"The first animal you saw had nearly complete hemiplegia for a considerable time after the operation, which consisted in an extensive but carefully localized lesion. The paralysis of the leg has in a great measure gone, but even now after seven and a half months he is distinctly lame in that leg, and is quite unable to grasp with his hand, the arm being held in the position of a paralyzed limb. Another animal which I had occasion to observe for just a year after operation was, until his death, perfectly blind, but showed no other sign of paresis of any kind. The retinae began to show signs of atrophy before his death. Now this result followed a carefully localized bilateral lesion of the posterior part of the brain, which was, however, much more extensive than Professor Munk has indicated as his idea of the centre of vision, as it included both posterior lobes and angular gyri.

"In the second animal I think there can be no doubt as to his deafness, and his great activity and ability in all other respects. I can testify as to the exact localization of the bilateral lesion of the cortex in this case.

"Having seen these animals, I feel sure Professor Goltz will modify his opinion as to the 'utter folly' of the view that special parts of the brain are peculiarly associated with certain functional departments, and, though I am far from endorsing the edicts of Munk, or accepting, without reservation, the views of Ferrier, I venture to hope that our friend from Strassburg will no longer think that the observations which describe any persistent functional disturbance, as the result of a local lesion of the brain-cortex, are *einfach falsch.*"[37]

The dog and the monkey with the motor lesion were sacrificed, and their brains were removed. Preliminary examination of the specimens was made within a few days by Dr. W. R. Gowers, Dr. E. Klein, Dr. E. A. Schäfer, and Mr. J. N. Langley.[21–24,29] This committee reported that the lesions in the monkey's brain corresponded exactly to the areas that Ferrier and Yeo had thought they had destroyed. In contrast, the destruction of the dog's brain was not as extensive as had been thought by Goltz, and some parts of the motor and sensory centers had remained normal. This, plus the lesser differentiation of function found in the lower animals, had permitted the dog to retain a surprising degree of motor and sensory function. The committee's statement therefore constituted an unequivocal triumph for Ferrier.[31]

Ferrier's "victory" provided a needed stimulus to cerebral surgery, and just three years later he watched Rickman Godlee remove the first brain tumor to be located solely by neurological examination.[33,34]

References

1. ANDERSON, E., and HAYMAKER, W. Friedrich Leopold Goltz (1834–1902). In: *The founders of neurology.* W. Haymaker, Ed. Springfield, Ill.: Charles C Thomas, 1953, xxvii, 479 pp. (see pp. 131–135).
2. BALLANCE, C. The Thomas Vicary lecture: being a glimpse into the history of the surgery of the brain. *Lancet,* 1922, *1:* 111–116, 165–172.
3. BOWMAN, A. K. The life and teaching of Sir William Macewen. A chapter in the history of surgery. *London: W. Hodge & Co., Ltd.,* 1942, x, 425 pp. (see pp. 250–288).
4. BRITISH MEDICAL JOURNAL. Summons under the Vivisection Act. *Brit. med. J.,* 1881, *2:* 752.
5. BRITISH MEDICAL JOURNAL. The antivivisection prosecution. *Brit. med. J.,* 1881, *2:* 785.
6. BRITISH MEDICAL JOURNAL. Dr. Ferrier's localisations; for whose advantage? *Brit. med. J.,* 1881, *2:* 822–824.
7. CORRESPONDENCE. Proposed subscription to Dr. Ferrier. *Brit. med. J.,* 1881, *2:* 834.
8. FERRIER, D. Experimental researches in cerebral physiology and pathology. *W. Riding Lunatic Asylum med. Rep.,* 1873, *3:* 30–96.
9. FERRIER, D. The functions of the brain. *London: Smith, Elder & Co.,* 1876, xv, 323 pp.
10. FERRIER, D. The localisation of cerebral disease, being the Goulstonian lectures of the Royal College of Physicians for 1878. *London: Smith, Elder & Co.,* 1878, 142 pp.
11. FERRIER, D. The Goulstonian lectures on the localisation of cerebral disease. *Brit. med. J.,* 1878, *1:* 399–402, 443–447, 471–476, 515–519, 555–559, 591–595.
12. FERRIER, [D.]. Discussion on the localisation of the functions in the cerebral cortex. *Brit. med. J.,* 1881, *2:* 588–589.
13. FERRIER, D. Discussion on the localization of function in the cortex cerebri. In: *Transactions of the International Medical Congress.* W. Mac Cormac, Ed. London: J. W. Kolckmann, 1881, 4 vols. (see *1:* 228–233; 237).
14. FERRIER, D. Discussion on cerebral localization. *Trans. Congr. Amer. Phys. Surg.,* 1889, *1:* 337–340.
15. FERRIER, D. The Croonian lectures on cerebral localisation. *London: Smith, Elder & Co.,* 1890, vi, 152 pp.
16. GARRISON, F. H. An introduction to the history of medicine. With medical chronology, suggestions for study and bibliographic data. *Philadelphia: W. B. Saunders Co.,* 1929, 4th ed., 996 pp. (see pp. 540–541).
17. GOLTZ, F. Beiträge zur Lehre von den Functionen der Nervencentren des Frosches. *Berlin: A. Hirschwald,* 1869, 130 pp.
18. GOLTZ, F. Ueber die Verrichtungen des Grosshirns. Gesammelte Abhandlungen. *Bonn: E. Strauss,* 1881, 177 pp.
19. GOLTZ, F. Discussion on the localization of function in the cortex cerebri. In: *Transactions of the International Medical Congress.* W. Mac Cormac, Ed. London: J. W. Kolckmann, 1881, 4 vols. (see *1:* 218–228; 234–237).
20. GOLTZ, B. Der Hund ohne Grosshirn. Siebente Abhandlung über die Verrichtungen des Grosshirns. *Pflügers Arch. ges. Physiol.,* 1892, *51:* 570–614.
21. KLEIN, E. Report on the parts destroyed on the left side of the brain of the dog operated on by Prof. Goltz. *J. Physiol.,* 1883, *4:* 310–315.
22. KLEIN, E., LANGLEY, J. N., and SCHÄFER, E. A. On the cortical areas removed from the brain of a dog, and from the brain of a monkey. *J. Physiol.,* 1883, *4:* 231–247.
23. LANGLEY, J. N. The structure of the dog's brain. *J. Physiol.,* 1883, *4:* 248–285.
24. LANGLEY, J. N. Report on the parts destroyed on the right side of the brain of the dog operated on by Prof. Goltz. *J. Physiol.,* 1883, *4:* 286–309.
25. LETTER FROM LONDON. The prosecution or persecution of Professor David Ferrier, F.R.S., M.D., by the antivivisectionists. *Boston med. surg. J.,* 1881, *105:* 552–554.
26. PARK, R. Surgery of the brain, based on the principles of cerebral localization. *Trans. Congr. Amer. Phys. Surg.,* 1889, *1:* 285–328.
27. PENFIELD, W. Neurosurgery yesterday, today and tomorrow. *J. Neurosurg.,* 1949, *6:* 6–12.
28. RIOCH, D. McK. Sir David Ferrier (1843–1928). In: *The founders of neurology.* W. Haymaker, Ed. Springfield, Ill.: Charles C Thomas, 1953, xxvii, 479 pp. (see pp. 122–125).
29. SCHÄFER, E. A. Report on the lesions, primary and secondary, in the brain and spinal cord of the macaque monkey exhibited by Professors Ferrier and Yeo. *J. Physiol.,* 1883, *4:* 316–326.
30. STOOKEY, B. A note on the early history of cerebral localization. *Bull. N. Y. Acad. Med.,* 1954, *30:* 559–578.
31. THORWALD, J. The triumph of surgery. R. Winston and C. Winston, Transl. New York: Pantheon Books, Inc., 1960, xi, 454 pp. (see pp. 3–40).
32. VIETS, H. R. West Riding, 1871–1876. *Bull. Hist. Med.,* 1938, *6:* 477–487.
33. WILKINS, R. H. Neurosurgical classic—I. *J. Neurosurg.,* 1962, *19:* 700–710.
34. WILKINS, R. H. Neurosurgical classics—II. *J. Neurosurg.,* 1962, *19:* 801–805.

35. WILKINS, R. H. Neurosurgical classic—XII. *J. Neurosurg.*, 1963, *20:* 904–916.
36. WILKINS, R. H. Neurosurgical classics—XIX. *J. Neurosurg.*, 1964, *21:* 424–431.
37. YEO, G. Discussion on the localization of function in the cortex cerebri. In: *Transactions of the International Medical Congress*. W. Mac Cormac, Ed. London: J. W. Kolckmann, 1881, 4 vols. (see *1:* 237–240).
38. YOUNG, A. The limitations of surgery, past and present. *Glasgow med. J.* 1924, *102:* 273–313.

* DR. FERRIER, London: I have listened with great interest to the facts and able arguments brought before us by Professor Goltz, on the question of the localization of functions in the cerebral hemispheres. If I cannot argue with him —and I must differ from him very widely—it is not because I dispute his facts. These, from Professor Goltz's character as a trustworthy observer, I should be prepared to accept without further verification. But, I reject his conclusions. It seems to me a matter of essential importance that in generalizing as to the functions of the cerebral hemispheres, we should be careful lest the hypothesis we adopt, however well it may seem to accord with the facts of experiment on one order of animals, should not stand in flagrant contradiction to facts equally well established obtained by experiment on others. For if the brains of animals are anatomically homologous, we may fairly assume that they are so also physiologically, and that any differences observable will be differences in degree only, and not in kind; and as a matter of fact, I hope to show you that Professor Goltz's hypothesis is irreconcileable with the facts of experiments on monkeys; whereas, the hypothesis of localization harmonizes not only with these facts, but also with those of Professor Goltz. He tells us that dogs, after extensive destruction of their cerebral cortex, though degraded as regards intelligence and mental capacity, yet retain in a greater or less degree all the sensory and motor powers possessed by the dog under normal conditions. He argues, therefore, that every portion of the cortex is in relation more or less with every function exercised by the hemispheres as a whole. He thus maintains essentially the doctrines advocated by Flourens. But not in their entirety. For he admits that the posterior part of the brain is more in relation with vision than the anterior; and the anterior more in relation with motor power than with sensation. This is to my mind a very significant concession, and is practically admitting the doctrine of localization, and I am hopeful that Professor Goltz may yet see his way to admitting it in a

* Reprinted from the *Transactions of the seventh session of the International Medical Congress*, 1881, *1:* 228–233.

more thoroughgoing manner. If the facts of experiment on dogs were the only data on which to form an opinion as to the question of localization, I do not see that we are at all obliged to adopt his hypothesis. He assumes that the capabilities manifested by his dogs are entirely dependent on the portions of the cortex he has not succeeded in destroying. But this is merely an assumption. To prove it, he ought to show us that all these faculties are entirely annihilated when the last portion of the cortex has been removed. He may say this is not practicable—and I do not say it is—but, if so, the question cannot be settled in this way, and we must therefore turn our attention to other methods and other experiments. Now we all know how comparatively little effect on the powers of locomotion and reaction to sensory stimulation, general and special, even complete extirpation of the whole cerebral hemispheres has upon such animals as frogs and pigeons, and animals low in the animal scale. Professor Goltz has now shown us how much, even dogs can do, when their cerebral hemispheres have been extensively destroyed. I have elsewhere particularly insisted on the necessity of recognizing the relative differences observable in different animals in respect to the parts taken by the higher and lower centres respectively in the ordinary modes of activity of the animal. The lower the scale, the greater the independence of the lower centres, and the less the necessity of the cerebral hemispheres in all that relates to station, locomotion, and reaction to sensory stimuli. Whereas, the higher we go in the animal scale, the greater the importance of the cerebral hemispheres in regard to these manifestations. Hence, in the frog, pigeon, rabbit, &c., the removal of the cerebral hemispheres produces comparatively slight and transient paralysis; whereas, in the monkey and man the paralysis is permanent. Now, I believe that by applying this principle we can satisfactorily account for all the facts brought before us by Professor Goltz. His dogs still retain their lower centres, and a portion, more or less considerable, of their cerebral cortex. The activity of these together will be found amply sufficient to account for the powers of movement, such as they are, possessed by his dogs, and the indications of sensation which they exhibit. But I am not so much concerned to-day with criticizing and explaining Professor Goltz's results—the subject I have discussed elsewhere (Functions of the Brain—Localization of Cerebral Disease). I am more desirous to bring before you some new facts of experiments on monkeys, the bearing of which on the question of localization will be readily seen. It was urged against my former observations, made some six years ago, that the time the animals were allowed to live after the establishment of lesions of their cortex, was not sufficiently long to differentiate between merely functional disturbances due to the operation, and loss or impairment of the function belonging to the part immediately injured. There is some force in this argument as regards the question of restitution. But the fact of localization is not affected, inasmuch as I showed that different results, however temporary, followed lesions of different parts. And as I was more particularly investigating the fact of localization, it was necessary to sacrifice the animal, after the phenomena were satisfactorily observed, in order to ascertain the exact amount of injury inflicted, before secondary extension of the lesion could be caused by encephalitis. This I found it impossible to prevent, following the older methods of operation. But all this has been changed; and the arguments founded on the mere temporary nature of the disturbances have ceased to have any weight. During the last two years I have had opportunities of observing animals operated upon by my colleague, Professor Gerald Yeo, in an investigation into the application of the principles of antiseptic surgery to lesions of the brain and its coverings. By this method it has been found to be possible to establish lesions in any part of the brain without the slightest risk of encephalitis or extension of the primary lesion. Unlike Professor Goltz, who does not restrict his lesions with any degree of accuracy, care is taken to expose and limit the lesion with the cautery in the part whose functions are to be determined. Some of the results we have observed I shall now place before you. In the month of October, the right hemisphere of a monkey was cauterized superficially over an area about a centimetre in diameter, in the middle of the ascending frontal and parietal convolutions— the centres for the flexion of the forearm and closure of the fist. (Centre (6) (*b*, *c*), "Functions of Brain," p. 142). The position and extent of the lesion you will see in the photograph, which I show you. And that the lesion was purely cortical you will see in the microscopical sections through the right hemisphere, which I also exhibit. The animal lived only two months, unfortunately, dying during the intensely cold winter season. But the result was paralysis of the left arm—and not of the left arm in all its movements, but only of the power of flexing the forearm and closure of the fist. It could advance its arm forwards, but could never lay hold of anything with its left hand, or raise its hand to its mouth. The animal was perfectly normal in every other respect; and as to the tactile sensibility of the left hand, it was most acute, the slightest touch with a heated point causing emphatic demonstrations of sensation, as much on the left as the right hand. The next case I mention is that of a monkey, in which an area of the cortex was cauterized at the upper extremity of the fissure of Rolando, in what I have termed the "leg centre" (1) (2) *op. cit.* The lesion does not embrace the whole of the leg centre, but a considerable extent of it. I show you a plaster cast, and also a photograph of the brain of this animal. There is visible also a superficial erosion just in advance of the lesion alluded to, occupying the position of centre (5)—that for extension forward of the arm. The result of this lesion was paralysis of the right leg, complete at first, excepting slight flexion and extension at the hip. There was also observable for a day or two slight spasm of the right arm during extension forward—due, without doubt, to the slight lesion of the centre for this movement which I have just mentioned. All other movements were intact, and the animal was able to use its right hand in grasping, and for all other purposes as well as the left. As time went on, the power of flexion and extension of the thigh, and of the leg in progression improved, but there remained great impairment of the movements of the foot. This, instead of improving, after the lapse of six months, became worse. This was found to depend on the development of contraction, or late rigidity in the right leg. When the leg was extended, the toe pointed, and the foot assumed the equino-varus position. Dorsal flexion of the foot caused great tenseness of the sural muscles, and a tendency to flexion of the leg on the knee, and the animal exhibited distinct signs of uneasiness when the muscles were so made tense. From the beginning this animal was in every other respect perfectly well. Its special sensory faculties were absolutely unimpaired, and its tactile sensibility normal. At the time the rigidity was specially noted—after six months—the patellar reaction was found to be exaggerated on the right side, and the plantar cutaneous reflex diminished, precisely as in similar conditions in man.

The animal was killed eight months after the operation. The brain and spinal cord of this animal were examined microscopically, and I show you a series of microscopical sections, beginning with the left hemisphere, vertically through the lesion; then horizontally, so as to exhibit the internal capsule; next, through the crura cerebri, the pons, and medulla; and lastly, sections of the spinal cord from the cervical to the lumbar region. And you will see with the naked eye very clear indications of descending degeneration, commencing underneath the cortex, and traceable in the left internal capsule, left crus, pons, and medulla, and in the right side of the spinal cord, throughout its whole length, in the posterior portion of the lateral tract external to the posterior horn. This case demonstrates the persistence of the motor monoplegia depending on a lesion purely cortical, and also, with a completeness never before reached, the Wallerian degeneration of the motor path from the cortex down to the point whence the nerves to the limb take their origin. The next case I mention is one in which, perhaps, you will take greater interest, inasmuch as the subject of experiment is still alive, and will be presented to you for a verification of the phenomena which I describe. The animal in question had the motor zone destroyed in its left hemisphere seven months ago. The area destroyed embraced, as nearly as we can judge, the ascending frontal, and bases of the three frontal convolutions, and also the ascending parietal. We are not quite sure if the whole of the postero-parietal or paracentral lobule was destroyed, as these parts could not be completely exposed to view conveniently. But the result of this operation was complete motor hemiplegia of the right side, the limbs being perfectly powerless, with the exception of feeble power of flexion of the right thigh. At first there was conjugate deviation of the eyes and head to the left side, lasting for a few days only. The facial paralysis of the right side, at first distinct, ceased also to be perceptible after a fortnight. The limb gradually gained greater power of flexion and extension of the thigh and leg, but it is even now still very feeble, and the foot is lifted as a piece with the leg, and is only moved in connection with the left. The right forearm is generally kept flexed; though during emotion, and during vigorous action of the left, it is also brought into associated action more or less. Particularly is this seen as regards the hand. This is kept usually with the thumb bent over the palm, and the fingers tend to flex over the thumb. But if the left hand is strongly used, the right will also clench; and if the animal scratches itself vigorously with the left, it sometimes does the same with the right, clawing the air, and continuing to do so occasionally after the left has ceased. As to any independent volitional action of the right arm and leg, we have not seen a single indication since the operation was made. The animal is in every other respect perfectly well; and as to its tactile sensibility there is not the slightest sign of impairment. It has exaggerated tendon reflexes, and somewhat diminished superficial reflexes on the right side, as in motor hemiplegia in man. This diminution of superficial reflexes in motor hemiplegia is perfectly familiar to clinical observers, but has been erroneously interpreted by some physiologists as an indication of defective sensibility. It exists with the most perfect tactile sensibility, as I have verified, and frequently demonstrated in clinical practice. Turn next to another series of facts. I show you the brain itself, and also some photographs of the brain of a monkey, in which the occipital lobes and angular gyri were removed completely and exactly on both sides. An examination of the specimen will convince you of this, and of the total absence of any sign of secondary extension by inflammation. The result of this operation was complete blindness, all other sensory faculties and the motor powers remaining absolutely unimpaired. Hearing was keen, tactile sensibility was acute, and the animal would grope with its hands, and pick up the minutest objects (grains of corn, &c.), thrown down in its cage. It walked about with a somnambulistic air, at first knocking its head against all obstacles. After the lapse of some months it could move about without doing this, unless under new conditions, and if it were not hurried or startled. The only thing that looked like vision was the fact that if an object were waved round and round, immediately in front of its eyes, it would turn its eyes and head accordingly. But it made no such signs if this were done at a distance, so as to exclude all sensation communicated by agitation of the air. But to the last the animal did not wince when a light was flashed in its eyes. Its pupils were large and sluggish, if not entirely inactive, to light, and the optic discs became pale and anæmic. The animal lived nearly eleven months; death occurring during the cold winter season. Six weeks ago, a monkey, which will also be presented before you for examination, had the superior temporo-sphenoidal convolution destroyed in both hemispheres —the region where I have localized the auditory centre. You will see that this animal is in perfect possession of its sight and other sensory faculties, and of all its motor powers. But it has ceased to give any indications of hearing sounds which formerly attracted its notice, and which invariably cause very manifest signs of hearing in other monkeys. We thought at first that the sound of a percussion cap exploded in its ears did cause something like a reflex start, but our subsequent examinations would indicate that this was more probably mere coincidence. For when it was tested in this manner a few days ago, it gave no indications whatever; whereas its companion, the hemiplegic monkey I have previously described, always started in a very emphatic manner. But the experiment will be repeated before you, so that you may judge for yourselves. Contrast this with an experiment on another animal, in which the temporo-sphenoidal lobe posterior to this region was ploughed up on both sides with the cautery. It is in this region that Herr Munk supposes the auditory centre is situated, and not in the superior temporo-sphenoidal, where I have localized it. But this animal from the very first gave the most clear indications of the possession of the sense of hearing; for it replied when called to, and responded to sounds of all kinds, precisely as before.

Indeed, we could not make out with certainty any inpairment whatever, either as regards its sensory or motor powers. This animal was very feeble, and died three weeks after the operation; I show you the brain and lesion which I have described. I might adduce many other similar facts, but these, I think, are sufficient to demonstrate that Professor Goltz's hypothesis is erroneous, and that such facts are explicable only on the theory of a distinct localization of faculties in definite cortical regions.

At the afternoon meeting of the Section, the hemiplegic monkey above alluded to I trust will be exhibited, and also the monkey in which the superior temporo-sphenoidal convolutions have been destroyed. The latter gives no reaction when a percussion cap is exploded close to it, while the hemiplegic monkey is emphatically startled. The brain will be exhibited before the Section subsequently, and awaiting the minute examination of the lesion after its removal from the animal, I do not hesitate to predict that it will be found that the whole of the motor area has been destroyed, with the exception, possibly, of some portions of the postero-parietal lobule and the ascending convolutions, which are very difficult to reach owing to their position in the cranial cavity.

Otfrid Foerster, like Clovis Vincent, was a neurologist who later gained enough surgical skill to perform the operations he recommended. Because of his basic interest in neurophysiology, his operations were designed to be informative as well as beneficial.[5,6] An example of this concerns Foerster's experience with the operation of posterior rhizotomy.[1-4] This procedure was first performed in 1888 by William H. Bennett for the relief of peripheral pain, and twenty years later Foerster adapted it to the treatment of spastic paralysis and gastric crises.[7] Foerster's subsequent extensive experience with the patients undergoing this operation resulted in a careful analysis of the sensory dermatomes in man—a major contribution to the understanding of the human nervous system.[3]

References

1. FÖRSTER, O. Ueber eine neue operative Methode der Behandlung spastischer Lähmungen mittels Resektion hinterer Rückenmarkswurzeln. Z. orthop. Chir., 1908, 22: 203–223.
2. FOERSTER, O. Resection of the posterior spinal nerve-roots in the treatment of gastric crises and spastic paralysis. Proc. roy. Soc. Med., 1911, 4, pt. 3: 226–246.
3. FOERSTER, O. The dermatomes in man. Brain, 1933, 56: 1–39.
4. FOERSTER, O., and KÜTTNER, H. Ueber operative Behandlung gastrischer Krisen durch Resektion der 7.–10. hinteren Dorsalwurzel. Beitr. klin. Chir., 1909, 63: 245–256.
5. RAY, B. S. The management of intractable pain by posterior rhizotomy. Res. Publ. Ass. nerv. ment. Dis., 1943, 23: 391–407.
6. WARTENBERG, R. Otfrid Foerster (1873–1941). In: The founders of neurology. W. Haymaker, Ed. Springfield, Ill.: Charles C Thomas, 1953, xxvii, 479 pp. (see pp. 422–425).
7. WILKINS, R. H. Neurosurgical classics—XXIII. J. Neurosurg., 1964, 21: 812–823.

THE DERMATOMES IN MAN*,[1]

BY PROFESSOR O. FOERSTER,
Breslau.

The nervous system preserves more than any other part of the human body the original division of the embryonic tube into metameres. The spinal cord is divided in segments, each segment being provided with a pair of anterior and posterior roots. The area of skin which is supplied by the fibres of a certain spinal root is called a dermatome.

The skin is innervated by the posterior roots as well as by the anterior. The former carry the afferent sensory fibres and efferent fibres subserving vasodilatation. The anterior roots carry efferent motor, sudorific, pilomotor and vasoconstrictor fibres, and also afferent sensory fibres. In this lecture I shall deal exclusively with the fibres passing by the posterior roots.

There exist two different methods for the determination of the area of skin subserved by a certain posterior spinal root, the anatomical method and the physiological method.

The anatomical method, used first by Herringham and later chiefly by Bolk, consists in following up the fibres of one single root by anatomical dissection through the plexus and the peripheral nerves into the skin. Fig. 1 shows the second, third and fourth cervical dermatomes as outlined by Bolk by this method, and Fig. 2 the areas of the roots supplying the arm, that is the fifth, sixth, seventh and eighth cervical and the first and second thoracic roots. Each of these dermatomes occupies a different area and these show very little or no overlap.

It is obvious that this method, used by Bolk, has the disadvantage that by anatomical dissection it is impossible to follow the terminal and finest ramifications of the sensory nerves in the skin. The areas outlined by it certainly show the shape and the position of the dermatomes, but not their full extent.

To Sir Charles Sherrington we owe our knowledge of the complete topography of the dermatomes in the monkey. The method used by him, and called the method of "remaining sensibility" or the "isolation method," consists in dividing a series of contiguous roots above and below a single root which is preserved. The area of the skin, the sensibility of which is preserved after this procedure, represents the sensory dermatome of the intact root.

Fig. 3 demonstrates the second, third and

---

* Reprinted from Brain, 1933, 56: 1–39, with the kind permission of the Editor.
[1] The substance of this article was included in the Schorstein Lecture delivered at the London Hospital, on October 13, 1932.

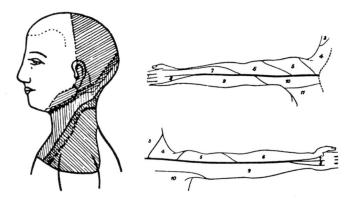

FIG. 1 (*left*). The 1st, 2nd and 3rd cervical dermatomes, according to Bolk.
FIG. 2 (*right*). Dermatomes of the upper extremity; the 4th to 8th cervical, and 1st and 2nd
thoracic (9 and 10), according to Bolk.

fourth cervical dermatomes of the monkey; these overlap to such a degree that the area of the third cervical root is supplied to its full extent by the second and the fourth cervical roots.

A similar condition exists in the upper extremity (Fig. 4). The fifth cervical dermatome, for instance, overlaps with the third and fourth on the one hand and with the sixth and the seventh on the other. The amount of the overlap of the different dermatomes is so considerable that division of a single root produces no loss of sensibility.

Another physiological method for the definition of the dermatomes is based upon local strychnine intoxication of the posterior roots. After segmental application of strychnine to the dorsal surface of the cord a sharply circumscribed skin field becomes hyperæsthesic, as Dusser de Barenne has demonstrated. The hyperæsthetic area is identical in shape, situation and extent with the dermatomes defined by the isolation method, and the same large degree of overlap of adjacent dermatomes is apparent.

Our knowledge of the dermatomes in man is chiefly based upon the work of Sir Henry Head,

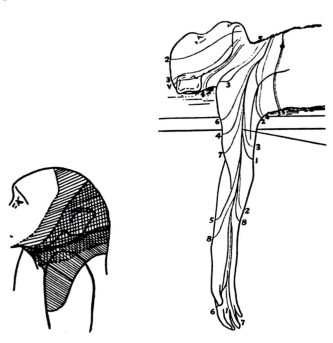

FIG. 3 (*left*). The 1st, 2nd and 3rd cervical dermatomes of the monkey, according to Sherrington.
FIG. 4 (*right*). Dermatomes of the upper extremity of the monkey, according to Sherrington.

who collected a large number of cases of herpetic eruption. Herpes is supposed to be an inflammatory lesion of the spinal ganglia, producing an eruption upon the skin in the corresponding cutaneous area. Head also contributed valuable information on the dermatomes in man by outlining carefully the borders of the hyperæsthetic skin areas in visceral disease, and the distribution of anæsthesia in traumatic lesions of the cord and the cauda equina. In Head's scheme (Fig. 5) the cutaneous root areas overlap very little, and in this respect it does not conform to the results of experimental physiology. How is this discrepancy to be explained? Do monkeys and men differ really from each other so much in regard to such a fundamental organization as metamery?

I have had the opportunity of defining a great number of dermatomes in man by exactly the same method as that used by Sherrington, that is by outlining the borders of the sensibility which remains after a large number of contiguous roots have been divided, and a single root in the middle of them has been left intact. I need not discuss here the circumstances under which such a selected procedure may be undertaken. By this method I have been able to define all dermatomes of the lower extremity and one dermatome of the upper extremity, namely the sixth cervical. In order to fill up the gap and to define the other cervical and the thoracic dermatomes we can use a method which I should like to call "the constructive method." It is obvious that when a series of contiguous roots is divided, the superior border of the resulting anæsthesia represents the inferior border of the dermatome which corresponds to the next higher intact root, while the inferior border of the anæsthetic area represents the superior border of the next lower dermatome. By such observations I have been able to map out nearly all dermatomes in man.

The other method which I have used for the definition of dermatomes is based upon the fact, first demonstrated by Stricker and Bayliss on animals, that faradic stimulation of the distal part of a divided posterior root is followed by vaso-dilatation. I have found the same in man. I have also observed that the vaso-dilatation following the electrical stimulation of a single posterior root is limited to a sharply circumscribed area similar in shape and situation to the dermatome as defined by means of the isolation method.

I have obtained vasodilatation by stimulation of nearly all cervical, thoracic, lumbar and sacral posterior roots. The area of vasodilatation resulting from the electrical stimulation of a single posterior root is not absolutely identical with the area of remaining sensibility; it is smaller and approximates in its extent much more to the area of herpetic eruption mapped out by Head.

For a long time it has been an open question whether the vasodilatation following faradic stimulation of a posterior root is due to antidromic conduction along the afferent nerve-fibres, as Bayliss believed, or whether it is the effect of stimulation of efferent fibres arising in the cord and passing outward by the posterior roots. In eight cases in which I had divided posterior roots in men we found a number of myelinated fibres preserved in the central part of the divided root. The root resection was performed in one of my cases five years before death (Fig. 6), and in another four and a half years before death. The fact that these fibres are preserved after the root had been totally divided proves that their ganglion cells do not lie in the spinal ganglia but in the cord, and that these fibres are really efferent. The calibre of these fibres is very fine as compared with the thick myelinated sensory fibres of the posterior root (Figs. 7 and 8). The results of these anatomical investigations prove, I believe, that the posterior roots carry, in addition to sensory fibres, efferent fibres and its seems to me admissible to assume that the vasodilatation following the electrical stimulation of a posterior root is the result of the stimulation of these efferent fibres.

After this short review of the methods of defining the dermatomes in man I shall describe the special dermatomery. I begin with the dermatomes of the lower extremity.

Lumbar and Sacral Dermatomes

First lumbar dermatome.—The first lumbar dermatome, that is the area of sensibility which remains after the eleventh and twelfth thoracic and the second to the fifth lumbar and all sacral roots having been divided, the first lumbar root alone being left intact, occupies the inferior part of the abdomen and the upper part of the anterior and lateral surfaces of the leg. At the dorsal side it forms a band, which reaches the spine of the fifth lumbar vertebra (Figs. 9 and 10). This area of remaining sensibility is very similar to the area outlined by Head (Fig. 5), but exceeds it to some extent, especially above its superior border. The extent of the herpetic eruption in a case of herpes of the first lumbar ganglion is shown in Fig. 11.

The constructive method defines the same borders for the first lumbar dermatome. In a case in which the eighth, ninth, tenth, eleventh and twelfth thoracic roots were resected, the inferior border of the anæsthesia, shown in Fig. 12, represents the superior border of the first lumbar dermatome; it conforms to the superior border of the remaining sensibility in the case described above. In another case, in which the second, third, fourth and fifth lumbar and all sacral roots were divided, the superior border of the anæsthesia shown in Figs. 13 and 14 was practically identical with the inferior border of the remaining sensibility in the case illustrated in Figs. 9, 10. In a case

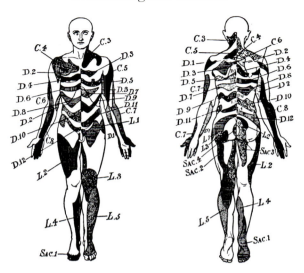

FIG. 5. Head's scheme of the dermatomes in man.

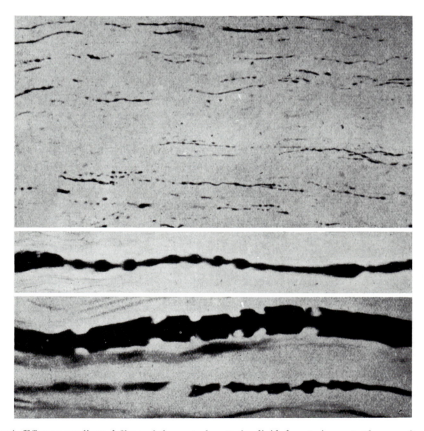

FIG. 6 (*above*). Efferent myelinated fibres of the central part of a divided posterior root, 4½ years after resection.
FIG. 7 (*middle*). A single myelinated efferent fibre of a posterior root; note its fine calibre.
FIG. 8 (*below*). A single myelinated sensory fibre of a posterior root; note its thick calibre.

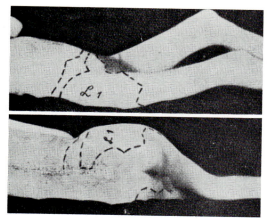

Figs. 9 and 10. The 1st lumbar dermatome defined by remaining sensibility after resection of 11th and 12th thoracic, and 2nd to 5th lumbar and 1st to 5th sacral roots.

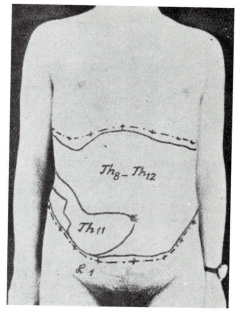

Fig. 12. The superior border of the 1st lumbar dermatome; resection of 8th to 12th thoracic roots.

of division of the second and third lumbar roots the superior border of the anæsthesia was similar to that of the preceding cases on the anterior aspect of the leg, but on the posterior aspect there was no anæsthesia, the sacral roots having been left intact (Figs. 15, 16).

Second lumbar dermatome was defined by the isolation method in a case in which the twelfth thoracic and the first lumbar, as well as the third, fourth and fifth lumbar and all sacral roots were divided (Fig. 17). It lies chiefly on the anterior aspect of the thigh, but there is also a small band on the dorsum of the trunk which is not continuous with the main area upon the anterior surface

of the leg (Fig. 18). We find exactly the same distribution in Head's scheme (Fig. 5).

The constructive method demonstrates the same borders for the second lumbar dermatome. In a case in which the third, fourth and fifth lumbar roots and the first sacral root were divided, the superior border of the anæsthesia corresponds to the inferior border of the second lumbar dermatome (Fig. 19), and in a case of

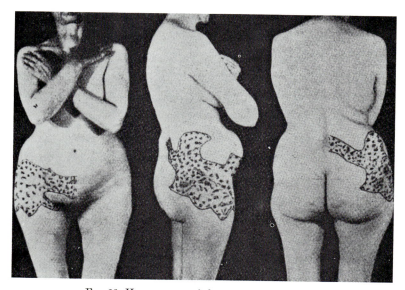

Fig. 11. Herpes zoster of the 1st lumbar ganglion.

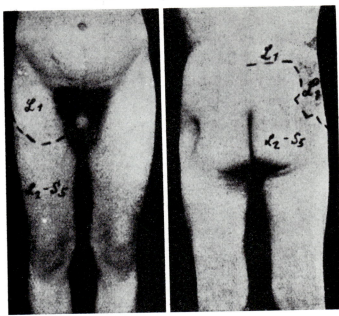

FIGS. 13 and 14. The inferior border of the 1st lumbar dermatome; resection of 2nd to 5th lumbar and 1st to 5th sacral roots.

resection of the eleventh and twelfth thoracic and the first lumbar roots the inferior border of the anæsthesia represents the superior border of the second lumbar dermatome (Fig. 20).

Third lumbar dermatome.—The third lumbar dermatome was outlined by the isolation method on the other leg of the same patient as the second lumbar dermatome (Fig. 17). On comparison of the legs the great extent of overlap becomes evi-

dent. The third lumbar dermatome has a characteristic shape; a central part around the knee, an upper prolongation along the anterior and internal surface of the thigh, and an inferior strip or band along the inner side of the leg reaching below as far as the internal malleolus. There is also a small band on the dorsal aspect of the trunk, which is not in continuity with the main area upon the lower limb (Fig. 18). Fig. 21 shows

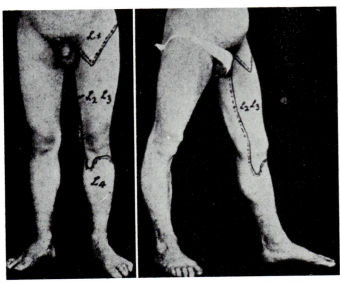

FIGS. 15 and 16. The inferior border of the 1st lumbar dermatome; resection of 2nd and 3rd lumbar roots.

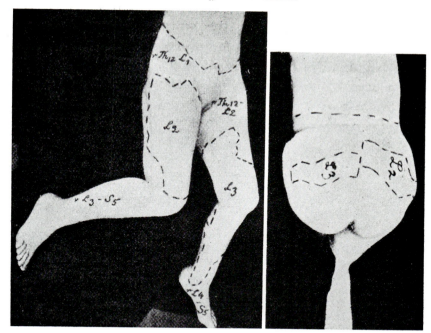

FIGS. 17 and 18. The 2nd lumbar dermatome; resection of Th12 and L1, and L3 to S5 on the right side. The
3rd lumbar dermatome; resection of Th12, L1 and L2, and L4 to S5 on the left side.

the third lumbar dermatome in another case. On comparing these cases it is seen that the extent of the same dermatome may present considerable individual variations. It is noteworthy that in the case represented by Fig. 21 the first sacral dermatome, which was also defined, had an unusually large extension. The situation and the extent of the third lumbar dermatome according to Head is shown in Fig. 5.

The constructive method confirms the results obtained by the isolation method. In a case in which all the roots between the ninth thoracic and the second lumbar were divided, the inferior border of the anæsthetic area corresponds exactly

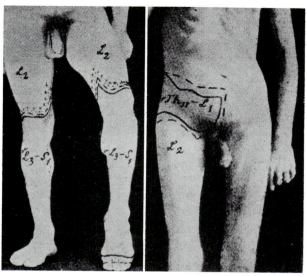

FIG. 19 (*left*). The inferior border of the 2nd lumbar dermatome; resection of L3 to S1.
FIG. 20 (*right*). The superior border of the 2nd lumbar dermatome; resection of Th11, Th12 and L1.

with the superior border of the dermatome demonstrated above by the isolation method (Fig. 22); and in another case in which the fourth and fifth lumbar and all sacral roots were divided, the superior border of the anæsthesia runs along the anterior side of the tibia down to the internal malleolus and then upwards along the internal side of the leg (Figs. 23 and 24).

The area of vasodilatation following electrical stimulation of the third lumbar root (Fig. 25) also coincides in situation and shape with the dermatome defined by the isolation method, but its extent is not quite as large as that of the area of remaining sensibility.

Fourth lumbar dermatome occupies the anterior side of the leg, the internal part of the dorsum of the foot and the great toe (Fig. 26). On the sole its border runs from between the first and second toes backwards behind the internal malleolus (Fig. 27), and upwards along the posterior-internal side of the leg. At the level of the knee it turns forwards, then bends behind the head of the fibula to the outer side of the leg (Fig. 28) and finally returns to the dorsal aspect of the foot where it reaches the interdigital space between the hallux and the second toe.

In the second case the situation, shape and extension of the fourth lumbar dermatome were almost identical (Figs. 29, 30 and 31). In a third case the extent was very similar (Figs. 32 and 25). The photograph (Fig. 25) shows the large overlap of the fourth and the third lumbar dermatomes, the latter of which was outlined by the vaso-dilatation excited by faradic stimulation of the third lumbar root. The topography of the fourth lumbar dermatome in a fourth case is shown in Fig. 33.

The fourth lumbar dermatome, as defined by the isolation method, has a markedly larger extent than Head determined. In Head's scheme the big toe is not included in it.

The fifth lumbar dermatome occupies the anterior side of the leg, the entire dorsum of the foot and of all toes (Figs. 34, 35 and 36). The border runs along the outer border of the foot behind the external malleolus, up the leg and then turns below the head of the fibula to the anterior aspect, from where it runs down along the internal side of the leg to the sole. The dermatome occupies the medial part of the sole, and the plantar surfaces of the first, second and third toes, but not that of the fourth and fifth toes (Fig. 37).

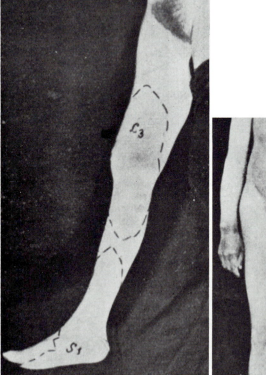

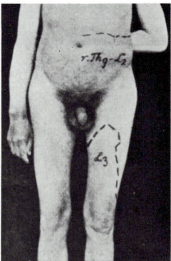

Fig. 21 (*left*). The 3rd lumbar dermatome of relatively small extent. The 1st sacral dermatome of large extent. Resection of Th11 to L2, L4 and L5, S2 to S5.

Fig. 22 (*right*). The superior border of the 3rd lumbar dermatome; resection of Th9 to L2.

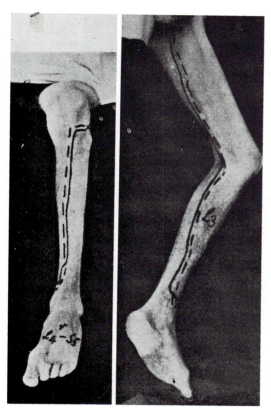

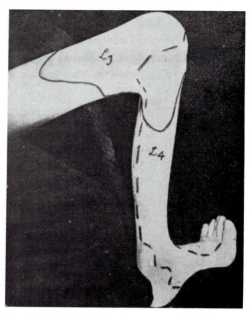

FIG. 25. The 3rd lumbar dermatome defined by vaso-dilatation following electrical stimulation of 3rd posterior lumbar root. The 4th lumbar dermatome defined in the same case by remaining sensibility after resection of all lumbar and sacral roots except the 4th lumbar. The continuous line represents the border of the 3rd dermatome, the broken line that of the 4th lumbar dermatome.

FIGS. 23 and 24. The inferior border of the 3rd lumbar dermatome; resection of L4 to S5.

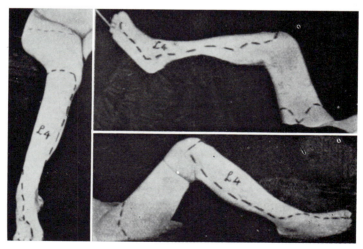

FIGS. 26, 27 and 28. The 4th lumbar dermatome; resection of L2 and L3, and L5 to S5.

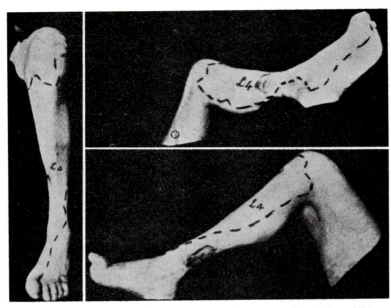

Figs. 29, 30 and 31. The 4th lumbar dermatome in a second case; resection of L2 and L3, and L5 to S5.

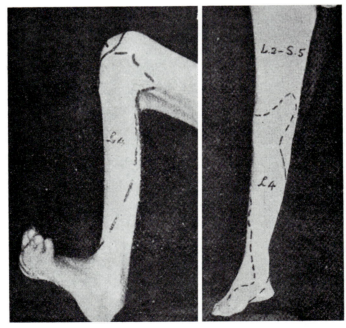

Fig. 32 (*left*). The 4th lumbar dermatome in a third case; resection of L2 and L3, and L5 to S5.
Fig. 33 (*right*). The 4th lumbar dermatome in a fourth case; resection of L2 and L3, and L5 to S5.

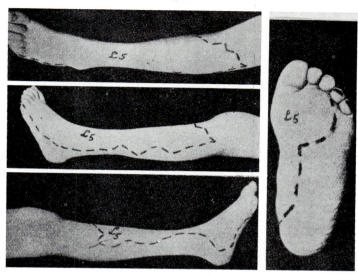

FIGS. 34, 35, 36 and 37. The 5th lumbar dermatome; resection of Th12 to L4, and S1 to S5.

The constructive method reveals the same borders for the fifth lumbar dermatome. In a case in which I resected the first, second and third sacral roots, the anæsthetic area on the posterior side is shown in Fig. 38. Its border runs along the external side of the foot, but the medial half of the sole and the first, second and third toes pre-

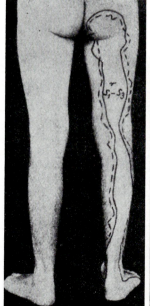

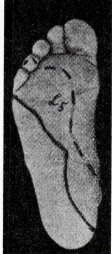

FIGS. 38 and 39. The anæsthesia following resection of S1, S2 and S3, showing the border of the 5th lumbar dermatome on the planta pedis; the tactile dermatome (continuous line) is of larger extent than pain dermatome (broken line).

served their sensibility (Fig. 39). In this photograph the continuous line indicates the limits of tactile anæsthesia, the broken line that of the analgesia; the extent of the latter is larger than that of the former. This is common in cases of root resection, and corresponds with the fact, pointed out by Sherrington, that the tactile dermatomes are larger than the pain dermatomes.

The first sacral dermatome occupies the sole and the plantar surfaces of the toes (Fig. 40); in some cases it extends even to the dorsal surfaces of the toes. From the sole the dermatome spreads upwards along the posterior side of the leg (Fig. 41). The size and shape of the first sacral dermatome, as defined by the isolation method, are very similar to the first sacral dermatome in Head's scheme (Fig. 5).

The second sacral dermatome occupies the posterior surface of the thigh and of the leg, the sole of the foot and the plantar aspects of the toes (Fig. 42). In another case the second sacral dermatome extended on to the dorsal surfaces of the toes (Fig. 19). The extent of the remaining sensibility in my cases was considerably larger than the area of the second sacral dermatome in Head's scheme (Fig. 5).

Thoracic Dermatomes

I have had no opportunity of defining the different thoracic dermatomes by the isolation method, but the constructive method has furnished all the details necessary for determining the inferior and superior borders of practically all of them. A full description of all these separate dermatomes is not necessary; their distribution and size can be seen in the diagram which I have worked out from the examination of a great

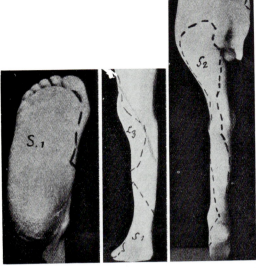

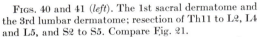

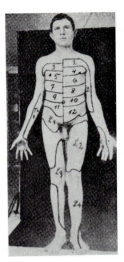

FIG. 43. Scheme of thoracic dermatomes.

FIGS. 40 and 41 (*left*). The 1st sacral dermatome and the 3rd lumbar dermatome; resection of Th11 to L2, L4 and L5, and S2 to S5. Compare Fig. 21.

FIG. 42 (*right*). The 2nd sacral dermatome; resection of Th11 to S1, and S3 to S5.

number of cases of division of posterior thoracic roots (Fig. 43). A few details are, however, worthy of notice.

The tenth thoracic dermatome has a typical situation around the umbilicus, and the superior border of the eleventh and the inferior border of the ninth thoracic dermatomes extend just to it. The mammilla lies within the fifth thoracic dermatome, and the inferior border of the fourth and the superior border of the sixth reach to a horizontal line through it.

The thoracic dermatomes, as defined by the vasodilatation excited by electrical stimulation of the posterior thoracic roots, conform closely to the areas obtained by the constructive method (Figs. 12, 44, 45, 46, 47, 48, 49, 50).

The area of vasodilatation following faradic stimulation of the third thoracic root includes a triangular patch in the axilla. In the case represented by Fig. 51 the latter was not continuous with the main area upon the thorax. I have found this lack of continuity of the areas of vasodilatation following electrical stimulation of the posterior roots in a good many other cases.

In another case the triangular area in the axilla was not so large (Fig. 52); there exist undoubtedly considerable individual variations in it. A similar

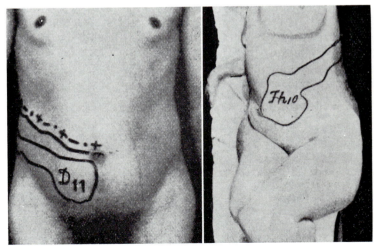

FIG. 44 (*left*). The 11th thoracic dermatome defined by vasodilation; resection of Th10 to S5.
FIG. 45 (*right*). The 10th thoracic dermatome defined by vasodilatation.

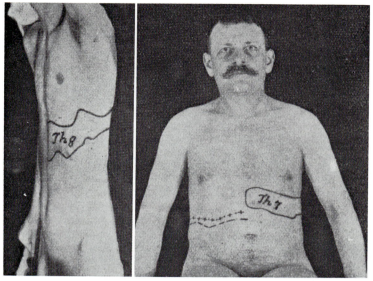

FIG. 46 (*left*). The 8th thoracic dermatome defined by vasodilatation.
FIG. 47 (*right*). The 7th thoracic dermatome defined by vasodilatation.

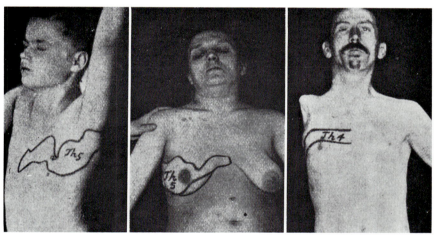

FIGS. 48 and 49 (*left*). The 5th thoracic dermatome defined by vasodilatation.
FIG. 50 (*right*). The 4th thoracic dermatome defined by vasodilatation.

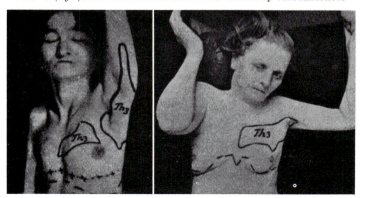

FIGS. 51 and 52. The 3rd thoracic dermatome defined by vasodilatation.

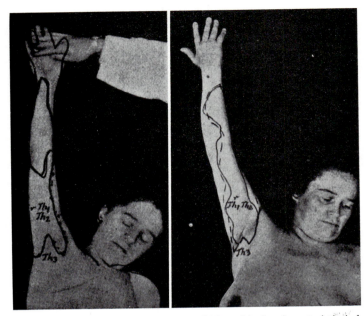

Fig. 53 (*left*). Anæsthesia following resection of Th1 and Th2 with the characteristic indentation of the 3rd thoracic dermatome in the axilla. Note the considerably larger extent of analgesia and thermanæsthesia $+-$. $+-$., than that of the tactile anæsthesia, ———.

Fig. 54 (*right*). Anæsthesia following resection of Th1 and Th2; indentation by the 3rd thoracic dermatome in the axilla. Analgesia and tactile anæsthesia of about the same extent.

triangular prolongation of the third thoracic dermatome into the axilla is demonstrable by the constructive method, as after division of the first and second thoracic roots the area of resulting anæsthesia shows the characteristic indentation due to its prolongation into the axilla (Fig. 53). In another case of resection of the first and second thoracic roots the characteristic triangular prolongation of the third thoracic dermatome also is visible (Fig. 54), and in another patient in whom the second and first thoracic, and the eighth and seventh cervical roots were resected, the triangular prolongation of the third thoracic dermatome into the axilla comes out very clearly (Fig. 55).

Sometimes this triangular prolongation of the third thoracic dermatome extends even further down the arm, as in a case of resection of the second and first thoracic roots and the fifth to the eighth cervical roots reported by Head (Fig. 56). In this case the triangular area of remaining sensibility resembles closely in size and shape the triangular prolongation delimited by the area of vasodilatation produced by electrical stimulation of the third thoracic root, which is shown in one of the illustrations (Fig. 51).

The second thoracic dermatome, as represented by the area of vasodilatation excited by faradic stimulation of the second thoracic root, occupies the inner side of the arm. It extends downwards

as far as the internal condyle of the humerus, and it is prolonged on to the anterior and posterior surfaces of the thorax (Figs. 57, 58). In the case illustrated by Fig. 58, vasodilatation reached as far as the wrist; this was due to the fact that the fibres of the first thoracic dermatome were also stimulated in consequence of an anastomosis between the second and the first thoracic roots. The two bands of the second thoracic dermatome which extend on to the thorax from the inner side of the arm form a characteristic angle (Fig. 58c), and consequently in all cases of division of the third, fourth and fifth thoracic roots the anæsthesia includes a triangular extension into the axilla (Fig. 59).

The first thoracic dermatome, as represented by the area of vasodilatation following electrical stimulation of the first thoracic root, occupies the internal side of the fore-arm as far down as the wrist (Fig. 57). Unfortunately the superior border of this dermatome could not be mapped out in this case, since the second thoracic root had been stimulated just before and the effect of this stimulation, which always lasts a considerable time, had not disappeared when the first thoracic root was stimulated.

That the second thoracic root, and probably the first thoracic root as well, take part in the innervation of the thorax, is demonstrated by the fact that after resection of the first and second

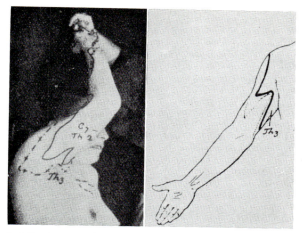

Fig. 55 (*left*). Anæsthesia following resection of C7, C8, Th1 and Th2, with characteristic indentation by the 3rd thoracic dermatome in the axilla. Analgesia and thermanæsthesia +−. +−. of larger extent than tactile anaesthesia, ———.

Fig. 56 (*right*). Tactile anaesthesia . . . . . and analgesia ——— following resection of C5 to Th2 reported by Head. The 3rd thoracic dermatome occupies the internal surface of upper arm.

thoracic roots a small band of anæsthesia is, in some cases, found on the thorax (Fig. 60).

Cervical Dermatomes

The eighth cervical dermatome, as represented by the area of vasodilatation following electrical stimulation of the eighth cervical root, occupies the fifth and fourth fingers, the ulnar half of the third finger, the ulnar part of the hand and to some extent the distal part of the fore-arm (Fig. 61). The overlap of the eighth cervical dermatome on the fore-arm is demonstrated by a case in which the first and second thoracic roots had been resected; the inferior border of the anæsthesia does not reach as far as the wrist (Fig. 62), and the sensibility preserved on the lower part of the fore-arm must be due to extension of the eighth cervical dermatome to the fore-arm. Individual variations in the distribution of the eighth cervical dermatome exist however, for in another case of resection of the first and second thoracic roots, already

demonstrated above, the anæsthesia reached distalwards as far as the wrist (Fig. 53).

I have no cases affording landmarks for the definition of the seventh cervical dermatome.

The sixth cervical dermatome, outlined by the remaining sensibility after resection of the first and second thoracic, and the eighth, seventh, fifth and fourth cervical roots, occupies the thumb, the index finger and the thenar eminence, and extends up the external side of the fore-arm and of the upper arm (Figs. 63, 64). The tactile dermatome is considerably larger than the pain dermatome.

In all cases in which the first, second, third, fourth and fifth cervical roots are divided, the inferior border of the anæsthesia outlines a triangular flap below the shoulder (Fig. 65). The borders of this area represent the superior limits of the sixth and seventh cervical dermatomes.

The fifth cervical dermatome, as shown by the vasodilatation following stimulation of the fifth

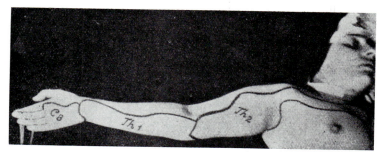

Fig. 57. The 2nd and 1st thoracic and 8th cervical dermatomes defined by vasodilatation. The 1st thoracic and the 8th cervical dermatomes do not show their full extent.

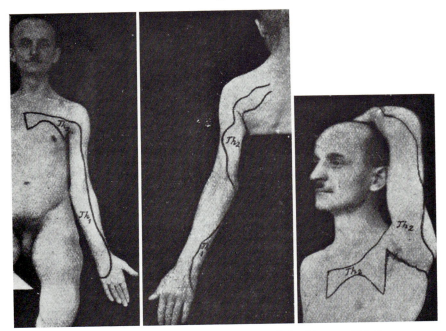

FIG. 58. The 2nd and 1st thoracic dermatomes defined by vasodilatation.

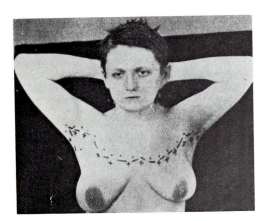

FIG. 59. The superior border of the anæsthesia in a case of chordotomy interrupting the pain and thermal fibres corresponding to the 3rd, 4th, 5th and 6th and lower thoracic roots.

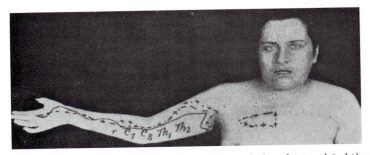

FIG. 60. The anæsthesia following resection of 7th and 8th cervical, and 1st and 2nd thoracic roots. Note the small band of analgesia and thermanæsthesia upon the chest.

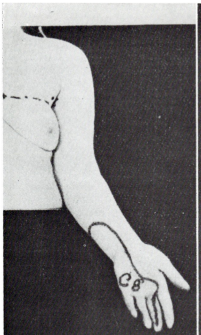

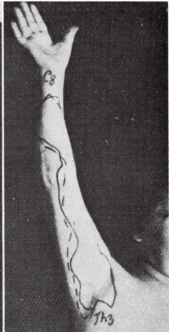

FIG. 61 (*left*). The 8th cervical dermatome defined by vasodilatation.

FIG. 62 (*right*). Anæsthesia following resection of Th1 and Th2. Note the conservation of sensibility in the interior part of the fore-arm. Compare Fig. 54.

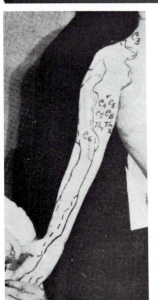

FIGS. 63 and 64. The 6th cervical dermatome; resection of C4 and C5, and of C7 to Th2.

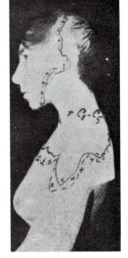

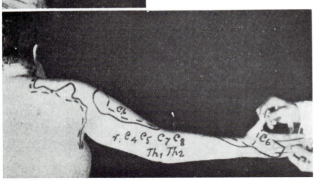

FIG. 65. The anæsthesia following resection of C1 to C5.

cervical root, covers a large area. It reaches from the shoulder along the lateral side of the arm downwards as far as the thumb (Figs. 66, 67, 68). The same case demonstrates very well the large overlap of the fifth cervical dermatome with the sixth and seventh dermatomes; the first, second, third, fourth and fifth cervical roots were resected, but the resulting anæsthesia does not extend further downwards than about 6 cm. below the shoulder; on the other hand the fifth dermatome reaches as far as the thumb.

The fourth cervical dermatome.—The inferior border of the area of vasodilatation following electrical stimulation of the fourth cervical root is shown in Fig. 69. Its superior border could not be outlined in this case as the skin of the neck had been coloured by a solution of iodine. In this case the first, second, third and fourth cervical roots were resected. Fig. 70 shows that the area of vasodilatation produced by faradic stimulation of the fourth cervical root extends much lower than the inferior border of the area of anæsthesia following the resection of the first to fourth cervical roots. This shows clearly the amount of overlap of the fourth cervical dermatome with the fifth, sixth

and seventh cervical dermatomes and the first and second thoracic.

The constructive method confirms the result obtained by the electrical stimulation of the fourth cervical root. In a case (Figs. 71 and 72) in which the fifth, sixth, seventh and eighth cervical, and the first, second and third thoracic roots were divided, the characteristic triangular area of the fourth cervical dermatome may be seen at the superior border of the resulting anæsthesia.

In a case reported by Cushing, in which the second and third cervical roots were resected, the inferior border of the anæsthesia marks the superior border of the fourth cervical dermatome (Fig. 73). My own cases of resection of the second and third cervical roots demonstrate a similar inferior border of the anæsthesia (Figs. 74, 75). The analgesia occupies a larger area than the tactile anæsthesia, that is to say the pain dermatome is considerably smaller than the tactile. The difference between the extent of analgesia and that of tactile anæsthesia is still greater in another case in which the second and third cervical roots were resected (Figs. 76, 77); the area of anæsthesia is exceptionally small, but the inferior border of the

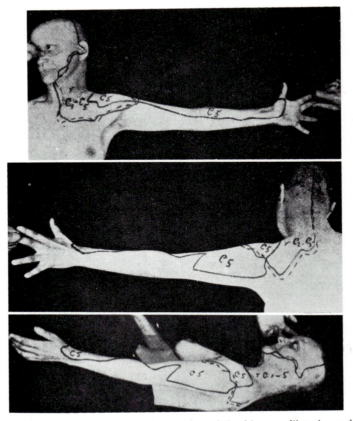

FIGS. 66, 67 and 68. The 5th cervical dermatome defined by vasodilatation and the anæsthesia following resection of C1 to C5.

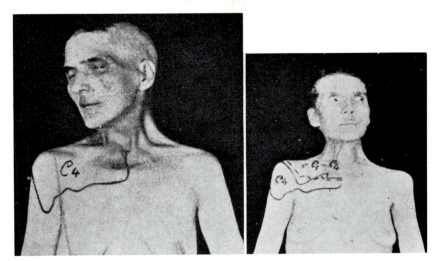

FIG. 69 (*left*). The inferior border of 4th cervical dermatome, defined by vasodilatation.

FIG. 70 (*right*). The inferior border of 4th cervical dermatome, defined by vasodilatation, and the inferior border of the anæsthesia following resection of C1 to C4. This figure demonstrates the large overlap of the 4th cervical dermatome on the adjacent dermatomes.

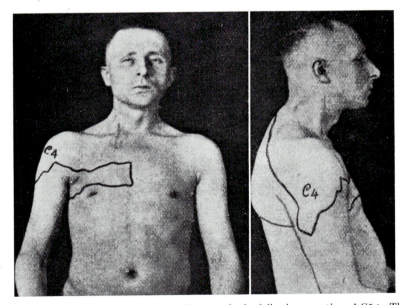

FIGS. 71 and 72. The superior border of the anæsthesia, following resection of C5 to Th4. It demonstrates the inferior border of 4th cervical dermatome.

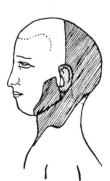

FIG. 73. The inferior border of the anæsthesia following resection of C2 to C3 (according to Cushing). It demonstrates the superior border of the 4th cervical dermatome.

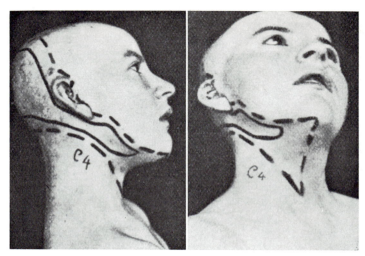

FIGS. 74 and 75. The anæsthesia following resection of C2 and C3. The inferior border of the anæsthesia indicates the superior border of 4th cervical dermatome. Note the much larger extent of the analgesia - - - than of the tactile anæsthesia ———.

analgesia and thermanæsthesia conforms to Cushing's observations.

The third cervical dermatome, as represented by the area of vasodilatation following electrical stimulation of the third cervical root, is shown in Fig. 78. It reaches upwards to the mandible, includes the ear and extends downwards as far as the clavicle. In the same case the fifth cervical root also was stimulated, and it can be seen how closely the two areas of vasodilatation come together.

The inferior border of the third cervical dermatome was also defined by resection of the fifth

and the fourth cervical roots (Fig. 79). The case is interesting in as far as there was no tactile anæsthesia; the resection of the two roots produced analgesia and thermanæsthesia only, further evidence of the larger extent of the tactile than of pain and thermal dermatomes. In another case in which the fourth, fifth, sixth, seventh and eighth cervical and the first to the fifth thoracic roots were resected the lower border of the third cervical dermatome was similar (Fig. 80), but sometimes the third cervical dermatome extended further downwards, as in a case in which the fourth, fifth, sixth, seventh and eighth cervical

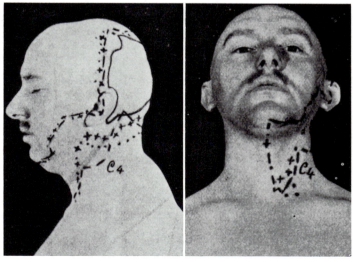

FIGS. 76 and 77. The anæsthesia following resection of C2 and C3. The inferior border indicates the superior border of the 4th cervical dermatome. Note the small extent of tactile anæsthesia ———, the much larger extent of the analgesia - - - , and of thermanæsthesia +. +. +.

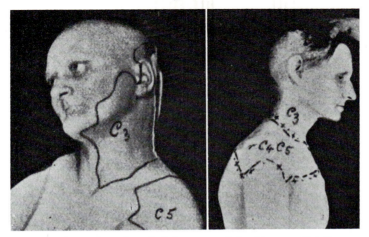

FIG. 78 (*left*). The 3rd cervical dermatome defined by vasodilatation.
FIG. 79 (*right*). The inferior border of the 3rd cervical dermatome defined by the superior border of the sensory loss following resection of C4 and C5. Note the complete absence of tactile anæsthesia in this case.

and the first to the fourth thoracic roots were resected (Fig. 81). This case demonstrates again the considerable individual variations in the extent of a single dermatome.

The second cervical dermatome occupies the occiput and the submental region, as may be seen in a case in which all cervical roots except the second were divided (Figs. 82, 83). The anæsthesia involves the ear and sends a triangular projection towards the temporal region. But there exist considerable individual variations in the extent of the second cervical dermatome, for in a case in which the same roots were resected and the second cervical root alone was left intact, the ear is partially included in the anæsthesia (Fig. 84); on the other hand the loss of sensation, at least as far as pain sensibility was concerned, ex-

tended into the submental region (Fig. 85). In a third case of resection of all cervical roots except the second, the second cervical dermatome occupied the occiput, a large area on the neck and the submental region (Figs. 86, 87). The distribution of the anæsthesia was similar in a further case in which the third, fourth, fifth and sixth cervical roots were divided; here the second cervical dermatome extends from the occiput far down on the neck and occupies a large area on its anterior surface (Figs. 88, 89).

The oral border of the second cervical dermatome is represented by the border of anæsthesia following resection of the fifth cranial nerve (Fig. 90). In the majority of my cases the line separating these two areas runs down from the vertex anteriorly to the ear, but the tragus is not included

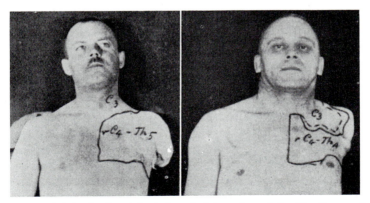

FIG. 80 (*left*). The inferior border of the 3rd cervical dermatome defined by the superior border of the anæsthesia following resection of C4 to Th5.
FIG. 81 (*right*). The inferior border of the 3rd cervical dermatome defined by the superior border of the anæsthesia following resection of C4 to Th4. Note the large extent of the 3rd cervical dermatome upon the thorax.

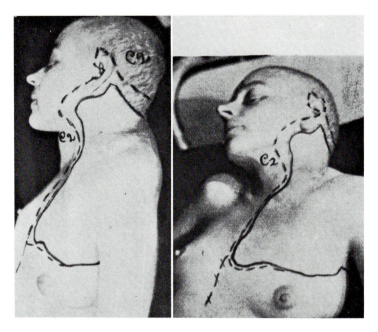

FIGS. 82 and 83. The 2nd cervical dermatome defined by the superior border of the anæsthesia
following resection of all the cervical roots except the second.

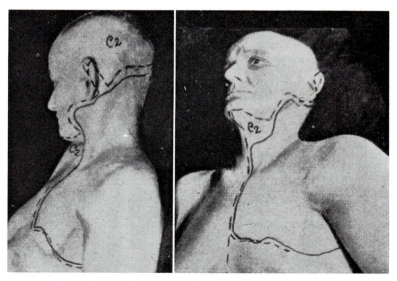

FIGS. 84 and 85. The 2nd cervical dermatome defined by the superior border of the anæsthesia
following resection of all the cervical roots except the second.

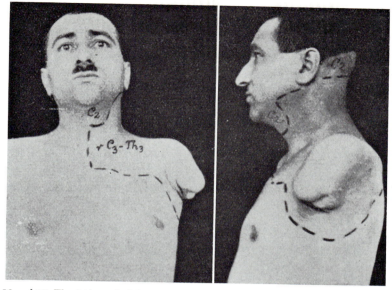

FIGS. 86 and 87. The 2nd cervical dermatome defined by the superior border of the anæsthesia following resection of all the cervical roots except the second.

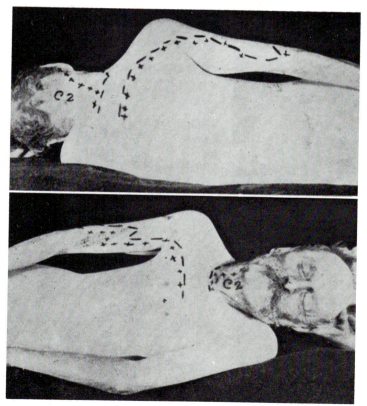

FIGS. 88 and 89. The 2nd cervical dermatome defined by the superior border of the anæsthesia following resection of C3, C4, C5 and C6.

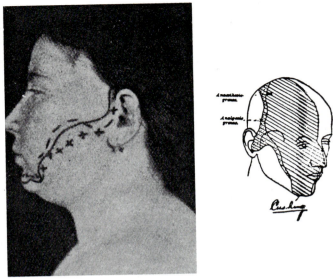

FIG. 90 (*left*). The superior border of the 2nd cervical dermatome defined by the caudal border
of the anæsthesia following resection of the 5th cranial nerve.
FIG. 91 (*right*). The tactile anæsthesia and analgesia following division
of the trigeminal root, according to Cushing.

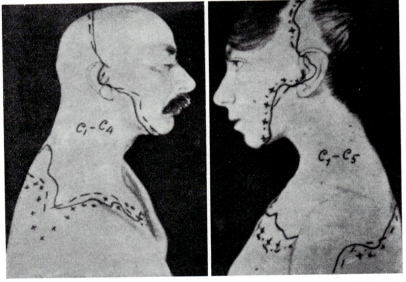

FIGS. 92 and 93. The superior border of the anæsthesia following resection of all the cervical
roots; it indicates the caudal border of the cranial nerve supply to the skin.

in the anæsthesia, and I have seldom found the helix anæsthetic. But the observations of other investigators indicate that individual variations exist. Fig. 91 shows the area of anæsthesia following section of the trigeminal root according to Cushing; the tragus is included within it.

The caudal border of the dermatomes corresponding to the cranial nerves. if such an expres-

sion be allowed, is represented, according to my experience, by a very typical line. I have been able to determine this in twelve cases in which I resected all the upper cervical roots (Figs. 92, 93). In all these cases the anæsthesia included the ear, but the external meatus and the skin around it were not anæsthetic. The individual variations are slight. I believe that it is not correct to say that this border is the caudal limit of the skin supply of the fifth cranial nerve, for we must bear in mind that the seventh, ninth and tenth cranial nerves participate to some degree in the supply of the ear.

Conclusions

From the material at my disposal several conclusions seem to me permissible.

(1) The dermatomes of man overlap to the same large degree as do those of the monkey. I never have found that resection of one single root in man was followed by loss of sensibility; at least by the usual clinical methods of examining sensibility no defect could be detected. When a single posterior root has been divided it is only by counting carefully the number of pressure and pain spots in the area innervated by that root, and by measuring exactly the threshold of the spots for mechanical or electrical stimuli, that a diminution in the number of root fibres connected with the skin can be demonstrated.

(2) The tactile dermatomes are larger than the pain and the thermal dermatomes. The area of analgesia and thermanæsthesia following resection of a number of contiguous roots is always larger than the area of tactile anæsthesia. Sometimes the resection of two contiguous roots produces analgesia and thermæsthesia, only, but no tactile anæsthesia.

(3) The areas of vasodilatation produced by electrical stimulation of posterior roots are similar to the dermatomes defined by the isolation method, but not identical with them. The former are very similar to the areas of herpetic eruption.

(4) One last word to illustrate the conformity between the dermatomes of man and monkey. A single dermatome is represented not only in the totality of the corresponding root, but in every single filament of the root. When all filaments except one of each of a number of roots are cut, no anæsthesia results, each of the corresponding dermatomes preserves its sensibility. This was demonstrated in animals by several investigators. The same is to be observed in man. I have resected in several cases about two-thirds and even more of each of all the lumbar and sacral roots, leaving intact a small filament only of each root. In these cases the sensibility was preserved.

(5) The difference between the results of experimental physiology in animals and clinical observation in man lies in the far greater difficulties presented by human material. The physiologist can do what he believes to be necessary for his investigation; the activities of the neurologist are limited to procedures which are necessary to help his patient, and he can do no more. This difference explains why the physiology of the nervous system of man lags far behind the experimental physiology of animals, and needs more time to achieve a result, which even when obtained will be a modest one.

The material which I have brought before you is the result of thirty years of neuro-surgery, and at the end I feel that I am at about the same milestone as at the beginning. I realize that all our present knowledge of the dermatomes in man has added little to the foundation which was laid just forty years ago by Henry Head in his doctorial thesis in Cambridge, June 1892.

It has given me much pleasure to be invited to deliver this lecture in memory of Dr. Schorstein, who was an eminent physician on the Staff of the London Hospital, more especially as it gives me the opportunity of paying a tribute to his colleague, Sir Henry Head, whose work on the dermatomes and other subjects has added distinction to English neurology.

Neurosurgical Classic—10

DECEREBRATE rigidity and similar phenomena in humans are periodically encountered in contemporary neurosurgical practice.[4,10] The understanding of these conditions is largely due to the efforts of one man—Charles S. Sherrington.[1-4, 7,9,11-16] Sherrington, who received a Nobel Prize in 1932 for his numerous contributions in neurophysiology,[15] devoted a major amount of his life's work to the study of spinal reflexes and their central control. During the course of these experiments, he discovered that prepontine transection of the brain stem in animals resulted in continuous spasm of the skeletal muscles, especially the extensors. Sherrington's analysis of the mechanisms involved in this phenomenon is one of the major milestones of modern physiology.[3,4]

"The phenomenon of decerebrate rigidity which is so conspicuous in a bulbospinal cat was no doubt observed by many early investigators, including Whytt, Rolando and Flourens, who all stated that animals may survive for varying periods following removal of the forebrain. The significance of the decerebrate posture, however, was not appreciated until Sherrington's well known paper was published on the subject in 1898. . . . For some 15 years prior to this Hughlings Jackson had been developing the concept of 'release' of function in order to account for various manifestations of injury to the higher parts of the brain in man. The concept of release is implicit in some of the writings of Charles Bell . . . , but Jackson was the first to give it general application. In hemiplegia, Jackson argued, the withdrawal of cortical influence and the accompanying loss of voluntary power led to the appearance of 'positive signs' which result from overactivity of certain lower centres normally restrained by the cerebral cortex. Spasticity is not due, as some had supposed, to irritation from a lesion, but rather to 'release' of lower centres from cortical control. Sherrington also interpreted the manifestations of decerebrate rigidity as 'release phenomena,' since they persist indefinitely; they cannot, he maintained, be attributed to irritation, for direct irritation of the cut surfaces of the brain stem does not increase the rigidity. . . .

"Decerebrate rigidity has often been reported in man, sometimes occurring in the form of tonic fits, but more often appearing as an enduring rigidity developing prior to death. Jackson's[5] (1870) 'cerebellar' seizures actually represent functional decerebration near the junction between the pons and medulla. Similar functional decerebration was reported by Cushing . . . , but prior to the work of Magnus and de Kleijn[8] (1912) the criteria of the decerebrate state in man had not been fully recognized. . . . "[4]

Despite the fact that rigidity following craniocerebral trauma in humans is frequently not the exact duplicate of decerebrate rigidity in animals,[4] and can be caused occasionally by supratentorial as well as midbrain lesions,[6,10] the pioneering studies of Sherrington have remained basic to the understanding of these conditions.

References

1. BRAZIER, M. A. B. The historical development of neurophysiology. In: *Handbook of physiology. A critical, comprehensive presentation of physiological knowledge and concepts.* J. Field, Ed. Washington, D.C.: American Physiological Society, 1959, Sect. 1, *1*: 1–58.

2. FEARING, F. Reflex action. A study in the history of physiological psychology. *Baltimore: Williams & Wilkins Co.*, 1930, xiii, 350 pp. (see pp. 220–222).

3. FULTON, J. F. Sherrington on neurophysiology. *Brit. med. J.*, 1947, *2*: 807–810.

4. FULTON, J. F. Physiology of the nervous system. *New York: Oxford Univ. Press*, 1949, 3rd ed., x, 667 pp. (see pp. 157–176).

5. JACKSON, J. H. A study of convulsions. *Trans. St. Andrews med. Grad. Ass.*, 1870, *3*: 162–204.

6. JEFFERSON, G. Bilateral rigidity in middle meningeal haemorrhage. *Brit. med. J.*, 1921, *2*: 683–685.

7. LIDDELL, E. G. T. The discovery of reflexes. *Oxford: Clarendon Press*, 1960, vi, 174 pp. (see pp. 98–143).

8. MAGNUS, R., and DE KLEIJN, A. Die Abhängigkeit des Tonus der Extremitätenmuskeln von der Kopfstellung. *Pflüg. Arch. ges. Physiol.*, 1912, *145*: 455–548.

9. SCHMIDT, J. E. Medical discoveries. Who and when. A dictionary listing thousands of medical and related scientific discoveries in alphabetical order, giving in each case the name of the discoverer, his profession, nationality, and floruit, and the date of the discovery. *Springfield, Ill.: Charles C Thomas*, 1959, ix, 555 pp. (see p. 120).

10. SCHNEIDER, R. C. Craniocerebral trauma. In:

Kahn, E. A., *et al. Correlative neurosurgery*. Springfield, Ill.: Charles C Thomas, 1955, xv, 413 pp. (see pp. 275–326).

11. SHERRINGTON, C. S. On reciprocal innervation of antagonistic muscles. Third note. *Proc. roy. Soc.*, 1897, *60*: 414–417.

12. SHERRINGTON, C. S. Experiments in examination of the peripheral distribution of the fibres of the posterior roots of some spinal nerves. II. *Philos. Trans.*, 1898, *190B*: 45–186.

13. SHERRINGTON, C. S. Decerebrate rigidity, and reflex coordination of movements. *J. Physiol.*, 1898, *22*: 319–332.

14. SHERRINGTON, C. S. The integrative action of the nervous system. *New Haven: Yale Univ. Press*, 1947, 2nd ed., xxiv, 433 pp.

15. STEVENSON, L. G. Nobel Prize winners in medicine and physiology, 1901–1950. *New York: H. Schuman, Inc.*, 1953, ix, 291 pp. (see pp. 154–164).

16. U. S. NATIONAL INSTITUTE OF NEUROLOGICAL DISEASES AND BLINDNESS. Great names in neurology. Bibliography of writings by Joseph Babinski, Victor Horsley, Charles Sherrington, and Arthur van Gehuchten. *Bethesda, Md.: U. S. Public Health Service*, 1957, v, 80 pp. (see pp. 39–65).

DECEREBRATE RIGIDITY, AND REFLEX COORDINATION OF MOVEMENTS.* By C. S. SHERRINGTON, M.A., M.D., F.R.S. (*University College, Liverpool*). (Three Figures in Text.)

1. Decerebrate rigidity.
2. Afferent nerve-roots and decerebrate rigidity.
3. Forms of extensor rigidity allied to decerebrate rigidity.
4. Inhibition of decerebrate rigidity by central stimuli.
5. Inhibition of decerebrate rigidity by peripheral stimuli.

1. *Decerebrate Rigidity.*

In a communication to the Royal Society in 1896[1] I described under the name *decerebrate rigidity* a condition of long-maintained muscular contraction supervening on removal of the cerebral hemispheres. The condition is one possessing considerable physiological interest, but I have not succeeded in finding any description of it prior to the above mentioned. Although continued experimentation still leaves me in doubt concerning the actual focus of origin of the rigidity, it will be useful to give here a further account of the phenomenon and of some points connected with it.

When in the monkey after ligation of the carotid arteries and under deep chloroformisation the cerebral hemispheres are removed, and little haemorrhage has occurred, the respiratory move-

* Reprinted from *The Journal of Physiology*, 1898, *22*: 319–332, with the kind permission of the Secretary of the Editorial Board.

[1] *Proc. Roy. Soc.* LX.

ments proceed, after a slight temporary check, regularly as before, and the chloroform narcosis can be somewhat relaxed because profound unconsciousness has resulted from the ablation itself. Then ensues, often almost at once, *i.e.* in a few minutes, sometimes however only after an interval of an hour or more, a status characterised by a peculiar rigidity of certain joints. The elbow joints do not allow then of the usually easily made passive flexion, the knee joints similarly are stiffly extended. The tail is stiff and straight instead of flexible and drooping. The neck is rigidly extended, the head retracted, and the chin thrown upward.

In my observations I have been accustomed to support the animal freely above the table. In that way opportunity is afforded for separate inspection and investigation of the individual parts of the trunk and limbs. The joints are then free to move with little hindrance. Moreover the existence of and even the degree of paralysis of different regions is indicated very valuably by the extent to which the attitude is determined by mere gravitation. If in a monkey or cat transection below or in the lower half of the bulb has been performed, the animal, artificial respiration when necessary being kept up, hangs from the suspension points with deeply drooped neck, deeply drooped tail, and its pendent limbs flaccid and slightly flexed. The fore-limb is slightly flexed at shoulder, at elbow and, very slightly, at wrist. The hind-limb is slightly flexed at hip, at knee and at ankle. On giving the hand or foot a push forward and then releasing it the limb swings back into and somewhat beyond the position of its equilibrium under gravity; and it oscillates a few times backward and forward before finally settling down to its original position.

To this condition of flaccid paralysis supervening upon transection in the lower half of the bulb the condition ensuing on removal of the cerebral hemispheres offers a great contrast. In the latter case the animal, on being suspended just in the same manner as after the former operation, hangs with its fore-limbs thrust backward, with retraction at shoulder joint, straightened elbow, and some flexion at wrist. The hand of the monkey is turned with its palmar face somewhat inward. The hind-limbs are similarly kept straightened and thrust backward; the hip is extended, the knee very stiffly extended, and the ankle somewhat extended. The tail in spite of its own weight, and it is quite heavy in some species of monkey, is kept either straight and horizontal or often stiffly curved upward. There is a little opisthotonus of the lumbosacral vertebral region. The head is kept lifted against gravity and the chin is tilted upward under the retraction and backward rotation of the skull. The differences in general attitude assumed after transection in the lower half of the bulb and after ablation of the cerebral hemispheres respectively is indicated in the diagrams Figure 1, *a* and *b*. When the limbs or tail are pushed from the pose they have assumed considerable resistance to the movement is felt, and unlike the condition after bulbar section on being released they spring back at once to their former position and remain there for a time more stiffly than even before.

The phenomenon of this decerebrate rigidity occurs with little variation in the monkey, dog, cat, rabbit and guinea-pig. In all these species the effect upon the fore-limb seems more intense than on the hind-limb. In the hind-limb the knee is the principal joint affected. In the rabbit the phenomenon in the hind-limb has so far as my observations go been particularly well seen. It is noteworthy that the wrist and ankle are comparatively slightly implicated in the rigidity, the ankle more than wrist. I have never in any instance been able to satisfy myself that the digits are implicated at all.

The rigidity is immediately due to prolonged spasm of certain groups of voluntary muscles. The chief of these are the retractor muscles of the head and neck, the elevators and dorsal flexors of the tail, and the extensor muscles of the elbow and knee, and shoulder and hip. This prolonged spasm I have seen maintained in young cats, with some intermissions, for a period of four days. It is increased, and even when absent or very slight may be soon developed, by passive movements of the part. For example, passive flexion and extension of the elbow will suffice to "develop" in a few seconds a high "extensor rigidity" of that joint. This will after continuing a short time then tend to slowly relax again and then again it can be recalled by repetition of the passive movements. There is no obvious tremor in the spasm in the earlier hours of its continuance; later it does sometimes become tremulant.

Administration of chloroform and ether, if carried far, quite abolishes the rigidity. On interrupting the administration the rigidity again rapidly returns.

Section of the dorsal columns of the spinal cord does not abolish the rigidity. Section of one lateral column of the cord in the upper lumbar region abolishes the rigidity in the hind-limb of the same side as the section. Section of one ventro-lateral column of the cord in the cervical region destroys the rigidity in the fore and hind-limbs of the same side.

It would be possible to ascribe these results to interruption of the pyramidal tract. The following however cannot be explained by appeal to the pyramidal system. Section of one lateral half of the bulb in the lower half of the floor of the fourth ventricle and quite above the level of the decussation of the pyramidal tracts abolishes the rigidity in the limbs *on the same side as the section.* And,

further, transverse severance of the lateral region only of this part of the bulb without interference to either pyramidal tract produces similar abolition of the rigidity of the homonymous limbs. Finally, excitation of this lateral region with rapidly alternating series of induction shocks reinforces the rigidity in the homonymous side.

If instead of both cerebral hemispheres one only, say, the right, be ablated, the decerebrate rigidity appears, though not with the same certainty as after double ablation, chiefly on the *same* side as the hemisphere removed. The monkey when slung after ablation of one, *e.g.* the right, hemisphere exhibits generally the following attitude. The right limbs are extended in the pose above-described as characteristic for decerebrate rigidity, the tail is strongly incurvated toward the right, that is, its concavity is toward the right and its tip is also toward the right. It resists passive movement to the left, and if displaced thither immediately on being released flies back. The head also is pulled toward the right and retracted. The left fore-limb—and the point will be returned to— is sometimes distinctly more flexed than would be expected in the paralysed condition of the animal; the left knee likewise. The same results are seen in the cat. The contrast between the attitude of the crossed and homonymous sides is very striking. They are indicated by the diagrams Figure 1, *b* and *c*. The retraction and bending of the head cannot however be well shown in a diagram taking the dorsal view.

Homonymous extensor rigidity consequent on ablation of one hemisphere is however neither so constant of production nor so persistent when it has appeared as the rigidity following bilateral ablation. After coming on it may totally subside and again reappear, and so on several times over. There would seem under these circumstances a struggle between two conflicting influences, as though a tonic influence from the still intact crossed hemisphere at times overcame and at times was overcome by another opposed influence from a lower centre. Some amount of extensor rigidity on the side opposite to the lesion is not uncommon.

2. *Afferent nerve-roots and decerebrate rigidity.*

If after ablation of both cerebral hemispheres, even when the rigidity is being maintained at its extreme height, the afferent roots, which have been previously laid bare and prepared, are carefully severed, the limb at once falls into flaccidity. From the stiffly extended position it drops into the slightly flexed position it assumes when flaccid under gravity. The result is quite local, as indicated in Figure 1, *d*.

A question arises; is this setting aside of the rigidity by severance of afferent spinal roots a result of their paralysis or of their irritation? Is it

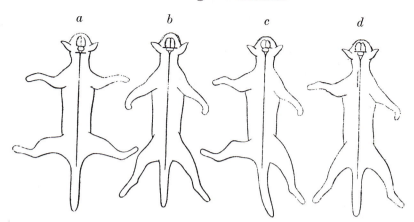

Fig. 1. *a.* Position of animal after transection at calamus scriptorius.
  b. Position of animal after ablation of cerebral hemispheres when decerebrate rigidity has developed.
  c. Position of animal after ablation of one cerebral hemisphere when decerebrate rigidity has developed.
  d. Effect on decerebrate rigidity of severance of afferent spinal roots of left fore-limb.

due to pure interruption of the afferent path leading from the periphery to the spino-cranial centres, or is it due to mere irritation of the afferent fibres by the mechanical process of severing them and the irritation of the injury set up in them? The former seems the explanation on the following grounds. Firstly, the abolition of the rigidity is long-lasting, *i.e.* persists for several hours, however the mechanical stimulation be minimised, the roots being cut through with as little disturbance as possible at the single closure of a sharp pair of scissors. Secondly, the rigidity develops either very imperfectly or not at all when the afferent roots have been severed some time, *i.e.* a number of days prior to carrying out the operation which produces the rigidity. Of this the following are examples.

Cat. The dorsal (afferent) roots of the 5th, 6th, 7th and 8th right cervical and of the right 1st thoracic nerves were severed in the vertebral canal. Marked ataxy of the right fore-limb ensued with obvious weakness of the right fore-paw (ankle). Ten days later under deep anaesthesia the cerebral hemispheres were removed. In the course of half-an-hour *decerebrate rigidity* fixed both knees and the left elbow in the extended position. The right elbow remained flaccid, although perhaps not quite so flaccid as is usual after transection at the calamus. After the animal had been subsequently killed, the onset of rigor mortis was much delayed in the extensors of the right elbow as compared with those of the left.

Cat. The dorsal (afferent) roots of the 6th, 7th and 8th right cervical and of the right 1st thoracic nerve were severed in the vertebral canal. There resulted distinctly less ataxy in movements employing the paw than in the above example; there appeared also less weakness at the wrist, but in the erect position the animal stood with its left wrist less dorsal-flexed than its right. In jumping the animal appeared always to alight on the left fore-foot a little before the descent of the right. In walking each step foward with the right fore-limb brought the foot far round, sometimes even to the left of, the left foot. Twelve days later the cerebral hemispheres were removed under deep anaesthesia. *Decerebrate rigidity* rapidly ensued, fixing in the extended position both the two knee-joints and the left elbow; but the right elbow remained flaccid. After killing the animal rigor mortis set in much later in the right than in the left triceps. Histological examination of the spinal cord revealed degeneration in the dorsal column of the right side but no further lesion. The ventral (motor) roots were quite intact.

Monkey. Macacus rhesus. The afferent (dorsal) roots of the 5th, 6th, 7th and 8th left cervical nerves and of the left 1st thoracic nerve were severed in the vertebral canal. Marked ataxy of the left arm ensued. The movement of 'grasp' by the left hand was lost. Twenty-one days later the cerebral hemispheres were removed under deep anaesthesia. *Decerebrate rigidity* rapidly supervened in both knees and in the right elbow, also to some extent in the ankles and in the right wrist. There was for some time no rigidity at all in the left elbow, which remained flaccid. In the course of three hours the rigidity increased considerably, and there were dubious traces of rigidity in the left elbow; although certainly there was no rigidity in the left wrist. After the killing of the animal subsequently the onset of rigor mortis was much later in the extensors of the left elbow than in those of the right. Histological examination showed the lesion to be confined to the afferent roots mentioned above, and the degeneration to their continuations in the dorsal column of the cord.

Monkey. Macacus sinicus. The dorsal (afferent) roots of the 5th, 6th, 7th and 8th left post-thoracic spinal nerves severed in the vertebral canal. There ensued the usual symptoms of ataxy and enfeebled grasp movement noted by Mott and myself. The left knee-jerk was abolished. As the animal ran about it kept its left limb flexed at hip and knee. There was no actual 'contracture' in the limb. Five weeks after the initial operation the cerebral hemispheres were removed under profound anaesthesia. *Decerebrate rigidity* soon developed in high degree. Both elbows became fixed in the extended position, as also the right knee. At first there was no rigidity in the left knee, and later even when the rigidity elsewhere was extreme it was doubtful whether at the left knee any developed; but I do not think the knee was so flaccid as it would have been after transection at the calamus. Subsequently after killing the animal rigor mortis set in much later in the left knee than in the right. Histological examination showed the lesion to implicate only the afferent roots above mentioned.

The decerebrate rigidity seems therefore in some way dependent on integrity of the afferent paths of the limbs. This dependence points to centripetal impulses from peripheral sense-organs of the limb as important for the production and maintenance of decerebrate rigidity in the muscles of the limb in question. Normal tonus of limb-muscles has been shown (Brondgeest, v. Anrep, & c.) to be similarly dependent on centripetal impulses from the limb; and in the case of tonus the afferent paths from the skin have been found less important (Mommsen[2]) than those from deep structures, and especially from the muscles themselves.[3] I find that similarly the afferent nerves from muscles can exercise a great local influence on decerebrate rigidity. Electrical excitation of the central end of a nerve-trunk distributed purely to muscles, *e.g.* the hamstring nerve of the cat,[4] produces immediate relaxation of the rigid extensors of the knee. On discontinuing the excitation the extensor rigidity of the knee returns. A ligature drawn tightly round this nerve keeps the knee of the homonymous side relaxed, presumably by acting as a continual slight stimulus. The extensor rigidity of the knee of the crossed side seems on the other hand somewhat increased. Mere section of the hamstring-nerve did not however in three experiments, made with a view to determining the point, prevent the development of the rigidity of the knee.

It is noteworthy that in the second example given above the sensory spinal roots severed in the

brachial plexus were exactly those in which exist the afferent nerve-fibres coming up from the triceps (extensor of the elbow) muscle itself—namely, from the muscle especially affected by the decerebrate rigidity. Also it should be stated that in all of the experiments performed the afferent roots cut were roots in which the extensor muscles—the seat of the rigidity—are represented.

These results are strikingly in accord with views that Mott and myself[5] have put forward, and especially with an argument advanced by Bastian[6] in discussing the condition of the limb in our experiments on the effect of severance of the sensory spinal roots upon the movements executed by the limb.

J. R. Ewald[7] has pointed out that destruction of the otic labyrinth reduces the tonus of the skeletal musculature of the homonymous half of the body. He also found[8] the onset of rigor mortis delayed in the muscles of the homonymous side. Similarly also I found[9] section of the afferent nerve-roots of a limb delay considerably the onset of rigor mortis in it. Decerebrate rigidity undoubtedly hastens the onset of rigor mortis in the muscles it involves. It seemed therefore desirable to enquire whether section of the nervus octavus would affect the development of decerebrate rigidity. In a monkey the VIIIth cranial nerve of the left side was accordingly cut intracranially between its surface origin and the internal auditory meatus. Nystagmus, lateral rolling movement, and other effects more or less striking ensued. Five hours later the cerebral hemispheres were removed under profound anaesthesia. Decerebrate rigidity then quickly set in and developed with about equal rapidity and in about equal degree on the left as on the right side.

3. *Forms of extensor rigidity allied to decerebrate rigidity.*

While attempting however to obtain as above some nearer view of the causation of decerebrate rigidity it must be added that other mutilations than ablation of the cerebral hemispheres induce phenomena of extensor rigidity bearing at least superficially much resemblance to that produced by removal of the cerebrum.

After median section of or ablation of the cerebellum a rigidity often, but not always, sets in somewhat similar to that ensuing on removal of the cerebral hemispheres. That the two conditions are identical I am not convinced. The uncrossed nature of the decerebrate rigidity suggests a causal connection between the cerebellum and the rigidity, perhaps through the nucleus of Deiters,

---

[2] Virchow's *Archiv*, 101, p. 22.
[3] Sherrington. *Proc. Roy. Soc.* LIII. 1893.
[4] *Proc. Roy. Soc.* LIII. 1893. *loc. cit.*

[5] *Proc. Roy. Soc.* LVII. p. 481. 1895.
[6] *Proc. Roy. Soc.* LVIII. p. 96. 1895.
[7] *Nervus Octavus.* Wiesbaden, 1892.
[8] *Pflüger's Archiv.* 1894.
[9] *Proc. Roy. Soc.* LIII. 1893.

which as first shown by Ferrier and Turner possesses large efferent connections from the side of the cerebellum. On the other hand the crossed cerebello-cerebral and crossed cerebro-cerebellar paths, in the anterior and middle peduncles on which Mingazzini's histological work has recently thrown more light, may form a circuit whose function is upset in much the same way whether cerebellar or cerebral ablation be performed. This might explain the supervention of a similar condition after either one of those injuries. Median section of the cerebellum also causes some extensor rigidity of the limbs. It will be remembered in this connection that the paths ascending by the inferior peduncle and reaching the superior vermis largely decussate there across the median line (Mott, Thomas, etc.).

It is significant that decerebrate rigidity sometimes persists after removal of the cerebellum, if the latter ablation be performed without any serious amount of haemorrhage.

These allied forms of extensor rigidity further resemble decerebrate rigidity in similarly being readily broken down by appropriate central and peripheral excitations, among the former of which are to be included excitations applied to the Rolandic area of the cortex cerebri.

4. Decerebrate rigidity inhibited by central stimuli.

One of the chief interests of decerebrate rigidity attaches to it as a field for examination of the play of inhibition. For this it gives a wider scope than can be usually obtained, and it has revealed to me an almost unexpectedly significant number of examples of depressor effect generally, perhaps always, in combination with pressor effects, that is to say, in the form of *reciprocal innervations*.

Electrical excitation of the *dorsal spinal columns* in the cervical region provokes such inhibitions. Similarly, as mentioned in my first paper, electrical excitation of the *crusta cerebri* sometimes inhibits the rigidity, evoking reciprocal innervation of antagonistic muscles at elbow, knee, etc. So also excitation of the *pyramidal tract*. In the monkey similar inhibition of the decerebrate rigidity can be produced by excitation of the anterior (cerebral) surface of the *cerebellum*,[10] as mentioned in my previous paper. Faradisation of points in a large area extending from near the middle line far out toward the lateral border of the cerebellar surface causes relaxation of the rigid neck and tail muscles, and relaxation of the rigid limbs, especially of the uncrossed side.

But the homonymous extensor rigidity which frequently ensues, as above mentioned, on ablation of one cerebral hemisphere presents an opportunity for examining the effect of excitation of the cerebral cortex itself (of the remaining hemisphere) upon the activity of the extensor muscles of the crossed elbow and knee. I find in the Rolandic region of the monkey a cortical area which gives, markedly and forthwith, inhibition of the contraction of the extensor of the elbow; and another cortical area which similarly when excited inhibits the contraction of the extensors of the knee. This is in accord with the results obtained under different conditions by H. E. Hering and myself.[11] Also, as Hering and myself in those other experiments noted, the areas of cortex whence inhibition of the active extensors is elicited are not the same areas as those whence contraction of the extensors is elicited, but on the other hand coincide with the areas whence contraction of the flexors can be excited.

5. Decerebrate rigidity inhibited by peripheral stimuli.

Besides the inhibitions from the central nervous system inhibition of decerebrate extensor rigidity can be evoked by excitations applied to the periphery.

Thus on excitation of the central end of the 2nd cervical nerve, or of a branch, even a small twig of that nerve, the high-held retracted head drops almost as if knocked down by a blow from above. The muscles causing the retraction can be seen and felt to relax at once under the excitation; the completeness and suddenness of the relaxation is surprising.

Similarly, after removal of the cerebral hemispheres, when it is easy to apply electrodes to the divisions of the trigeminus on the floor of the middle fossa of the cranium, a touch with the electrodes is enough to cause the relaxation of the rigid neck muscles: and the stimulation need not be strong in order to similarly evoke relaxation in the fore-limb, the hind-limb, and in the tail. Indeed the erected tail drops almost as easily and suddenly as the retracted neck. Excitation of even small twigs of distribution of the 5th effects the same; even the faradisation of certain spots of the dura mater suffices. Stimulation of a digital nerve or of the radial trunk causes relaxation of a similar kind, but commencing in the limb. Stimulation of the saphenous nerve as mentioned in my previous paper[12] similarly causes relaxation commencing in the hind-limb and tail.

Electric stimulation of the optic nerve is less effectual.

Excitation of the skin itself produces similar results, and here it is easier to obtain more restricted play of the inhibitions, and therefore results more instructive in regard to the mutual dis-

[10] In the following year its occurrence in the dog and cat was reported by Loewenthal and Horsley, *Proc. Roy. Soc.* LXI. 1897.

[11] *Proc. Roy. Soc.* LXI. 1897. *Pflüger's Arch.* LXVIII. 1897.

[12] *Proc. Roy. Soc.* LX.

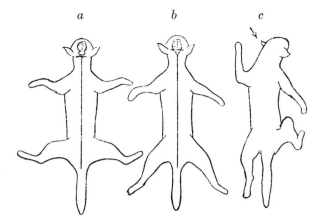

Fig. 2. *a.* Position of animal after transection at calamus scriptorius.
b. Position under decerebrate rigidity.
c. Change of attitude from *b* evoked by stimulation of left pinna.

tribution and cooperation of depressor and pressor reactions.

On excitation of the pinna of the ear, *e.g.* the left—whence the afferent paths are 5th cranial and 2nd cervical (in dog, cat and rabbit 1st cervical also) admixed—a complex reflex reaction to the following effect occurs.

The head high-held and retracted, is somewhat dropped and turned away toward the right, the stiffly extended left fore-limb is flexed at elbow, extended at wrist, and brought forward. The left hind-limb is thrust backward, its existing extension at hip and knee being increased. The right fore-limb is thrust backward, its existing extension at elbow and shoulder being increased. The right hind-limb is flexed at hip and knee and ankle. The erected tail is dropped. (Fig. 2, compare *b* and *c*.)

In this reaction there occurs (1) inhibition of the rigid left triceps, with contraction of the antagonistic pre-brachial muscles, (2) further increase of the maintained spasm of the extensors of the left knee and hip, (3) further increase of the maintained spasm of the right triceps brachii with relaxation of the antagonistic pre-brachial muscles, (4) inhibition of the rigid maintained spasm in the extensors of the right knee and hip with contraction of the hamstring and tibialis anticus muscles of the right hind-limb.

In this reflex the turning of the head away from the stimulus forcibly gives the impression of an attempt to escape from the irritation; and the concomitant raising and moving forward of the left fore-paw forcibly gives the impression of an attempt to remove the source of irritation.

If instead of the left pinna the skin of the left hand (or in cat the pad of the fore-foot) be the site of stimulation reaction occurs to the following effect. (Figure 3, *b*.)

The high-held retracted head is let fall some-

what and turned *toward* the side stimulated. The stiffly extended left fore-limb is flexed at elbow, extended at wrist and brought forward. The left hind-limb already extended is extended even further, especially at the hip. The right fore-limb is thrust backward and its already existing extension at elbow and shoulder is increased. The right hind-limb is flexed at hip and knee and ankle, its preexisting extensor rigidity being broken down. The erected tail is dropped.

Between this reaction and the foregoing the chief difference is in regard to the movement of the head. In the foregoing the movement resembled one employing the left sternomastoid—but inspection proves that at least other muscles besides the sternomastoids are involved in it. In the latter the movement seems due to lateral flexors of the neck in combination with relaxation of some of the retractors of the head.

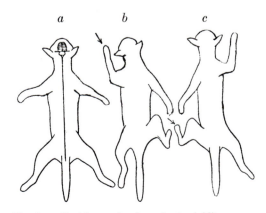

Fig. 3. *a.* Position under decerebrate rigidity.
b. Change of attitude from *a* evoked by stimulation of left fore-foot.
c. Change of attitude from *a* evoked by stimulation of left hind-foot.

If the cutaneous point excited instead of being in the hand be in the left foot (*i.e.* be in cat the left hind-pad) the reaction which occurs is to the following effect. The extensor spasm in left hind-limb at knee and hip is broken down, and flexion at hip, knee and ankle occurs. The tail is drooped from the stiff erect position. The left fore-limb has its extensor rigidity not diminished but increased. The right hind-limb also undergoes not a relaxation of its extensor spasm but an increase. In the right fore-limb the extensor spasm is broken down, and the limb is advanced with flexion at elbow, extension at wrist and advancement at shoulder. The head is somewhat drooped. These results as illustrated in the cat are indicated in Figure 3, c. Here again the movement is forcibly suggestive of a *purpose*, namely, the withdrawal of the limb from the place of an irritation.

In this reaction the relaxation of the extensors of the left knee and hip is accompanied by active contraction of the hamstring muscles, of the part of the quadriceps cruris which flexes the hip, and of the tibialis anticus and pretibial flexors, also in some cases of the peroneus longus. The relaxation of the right triceps brachii is accompanied by active contraction of the pre-brachial flexor.

Further examples of local restriction of the inhibitory effect are those which I gave in my first communication: a touch on the skin of the perineum producing inhibition often confined to relaxation of the spasm of the extensors of the stiffly elevated and tonically upcurved tail; rubbing of the check producing inhibition of the spasm of the muscles retracting the neck and head.

Regarding the inhibition of triceps brachii and quadriceps cruris, and to a less extent of the gastrocnemius, it is interesting to note that these muscles, which among the limb muscles are particularly difficult to provoke to action by local spinal reflexes, are seen in these experiments to be easily accessible when inhibition and not merely augmentation is taken into account. The well-known observation, first established I believe by Sanders Ezn, that the extensors of the knee are very inaccessible to spinal reflex action, has as I have recently shown[13] certain important limitations. But at the same time so long as the transection is spinal—even when carried out so as to isolate not merely a portion of the spinal cord, but the whole cord entire from bulb to filum terminale—does apply really very strictly to excitations arising in its own local region proper. And the spinal reflex relations of triceps brachii in this respect, and also of gastrocnemius somewhat resemble, as I have elsewhere pointed out, those of the distal portion of the quadriceps extensor of the leg. The difference between the accessibility

of the quadriceps and triceps to reflex action after infrabulbar and after suprabulbar transection it seems to me is a matter of superficial rather than fundamental distinction. The *manner* of reply of triceps brachii and quadriceps cruris seems not different in the two conditions. When the conduction across a nexus is signalised by a minus sign instead of a plus, the former, to find expression, must predicate an already existent quantity of contraction—tonus or spasm—to take effect upon. Against a background of maintained contraction effects otherwise invisible, because in the nature of inhibition and therefore finding expression as relaxation, become visible. It seems likely enough that even when transection is infrabulbar, and therefore when merely spinal mechanisms remain in force, the same nexus obtains but that then, since that background of maintained contraction is lacking, the play of inhibitions remains invisible, never coming within the field of ordinary methods of observation.

When the rigidity is developed after ablation of one cerebral hemisphere only, besides the extensor spasm on the uncrossed side there is usually some flexion on the crossed side, and this especially, I think, when the cortex is inexcitable, owing to anaemia, etc. In connection with this I would add that, in conformity with results in the dog recently reported by Wertheimer and Lepage, I have in examining in repeated experiments the movements obtainable from the *homonymous* limbs by excitation of the cerebral cortex never seen flexion of the limbs but always extension, whereas from the crossed limbs it is easy, as is well-known, to obtain both flexion and extension, separately.

The results arrived at in the above communication can be shortly summarised thus:—

"Decerebrate rigidity" is but a type of extensor spasm of which allied examples follow various other lesions of the cerebello-cerebral region.

The development of "decerebrate rigidity" in a limb is largely determined by centripetal impulses coming from the limb in question.

The contraction of the muscles active in "decerebrate rigidity" can be readily inhibited by stimulation of various regions of the central nervous system, and, among others, of the sensori-motor region of the cerebral cortex.

The activity of the rigid muscles can be readily inhibited by stimulation of various peripheral nerves, and, among others, of the afferent nerve-fibres proceeding from skeletal muscles.

Reflexes obtained from the decerebrate animal exhibit contraction in one muscle-group accompanied by relaxation, inhibition, in the antagonistic muscle group ("reciprocal innervation"), and this in such distribution and sequence as to couple diagonal limbs in harmonious movements of similar direction.

[13] *Proc. Roy. Soc.* LX. 1896.

Neurosurgical Classic—11

I N RECENT years, stereotaxic techniques have been used extensively to plot the locations and study the functions of areas within the brain.[1,4,6,7,15] By employing similar techniques for the production of localized intracranial lesions, neurosurgeons have created the relatively new field of stereotaxic surgery. In 1947, Spiegel *et al.*[14] introduced a stereotaxic apparatus for operations on the human brain, and since then these procedures have been devised for the relief of certain psychiatric symptoms, pain, and involuntary movements.[2,5,8,12,13]

It is interesting, in view of the recent nature of these developments, to realize that the forerunner of modern stereotaxic instruments was developed and used by Clarke and Horsley before 1908.[3,9–11] Portions of their first full report are reproduced below.

References

1. AMADOR, L. V., BLUNDELL, J. E., and WAHREN, W. Description of coordinates of the deep structures. In: *Introduction to stereotaxis with an atlas of the human brain.* G. Schaltenbrand and P. Bailey, Ed. Stuttgart: G. Thieme, 1959, *1:* 16–28.
2. BAILEY, P. Diseases to be treated by stereotaxic methods. In: *Introduction to stereotaxis with an atlas of the human brain.* G. Schaltenbrand and P. Bailey, Ed. Stuttgart: G. Thieme, 1959, *1:* 489–493.
3. CLARKE, R. H., and HORSLEY, V. On a method of investigating the deep ganglia and tracts of the central nervous system (cerebellum). *Brit. med. J.,* 1906, *2:* 1799–1800.
4. COOKE, P. M. Effects of electrical stimulation of deeper cell masses within the brain. In: *Introduction to stereotaxis with an atlas of the human brain.* G. Schaltenbrand and P. Bailey, Ed. Stuttgart: G. Thieme, 1959, *1:* 372–400.
5. COOPER, I. S. Parkinsonism. Its medical and surgical therapy. *Springfield, Ill.: Charles C Thomas,* 1961, xii, 239 pp. (see pp. 20–23).
6. DELGADO, J. M. R. Electroencephalography of the deeper cell masses of the brain. In: *Introduction to stereotaxis with an atlas of the human brain.* G. Schaltenbrand and P. Bailey, Ed. Stuttgart: G. Thieme, 1959, *1:* 401–420.
7. DELMAS, A., and PERTUISET, B. Cranio-cerebral topometry in man. Location and variation in position of cerebral subcortical structures with special reference to neurology, neurosurgery, and neuro-radiology. *Springfield, Ill.: Charles C Thomas,* 1959, 436 pp. (see pp. 5–10).
8. HASSLER, R. Stereotactic brain surgery for extra-pyramidal motor disturbances. In: *Introduction to stereotaxis with an atlas of the human brain.* G. Schaltenbrand and P. Bailey, Ed. Stuttgart: G. Thieme, 1959, *1:* 472–488.
9. HORSLEY, V., and CLARKE, R. H. The structure and functions of the cerebellum examined by a new method. *Brain,* 1908, *31:* 45–124.
10. RIECHERT, T., and MUNDINGER, F. Stereotaxic instruments. In: *Introduction to stereotaxis with an atlas of the human brain.* G. Schaltenbrand and P. Bailey, Ed. Stuttgart: G. Thieme, 1959, *1:* 437–471.
11. SACHS, E. Fifty years of neurosurgery. A personal story. *New York: Vantage Press,* 1958, 186 pp. (see pp. 50–51).
12. SPIEGEL, E. A., and WYCIS, H. T. Stereoencephalotomy (thalamotomy and related procedures). Part I. Methods and stereotaxic atlas of the human brain. *New York: Grune & Stratton,* 1952, viii, 176 pp.
13. SPIEGEL, E. A., and WYCIS, H. T. Stereoencephalotomy. Part II. Clinical and physiological applications. *New York: Grune & Stratton,* 1962, viii, 504 pp.
14. SPIEGEL, E. A., WYCIS, H. T., MARKS, M., and LEE, A. J. Stereotaxic apparatus for operations on the human brain. *Science,* 1947, *106:* 349–350.
15. TALAIRACH, J., DAVID, M., TOURNOUX, P., CORREDOR, H., and KVASINA, T. Atlas d'anatomie stéréotaxique. Repérage radiologique indirect des noyaux gris centraux, des régions mésencéphalo-sous-optique et hypothalamique de l'homme. *Paris: Masson & Cie,* 1957, 293 pp.

THE STRUCTURE AND FUNCTIONS OF THE CEREBELLUM EXAMINED BY A NEW METHOD.*

By SIR VICTOR HORSLEY, F.R.S., F.R.C.S.,
AND
R. H. CLARKE, M.A., M.B.
(From the Laboratory of Pathological Chemistry,
University College, London.)

PART I.—METHODS.

I.—INTRODUCTION.
II.—RECTILINEAR TOPOGRAPHY.
III.—STEREOTAXIC INSTRUMENT.
IV.—ELECTROLYSIS.
V.—EXCITATION.

I.—INTRODUCTION.

THE methods and experiments described in the following pages are the direct outcome of an investigation into the anatomical relations of the cortex of the cerebellum to its nuclei and peduncles, and to the rest of the brain and spinal cord. An

---

* Reprinted in part from *Brain,* 1908, *31:* 45–124, with the kind permission of the Editor.

account of that research was published in *Brain* in the spring of 1905.

When we began that work (1903) the view had been gaining ground that there was no direct path from the cortex of the cerebellum to the peduncles or to the spinal cord, and had been advanced by distinguished observers, especially Ferrier and Turner, Risien Russell and Thomas, who expressed themselves more or less definitely in favour of this opinion, and supported it with observations furnished by their own experiments. But although the evidence adduced established a strong probability we did not consider that it amounted to proof, as the conclusions were founded on lesions involving both cortex and nuclei, or complicated with injuries to other parts. Nor were all the conclusions of the authors absolutely definite. Marchi originally described a direct descending path in the spinal cord derived from the cerebellum. Ramon y Cajal spoke of this tract in a rather ambiguous way, leaving the reader in some doubt whether he recognized the tract himself or was merely quoting Marchi by calling it the *via descendente*. Ramon y Cajal also described some fibres passing from the cerebellar cortex to the superior peduncle. Thomas in his classical work ("Le Cervelet"), though generally supporting the view that no direct cerebello-spinal path existed, yet gave illustrations of a case of cerebellar lesion exhibiting degenerated (tecto-spinal) fibres in the spinal cord; and though he stated that there was an accidental lesion of the posterior colliculus which might have produced degeneration of such a spinal tract, Thomas was of opinion that these fibres were derived from the cerebellum.

The later illustrations of Probst all showed more or less injury to the nuclei, and though he made the deduction that the amount of degeneration seen in the peduncles or beyond them was proportional to the amount of injury to the nuclei, and was therefore derived entirely from them, the lesions were not sufficiently defined to justify these conclusions.

Considering this position of the subject was unsatisfactory, and that besides the anatomical question the much broader one of the respective functions of the cerebellar cortex and nuclei was as yet wholly undetermined, we resolved to try and find some more conclusive evidence by which to decide these points. The failure of previous experiments to afford absolute proof appeared to be due in all cases to the fact that the lesions had not been sufficiently limited, and it seemed most probable that if special precautions were observed to avoid this defect in a series of cortical lesions, following the resulting degenerations by Marchi's method, definite information regarding the course and destination of the cortical fibres would be afforded.

The results justified these anticipations. Small lesions of the cortex were made by one of us (V. H.) in anaesthetized animals—monkeys, dogs and cats. In thirteen cases the cerebellar nuclei were absolutely untouched, the lesions being strictly confined to the cortex; and of these cases, though there were abundant well-stained fine fibres passing to the adjacent folia (arcuates) and to the intrinsic nuclei, none showed degenerated fibres in any of the peduncles or in the spinal cord; this evidence appeared to us conclusive.

We did not think it necessary to perform any more experiments for the purpose of accumulating evidence on this question, but accepting the data as correct have endeavoured to follow up the indications they afforded. This view was corroborated by the appearance (after the publication of our paper) of an important research by van Gehuchten, who quite independently came to the same conclusion from experiments on another species of animal, viz., the rabbit.

As a result of these experiments we were led to the conclusion that the cerebellar cortex is essentially a recipient organ (Edinger); its efferent fibres passing to neighbouring folia and to the cerebellar nuclei, the latter being regarded as stations interposed between the efferent cortical fibres and the rest of the nervous system. Collectively, therefore, these nuclei might be considered the focus of cerebellar activity, and regarding this as the standpoint from which further investigations of their structure and function must proceed, we resolved upon a systematic inquiry into the function of the cerebellar cortex and nuclei respectively.

On making a general survey of the subject before us, and considering the most promising methods of research, we were confronted with the following preliminary difficulty: The nuclei of the cerebellum in monkeys, dogs, and cats are small, deeply situated, and not very accessible for excitation experiments, while it is evident that to get results of any value by Marchi's degeneration method, lesions must be precisely limited to the nuclei, or, if possible, to parts of them, and that such lesions must not only be accurately localized but also produced without noteworthy injury to other structures, for we had already observed the difficulties and confusion which such complications have introduced into the discussion of the subject. An essential preliminary, therefore, to further progress was to find some method which would satisfy these conditions, viz., a means of producing lesions of the cerebellar nuclei which should be accurate in position, limited to any desired degree in extent, and involving as little injury as possible to other structures. . . . Neither puncture with a small knife, nor galvano-cautery, nor the injection of acids or other fluids appeared to us to fulfil these conditions adequately, and we therefore discarded them. At this time (1904) we were unaware of the experiments of Sellier and Verger . . . , in which insulated needles were used for the production of electrolytic lesions in the brain, and we arrived independently at the same point after a number of preliminary experiments which will be referred to presently. At first, although the application of an electrical current to the nuclei by means of needles insulated to within a short distance of their points appeared most likely to serve our purpose, we were doubtful whether it would be better to employ two insulated needles and a current of high tension, thus obtaining destruction by sparks, or to use a single needle and a surface electrode with faradism or electrolysis; it is sufficient to say here we soon abandoned both the spark and faradism. The former was too violent and difficult to regulate, and the latter set up vigorous convulsive movements which are too severe to allow the application being maintained long enough to produce an effective lesion; but the electrolytic method appeared promising from the first, and after several years experience we regard it as satisfactory. The conditions under which a lesion should be made, and which we have enumerated already, are not very exacting, but, such as they are, electrolysis fulfils them in a way which leaves little to be desired. As we shall explain more fully later, electrolytic lesions of the brain, especially anodal ones, are quickly and easily produced with very slight injury to any other parts; their size can be accurately regulated, their form depends on the nature of the electrode, they are precisely defined, and the necrosed tissue passes in all directions almost abruptly into the uninjured tissues, which do not appear to be even temporarily affected by the lesion; while, finally, with the stereotaxic instrument we are going to describe, we are able to direct a protected stimulating and electrolytic needle to any desired part of the brain with very fair accuracy. All these particulars are included in the method which in this paper we propose to explain fully before giving in a separate communication the results we have obtained with it on the cerebellum. We shall begin with an account of our method of cranio-encephalic topography and measurement, followed by a brief discussion of the subject of electrolysis of central nerve tissue, including the physical and chemical characters and microsopical structure of the lesions, the different effects of anode and cathode, concluding with a discussion of the methods of electrical stimulation we have employed on the cerebellum. In a second communication we shall describe the results obtained by these methods on the structure and functions of the various parts of the cerebellum and cognate centres; this will include an account of the anatomical position of a great number of lesions, the course of the degenerated fibres and tracts they have produced, and an analysis of the functional changes and clinical symptoms which have been associated with them.

A preliminary account of our methods and of the stereotaxic instrument was published by one of us (V. H.) at the meeting of the British Medical Association at Toronto, August, 1906.

II.—RECTILINEAR CRANIO-ENCEPHALIC TOPOGRAPHY.

The first requirement in a research of this kind is the establishment of the relations existing between the exterior of the head in animals and its encephalic contents, especially in the monkey, but also in orders as far apart as the carnivora, insectivora, and birds.

As yet relatively little information exists on this question, although it is of fundamental importance in anatomy.

For the higher vertebrates the valuable drawings (especially fig. 9, p. 69) in the text-book by Flatau and Jacobson [3] are useful indications, but for our purpose, it was necessary to have not only a precise knowledge of the proportionate relations, but a means of reaching any definite spot in the encephalon, and we were therefore compelled to begin de novo, and, as will be seen directly, have adopted a method in which the objective is determined by measurement from a zero inside the encephalon, and not by the usual projection on the exterior and measurement from it.

On the question of correct technique in making cutting lesions in the central nervous system, the most important communication that has recently appeared is that by Wilhelm Trendelenburg [24]. After quoting the well-known methods of Longet, Nawrocki, Dittmer, Cyon, Woroschiloff, Probst, and Corona he points out that it is possible to devise an apparatus which consists of two parts: first, a model in brass foil of a sagittal section of that portion of the nervous system in which it is desired to make a lesion; and, second, a knife ingeniously devised of stout steel wire, so that it is possible to guide its one extremity by a hole in the brass plate (such hole representing the desired lesion), while the other extremity enters the brain. It will be understood that the model is fixed above the brain in which the lesion is to be made, that the knife is made to follow the outline in the model, and that its parallel movements and adjustment are cleverly obtained by a lazy-tongs arrangement, for movements in two planes, frontal and horizontal, that in the vertical plane being provided by sliding up and down an upright. It will be seen, of course, that this myelotom, as Trendelenburg names it, does not fulfil the conditions we feel must be satisfied. It is, however, a great advance on the cannulae and hook-like stilettes, devised by Veyssière and subsequently employed by Bechterew, Probst, and other workers, since it includes an accurate control of the cutting point during the whole operation.

To meet our immediate necessities, and at the same time to provide a plan of general application to the whole encephalon, a method of rectilinear topography and a stereotaxic instrument for applying it to direct an insulated needle to any desired point in the brain for excitation or electrolysis were devised by one of us (R. H. C.), and we have employed them for the last three years for the study of the structure and functions of the cerebrum and cerebellum in various animals.

Topographical Data and Measurements.

The difficulty of arriving at the precise localization of a point in the deep structures of the brain is due to several causes which have been generally recognized but not hitherto satisfactorily met. The first and most obvious one is that of making accurate measurements of the curved surface of an irregular sphere, like the head, especially when there are few constant and trustworthy features to serve as fixed points, while of these the precise definition is obscured, and their value more or less impaired by the mobile integument and muscles which cover the cranium. The initial difficulties are much enhanced when the ultimate objective to be localized is not on the surface, but deeply situated and probably at an uncertain distance within the cavity of the skull, and when allowance must be made for variations of thickness of the bones and their coverings, and of the size, shape, and symmetry of the structures concerned. We find, however, that a practicable and, on the whole, satisfactory solution of this problem may be attained by dividing the cranium into eight segments, by three section planes at right angles to each other, e.g., sagittal, horizontal, and frontal. As a result of these sections, each segment presents the three internal surfaces of a cube, and every point in it can be identified by rectilinear measurements from those surfaces or section planes, i.e., from their *internal* boundaries. By this means the irregular curved surface, which corresponds to the three outer sides of the cube, is not involved in any way and needs no further consideration.

In short, instead of employing the usual method of endeavouring to project the detailed stucture of the interior of the encephalon on to the surface of the head, we measure the position of the deep parts of the brain by their relation to three section planes.

The advantage of applying this principle, which, so far as we know, is new in the topography of the brain, to the localization of structural detail for the identification and record of lesions, and for the mechanical direction of an insulated needle

for excitation or electrolysis, is obvious, and its utility will become more evident as we proceed to consider the details of its practical application.

The essential points of this principle may be briefly summarized as follow:—

(1) Any irregular solid may be divided by three section planes in three dimensions into eight segments, in each of which the three internal surfaces are those of a cube.

(2) In any solid body a constant point which can be measured from plane surfaces, representing the three dimensions of a cube, can be identified by three perpendiculars of correct length dependent from those surfaces, and it is the only point where those perpendiculars can meet.

(3) A needle may be substituted for any of these perpendiculars, and in order that it may be directed mechanically to any required point in any of these rectilinear segments, an instrument is necessary which will introduce it in a direction perpendicular to one surface, and therefore parallel to the other two, to any required distance from the first surface, any required distance from the others, i.e., the needle must have a regulated movement in three dimensions.

The Determination of the Three Section Planes of the Head.

These principles are applicable to the identification of any point within the brain of a living animal and to the direction of a needle to it, provided that the conditions as defined are fulfilled. Now it is obviously practicable to divide the cranium by three section planes, which in the living animal are imaginary (definition 1). We can construct an instrument which meets the requirements of definition 3. The only difficulty lies in the determination of "constant points which can be measured from plane surfaces representing the three dimensions of a cube" (definition 2). This measurement cannot be effected in the living animal; the distance of a selected point must therefore be known from the measurement of other heads, and can be trusted only so far as these data are constant. Hence it is essential to find a method of determining section planes, which are themselves constant and can be proved by experiment to have a constant relation to any selected point within the brain.

The simplest method of selecting section planes of the cranium would be to bisect its longest diameters in three dimensions by planes perpendicular to them. This is not practicable in the case of the vertical diameter because of the structures of the neck, and in order to determine the frontal and median sagittal planes, by bisecting the longitudinal and transverse diameters of the cranium, we must first define those diameters. But there are no landmarks on the surface of the skull beneath the integuments which are sufficiently clear and precise to determine an accurate longitudinal diameter, though for transverse diameters we can utilise such prominent features as the eye and ear. The simplest method, therefore, is to begin with these stuctures and adopt the centre of the external auditory meatus and the centre of the lower margin of the orbit on both sides for the definition of the horizontal plane, or a basal plane to which the horizontal section plane is parallel but about 10 mm. nearer the vertex.

Beginning with this basal plane we can define the frontal section plane as perpendicular to the horizontal and passing through the centres of both meatus, and the sagittal section plane as bisecting the cranium perpendicular to the other two (section planes).

It will be seen . . . that this order will be followed in the application of Clarke's sterotaxic instrument. The horizontal frame is adjusted and fixed to the four points (eyes and ears) of the basal plane. By the same process the frontal zero plane is brought into place perpendicular to the horizontal plane and cutting the centres of both meatus, and the sagittal zero plane, perpendicular to the other two, is made to correspond with the median sagittal plane of the cranium by four graduated lateral clamps.

We consider the above are the most satisfactory section planes; we have verified them by the methods of drilling and passing ivory needles and making frozen sections as described elsewhere . . . and, as far as our experience goes, their relations to the most important structures of the brain are constant, with such corrections for size and symmetry as are necessary, and also quite practicable. . . .

Various anatomical features, such as sutures of the cranial and facial bones and surface markings of the brain, will be found useful for verification of the accuracy of adjustment of the instrument.

It will be noticed that the centre of the external auditory meatus corresponds to the auricular point of anatomists, and the basal plane differs very slightly from the Frankfort-Munich plane, the latter being determined by the upper margins instead of the centres of the external auditory meatus.

Reference has been made to the situation of the zero horizontal section plane being about 10 mm. above the basal plane; the object of this is to make it more central. The advantage of making the section planes as central as possible is not only that it brings them into closer relation with the most important structures of the brain, but as all measurements are made in both directions from each of the three section planes which count as zero, the margin of error in measurement is reduced.

The precise position of the zero horizontal section plane is therefore a level determined by what has been found convenient in practice in the animals we have used. Thus in the average *Macacus rhesus* the distance from the centre of the auditory meatus to the vertex, perpendicular to the base line, is 40 mm.; in the cat it is about 30 mm.; in the hedgehog about 20 mm. But whilst in the *Macacus rhesus* the inter-aural line (that is a line passing from the centre of one meatus to the other) passes through the pons, in the cat it touches the inferior surface of the pons, while in the hedgehog it is still further ventral and lies in the basi-occipital bone. This has suggested to us that the zero-horizontal section plane in the *Rhesus* should be placed at one-fourth of the distance from the meatus to the vertex, that is 10 mm. on the average above the basal plane (passing through the auricular point in the meatus and the orbital border). In the cat one-third of the distance from the meatus to the vertex, and in the hegehog one-half the distance, places the zero horizontal plane at proportionately the same region of the encephalon. In all these animals the horizontal section plane will then be about 10 mm. above the base line and convenient for measurements above and below it. For these animals, therefore, we have adopted this arrangement, but possibly future investigators employing different animals may find other proportions more convenient.

The Subdivision of the Encephalic Segments into Lamellae and Cubic Millimetres.

As already described, the whole encephalon is divided by the three zero section planes into eight segments, which are, we designate, right and left frontal, occipital, temporal and cerebellar, and each segment of the encephalon presents on its inner aspect three rectilinear surfaces corresponding to the three section planes—sagittal, frontal, and horizontal. On frozen sections of an animal's head, the preparation of which will be presently described, the distance from any point of these three surfaces of any segment can be measured and then, for an actual experiment, by means of the stereotaxic instrument, which is adjusted by these indications and carries an excitation and electrolyzing needle travelling on graduated guides in each of the three planes, it is easy to direct the latter to a similar point in an intact head. The identification of the desired point and the direction of the needle are made practicable by finally subdividing the segments into cubic millimetres as follows: Each segment is theoretically subdivided into slices or lamellae 1 mm. thick in each plane, and each lamella is divided by lines parallel to the other two planes into millimetres. For the study of the topographical detail and structure of each lamella working "charts" are made by cutting frozen heads in a special

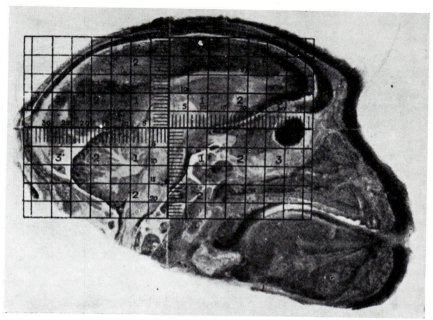

FIG. 1.

Sagittal section of frozen head of Rhesus, and millimetre glass plate.

instrument into lamellae in all three planes. To secure the identification of the section planes perpendicular to the lamellae thus prepared fine ivory knitting needles are previously introduced by a drill. For instance, for lamellae in sagittal sections, two fine ivory rods are passed transversely from the auditory meatus and orbital margin of one side to the corresponding points on the other; each sagittal lamella therefore shows a section of the two ivory needles, a line joining which is our base line. A glass plate (fig. 1), divided by ruled lines into square millimetres and by two bold lines crossing in the middle into four parts, is then placed on the surface of the lamella, and with the aid of the centres of the ivory points the glass plate is adjusted so that the two bold lines coincide with the frontal and horizontal lines or section planes. The distance of any point in the lamella from these lines can then be directly read off, and as the number of the lamella indicates the number of millimetres from the median section plane, the exact[1] distance of the selected point from the three inner surfaces of the segment in which it lies is known. Though it is useful to have several series of lamellar sections cut in all three planes, it is best to make records and references as far as possible to one plane only, and the sagittal plane is the most convenient for this purpose.[2] Further advantages of such limitation

are: much less confusion and greater brevity of reference. If it is understood that all lamellae not otherwise specified are situated in the sagittal plane, the word sagittal is superfluous. Lamella vi. then signifies a lamella in the sagittal plane 6 mm. from the median sagittal plane. It is also convenient to indicate the ordinates, *i.e.*, distances above or below the zero horizontal plane in the ruled plate, and so in the lamellae by letters of the alphabet, while the abscissae or distances in front or behind the zero frontal (inter-aural) plane are denoted by numerals. If the sagittal plane is adhered to, one soon learns that letters refer to millimetres above and below the horizontal line and numerals to millimetres before and behind the frontal line. At first the use of letters to indicate numbers is rather confusing, but after a little practice one remembers the numbers the letters correspond to without much difficulty. The advantage of having a short and easily recognized reference to any cubic millimetre will be appreciated in practice. Thus a rhesus' brain contains about 200,000 c.mm., and yet by the method described any given cubic millimetre can be identified by a reference as short as the following: *Left*

encephalon sagittally, *i.e.*, as a lateral view, the head being in the anatomical position with the visual axes horizontal, although it has unfortunately been the stereotyped custom to make the large majority of anatomical researches by sections in the frontal plane only.

[1] For corrections due to size, &c., see p. 124.

[2] Probably, too, most investigators visualize the

frontal segment, lamella v. *J.* 6. Such a statement refers to a cubic millimetre in the left frontal segment 5 mm. to the left of the median sagittal plane, 10 mm. above the zero horizontal plane, and 6 mm. in advance of the inter-aural or zero frontal plane. With that reference it is easy to select from the frozen sagittal sections lamella v., and by applying the ruled glass plate with the help of the points marked by the ivory, so that the cross coincides with the frontal and horizontal lines, to identify the deep structures which correspond to J. 6.

This sketch of the principles of what may be called rectilinear topography may serve to explain the measures required for its application, which must now be rather more fully described.

Working "charts."—These consist of a series of sections of the frozen head of an animal of the same species, and as nearly as possible of the same size as that which is to be used for the experiment. These sections are cut with a saw in a special instrument (Clarke) (*see* fig. 2) 2 mm. thick, parallel to one of the section planes, and mounted in glycerine jelly between glass plates. Each section shows two lamellae, one surface of each lamella being visible under the glass plate which covers it. The lamellae are measured and numbered from the section plane to which they are parallel. Thus they will be right and left sagittal, superior and inferior horizontal, anterior and posterior frontal lamellae in their respective planes, and the number of any lamella indicates the number of millimetres from the zero section plane to its distal surface, *i.e.,* lamella-i. lies between the section plane and a section 1 mm. from it. It is convenient to have a series of lamellae in each plane, but the sagittal is most important, since we make, as already stated, all records and references in it unless otherwise indicated.

Preparation of the head.—Heads of different sizes are injected with warm 10 per cent formalin, or equal parts of this and Müller's fluid. If not injected before the vessels have time to contract, the injection should be put off for several hours till the contraction of the vessels has begun to pass off; only moderate pressure should be employed, 0.5 to 1 metre of water is sufficient. After the injection is completed two or three holes are trephined in the skull, and the head is suspended in equal parts of 10 per cent formalin solution and Müller's fluid of double strength; it is ready to cut in a few days.

Drilling.—It has been explained already that the directions of the section planes are identified by passing two ivory knitting needles (size No. 13 or 14) in one of the section planes perpendicular to that in which the sections are made. For this purpose, and for the attachment of the stereotaxic apparatus later, it is necessary to obtain an accurate centreing of the external auditory meatus, which is accomplished as follows. Fig. 3 represents the drill, which is passed through the auditory meatus in the following manner: The same ear plugs which are used for subsequently adjusting the head in the stereotaxic instrument are employed for the drilling, being bored for this purpose. These ear plugs are made by modelling from casts of the external auditory meatus, conical plugs of different sizes so as to fit different meatus, and bent 3 mm. or 4 mm. from the base at an angle of about 20°. The floor of the meatus in the rhesus and in most animals forms a slight elevation a little internal to the external orifice and, in the rhesus, is then directed downwards and forwards. The bend in the conical plug divides it into two parts, an inner conical part (the cone) and a short outer cylinder, the barrel (fig. 4). A disc and flange are attached 3 mm. or 4 mm. from the bend, and the barrel is continued and expands slightly to a few millimetres beyond the external surface of the disk to form the funnel (fig. 4), which admits the cylindrical end of the aural pivots in the stereotaxic instrument or the nipples of the drilling apparatus. For passing the ivory needle and marking the inter-aural line, the ear plugs are introduced into the meatus and the two inner uprights of the drilling apparatus (*see* fig. 3) are brought together in the slide till the nipples enter the funnels of the ear plugs; they are then pushed home and clamped, the head being supported by the ear plugs and nipples on the two inner uprights. The drill is passed first on one side and then on the other through the perforation in the two uprights, by which accuracy of direction is secured, the petrous bone being drilled through on each side to the middle line; then a steel needle is passed the whole distance from one outside upright to the other (fig. 3), and finally the ivory needle. For drilling between the malar margins of the orbit the points are marked on each side, then the head is fixed in a clamp between the two uprights and drilled from each side as before, and the ivory needle can then be passed in the place of the drill. The points at which the drills are entered for different section planes should be marked by putting the head in the stereotaxic instrument, and it is desirable to do this and to drill when the head has been but recently fixed (*i.e.,* before it has been rigidly hardened), so that the soft parts of the auditory meatus are practically in a natural condition.

Cutting.—The instrument for cutting frozen sections has been altered from time to time, but its general construction can be seen in the illustration (fig. 2). It consists of a hack-saw working in vertical (2) and horizontal guides (3), the saw being raised or lowered by a screw which can be released by a catch (4). The head is carried on a travelling stage which is moved in guides at

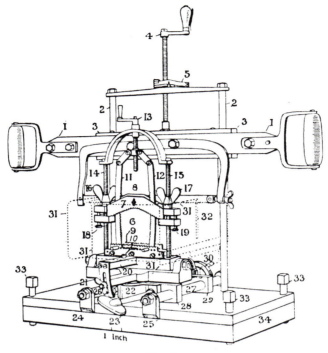

FIG. 2.

Clarke's Saw for cutting sections of frozen heads 1 mm. or 2 mm. thick.

	1	Hack saw working on horizontal and vertical guides.
	2	Vertical guides for saw.
	3	Horizontal guide for saw.
	4	Screw for raising and lowering saw.
	5	Grip with spring catch, in which screw 4 works.
	6	Placed in centre of head vice.
	7	Posterior blade of upper jaws of head vice.
	8	Anterior blade of upper jaws of head vice.
9	10	Anterior and posterior lower jaws of head vice.
11	12	Vertical jaws of head vice.
	13	Screw for approximating vertical jaws of head vice.
14	15	Screw guides for upper jaws of head vice.
16	17	Fly nuts for depressing upper jaws of head vice on screw guides (14, 15).
18	19	Screw for adjusting upper jaws of head vice.
	20	Rocking adjustment of head vice.
	21	Fly nut for clamping rocking adjustment (20).
	22	Rotatory adjustment of head vice.
	23	Screw for clamping rotatory adjustment (22).
24	25	Fixed brackets supporting guides of travelling stage of vice.
	27	Right guide of travelling stage of vice.
28	29	Travelling stage of head vice.
	30	Graduated wheel for moving travelling stage of vice on guides—One complete turn=2 mm. movement of stage.
	31	Zinc tray (shown by dotted lines) to confine CO_2 snow.
	32	Dotted lines show gap in sliding side of tray for saw.
	33	Levelling screws of foot-plate.
	34	Foot-plate.

right angles to the saw by a graduated wheel (30), one complete turn of which moves the block 2 mm. The stage (28) carries a head vice (6) on a plate with rotating and rocking adjustments (20–22) by which the head can be adjusted in two dimensions after it is fixed in the clamp. Two zinc plates (31) are fixed to the front and back of the travelling stage (28), and two lateral ones, attached by a sliding movement to its sides (32), confine the frozen CO_2 which is used to freeze the head, and the lateral plates have a gap (32) directly beneath the saw in which it descends. Some of the frozen snow escapes through these gaps, but not much. The head can be gripped in the clamp by one side, by the face, or by the base for sections in the sagittal, frontal, or horizontal planes. Having been secured it is next aligned by the adjustable plate guided by plummets suspended from the ends of the saw and by the surface markings on the head. A superficial saw cut is made to begin with in the median section plane, *i.e.*, for sagittal sections in the median sagittal line, and the distance from this line to the limit of the furthest sections to be cut is measured and marked. The head is then packed with frozen CO_2 moistened with ether. Freezing usually takes about half an hour. If frozen too hard the sections are too brittle and apt to break. If too soft they are apt to bruise and tear, but the right degree is soon learned with a little practice. When freezing is apparently complete the screw is worked till the position chosen for the first saw cut is brought directly under the saw and the first slice removed. If the surface, which can now be seen, is properly

frozen its distance from the median section plane is measured with a depth gauge, the plate of which is applied to the cut surface, while the sliding bar of the gauge terminates in a knife edge which fits into the superficial saw cut previously mentioned, and gives the distance in millimetres of the cut surface from the section plane, that is to say, the number of the lamella which that surface represents. A glass plate is then smeared with gum and applied to the cut surface, to which it immediately freezes and protects the next section while it is being cut. The block is now moved forwards 3 mm. by the screws, so that the saw cut and *débris* being equivalent to 1 mm., the section will be 2 mm. thick. As soon as it is sawn through it is placed in a dish of water, the number of the section and the distance of its surface being written on the glass plate. The same operation is repeated till all the sections are cut. They must then be carefully cleaned from the saw dust and *débris* in water, and left for a couple of days in equal parts of glycerine and water to dissolve out some of the formalin and chromates, as these have a tanning effect on the gelatine of the glycerine jelly which is apt to be troublesome. The sections are permanently mounted in glycerine jelly.

It is right to mention that there is a difficulty in mounting in glycerine jelly owng to the shrinking of gelatine produced by formalin and chromates, even after soaking the sections in glycerine and water. The most convenient way of mounting them is to make cells with glass plates large enough to include the section, and walls of square

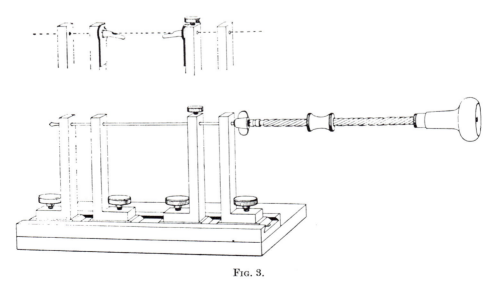

Fɪɢ. 3.

Clarke's drilling instrument.—For defining the relation of external to internal structures and determining section planes by means of ivory needles passed through corresponding points on opposite sides of the cranium and cut in frozen sections.

glass rods 3 mm. or 4 mm. diameter. When dry the cell is filled with warm glycerine jelly, and the section introduced with care to avoid bubbles. After a time the gelatine shrinks, air may find its way in, and occasionally the shrinkage breaks the glass plates and the sections have to be re-mounted. The number of the lamella should always be immediately written on the glass covering the section with enamel paint.

General Conclusions on the Topographical Relations of the Encephalon in the Macacus rhesus.

From a large series of measurements of heads of *Macacus rhesus* and in a few cases of *Macacus cynomologus* we have been able to construct a scale of averages for the former animal, and before describing the stereotaxic instrument we use for excitation and electrolysis we may perhaps with advantage first recount the general dimensions of the head in a *Macacus rhesus*, whose total body (head and trunk) length is about 320 mm. This being the commonest and most convenient size, we have as far as possible employed it only.

In fig. 5 is a reduced outline from a drawing on millimetre ruled paper showing the dimensions of a rhesus' head taken from an average of between thirty and forty specimens (avoiding fractions of 1 mm.). The base line passes through the centre of the lower margin of the orbit and the centre of the auditory meatus. Its length longitudinally is not used for calculation. Perpendicular to the base line is the frontal line, representing the (inter-aural) frontal section plane and erected from the centre of the meatus to the vertex; in the average rhesus it is 40 mm. in length. The greatest vertical diameter of the orbit is next taken and found to be 20 mm. on the average, or exactly half the height of the frontal line. On this point the constancy of the dimensions of the orbit in *Macacus rhesus* deserves some attention in view of opinions prevailing among craniologists on the value of orbital measurements. It is not a little remarkable that in examples of this species of monkey about 320 mm. long, the greatest vertical height of the orbit should rarely vary more than 0.5 mm., or at the outside 1 mm. from a total (greatest depth) of 20 mm., and in the large majority of cases not at all.

Further as regards symmetry any difference between the two orbits when present (and this is extremely rare) never exceeds 0.5 mm. It follows, therefore, that the determination of the lowest point in the lower margin of the orbit gives very satisfactorily the anterior point for the construction of the base line. To obtain the next convenient dimension, namely, the horizontal zero section plane, it will be seen that half the orbital height and one-fourth of the average frontal line

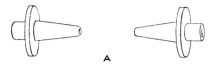

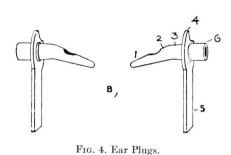

FIG. 4. Ear Plugs.

1, cone; 2, angle; 3, barrel; 4, disk; 5, flange; 6, funnel.

are in both cases 10 mm. on the average. At this level, therefore, viz., one-fourth of the frontal line, we draw parallel to the base line the horizontal line representing the zero horizontal section plane, which extends from about the nasion to the occiput. Level in front with a line joining the two inner canthi, from nose to inter-aural plane it measures 47 mm. on an average, and from this plane to occiput 33 mm., making an average total length of 80 mm. Finally the greatest transverse diameter of the frontal plane is taken with callipers and found to be maximal at about the level of the horizontal plane and 64 mm. on the average. The point where these section planes meet in the median plane is zero, and all measurements are reckoned from it, as we have already indicated. . . . Two interesting points may be noticed in the above measurements: one is that the frontal line (the median section of the inter-aural plane) is exactly double the vertical diameter of the orbit, the other is the relation of the number 16 to several of the average measurements; thus it is one-fifth of the longitudinal and one-fourth of the transverse diameter in the horizontal plane. In some animals with the same total longitudinal measurements the frontal line is 1 mm. further back, making the division of the longitudinal diameter 48 and 32 instead of 47 and 33 mm., these being also multiples of 16 in the proportion of 3:2, and in the horizontal section plane itself the relations of this number are still more striking, for the section of the skull at this level is almost exactly represented by one circle with a radius of 32 mm. and its centre at

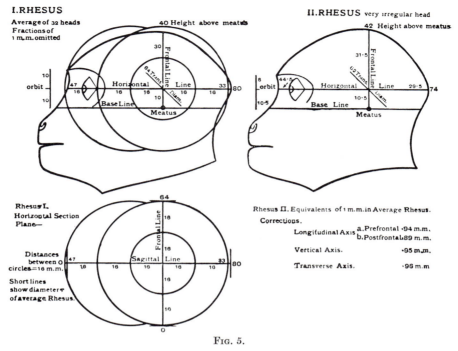

FIG. 5.

Drawing of sagittal sections of heads of two Rhesus. I. Average size,
and II. an irregular head. To illustrate measurements.

zero and half a circle with the same radius at a
point 16 mm. further forward on the median
sagittal line. Probably the average of a still larger
number of (320 mm.) rhesus monkeys will differ
a little from this, but the relative proportions are
not likely to alter much, and accumulated experience proves that the above-stated figures will
continue to be accurate guides.

III.—Description of Clarke's Stereo-
scopic Instrument Employed for
Excitation and Electrolysis.[3]

The application of the foregoing facts to our
experimental investigations has been effected by
an instrument, the general plan of which will be
most easily obtained by an examination of the
illustrations. It would be very tedious to follow a
minute description of every screw and detail,
and the purport of any of these can be ascertained
by referring to the figures and letterpress, consequently no more will be attempted in the text
than a short explanation of the essential features
and their direct application to the animal's head.

The foundation of the stereotaxic instrument
is a rigid quadrilateral rectangular frame (the
"horizontal frame") the ends of which (the
"nasal" and "occipital" bars) can be approxi-

[3] The instruments were made by Messrs. Swift and
Son, Tottenham Court Road.

mated by joints which slide on the lateral bars.
The lower border of this frame, which is in the
same plane on all four sides, is adjusted so as to
correspond accurately with the zero horizontal
section plane of the head and is fixed in this position on the skull by four lateral screw points all
furnished with millimetre scales, so that in addition to fixing the frame they make the median
sagittal line of the frame coincide with the sagittal
section plane of the head. It will be seen directly
that the horizontal pivot bars articulating with
the ear plugs in the auditory meatus, on which
the topographical adjustment of the horizontal
frame primarily depends, also indicate the points
of incidence of the perpendiculars to the horizontal frame which coincide with the frontal
section plane. When, therefore, the horizontal
frame is accurately adjusted, by erecting two
perpendiculars of equal length on the centres of
the nasal and occipital bars and joining their upper and lower extremities with two straight lines,
we can obtain a rectangular quadrilateral figure
which represents the sagittal section plane. A
similar figure representing the frontal section
plane can be constructed from perpendiculars to
the lateral bars which fall through the centres of
the auditory meatus; in short, by the adjustment
of the horizontal frame we secure data for con-
structing a rectilinear framework or cage corresponding to the three section planes of the head,

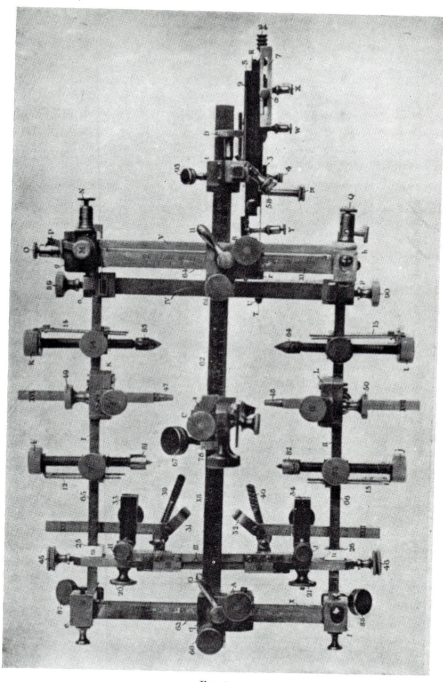

FIG. 6.

I.—*Clarke's stereotaxic apparatus for directing an insulated needle
by graduated movement in three planes.*

(Legend for Figure 6 continued on next page)

I.—Plan.

No. I. Plan.—Roman Numerals.

I & II	Right and left lateral bars of horizontal frame.
III	Frontal bar, comprising nasal and orbital plates.
IV	Occipital bar.
V	Occipital stay.
X XI	Anterior and posterior transverse guides.
XII	Sagittal guide.
XVI XVII	Right and left aural pivots, horizontal.
XXI XXII	Right and left infra-orbital bracket bars.

Capital Letters.

A & B		Anterior and posterior pinions for racking sagittal guide on transverse guides.
	C	Pinion for racking needle carrier on sagittal guide.
	D	Pinion for racking sheath on vertical guide.
	E	Pinion for racking bed of needle forward on sheath.
F	G	Right and left screws for aural adjustment of horizontal frame.
H	J	Right and left screws for orbital adjustment of horizontal frame.
K	L	Right and left aural adjustment fitting.
	M	Terminal for cathode lead from battery or coil.
	N	Terminal for cathode lead to needle.
	O	Terminal for cathode lead to live stop.
	P	Switch.
	Q	Terminal for anode leads, battery and needle.
	R	Vulcanic bed of needle holder.
	S	Sheath of needle holder.
	T	Needle.
	U	Stop.
	W	First needle terminal.
	X	Second needle terminal.
	Y	Live stop terminal.

Small Letters.

e	f	Right and left terminal joints of anterior transverse guide.
g	h	Right and left terminal joints of posterior transverse guide.
i	j	Right and left anterior lateral frame clamps.
k	l	Right and left posterior lateral frame clamps.
m	n	Right and left sliding joints of nasal plate.
o	p	Right and left sliding joints of occipital bar.
q	r	Two-way travelling joints of anterior and posterior transverse guides.
	s	Needle carrier travelling joint.
	t	Vertical guide two-way joint rack and slide.

Ordinary Numerals.

	3	Vulcanite clamp on needle holder.
	4	Screw for vulcanite clamp.
	7	Adjustable index on bed of needle.
	8	Screw for fixing index on bed of needle.
	9	Millimetre scale on sheath graduated 40–0 mm.
10 & 11		Clamps to lock travelling joints on anterior and posterior transverse guides.
12	13	Millimetre scales on right and left anterior lateral frame clamps.
14	15	Millimetre scales on right and left posterior lateral frame clamps.
18	19	Right and left millimetre scales of orbital adjustment.
20	21	Right and left screws for fixing orbital adjustment.
	24	Screw to adjust vulcanite bed for second needle.
25	26	Right and left bevelled edge indices on slots of nasal plate.
31	32	Right and left infra-orbital brackets.
33	34	Right and left sliding clamps for infra-orbital bracket bars.
39	40	Right and left horizontal maxillary rods.
45	46	Right and left screws for clamping sliding joints of nasal plate.
47	48	Tapered ends of right and left aural pivots.
49	50	Right and left fixing clamps of aural adjustment.
	58	Clamp for fixing rack movement of vertical guide.
60	61	Right and left clamps to fix sagittal guide in longitudinal slots of travelling joints of transverse guides.

(Legend for Figure 6 continued at the bottom of the next page)

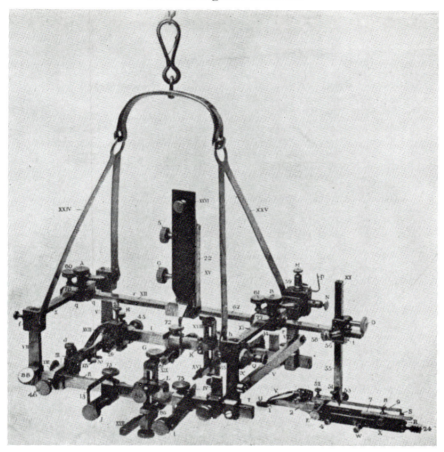

FIG. 7.

Side Elevation of Clarke's instrument.

Roman Numerals.

I II	Right and left lateral bars of horizontal frame.
III	Frontal bar.
IV	Occipital bar.
V	Occipital stay.
VI VII VIII IX	Right and left anterior and right and left posterior corner columns.
X XI	Anterior and posterior transverse guides.
XII	Sagittal guide.
XIII	Nasal plate.
XIV	Orbital plate.

(*Legend for Figure 7 continued on next page*)

	62	Millimetre scale on sagittal guide.
63	64	Millimetre scales on anterior and posterior transverse guides.
65	66	Millimetre scales on lateral bars of horizontal frame.
	67	Clamp to fix travelling joint of needle carrier (vertical).
72	73	Right and left fixing screws for sliding joints of anterior lateral frame clamps.
	78	Bevelled edge index of travelling joint of needle carrier for scale on sagittal guide.
81	82	Terminal points of right and left anterior lateral frame clamps.
83	84	Terminal points of right and left posterior lateral frame clamps.
87	88	Right and left anterior corner clamps for horizontal frame.
89	90	Right and left clamps for occipital sliding bar.
	93	Clamp for posterior sliding joint on sagittal guide.

XV   Needle carrier, vertical.
XVI XVII   Right and left aural pivots, horizontal.
XVIII XIX   Right and left aural pivots, vertical.
XX   Vertical guides.
XXIII   Supra-orbital stay.
XXIV XXV   Anterior and posterior slings.
XXVI   Dummy needle.

Capital Letters.

A   B   Pinions for racking sagittal guide on anterior and posterior transverse guides.
    C   Pinion for racking needle carrier on sagittal guide.
    D   Pinion for racking vertical guide.
    E   Pinion for racking needle bed on sheath.
    G   Screw of left aural adjustment of horizontal line.
H   J   Right and left screws of orbital adjustment of horizontal line.
K   L   Right and left aural adjustment fitting.
    M   Terminal for battery lead; cathode.
    N   Terminal for needle lead; cathode.
    P   Switch.
    Q   Terminal for battery and needle leads; anode.
    R   Vulcanite bed of needle holder.
    S   Sheath of needle holder.
    T   Needle.
    U   Stop.
    V   Live stop.
    W   Needle terminal, first.
    X   Do.   do.   second.
    Y   Terminal for live stop.

Small Letters.

e   f   Right and left terminal joints of anterior transverse guides.
    h   Left terminal joint of post, transverse guide.
    j   Left anterior lateral frame clamp.
    l   Left posterior lateral frame clamp.
q   r   Two-way travelling joints on anterior and posterior transverse guide.
    t   Two-way joint rack and slide on vertical guide.

Ordinary Numerals.

    1   Neck of sheath of needle holder.
    2   Shoulder of sheath of needle holder.
    4   Screw of vulcanite clamp on needle holder.
5   6   Screw for clamping needle holder in vertical carrier.
    7   Adjustable index on bed of needle.
    8   Screw for fixing adjustable index.
    9   Millimetre scale on sheath of needle holder.
    13   Millimetre scale on left anterior lateral frame clamp.
    14   Millimetre scale on left posterior lateral frame clamp.
    22   Millimetre scale on needle carrier.
    23   Screw to depress forehead on supra-orbital brackets.
    24   Screw to adjust sliding bed of second needle.
29   30   Right and left supra-orbital brackets.
45   46   Screws for clamping right and left sliding joints of nasal plate.
    50   Fixing clamp of left aural vertical adjustment.
51   52   Screws for fixing needle pinion.
    53   Screw for attaching needle holder to vertical guide.
    55   Millimetre scale on vertical guide.
    56   Bevelled edge of index millimetre scale of vertical guide.
    58   Clamp for fixing rack motion of vertical guide.
    59   Vulcanite insulator of cathodal terminal.
60   61   Clamps to fix sagittal guide in sliding joints of anterior and posterior transverse guides.
    62   Millimetre scale on sagittal guide.
72   73   Fixing screws for sliding joints of right and left anterior lateral frame clamps.

(Legend for Figure 7 continued at the bottom of the next page)

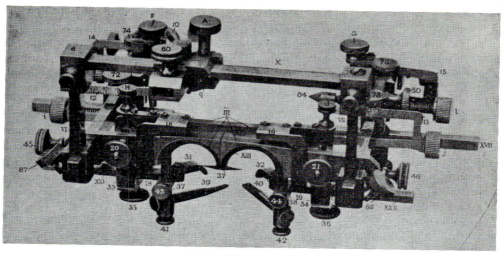

FIG. 8.

Front Elevation (anterior half) with orbital adjustment for various animals.

Roman Numerals.

III   Frontal bar.
VI VII   Right and left anterior corner columns.
X   Anterior transverse guide.
XIII   Nasal plate.
XIV   Orbital plate.
XVII   Left aural pivot, horizontal.
XXI XXII Right and left infra-orbital bracket bars.

Capital Letters.

A   Pinion for racking sagittal guide on anterior transverse guide.
F   G   Screws for right and left aural adjustment of horizontal line.
H   J   Screws for right and left orbital adjustment of horizontal line.

Small Letters.

e   Right terminal joint of anterior transverse guide.
i j Right and left anterior lateral frame clamps.
l   Left posterior lateral frame clamp.
q   Two-way travelling joint of anterior transverse guide.

Ordinary Numerals.

10   Clamp to lock travelling joint on anterior transverse guide.
12 13 Millimetre scales on right and left anterior lateral frame clamps.
14 15 Millimetre scales on right and left posterior lateral frame clamps.
18 19 Right and left millimetre scales of orbital adjustment.
20 21 Right and left screws for fixing orbital adjustment.
27   Needle indicating lower border of nasal plate, and therefore anterior limit of horizontal frame.

(*Legend for Figure 8 continued at bottom of next page*)

75   Fixing screw for sliding joint of left posterior lateral frame clamp.
76 77 Bevelled edge indices for scales on anterior and posterior transverse guides.
81   Terminal point of right anterior lateral frame clamp.
85 86 Right and left slots for posterior lateral frame clamps for small animals.
88   Right and left anterior corner clamps for horizontal frame.

which can be used for measurement and to direct a needle to any depth perpendicular to any section plane and at any distance from the other two, or, in other words, to any point of known distance from the three inner surfaces of any of the segments into which the head is divided by the three section planes.

These considerations show that the adjustment of the horizontal frame is of primary importance, and the means by which it is effected require some explanation. It has been mentioned that the base line is drawn through the middle of the lower margin of the orbit to the centre of the auditory meatus on each side and that the zero horizontal line is drawn parallel to the base line but at a convenient distance above it, namely, one-fourth of the height of the inter-aural frontal line. The adjustment of the horizontal frame to the zero horizontal plane is effected by two little pieces of mechanism called the aural and orbital adjustments, which enable the operator to bring the lower border of the horizontal frame to the correct height above the base line at these two points without difficulty.

(1) *The Aural Adjustment.*—In the illustration (fig. 7) two upright columns will be seen on the upper surface of the lateral bars. Each of them has a screw (G) at the top which raises and lowers a short vertical rod graduated in millimetres on its outer surface (XIX); this is the vertical bar of the aural pivot. Its lower end terminates in a clamp which carries another graduated rod at right angles to it, the horizontal bar of the aural pivot (XVI XVII); this bar slides in the clamp perpendicularly to the sagittal plane and can be fixed by a screw in the clamp. Its inner extremity tapers slightly (fig. 6, 47) and fits accurately into the funnel of the ear plug. These conical plugs have been described on . . . ; they are fitted into the meatus, and the frame lowered over the head of the animal sufficiently

to allow the horizontal aural pivots to engage the ear plugs. They are pushed into the funnels to exactly the same distance measured by the millimetre scales on the horizontal bars of the pivots, and when these are the same length they are fixed by the screws. Thus in practice these are the first lateral adjustments made, and by their equality these pivots first approximately centre the head in the sagittal plane. If the height of the horizontal line above the base line is known—suppose it is 10 mm.—the vertical aural pivot bar is set at 10 mm. by its scale and screw, and this brings the lower border of the frame 10 mm. above the centre of the meatus; but generally the height of the vertex above the meatus is not known and has to be measured in the apparatus, and the first adjustment of the vertical height of the aural pivots is only approximate and provisional. The measurement of the frontal line is made by provisionally fixing the aural pivots at 10 mm. and then dropping a dummy needle (fig. 7, XXVI) vertically by the needle carrier (fig. 7, XV) on to the vertex. The scale on the needle carrier gives the distance from the vertex to the horizontal plane, and this, plus the provisional setting of 10 mm., gives the whole height. If this exceeds or is less than 40 mm. then corrections are made accordingly in the aural and orbital adjustments (*see* figs. 5 and 7).

(2) *The orbital adjustment* for the monkey is somewhat different from that which is employed for other animals, and will be described first.

The front of the horizontal frame is formed by the frontal bar, which consists of two thin plates, one in front of the other, and held together by two screws (fig. 10, 20 21). They are called nasal (the front one, XIII) and orbital plates (the rear one, XIV) respectively; their connection permits a vertical sliding movement between them, regulated by the screws (fig. 10, H J) and indicated by the millimetre scales (18–19) on the face of the

31	32	Right and left infra-orbital brackets.
33	34	Right and left sliding clamps for infra-orbital bracket bars.
35	36	Screws for clamping right and left sliding clamps for infra-orbital bracket bars.
37	38	Right and left vertical maxillary rods.
39	40	Right and left horizontal maxillary rods.
41	42	Screws for clamping right and left horizontal maxillary rods.
43	44	Screws for clamping right and left vertical maxillary rods.
45	46	Screws for clamping right and left sliding joints of nasal plate.
	50	Fixing clamp of left aural adjustment vertical.
	60	Clamp to fix sagittal guide in travelling joint of anterior transverse guide.
72	73	Right and left screws for fixing sliding joints of anterior lateral frame clamps.
74	75	Right and left screws for fixing sliding joints of posterior lateral frame clamps.
	84	Terminal point of left posterior lateral frame clamp.
87	88	Right and left anterior corner screws of horizontal frame.

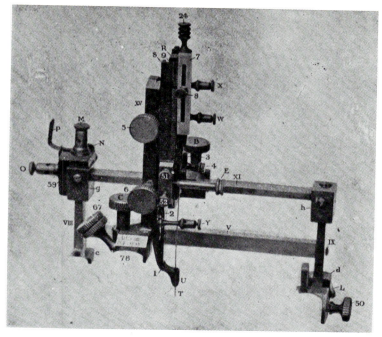

FIG. 9.

Front Elevation (posterior half), with needle mounted for vertical insertion.

Roman Numerals.

V   Occipital stay.
VIII IX   Right and left posterior corner columns.
   XI   Posterior transverse guide.
   XV   Needle carrier, vertical.

Capital Letters.

B   Pinion for racking sagittal guide on posterior transverse guide.
C   Pinion for racking needle carrier on sagittal guide.
E   Pinion for racking bed of needle holder in sheath.
L   Left aural adjustment fitting.
M   Terminal for battery lead; cathode.
N   Terminal for needle lead; cathode.
O   Terminal for live stop lead; cathode.
P   Switch.
R   Vulcanite bed of needle holder.
S   Sheath of needle holder.
T   Needle.
U   Stop.
W   Terminal of first needle; anode.
X   Terminal of second needle; cathode.
Y   Live stop terminal.

Small Letters.

c d   Right and left posterior corner joints of horizontal frame.
g h   Right and left terminal joints of posterior transverse guide.

Ordinary Numerals.

1   Neck of sheath of needle holder.
2   Shoulder of sheath of needle holder.
3   Vulcanite clamp on bed of needle holder.

(Legend for Figure 9 continued on next page)

nasal plate. The latter is extended laterally and slotted near its extremities, which thus form sliding joints on the lateral bars (fig. 10, m n). As the upper surfaces of these latter are graduated in millimetres backwards and forwards from a point opposite the centre of the auditory meatus, which is marked zero (and the posterior edges of the slots are bevelled as indices), the distance of the posterior surface of the oribtal plate from the inter-aural frontal line is read off at once. The orbital plate is brought into contact with the forehead by sliding the whole adjustment backwards on the lateral bars, to which the nasal plate is fixed by the clamping screws as described (fig. 10, 45 46). The lower border of the nasal plate, of course, has, with the rest of the horizontal frame, to coincide with the horizontal section plane. This is effected as follows: Where the orbital plate is in contact with the forehead there are attached to it on each side small horizontal slightly convex plates, the superior orbital brackets (fig. 10, 29–30), which project backwards about 6 mm. beneath the supra-orbital arches. An arm (XXIII), the "supra-orbital stay," which extends back about 2 cm. over the forehead and carries a vertical screw (fig. 10, 23), affords a simple means by which the supra-orbital arches are kept in contact with the orbital brackets on which they rest. The brackets and stay, therefore, like the blades of a pair of forceps, hold the frontal bone to the orbital plate, and the vertical movement and millimetre scales between this and the nasal plate enable the operator to see and regulate the height of the supra-orbital arch above the lower edge of the horizontal frame, i.e., of the nasal plate. As the vertical diameter of the orbit is taken beforehand with callipers (in the average Rhesus, as already stated, it is 20 mm.), if the distance of the edge of the frame below the supra-orbital arch is known its distance above the lower margin of the orbit is known also. The lower border of the horizontal frame is therefore made to coincide with the horizontal section plane at the specified height (one-fourth of the frontal line) above the lower

margin of the orbit by the screws (fig. 10, H J) and then fixed by the screws (20 21). The orbital adjustment being thus completed, the bevelled edges (fig. 6, 25 26) behind the nasal bar slots will now on the average read 47 mm. on the pre-aural scales of the lateral bars on both sides, and the nasal plate is fixed by the screws (fig. 10, 45 46). The occipital bar (fig. 6, IV) is next brought forwards into contact with the occiput, the bevelled edges of its sliding joints (fig. 6, o p) reading on the average 33 mm. on the post-aural scale of the horizontal frame bar, and it is also clamped.

The scale of the aural (fig. 7, XVIII XIX) adjustments is set at 10 mm. (if this be one-fourth of the frontal line), and then the four lateral frame clamp points (fig. 6, 81 82, 83 84) are screwed in sufficiently to secure the head firmly in its position. Each clamp is provided with a millimetre scale to ensure that the corresponding pairs, pre-aural and post-aural, are screwed into the same distance on each side. Since the same precaution was observed in adjusting the aural pivots the sagittal centreing of the head is adequately provided for by these six lateral supports thus accurately measured to corresponding lengths. After the clamping points have been fixed the occipital bar can be removed to give free access to the cerebellum. The horizontal frame has thus been accurately adjusted so that its lower border coincides with the zero horizontal line, and it now constitutes the foundation of a frame which corresponds with the three section planes and provides for directing a needle by them. Before describing the needle mechanism a few words are required on the adjustments for various other animals besides monkeys and on corrections for size, for hitherto we have only considered the average rhesus. As the measurement of the head in the apparatus, in correcting for size, &c., involves the use of some parts which have not been described it will be best to complete the description of the instrument and then consider the remaining questions of measurement.

Adjustment for animals below primates.—The

---

4   Screw for clamp on bed of needle holder.
5   6   Screws for clamping needle holder in vertical carrier.
7   Adjustable index on bed of needle.
8   Screw for fixing index on bed of needle.
9   Millimetre scale on sheath of needle holder.
24   Screw to adjust sliding bed for second needle.
50   Fixing clamp for left aural adjustment.
59   Vulcanite insulator of cathodal terminal
67   Clamp to fix travelling joint of needle carrier.
78   Bevelled edge index on travelling joint of vertical needle carrier for
      scale on sagittal guide.

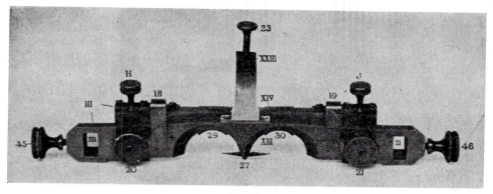

FIG. 10.

Orbital Adjustment for Monkey.—Front Elevation.

Roman Numerals.

III	Frontal bar.
XIII	Nasal plate.
XIV	Orbital plate.

Capital Letters.

H   J   Right and left screws for orbital adjustment of horizontal frame.

Small Letters.

m   n   Right and left sliding joints of nasal plate.

Ordinary Numerals.

18	19	Right and left millimetre scales of orbital adjustment of horizontal frame.
20	21	Right and left screws for fixing nasal and orbital plates.
	23	Screw to depress forehead.
	27	Needle indicating lower border of nasal plate, and therefore horizontal frame.
29	30	Right and left supra-orbital brackets.
45	46	Screws for clamping right and left sliding joints of nasal plate.

instrument can be applied to any moderately sized mammals and to the larger birds, such as geese and ducks. We have not attempted to enlarge it so as to include dogs because in almost every respect the cat's brain is superior to the dog's for elementary neurological purposes; the nerve tracts are better marked, the size of the encephalon is more convenient for serial sections, and, most important of all, cats' heads are of much more uniform size and shape than those of dogs; in fact, the endless variations in the size and shape of dogs' heads make them unsuitable for a research involving accurate cranio-encephalic topography. The orbital adjustment is the only one that needs modification to suit the heads of animals below the primates, for in all cases the range of movement in other parts of the apparatus is sufficient for any variation of size that is required, the aural adjustment fitting the form of ear plug which may be required for any species of animal.[4]

[4] It should be mentioned that in the cat the orifice of the meatus is so covered by the pinna that division of

Though the modification of the orbital adjustment we suggest as more useful[5] for animals below the monkey looks different (*see* fig. 11), anyone who has followed the description of the adjustment for the monkey will find the principle the same and the modifications easy to understand. The head, and therefore the lower border of the orbit, is raised and lowered in relation to the lower border of the frame (*i.e.*, of the nasal plate, fig. 11, XIII) by a vertical sliding motion between the nasal and orbital plates regulated by screws (fig. 11, H J) and indicated by millimetre scales (fig. 11, 18 19) on the face of the nasal plate—all this is the same in plan as before. The only difference is that while the orbital plate is connected to the forehead of the monkey by the superior orbital brackets and stay, which grasp the frontal bone like the blades of a pair of forceps, in this pattern

the latter is necessary to admit the ear plugs; the incision should be made in the line of the postero-inferior edge of the tragal portion of the pinna.

[5] Possibly for any species.

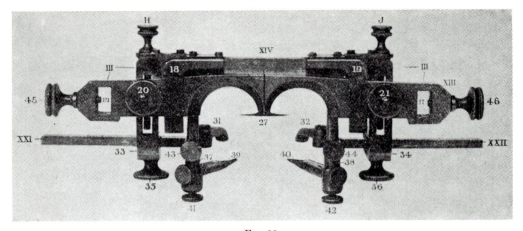

Fig. 11.

Orbital Adjustment for Various Animals.—Front Elevation.

Roman Numerals.

III   Frontal bar.
XIII   Nasal plate.
XIV   Orbital plate.

Capital Letters.

H   J   Right and left screws for orbital adjustment of horizontal frame.

Small Letters.

  m   n   Right and left sliding joints of nasal plate.

Ordinary Numerals.

18   19   Right and left millimetre scales of orbital adjustment of horizontal frame.
20   21   Right and left screws for fixing nasal and orbital plates.
      27   Needle indicating lower border of nasal plate, and therefore horizontal frame.
31   32   Right and left infra-orbital brackets.
33   34   Right and left sliding joints for infra-orbital bracket bars.
35   36   Right and left screws for fixing sliding joints (33 34)
37   38   Right and left maxillary rods, vertical
39   40   Right and left maxillary rods, horizontal.
41   42   Right and left screws for clamping horizontal maxillary rods.
45   46   Right and left screws for clamping sliding joints of nasal plate.

the orbital plate is attached to the superior maxilla by inferior orbital brackets (fig. 11, 31 32) and horizontal maxillary bars (39–40). The former project a few millimetres into the orbit over its lower edge, the latter similarly into the mouth, and both together hold the superior maxilla, grasping it like a pair of forceps by the lower edge of the orbit and the upper teeth. In birds the horizontal maxillary bars pass under both mandibles instead of between them. The maxillary bars consist of vertical (fig. 11, 37 38) and horizontal (39 40) portions freely adjustable in all directions; they and the orbital brackets are supported on graduated arms (fig. 11, XXI XXII), supported and sliding in clamps (fig. 11, 33 34) which allow them a transverse motion; the clamps are fixed to the orbital plate, and thus, being attached to the nasal plate, have a longitudinal motion on the lateral bars. Both infra-orbital brackets and maxillary bars have therefore a transverse and longitudinal movement by which they can be adjusted to heads of any size.

Mechanism for Directing the Excitation or Electrolytic Needle.

We have pointed out the data for the mechanical direction of a needle in any plane by the adjustment of the horizontal frame, and the illustrations (fig. 6 and 7) show how one method of giving effect to the principles of localization we have described are carried out in the instrument. Four rigid perpendiculars, the corner columns (fig. 7, VI VII VIII IX), are fixed to the corners of the horizontal frame and joined in pairs by two transverse graduated bars, the anterior and posterior transverse guides (figs. 6 and 7, X XI); the centre of each bar corresponding to the median sagittal plane is marked zero and graduated in millimetres from that point on each side. Each transverse guide carries a travelling two-way joint (figs. 6 and 7) with rack and pinion motion. These joints travel on the transverse guides and at the same time support and carry with them a long graduated bar, the sagittal guide (figs. 6 and 7, XII). This bar is fixed in the slots of the two-way joints in such a position that the zero marked on it corresponds to the inter-aural frontal line, and the sagittal guide is graduated forwards and backwards from this point. The only movement of the sagittal guide is a lateral one, by means of the travelling joints on the transverse guides; longitudinally it is a fixed base on which the arm carrying the horizontal needle slides by a simple joint and on which also the vertical (see fig. 7, XV) needle carrier connected perpendicularly to it by a travelling joint moves forwards and backwards from the zero inter-aural frontal plane. The excursions of the needle carriers are indicated by the millimetre scale on the sagittal guide.

The Needle Holder and its Movements.

(1) The needle, which may be single or double, consists of an iridio-platinum wire insulated nearly to the point in a capillary glass tube, and is clamped on a vulcanite plate, the bed. The glass is held by a vulcanite clamp, from which it is separated by a small piece of soft rubber. The proximal end of the projecting wire is fixed in a metal clamp secured by the terminal, which is screwed firmly down upon it, and electrically connects the needle with the lead from the coil or battery as the case may be. The bed slides by a bevelled edge on each side on a sheath, which tapers in front into a shoulder and neck, and the latter terminates in a small flattened vulcanite cylinder, the stop, perforated to permit the passage of the needle, which can be advanced and withdrawn through the stop by a rack and pinion movement of the bed on the sheath, registered by an adjustable index on the bed, and a graduated millimetre scale on the sheath. This gives the needle an excursion of 40 mm. The perforation in the stop is formed by a lateral slit open on one side to admit the needle and then closed by a fine brass rod which projects a little beyond the stop, and at its proximal end is attached to the shoulder of the sheath by a terminal which receives a lead if required and makes contact with the rod; this rod then constitutes what we call a "live stop," and may be used for so-called unipolar excitation. It also serves the purpose of exercising slight pressure on the needle in its groove, steadying it, and serves as an electrode when required. It is convenient when a single wire is employed. As we show later, in deep punctures faradization of the

brain by a long arc stimulation is highly objectionable, since if one electrode is formed by a needle point and the other by some form of surface contact the current traverses many excitable areas and may produce confused and misleading results, but in making electrolytic lesions the single needle is almost indispensable, and as we never electrolyze without at least one faradic excitation, and generally several, the difficulty is to get a satisfactory stimulation when the single needle is used. It was to meet this that the "live stop" was devised, and in practice we find that as it makes a small surface contact close to the needle, the current is notably confined to its track, thus very much diminishing the escape of current and irregular effects of wider and more distant surface contacts. The disadvantage electrolytically is the exaggeration of the needle track.

The essential parts of the needle holder are thus the bed and the sheath, the latter including the neck and stop. As the needle is carried forwards through the stop the adjustable index attached to the bed indicates the excursion of the needle on a scale on the sheath, which is so graduated that as the needle is advanced the index approaches zero. The object of this is that as the needle penetrates the brain perpendicular to either the horizontal or frontal zero section planes, it is convenient that the index should arrive at zero when the point of the needle reaches the zero plane.

The instrument is constructed to direct the needle at will into any part of the brain from two positions: (1) Vertical from above, and (2) horizontal from behind.

(1) In the vertical position the sheath of the needle bed slides in a slot in the carrier, where it can be fixed with two screws. It is perpendicular to the sagittal guide, and, of course, to the horizontal section plane. It has been explained that the carrier travels longitudinally on the sagittal guide from a zero, which corresponds with the inter-aural frontal section plane, and laterally on the transverse guides to right and left of the median sagittal plane. By these two movements the needle can be brought over any square millimetre in the horizontal plane. For the vertical movement the connection between the sheath and the carrier is used as a coarse adjustment. For this purpose there is a scale on the carrier and an index on the sheath (figs. 9 and 7). The scale is originally graduated as follows: The sheath is pushed downwards till the distal surface of the stop is level with the lower border of the horizontal frame. This point is marked zero on the scale, and the graduation is made as the sheath is drawn up. This scale therefore always indicates in millimetres the distance of the stop above the zero horizontal line. In use the sheath is pushed down

till the stop is at a convenient point, commonly the surface of the brain, and it is fixed there; the scale on the carrier (XV) then shows how many millimetres separate the stop from the horizontal line. The needle is then advanced till its point is exactly flush with the surface of the stop, and the adjustable index on the bed is set at the same figure on the scale on the sheath. If the stop, according to the scale on the carrier, is 30 mm. above the horizontal line, and the ivory index is set at 30, then as the needle penetrates the brain the figure on the sheath scale will always show the distance of the point from the horizontal section plane, and when it arrives there the index will be at zero.

(2) In the second or horizontal position the needle holder is connected to the sagittal guide in a different way. In the illustration it is shown connected to the hinder end of the sagittal guide as follows: The sheath carrying the bed and needle is fixed at right angles to the lower end of a vertical guide (fig. 7, XX) by two screws (fig. 7, 53). The vertical guide is connected with the sagittal guide by a two-way joint, one slot of which (horizontal) slides over the sagittal guide and can be fixed at any point by a screw (fig. 6, 93). The other slot of the joint is vertical and the vertical guide is worked up and down in it by a rack and pinion (fig. 7, D). The vertical guide is graduated in such a way that when the point marked zero is opposite the bevelled edge of the joint (fig. 7, 56) which serves as the index, the needle is on the horizontal line, and the graduations above and below zero show the vertical distance of the needle above or below the horizontal line.

The transverse movements of the sagittal guide to right and left of the median sagittal plane convey the same motion to the needle, and the vertical and sagittal guides in this way afford the two movements required to bring the needle opposite any square millimetre on the frontal plane. The third movement, that of the needle towards the frontal plane, is a double one as in the first position, but differently arranged. The coarse adjustment is the movement of the whole needle holder and stop towards the frontal section plane. This is effected by the sliding joint (fig. 6, t) on the sagittal guide. The bevelled edge of the joint is an index for the graduated scale on the guide and indicates the distance of this edge from the interaural plane, i.e., zero on the sagittal guide. The distal surface of the stop (U) is 50 mm. in front of the bevelled edge. As the distance of the bevelled edge from the frontal line is known, that of the stop from this line is known also. For example, if the bevelled edge is at 80, the anterior surface of the stop is 30 mm. behind the frontal section plane. The point of the needle is racked flush with the surface of the stop and the adjustable index (fig. 6, 7) set at 30. As the needle advances towards the frontal line the index travels towards zero on the scale on the sheath (fig. 6, 9), and when it reaches zero the point of the needle arrives at the zero frontal inter-aural plane. . . .

Corrections for Size and Symmetry.

In describing the adjustment of the instrument to the head of the rhesus it was assumed that the animal was a typical example of average measurements. In practice there are nearly always some variations, and they may be considerable; every head, therefore, must be carefully measured and corrections made for irregularities. The procedure we have adopted is as follows: We first take the maximal longitudinal and transverse diameters of the cranium, i.e., above the level of the zygomatic arch as well as the greatest vertical diameter of the orbit, with callipers before applying the instrument; an outline drawing of the head is made to scale on millimetre paper, and all the measurements filled in as they are taken (see specimen of such outline, fig. 5). The callipers are necessarily not as accurate as the apparatus, and the preliminary measurements with them are checked by reading on the instrument after the head is fixed. The measurements, including the true height (fig. 5, I and II) of the horizontal line shown in the outline sketch, are all filled in, and a chart frozen section which shows the required lamella is selected, and the dimensions of each segment in the experimental animal and the chart section compared. If the error of difference is less than 10 per cent, we usually treat it as negligible, but if it amounts to 1 in 10 or more we make the necessary correction according to a table of equivalents. With such corrections and careful adjustment of the apparatus the results are generally accurate in the rhesus. If there is a great difference between the absolute dimensions of the animal's head and the chart section, there is, of course, more likelihood of error, but discrepancies can be in a great measure avoided; thus if there is only one series of frozen sections to work by, animals must be selected which approach it in size, and, of course, if two or three series of sections of different sized animals are available the operator is less restricted. On the question of symmetry the measurements depend on the assumption that the positions of the bony landmarks, i.e., the meatus and orbits, are generally symmetrical. Moderate variations of proportional measurement can be corrected, and though, of course, the fewer such necessary amendments are the better, they are not necessarily inconsistent with accuracy provided they balance, but an irregularity which prevents the inter-aural plane being perpendicular to the sagittal plane is a grave fault. We do not find that such serious forms of asymmetry occur in monkeys. Of other animals we cannot speak from much experience, but cats' skulls are less regular than monkeys, and more care will be necessary in their selection. . . .

BIBLIOGRAPHY.

[1] FERRIER "Functions of the Brain," 1886.

[2] *Ibid. West Riding Asylum Reports*, 1873.

[3] FLATAU and JACOBSON. "Handbuch der Anatomie und vergleichenden Anatomie des Centralnervensystems der Saügethiere," Berlin, Karger, 1899.

[4] HITZIG. "Untersuchungen über das Gehirn," Berlin, 1874.

[5] HORSLEY, *Brain*, 1898, vol. xxi., p. 547.

[6] HORSLEY and CLARKE. *Brit. Med. Journ.*, 1906, vol. ii., p. 1799.

[7] *Ibid. Brain*, 1905, vol. xxviii., p. 13.

[8] LEDUC. "Les Ions," *Monographies Cliniques*, No. 48, January, 1907.

[9] LEWANDOWSKY. *Arch. f. Anat. u. Physiol.*, 1903.

[10] LOURIÉ. *Neurol. Centralbl.*, 1907, Bd. xxvi., S. 652; also *ibid.*, 1908, p. 102.

[11] LÖWENTHAL and HORSLEY. *Proc. Roy. Soc.*, 1897, vol. lxi., p. 20.

[12] NOTHNAGEL. *Virchow's Archiv.*, 1868.

[13] PAGANO. *Arch. Ital. de Biol.*, 1902, T. xxxviii., Fasc. 2.

[14] PRUSS (quoted by LOURIÉ). *Poln. Arch. f. d. med. u. biolog. Wissenschaft*, 1901.

[15] RIJNBERK, V. *Arch. di Fis.*, 1904.

[16] *Ibid.* "Lokalisation im Cerebellum," 1907. (Preischrift.)

[17] ROUSSY. "La Couche Optique," Paris, 1907.

[18] RUSSELL, RISIEN. *Brain*, 1897, vol. xx., p. 35.

[19] SELLIER et VERGER. *Arch. de Phys. norm. et path.*, 1898, p. 706.

[20] *Ibid. Comptes rendus de la Soc. de Biol.*, Paris, 1903, p. 485.

[21] SHERRINGTON. *Proc. Roy. Soc.*, 1897, vol. lxii., p. 183.

[22] *Ibid. Journ. of Physiol.*, 1902, vol. xxviii., p. 14.

[23] THOMSON, J. J. "The Electrolysis of Steam," *Proc. Roy. Soc.*, 1893, vol. liii., p. 93.

[24] TRENDELENBURG. "Studien zur Operationstechnik am Zentralnervensystem," *Arch. f. Anat. u. Phys.*, 1907, S. 83.

[25] "Verständigung über ein gemeinsames craniometrisches Verfahren" (Frankfurt-München), *Arch. f. Anthropol.*, 1884, Bd. xv., S. 1.

[26] WEIR-MITCHELL. *Amer. Journ. Med. Sci.*, 1869, p. 320.

Neurosurgical Classic—12

HEAD injuries have presented a problem to physicians since prehistoric times.[10,16] Most of the important works on surgery, from the first written record—the Edwin Smith papyrus,[21] have contained methods for their treatment.[17] Until the nineteenth century, however, the main emphasis in the treatment of skull fractures was placed on the care of the injured skull and scalp.[1,10,17] Hippocrates had proposed prophylactic trepanation, but the rational for this was not clearly expounded, and later surgeons argued its merits.[10,17] It appears that the principle expressed by Rhazes in about 900 A.D.—that in head injuries compression of the brain is more important than damage to the skull—was overlooked until relatively recent times.[17] In fact, according to Silvester O'Halloran,[11] an Irish surgeon (1728–1807), murder by blows to the head was not usually considered punishable in the British Isles in the eighteenth century unless a skull fracture could be demonstrated.[10]

By the end of the nineteenth century it was recognized that cerebral contusion and edema could cause increased intracranial pressure without coexisting hematomas.[17] Decompressive trephining was proposed by Jaboulay[9] in 1896, and in 1908 Cushing[3] advised subtemporal decompression in such cases. However, as experience accumulated, decompression was performed less often.[17]

Also at the end of the nineteenth century, surgeons began to perform major operations on the brain, and cerebral edema was frequently encountered.

"The relief of increased intracranial pressure during operative procedures was a problem met by various techniques. Ventricular puncture and drainage early used by surgeons was one of the most important aids in operating upon the hypertensive brain. Other less dramatic practices consisted of the use of continuous lumbar puncture drainage or the mere milking of cerebrospinal fluid from the opened arachnoid in the operative wound.[2,4] The posterior cistern was opened in procedures where lumbar puncture was inadvisable[4] . . . ."[7]

Bleeding and purging had been performed in the treatment of craniocerebral injuries for centuries, and during the early development of neurosurgery various indirect methods of reducing intracranial pressure were introduced—repeated lumbar puncture,[12] dehydration,[6] and the administration of hypertonic solutions.[14]

In 1919 the important pioneering work of Weed and McKibben[18–20]

" . . . demonstrated the effects of intravenous solutions upon brain bulk and cerebrospinal fluid pressure. In this same year perhaps the earliest account of the clinical use of hypertonic solutions (25 per cent glucose by vein) to decrease brain volume was given by Haden.[8] The oral use of hypertonic salt solutions received brief notice by Cushing and Foley[5] in 1920, and in this same year Sachs and Belcher[15] reported the use of intravenous salt solutions to control excessive swelling of the brain at the time of craniotomy. Further studies of the use of other salts and solutions followed."[7]

Since that time it has become recognized that the temporary reduction in intracranial pressure by the use of various hypertonic solutions is frequently followed by a later "rebound overshoot" in pressure when the effect of the solution becomes dissipated.[13,22] However, hypertonic solutions have become widely employed in the treatment of intracranial hypertension, and the search for better agents continues.

References

1. COURVILLE, C. B. The "wound man" and craniocerebral injury. A transitional figure bridging the gap between medieval astrological theories and scientific concepts of the Renaissance. *Bull. Los Angeles neurol. Soc.*, 1961, *26*: 47–61.
2. CUSHING, H. Technical methods of performing certain cranial operations. *Surg. Gynec. Obstet.*, 1908, *6*: 227–246.

3. CUSHING, H. Subtemporal decompressive operations for the intracranial complications associated with bursting fractures of the skull. *Ann. Surg.* 1908, *47:* 641–644.

4. CUSHING, H. Some principles of cerebral surgery. *J. Amer. med. Ass.*, 1909, *52:* 184–192.

5. CUSHING, H. and FOLEY, F. E. B. Alterations of intracranial tension by salt solutions in the alimentary canal. *Proc. Soc. exp. Biol., N. Y.*, 1920, *17:* 217–218.

6. FAY, T. The administration of hypertonic salt solutions for the relief of intracranial pressure. *J. Amer. med. Ass.*, 1923, *80:* 1445–1448.

7. GREEN, R. E., and STERN, W. E. Techniques of cranial surgery. In: *A history of neurological surgery.* A. E. Walker, Ed. Baltimore: Williams & Wilkins Co., 1951, xii, 583 pp. (see pp. 40–76).

8. HADEN, R. L. Therapeutic application of the alteration of brain volume by the intravenous injection of glucose. *J. Amer. med. Ass.*, 1919, *73:* 983–984.

9. JABOULAY. La trépanation decompressive (la mobilisation de la voûte du crâne). *Lyon méd.*, 1896, *83:* 73–75.

10. METTLER, F. A., and METTLER, C. C. Historic development of knowledge relating to cranial trauma. *Res. Publ. Ass. nerv. ment. Dis.*, 1945, *24:* 1–47.

11. O'HALLORAN, S. A new treatise on the different disorders arising from external injuries of the head; illustrated by eighty-five (selected from above fifteen hundred) practical cases. *London: G. C. & J. Robinson*, 1793, 335, iv pp. (see p. 24).

12. QUINCKE, H. Die diagnostische und therapeutische Bedeutung der Lumbalpunktion. Klinischer Vortrag. *Dtsch. med. Wschr.*, 1905, *31:* 1825—1829; 1869–1872.

13. ROSOMOFF, H. L. Distribution of intracranial contents after hypertonic urea. *J. Neurosurg.*, 1962, *19:* 859–864.

14. SACHS, E. The care of the neurosurgical patient before, during and after operation. *St. Louis: C. V. Mosby Co.*, 1945, 268 pp. (see p. 186).

15. SACHS, E., and BELCHER, G. W. The use of saturated salt solution intravenously during intracranial operations. Preliminary report. *J. Amer. med. Ass.*, 1920, *75:* 667–668.

16. STENDAHL, A., and COURVILLE, C. B. Development and use of helmets as a means of protection against craniocerebral injury. I. Among the prehistoric peoples of central and southern Mexico. *Bull. Los Angeles neurol. Soc.*, 1954, *19:* 1–17.

17. WALKER, A. E. Surgery of craniocerebral trauma. In: *A history of neurological surgery.* A. E. Walker, Ed. Baltimore: Williams & Wilkins Co., 1951, xii, 583 pp. (see pp. 216–247).

18. WEED, L. H., and McKIBBEN, P. S. The effect of intravenous injections of various concentration upon the central nervous system. *Anat. Rec.*, 1919, *16:* 167.

19. WEED, L. H., and McKIBBEN, P. S. Pressure changes in the cerebrospinal fluid following intravenous injection of solutions of various concentrations. *Amer. J. Physiol.*, 1919, *48:* 512–530.

20. WEED, L. H., and McKIBBEN, P. S. Experimental alteration of brain bulk. *Amer. J. Physiol.*, 1919, *48:* 531–558.

21. WILKINS, R. H. Neurosurgical classic—XVII. *J. Neurosurg.*, 1964, *21:* 240–244.

22. WISE, B. L., and CHATER, N. The value of hypertonic mannitol solution in decreasing brain mass and lowering cerebrospinal-fluid pressure. *J. Neurosurg.*, 1962, *19:* 1038–1043.

EXPERIMENTAL ALTERATION OF BRAIN BULK*

LEWIS H. WEED, *Capt., Med. Corps*

AND

PAUL S. McKIBBEN, *1st Lt., San. Corps*
From The Army Neuro-Surgical Laboratory, Johns Hopkins Medical School, Baltimore, Maryland

Received for publication March 22, 1919

In the early stages of an investigation of the factors underlying the swelling (edema) of the brain in acute infections or injuries, attention was directed to the possible relationship between the volume of the brain and the alteration in the pressure of the cerebro-spinal fluid, following intravenous injections of solutions of various concentrations (1). For in the study of cerebral edema, but little progress has in the past been made on account of the difficulty of experimental approach. This condition remains today one of the great problems in pathology of the central nervous system.

The marked changes in the pressure of the cerebro-spinal fluid, reported in the foregoing paper, were quickly found to have a definite relation to the resultant volume of the brain. Thus, following intravenous injections of strongly hypertonic solutions which markedly lowered the pressure of the cerebro-spinal fluid, definite shrinking of the brain occurred. And conversely the brain bulk was appreciably increased by the intravenous injection of hypotonic solutions, which raised the pressure of the cerebro-spinal fluid. Such changes in the size of the brain are rapidly and uniformly brought about, giving definite information as to one phase of the physiological regulation of the volume of this organ.

METHODS

Cats were used entirely in this work. Intravenous injections of the various solutions were given with a syringe or with a burette connected directly with a fore-leg vein. For the hypertonic solutions, 30 per cent sodium chloride or saturated sodium bicarbonate in distilled water were given, as previous work had demonstrated their

* Reprinted from *The American Journal of Physiology*, 1919, *48:* 531–558, with the kind permission of the American Physiological Society.

efficacy in lowering the pressure of the cerebro-spinal fluid. Ringer's solution (NaCl, 0.9 per cent; KCl, 0.042 per cent; CaCl$_2$, 0.025 per cent) was injected intravenously to give data regarding the possible alteration in the circulation and in the volume of the brain brought about by the introduction of an increased volume of fluid, while distilled water was used as the hypotonic solution. Cats which had been given the custo-mary intravenous injections of these solutions and then allowed to recover from the anesthetic, were usually a little slow for six hours but became normal and active within twelve hours. For the most part the observations were carried out on cats with unopened skulls, but in two series, subtemporal trephine openings were made, not only to relieve the intracranial tension but also to permit direct observation of the brain.

All animals used in these observations were anesthetized with ether, usually by intratracheal insufflation but in the earlier experiments by cone. The body temperature of the animals was maintained throughout. After the lapse of time necessary for the maximum action of the solution intravenously introduced, the animals were killed by ether. In the routine experiment, 10 per cent formalin was injected, immediately after death, through the aorta at a pressure of not more than 800 mm. of water. When the cranial vessels were well filled, the central nervous system was removed (the skull and vertebral canal being partially opened) and the whole immersed in 10 per cent formalin. In spite of all the care it was possible to exercise, it was soon very evident that by this method of fixation, the form and size rela-tions of the central nervous system prevailing prior to the death of the animal were not being accurately preserved. Brains markedly shrunken during life or at death of the animal approached almost normal proportions after such fixation, and brains markedly herniated at death often sub-sided perceptibly during preservation. The brains of other animals were fixed by direct immersion in formalin; the results of this method were sim-ilar in regard to alteration in volume. The addi-tion of a suitable amount of sodium chloride to the formalin solution did not prevent these changes in brain bulk during preservation and was as unsatisfactory as other solutions.

Although the method of fixation used is inade-quate, still it enables one to make general com-parisons of the brains after various intravenous injections, even though it does not preserve the volume relations accurately. It is hoped there will be found a means of fixation which will preserve more exactly the form and size relations and at the same time make possible a study of the histology and cytology of these brains with reasonable confidence.

EXPERIMENTS WITH UNOPENED SKULL

The majority of these experiments were car-ried out on animals without opening of the skull. Some of this series, however, were used for deter-minations of the pressure of the cerebro-spinal fluid; in these the subarachnoid space was entered by a needle through the occipitoatlantoid liga-ment for connection with a manometer. In this limited manner the pressure relations within the cranium may be considered to have been altered; other animals of this series were carried through with intact cranial cavities.

Normal. Under this heading it is purposed to discuss the normal bulk of brains as found in cats killed without experimentation, and in those given Ringer's solution in such amounts as to control the volume of the other intravenous in-jections. The intravenous injections of Ringer's solution in these quantitites did not alter the volume or appearance of the brain, so that, as far as our observations go, the brains of these ani-mals are to be classed as normal.

When removed from the skull after routine fixation with formalin, the normal brain sur-rounded by unopened dura presents in the cat typical appearances. The dura over the convex-ities is only fairly well filled out and is under no appreciable tension, falling slightly between the adjacent gyri. On looking through the dura, a definite rounding of the convolutions and the fairly well-defined edges of the sulci are apparent. On transverse section of the normal brain (fig. 3), differentiation between gray and white matter is obvious. At the periphery of the section, the dura is seen to fall slightly between adjacent gyri. The surfaces of the gyri present smoothly-rounded curves, dipping into well-defined sulci of appreci-able width. The median longitudinal fissure is clear cut and the adjacent gyri definitely sepa-rated. A line formed by the arachnoid membrane can be made out, bridging the larger sulci. Quite similar appearances are presented by the brains of animals receiving intravenous injections of Ringer's solution (fig. 4).

Examination of a large series of cats' brains fixed under similar conditions has shown that considerable individual variation exists. In brains of old animals, the gyri appear more rounded and the sulci deeper than in the younger cats. The dura in such older animals seems looser and denser, suggesting the various phenomena of old age exhibited by the brain in man. In very young cats and kittens, there seems to be a tendency toward swelling following formalin fixation. These individual variations, according to age, must be constantly borne in mind while interpret-ing the results of the experimental modification of the volume of the brain.

Hypotonic solutions. The intravenous injection

of water, which has been found to produce a definite increase in the pressure of the cerebro-spinal fluid, causes also a frank swelling of the substance of the brain. Amounts varying from 20 cc. to 100 cc. were injected intravenously; the degree of the reaction was apparently not dependent upon the absolute quantity of water injected, for the maximum effect observed occurred in a cat receiving only 20 cc. of water intravenously. Figure 1 gives the gross appearance of the formalinized brain of a cat which had been subjected to an intravenous injection of 35 cc. of distilled water, and sacrificed thirty-five minutes after completion of injection. The dura over the cerebral hemispheres is markedly tense as in all others similarly treated. The convolutions appear flattened when viewed through the dura and the sulci are traced with greater difficulty than in the normal. On passing the finger over the dura covering the upper surface of the brain, one receives an impression of marked tenseness of dura and brain, and recognizes the gyri and intervening sulci with difficulty.

On section, such brains (figs. 5 and 7) exhibit the same tenseness of dura previously noted. The normal differentiation between the gray and white matter has been diminished (figs. 3, 5 or 7). The convolutions appear definitely flattened, adjacent gyri being pushed together so as to make the identification of the intervening sulci difficult. This is particularly true of the smaller sulci. The surfaces of the gyri are no longer gently convex but acute angles in the curve are found where the surface dips into the sulci. The superior longitudinal fissure is narrow and the bounding gyri press tightly against the falx. The cut surface of the brain appears definitely turgid and gives the impression of having been subjected to increased tension.

An increase in the volume of the brain following the intravenous injection of water is therefore definite, marked and readily apparent.

Hypertonic solutions. The intravenous injection of strongly hypertonic solutions, which has been found to cause a profound lowering of the pressure of the cerebro-spinal fluid, has been observed to produce also a decrease in the bulk of the brain. This alteration in the volume of the brain has been brought about by intravenous injections of from 8 cc. to 20 cc. of 30 per cent sodium chloride or saturated sodium bicarbonate. As reported elsewhere under the subject of alterations in the cerebro-spinal fluid pressure, a marked individual variation in reaction to hypertonic solutions has been found to exist. The dose bringing about the maximal cerebral shrinkage varied, but in general the larger doses, approaching the limit of the animal's tolerance, seemed to cause the most marked effect. Some of the cats were given single injections of as much of the

hypertonic solution as they seemed able to stand at one administration. Other animals were given a series of 5 cc. doses of 30 per cent sodium chloride at half-hour intervals, until a total of 20 cc. was injected. The animals, except when given the divided doses at half-hour intervals, were kept under ether anesthesia until sacrificed.

The time necessary for the maximum action of the fluid injected could not be determined accurately for the cats with unopened skulls. Assuming however, that the maximum lowering of the pressure of the cerebro-spinal fluid after such an injection coincides with the maximal diminution of brain-volume, it is probable that an interval of fifteen to twenty minutes suffices for the maximum change. Within certain limits, these observations substantiate this assumption, namely that the amount of fall in pressure of the cerebro-spinal fluid is an index of the extent to which the volume of the brain has been reduced.

The brain of a cat after the intravenous injection of a strongly hypertonic solution shows, on routine formalin fixation, a marked decrease in volume. As seen through the dura (fig. 2), which is very loosely applied, the brain seems comparatively small, occupying only a part of the intradural space. The gyri appear markedly rounded and the sulci wide and deep, so that individual convolutions appear throughout their extent. In the medulla oblongata and spinal cord there is also evidence of marked decrease in size. The dura here is very much more loosely applied than in the normal and the markings of the medulla oblongata and spinal cord seem sharp and accentuated. The general impression received from such an uncut brain is that it is quite small in comparison to the dural sac.

When cut transversely, the brain from a cat subjected to this experimental procedure presents an appearance quite different from the normal. The gray and white matter are far more sharply contrasted. Furthermore, the gray matter, particularly that of the thalamus and corpus striatum, appears dark with a brownish tinge, clearly outlining the nuclei from the adjacent white fibers. This phenomenon has been noted quite uniformly in this sereis. On such a section, the dura is very loosely applied (fig. 6), touching on the dorsal surface only the highest points of the gyri. Each individual gyrus stands out cleanly separated from adjacent gyri by widely opened sulci. The curve presented by the upper surface of each gyrus is of smaller radius than the normal, and may be followed deeply into each sulcus. The superior longitudinal fissure gapes widely and the falx seems to hang loosely within this space.

Similar shrunken brains have been obtained by the intravenous injection of saturated solutions of sodium bicarbonate. A section of such a brain is shown in figure 8, which presents in general the

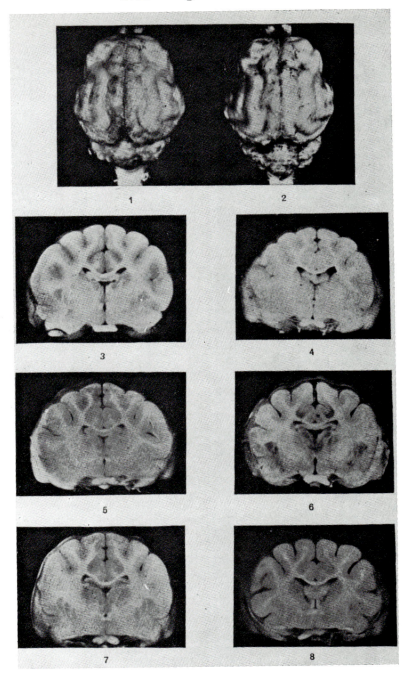

PLATE I

Fig. 1. Photograph ×¾. Cat no. 1304. Adult female. Occipito-atlantoid puncture. Continuous observation of pressure of cerebro-spinal fluid for 75 minutes, with intravenous injection of 35 cc. sterile distilled water. Pressure rose from 105 mm. to 175 mm. following injection. Sacrificed with ether 30 minutes after completion of injection. Fixed by injection with 10 per cent formalin. Dura not removed.

Fig. 2. Photograph ×¾. Cat no. 1371. Adult male. Intravenous injection of 20 cc. 30 per cent NaCl (Squibb)

⟫⟫→

characteristic features noted above. The decrease in volume is, however, not so striking as in the brain reproduced in figure 6.

It was thought possible that the action of these hypertonic solutions might be enhanced by depriving such animals of all fluid for a sufficient length of time before experimentation to insure the exhaustion of a considerable quantity of the water available in the body. Two series of animals were thus prepared and injected with 30 per cent sodium chloride in 5 cc. doses at one-half hour intervals. While the cats receiving four 5 cc. doses showed the effects of the injection in a very marked way (gross clonus of whole body, mild mania, etc.), the brains failed to show any more, if as much shrinkage as is shown by the brains of animals not denied water. These observations indicate that deprivation of water for twenty-four hours in the cat is not sufficient to alter the fluid-volume of the body tissues available for reaction with hypertonic solutions.

In the unopened skull, then, a definite decrease in the bulk of the brain may be brought about by intravenous injection of strongly hypertonic solutions.

The supply of a foreign solution to subarachnoid space. At the end of a number of the experiments in which an intravenous injection of hypertonic sodium chloride was given, a mixture of sodium ferrocyanide and iron-ammonium citrate was allowed to flow into the subarachnoid space. This was done at a time when the pressure of the cerebrospinal fluid was about zero or falling rapidly. Two or three cubic centimeters were usually so introduced. At the end of the experiment the animal was injected through the aorta with 10 per cent formalin, to which 5 per cent hydrochloric acid had been added, and when the vessels were well filled the central nervous system was quickly removed and immersed in the acid

formaldehyde. By this procedure, Prussian blue was precipitated at the points to which the solutions of sodium ferrocyanide and iron-ammonium citrate had penetrated prior to fixation. The Prussian blue in almost every case was found to have passed from the subarachnoid space along the perivasculars into the substance of the nervous system, reaching the interfibrous spaces in the white matter and the pericellular spaces in the gray. These observations may be interpreted as indicating that the hypertonic solution of sodium chloride, injected intravenously, had caused the dislocation of a considerable quantity of the cerebro-spinal fluid into the nervous system.

EXPERIMENTS WITH THE OPENED SKULL

The experiments dealing with the alteration of brain bulk by intravenous injection of solutions of varying concentrations were, in the earlier part of this investigation, carried out with the unopened cranial cavity, in which a fairly constant fluid volume was necessarily maintained. Even with such limitation to change in the volume of the brain, these solutions of various tonicities caused marked modification in its size. It was therefore thought desirable to carry out similar observations but with opening of the skull to permit expansion or contraction of the brain— changes impossible under the physical conditions imposed by the closed cranium. The rate of reaction to the intravenous injection and the appearance of the brain throughout the experiment could also, under these conditions, be determined by direct observation.

The opening of the skull was accomplished in the subtemporal region. In the etherized animal, through a midline incision, the temporal muscle on one side was freed from its origin, and a trephine opening of 2 cm. made in the skull be-

---

in 5 cc. doses given at 30 minute intervals. Sacrificed with ether 2 hours after first and 30 minutes after last dose Fixed by injection with 10 per cent formalin. Dura not removed.

Fig. 3. Photograph ×1. Cat no. 1402. Adult female. Control. Well-nourished, normal animal. Sacrificed with ether. Transverse section through optic chiasma. Fixed by injection with 10 per cent formalin.

Fig. 4. Photograph ×1. Cat no. 1309. Young adult female. Occipito-atlantoid puncture. Continuous observation of pressure of cerebro-spinal fluid for 81 minutes, with intravenous injection of 12 cc. Ringer's solution. Initial pressure 90 mm., final pressure 110 mm. Sacrificed with ether 1 hour after completion of injection. Transverse section through optic chiasma. Fixed by injection with 10 per cent formalin.

Fig. 5. Photograph ×1. Cat no. 1304. Transverse section through optic chiasma of brain shown in figure 1.

Fig. 6. Photograph ×1. Cat no. 1371. Transverse section through optic chiasma of brain shown in figure 2.

Fig. 7. Photograph ×1. Cat no. 1303. Adult female. Occipito-atlantoid puncture. Continuous observation of pressure of cerebro-spinal fluid for 84 minutes, with intravenous injection of 20 cc. sterile distilled water. Pressure rose from 106 mm. to 195 mm. Sacrificed with ether 1 hour after completion of injection. Transverse section through optic chiasma. Fixed by injection with 10 per cent formalin.

Fig. 8. Photograph ×1. Cat no. 1364. Young adult female. Occipito-atlantoid puncture. Continuous observation of pressure of cerebro-spinal fluid for 90 minutes, with intravenous injection of 10 cc. saturated aqueous solution of sodium bicarbonate. Pressure fell from 115 mm. to below zero. Sacrificed with ether 70 minutes after completion of injection. Transverse section through optic chiasma. Fixed by injection with 10 per cent formaldehyde.

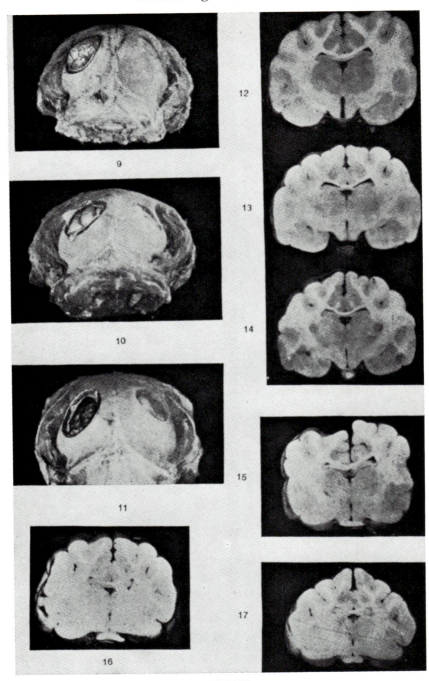

PLATE II

Fig. 9. Photograph ×¾. Cat no. 1524. Adult female. Weight 2,350 grams. Temporal decompression on left side. Intravenous injection of 100 cc. sterile distilled water. Marked hernia of brain through trephine opening 3 mm. beyond outer table of skull beginning with the injection and persisting until animal was sacrificed with ether 35 minutes after completion of injection. Fixed by immersion with 10 per cent formalin. Trephine opening made on right side after the beginning of fixation.

Fig. 10. Photograph ×¾. Cat no. 1531. Adult male. Weight 2,330 grams. Temporal decompression on left side.

≫≫→

neath the muscle. The upper border of this opening came within 3 mm. of the mid-sagittal line of the skull. In another series bilateral subtemporal decompression openings were made. In every case the dura was freely opened by cruciate incisions. Injury to the underlying arachnoid and brain was carefully avoided.

Normal. Control experiments with single and bilateral decompressions were carried out. Following the opening of the skull, the animal was kept under ether until sacrificed at the expiration of about the same length of time as was consumed in the experiments where intravenous injections were given. In these control animals under such conditions the brain lay slightly convex beneath the trephine opening, pulsating freely, and did not change perceptibly in any way during the period of observation. The dural flaps were allowed to lie loosely on the exposed surface of the brain and throughout the experiment the edges of these flaps were separated from 1 to 2 mm. in the center of the trephine opening. At the end of these observations the animals were sacrificed with ether and the brains immediately preserved in 10 per cent formalin. On section, these brains appear quite normal with evidence of slight dis-

location of brain substance toward the site of the trephine openings. Figure 13 shows a section of such a brain which was relieved by a single opening in the skull and dura; figure 16 represents the condition prevailing after a bilateral subtemporal decompression. It may be concluded, then, that under the conditions of experimentation the volume of the brain has been but little changed by the anesthesia and operative procedures employed.

Further control of the observations of brain bulk, following intravenous injection of solutions of various concentrations, is afforded by several experiments in which Ringer's solution was injected intravenously after single or bilateral openings had been made in the skull and dura. The injection of Ringer's solution was from a burette, and the rate of fluid-introduction was regulated to coincide with that used in the injection of similar amounts of hypotonic solutions. During and after the injection of Ringer's solution, in amounts up to 100 cc., the brain lay slightly convex in the trephine openings, pulsating freely, and showed no evidence that it had been affected in volume by the intravenous injection. The appearance of the cortex viewed through

---

Intravenous injection of 100 cc. Ringer's solution. Brain lies convex with no hernia or evidence of swelling o shrinkage throughout the experiment. Sacrificed with ether 36 minutes after completion of injection. Fixed by immersion with 10 per cent formalin. Trephine opening made on right side 45 minutes after the beginning of fixation.

Fig. 11. Photograph ×¾. Cat no. 1506. Adult male. Weight 2,100 grams. Temporal decompression on left side. Intravenous injection of 16½ cc. 30 per cent NaCl (Squibb). Brain rises slightly with beginning of injection but falls away from skull before injection is finished. Thirty minutes later lies concave, 3 mm. below inner table of skull at forward edge of opening. Sacrificed with ether 33 minutes after completion of injection. Fixed by immersion with 10 per cent formalin. Trephine opening made on right side after the beginning of fixation.

Fig. 12. Photograph ×1. Cat no. 1501. Adult female. Weight 2,400 grams. Temporal decompression on left side. Intravenous injection of 100 cc. sterile distilled water. Brain rises as injection begun; hernia increases during injection; brain bulges markedly through trephine opening with protrusion in center about 8 mm. beyond outer table of skull, 35 minutes after injection finished. Sacrificed with ether 37 minutes after completion of injection. Fixed by injection through aorta with 10 per cent formalin. Transverse section just behind optic chiasma. Dura removed.

Fig. 13. Photograph ×1. Cat no. 1503. Adult female. Weight 2,260 grams. Control. Temporal decompression on left side. No intravenous injection. Brain lies convex about level with the outer table of the skull throughout experiment. Sacrificed with ether 35 minutes after completion of decompression. Fixed by injection through aorta with 10 per cent formalin. Transverse section just behind optic chiasma. Dura removed.

Fig. 14. Photograph ×1. Cat no. 1505. Adult female. Weight 2,050 grams. Temporal decompression on left side. Intravenous injection of 16½ cc. 30 per cent NaCl (Squibb). Brain bulges markedly during injection, but immediately begins to subside on completion of injection until in 30 minutes it lies concave 1 mm. below inner table of skull. Sacrificed with ether 36 minutes after completion of injection. Fixed by injection through aorta with 10 per cent formalin. Transverse section just behind optic chiasma. Dura removed.

Fig. 15. Photograph ×1. Cat no. 1536. Adult female. Weight 2,430 grams. Double temporal decompression. Intravenous injection of 100 cc. sterile distilled water. Beginning with the injection brain rises in a tense hernia on both sides. Sacrificed with ether 31 minutes after completion of injection. Fixed by injection through aorta with 10 per cent formalin. Transverse section through optic chiasma. Dura removed.

Fig. 16. Photograph ×1. Cat no. 1532. Adult male. Weight 2,250 grams. Control. Double temporal decompression. No intravenous injection. Throughout experiment brain lies convex with no bulging. Sacrificed with ether 20 minutes after completion of decompression. Fixed by injection through aorta with 10 per cent formalin. Transverse section through optic chiasma. Dura removed.

Fig. 17. Photograph ×1. Cat no. 1541. Young male. Weight 1,500 grams. Double temporal decompression. Intravenous injection of 16 cc. 30 per cent NaCl (Squibb). Beginning with injection brain falls away from skull lying about 3 mm. below inner table 20 minutes after injection stopped. Sacrificed with ether 55 minutes after completion of injection. Fixed by injection through aorta with 10 per cent formalin. Transverse section through optic chiasma. Dura removed.

the trephine opening was exactly that of the brain of an animal receiving no intravenous injection, but subjected to the other operative procedures. In figure 10 is shown the result (after fixation in formalin) of an experiment in which a single opening was made in the skull and 100 cc. of Ringer's solution injected intravenously. As pointed out previously, we have been unable with our present methods to preserve, by fixation in formaldehyde, the form and size relations prevailing in the brain at the end of experimentation. This figure shows a slightly more marked bulging of the brain in the trephine opening than was present at the end of the experiment. In spite of this slight swelling due to fixation it presents a fairly normal appearance, particularly when compared with more swollen or shrunken brains as shown in figures 9 and 11. In this and in all of our observations in which Ringer's solution was injected, the anesthesia, the operative procedures, the time consumed by the intravenous injection and the interval of time from the end of the injection to the sacrifice of the animal, were similar to those in the experiments in which solutions of various concentration were injected.

It may be concluded, then, that in etherized animals with the skull opened, the intravenous injection of Ringer's solution in amounts up to 100 cc. causes no appreciable change in the volume of the brain. The protocol of a typical experiment in which there was a bilateral opening of the skull and the intravenous injection of 100 cc. of Ringer's solution, is given below:

No. 1537. Adult male cat. Weight 2,500 grams. Control intravenous Ringer.

9.46 a.m.   Ether with intratracheal tube.

10.15 a.m.   Double subtemporal decompression. Dura opened. Brain lies with normal convexity, pulsation and circulation good.

10.20 a.m.   Cannula in vein of fore-leg connected with burette containing Ringer's solution.

10.25 a.m.   Injection begun. Brain as before.

10.33 a.m.   25 cc. in. Brain as before.

10.38 a.m.   50 cc. in. Brain slightly more convex.

10.45 a.m.   90 cc. in. Brain as before.

10.50 a.m.   100 cc. in. Brain normally convex, shows no bulging. Pulsation free, circulation good. Injection stopped.

11.10 a.m.   Brain lies normal as before. Pulsation free.

11.26 a.m.   Brain lies normal as before. Ether to death. Immediately injected with 10 per cent formaldehyde until vessels well filled, then head cut off and immersed in same solution. Original relations fairly well preserved after fixation.

With the control afforded by these experiments in which the skull was opened and in which there was no intravenous injection, or else the introduction of Ringer's solution, an interpretation of the results of the intravenous injection of hypotonic and hypertonic solutions may be safely attempted.

Water. A number of observations on cats with single and bilateral openings of the skull have been made, during and following the intravenous injection of sterile distilled water which, as noted in a previous section of this paper, has been shown to bring about an increase in the volume of the brain in the unopened skull. The conditions prevailing in these experiments were similar to those maintained during the injection of Ringer's solution. In all these animals the brain, which lay normally convex in the trephine openings, began to protrude very soon after the intravenous injection of distilled water was started. This bulging increased throughout the period of injection and reached its maximum usually in from ten to twenty minutes after the completion of the introduction of water. Tense herniae of the brain through the trephine openings were thus produced. The tension was in all cases so great that cerebral pulsation ceased before the swelling reached its maximum. The pressure of the brain on the dura at the edges of the trephine openings was usually marked enough to stop the circulation in the dural flaps. These triangular flaps were stretched, pulled and rolled back into the interval between the hernia and the cut edge of the trephine opening. Figure 9 shows the result of such an experiment and presents fairly well the appearance of the cerebral hernia before the sacrifice of the animal, although fixation in formaldehyde at death of the animal caused some subsidence of the hernia. When observed just before the death of the cat, usually thirty minutes after the completion of the injection of water, the brain protruded, in most of our experiments, at least 4 mm. beyond the outer table of the skull; in one animal which gave a very marked reaction, the height of the hernia at the end of the observation was 8 mm.

The protocol of an experiment in which there was a bilateral opening of the skull and the intravenous injection of 100 cc. of sterile distilled water, is given below:

No. 1536. Adult female cat. Weight 2,430 grams. Intravenous water.

3.50 p.m.   Ether with intratracheal tube.

4.00 p.m.   Double subtemporal decompression.

4.15 p.m.   Dura opened. Brain lies with normal convexity, pulsating freely. No trauma to brain or membranes.

4.18 p.m.   Cannula in vein of fore-leg connected with burette containing sterile distilled water.

4.19 p.m.   Injection begun. Brain bulges immediately after beginning of injection.

4.25 p.m.   Brain bulges more.

4.31 p.m.   50 cc. in. Brain bulges markedly with pulsation; circulation good.

4.35 p.m.   75 cc. in. Brain bulges markedly. Pulsation slight, circulation good.

4.45 p.m. 100 cc. in. Injection stopped. Brain in tense hernia. Pulsation slight on left side. No pulsation on right side.

5.00 p.m. Brain markedly herniated. No pulsation on either side.

5.15 p.m. Brain in tense hernia on both sides—stops circulation in dural flaps.

5.16 p.m. Ether to death. Immediately injected through the heart with 10 per cent formalin and when vessels filled, head cut off and immersed in same solution. After immersion hernia remains about as before. Convolutions slightly more rounded and whole hernia slightly flatter.

On section, these brains present the appearance seen in figure 12 (after single decompression) and in figure 15 (after bilateral opening of the skull). A considerable dislocation of brain substance is apparent with some flattening of the gyri and narrowing of the sulci; but the general impression gained from an examination of these sections is different from that resulting from observation of sections, as shown in figures 5 and 7, of brains obtained from animals subjected to the intravenous injection of water, but with unopened skulls. In the sections of the brains which were allowed to herniate, the impression of extreme tenseness and turgidity is not outstanding as is the case with the brains which were restrained by unopened dura and skull. The difference is undoubtedly to be explained by the different mechanical limitations to expansion present in the two types of experiment.

It is apparent from the foregoing that, under experimental conditions similar to those prevailing in the control observations on brains with opened skull (with or without the intravenous injection of Ringer's solution), the intravenous introduction of water causes a marked herniation of cerebral substance resulting from the increase in the volume of the brain. It is also worthy of note that the gross appearance of sections of such brains is different from that previously observed in section of brains of animals receiving water intravenously but with unopened skulls.

Salt. Intravenous injections of a hypertonic solution (30 per cent sodium chloride), which produced a marked reduction in volume of the brain in animals with unopened skulls, have been given to a number of cats in which openings in the skull and dura were made on one or both sides. The conditions prevailing in these experiments were similar to those already described for the control observations. Following the intravenous injection of 30 per cent sodium chloride, the normal convexity of the brain in the trephine opening disappears soon after the injection is begun, so that the brain is seen to lie flat. As the intravenous injection of the salt is continued, the brain falls away from the skull until the surface presented becomes concave. The maximum shrinkage has been observed usually in from fifteen to thirty minutes after the completion of the injection, when the brain lies flaccid, 3 to 4 mm. below the inner table of the skull, with only very slight visible pulsation. In figure 11 is shown the result of an experiment in which a single opening was made in the skull, and 16½ cc. of a solution of 30 per cent sodium chloride injected intravenously. The photograph reproduced in this figure was taken after the fixation of the head in 10 per cent formalin and does not show the marked shrinkage which was so striking at the end of the experiment. As has been emphasized, the methods of fixation employed do not preserve, with the accuracy desired, the relations existing during life; in spite of this difficulty it is readily apparent, from figure 11, that here the skull is only partially filled by this markedly shrunken brain.

The individual reaction and tolerance of cats to intravenous injections of a hypertonic solution of sodium chloride and the quantities most effective in producing a decrease in the volume of the brain, have been discussed in a preceding section of this paper. In these observations with the opened skull, doses approaching the limit of the animal's tolerance (16 to 20 cc.) have been administered; the same differences in individual reaction and tolerance, noted before, have been observed.

There is given below the protocol of a typical experiment in this series, in which there was a bilateral opening of the skull and dura and an intravenous injection of 20 cc. of a hypertonic solution of sodium chloride:

No. 1535. Adult female cat. Weight 2,250 grams.
Intravenous NaCl.

9.35 a.m. Ether with intratracheal tube.

10.10 a.m. Double subtemporal decompression.

10.15 a.m. Dura opened. Brain lies with normal convexity, pulsating freely. No injury to brain or membranes.

10.20 a.m. Cannula put in vein of fore-leg and connected with burette containing 30 per cent NaCl (Squibb).

10.23 a.m. Injection begun. Convexity of brain normal.

10.30 a.m. Brain as before. No hernia.

10.35 a.m. 11 cc. in. Both sides of brain receding—lie flat.

10.40 a.m. 14 cc. in. Brain fallen more—lies concave.

10.45 a.m. 16 cc. in. Brain fallen more.

10.50 a.m. 19 cc. in. Brain fallen still more.

10.54 a.m. 20 cc. in. Injection stopped. Brain markedly fallen. Circulation good, pulsation slight.

11.05 a.m. Brain markedly shrunk. Pulsation slight. Animal in good shape.

11.25 a.m. Brain far receded, pulsation slight. Brain lies 3 to 4 mm. away from the inner table of the skull.

11.26 a.m. Ether to death. Immediately injected through the heart with 10 per cent formaldehyde plus 1.5 per cent NaCl with cat lying on belly. Head cut off when vessels well filled and immersed in same solution. Within a few minutes after immersion brain rose in skull almost level with trephine opening.

After fixation in formalin and section, these brains, taken from animals with opened skulls and with intravenous injection of 30 per cent sodium chloride, are characterized by the condition shown in figure 14 (single skull opening) and figure 17 (bilateral subtemporal decompression). That there has been a decided decrease in the volume of the brain in both these cases is quite evident. Figures 12, 13 and 14 show sections of a series of brains taken from animals in which there was a single subtemporal decompression. In one animal (fig. 12) water was injected intravenously; in another (fig. 14) 30 per cent sodium chloride, while in the third (fig. 13), no injection was given. Figures 15, 16 and 17 show sections of brains from another series of animals in which bilateral openings were made in the skull and dura. Intravenous water was given in one animal (fig. 15), intravenous 30 per cent sodium chloride in another (fig. 17), but in the control (fig. 16) nothing was injected. A glance at these figures is quite sufficient to show that in the animal receiving the intravenous injection of a solution of hypertonic sodium chloride in both series, the brain has been markedly decreased in volume. A close examination of figures 14 and 17, and a comparison of these figures with figures 6 and 8, which resulted from experiments in which hypertonic solutions were injected intravenously but with the skull unopened, is extremely interesting in that, while there is evident shrinkage in both types of experiment, the way in which the brain was affected is different in the two. From figures 14 and 17 (opened skull) one gets an impression of marked compactness of the brain as a whole; this phenomenon is not so apparent in figures 6 and 8 (unopened skull). The well rounded gyri and the clearly apparent sulci, previously described as characteristic (following intravenous injections of hypertonic solutions) of brains arising from experiments in which the skull was unopened, are not to be found in brains after similar experimental procedures but with the skull opened. It is evident, then, that with the operation of the same factor which tends to produce a decrease in the volume of the brain, the form of the end result in the two cases is altered by the mechanical conditions imposed by the opened or unopened skull. It is thus apparent that when the brain is allowed by an opened skull to shrink and contract freely, the appearance of a greater decrease in total volume is obtained than in experiments where the force producing the reduction in volume must, as it were, pull against a partial vacuum furnished by the intact skull.

These observations make it clear that in brains unrestrained by the physical limitation of the closed cranium there is a marked decrease in volume after intravenous injection of hypertonic solutions of sodium chloride; but the resulting picture is different from that described for brains shrunken, after similar injections, within an intact skull.

In the course of the above experiments the failure of the brain of a very old cat to show marked swelling after the intravenous injection of water led to several observations on decidedly old animals. Two very old cats, following double temporal decompression, were given intravenous injections of 100 cc. of water. The brain of neither cat herniated markedly from increase in bulk. Another old cat, after double temporal decompression, was given an intravenous injection of 20 cc. of 30 per cent sodium chloride. The brain shrank away from the skull to a considerable extent, although not so far as is usually the case in younger individuals. It has been frequently noted that when exposed to view by operative procedure, the brains of these old cats look different from those of younger individuals. While they pulsate freely in the decompression openings, they lie flat and do not show so much convexity as is characteristic of the brains of younger individuals. The sulci of these brains of old cats seem wider and the gyri more rounded than those characteristic of younger cats. That the brains of these old animals react less readily to intravenous injections by changes in bulk than the brains of younger individuals seems certain from these observations; that increase in volume should be more difficult than decrease seems reasonable, in view of certain mechanical and other conditions existing within the cranium in old individuals.

Two very young cats weighing 1,300 and 1,500 grams, were selected as typical young adults, in which changes in brain bulk should be outspoken. Following double subtemporal decompression, one received an intravenous injection of 100 cc. of water, the other 16 cc. of 30 per cent NaCl. Both showed very well marked reactions, developing relatively as great swelling or shrinkage as has been seen in any animal.

HISTOLOGICAL EXAMINATION

The pronounced swelling, which occurs in the cat's brain after the intravenous injection of water, and the marked shrinkage which follows the intravenous injection of strongly hypertonic solutions, has led to the desire to correlate, if possible, these gross alterations with histological changes in the cerebral substance.

Mention has already been made in this paper of the fact that fixation with formaldehyde does not preserve accurately the gross form and size relations of the brain as seen prior to death of the animal, so that the preliminary observations here recorded may represent only very roughly the histological picture accompanying the various modifications of brain bulk. That there are marked histological changes is readily seen but their exact interpretation, particularly in regard to the representation of conditions prevailing prior to fixation, is a matter requiring further study. It is hoped that when a method of fixation is devised which will preserve the form and size relations accurately, more intelligent histological and cytological observations may be made. The present findings are reported tentatively, pending an attempt to control the artifacts probably introduced by the technical methods employed.

The material available for this study was that resulting from the experiments described in the preceding parts of this paper. This material was preserved in formaldehyde, which was in most cases injected through the aorta immediately after the death of the animal. One series of brains fixed by Formaline-Zenker's fluid was used in an attempt to control the material preserved in formaldehyde. Sections were cut in paraffin, 10 μ thick; stained with haematoxylin and eosin, toluidine blue and fuchsin S, and with Mallory's and Van Gieson's connective tissue stains. All sections were made from blocks of cortex including the sulcus lateralis and parts of the two adjacent gyri, taken from the dorsal surface of the brain in the same transverse plane as the optic chiasma. In the animals where the skull was opened during the experiment, this block of cortex was found to be in the upper part of the trephine opening. Examination of sections of cortex taken from animals used in this study quickly showed that, when judged by the histological changes which accompany or follow gross shrinkage or swelling, these animals may be divided into two groups; those in which the skull and dura were opened during the experiment and those in which the cerebral cavity remained intact. The histological changes seen in sections of non-decompressed brains following various intravenous injections are quite marked and constant in the material studied, but sections from decompressed brains fail to exhibit the same marked differences from the control. It is quite evident, then, that following decompression the brain may adjust its volume; it may herniate, being only partially restricted by the dura, or collapse freely. This comparative freedom to contract or expand probably explains the finding of similar histological pictures in the normal decompressed controls, and in the decompressed brains following intravenous injection of water or salts. All the specimens tended to approach the normal when the brains were allowed to contract or expand with freedom, but when the alterations in cerebral volume were limited by the closed cranium, the factors responsible for the macroscopic changes in brain bulk produced also marked microscopic changes. Although these histological changes as observed have doubtless been altered by the technical methods employed in the preservation of these brains, their constancy is ample evidence that they are indicative of certain fundamental changes in the brain substance, even though they may represent very inaccurately the actual conditions prevailing prior to death. The technical procedures employed have been practically uniform for all brains, so that the artifacts produced may be considered as constant.

Skull unopened

Normal. Control sections were made from blocks of cortex taken from animals receiving no intravenous injection and from animals in which Ringer's solution was introduced intravenously. While it is apparent that there are artifacts in these sections, due probably to the method of fixation, they furnish a reasonable control for sections of brains taken from animals receiving intravenous injections of various concentrations. An examination of sections made from brains of animals in which Ringer's solution was introduced intravenously and a comparison of these sections with normal controls shows no fundamental differences in the two, so far as our observations go. These sections, then, furnish a reasonable standard with which the sections from animals subjected to other experimental procedures may be compared.

Water. The general appearance of sections of the cortex made from non-decompressed brains following the intravenous injection of water, is that of a swollen tissue. The sulci are quite narrow and the gyri tend to be flat. The smaller vessels seem, if different from normal, contracted within normal or slightly expanded perivascular spaces. The intercellular material of the gray matter seems inflated, the spaces found among the interlacing cell processes appearing larger than in control sections. Many of the large dendrites which rise perpendicular to the free surface of the gyrus are apparently larger than in the normal. Under higher magnifications the nuclei of nerve cells seem compact, the whole nucleus being perhaps slightly contracted. About the cells in most of the water brains examined, there is an evidently enlarged pericellular space, the general impression being that the cell itself is contracted away from the surrounding tissue. The occurrence of enlarged pericellular spaces in the gray matter of the cortex, following the intravenous injection of water, is most striking and constant. Pericellular spaces are apparent in sections of normal cortex, particularly about the larger cells, but following the introduction of water intravenously these spaces, even about the smaller cells, are evidently considerably enlarged. In this material the enlarged pericellular spaces and other histological evidences of change may be interpreted as due to conditions within the brain, different from those existing normally, and produced by the intravenous injection of a hypotonic solution.

Salt. Sections of the cortex taken from brains following intravenous injection of 30 per cent sodium chloride, under low magnification, show in general an appearance of tissue contraction, the sulci being wide and the substance of the brain condensed. In practically all of the salt brains examined, the cortical capillaries seem distended. This distension may be explained partially, perhaps, by the arterial injection with formaldehyde (a procedure carried out with the normal and water brains) but it is a constant finding in the salt brains and may be taken as an indication of some constant factor in the fluid concentration within the nervous tissue. In most of the salt brains the perivascular spaces are apparent but not enlarged. The intercellular felt-work in the gray matter seems compacted and denser than in normal sections. The outstanding feature of the histological picture presented by these sections of salt brains concerns the occurrence of a marked clear space about the nuclei of many cells. These clear spaces vary in size from a slight space about a well-rounded nucleus to a wide space around a markedly crenated nucleus. These spaces increase in size in the gray matter from the medullary core out to the surface layers of each gyrus. The nuclei appear condensed, the chromatin being aggregated. The Nissl substance in the cytoplasm is at the periphery of the cell, the perinuclear spaces being between the nuclear membrane and a marginal ring of Nissl substance. In sections stained with toluidine blue and fuchsin S, these spaces are seen to be partially filled with a fluid-coagulum which stains with fuchsin. This coagulum in most cases has shrunk away from the nucleus toward and against the ring of Nissl substance. No pericellular spaces are usually apparent about the cells showing such perinuclear spaces. The pericellular spaces may be observed occasionally however in the deeper layers of the gray matter about the larger cells. As noted above, the perinuclear spaces are more marked and the nuclei more crenated in cells of the surface layers of the cortex. It seems evident, then, after a comparison of these sections with normal control sections, that in these brains the intracellular perinuclear spaces and other histological evidences of change in the brain substance may be attributed to changes brought about by the intravenous injection of a hypertonic solution.

Skull opened

Examination of sections of brains following intravenous injections of solutions of various concentration in animals with opened skulls reveals a histological picture quite similar in all. There are, of course, minor differences in the sections examined, but such differences do not seem to be due to any changes brought about by the intravenous injection. The decompression has evidently allowed each brain to expand or contract freely and to adjust its fluid distribution so that no essential histological differences are noticeable, all retaining very nearly a normal appearance. That there may be in these brains fundamental histological and cytological differences not revealed by the methods employed, is probable, but further work is necessary to establish such differences. With the methods employed it is certain that the decompressed brains do not show the histological characteristics which are so evident in the non-decompressed brains.

An exact interpretation of the above observations on the histological changes in the cortex of the brain following intravenous injections of hypotonic and hypertonic solutions can not now with reason be attempted. That there are histological changes in brains unrelieved by decompression is certain, but these changes need more accurate study and control before any sane effort can be made to explain them accurately. The changes described have no doubt been influenced by the technical methods employed; these methods may have, in addition, masked or destroyed other histological evidences of changes produced by the intravenous injections. Until one finds a method of fixation which will preserve the form and size relations of the brain accurately and at the same time will make possible accurate histological study, the above observations may be accepted tentatively as an indication that changes in the brain substance, recognizable histologically, do occur following intravenous injections of solutions of various concentrations.

DISCUSSION OF RESULTS

The experimental alteration of the volume of the brain by intravenous injections of hypotonic and hypertonic solutions has not, so far as we have been able to find, been previously recorded in the literature. The ease and rapidity of these changes in brain volume are of considerable interest in view of the old idea of the incompressible character of the brain and its relation to the conception of a constant vascular volume within the cranial cavity.

The hypothesis that the volume of the blood circulating within the cranium must at all times be constant was first brought forward by Alexander Monro, the younger (2) in 1783. At this time he wrote that

as the substance of the brain, like that of other solids of our body, is nearly incompressible, the quantity of blood within the head must be the same at all times, whether in health or disease, in life or after death, those cases only excepted in which water or other matter is effused or secreted from the blood-vessels; for in these cases, a quantity of blood equal in bulk to the effused matter, will be pressed out of the cranium.

This viewpoint advanced by Monro was accepted and elaborated by Kellie (3) in 1824, who based his ideas upon observations on men frozen to death and upon experiments on animals. His conclusions were that a state of bloodlessness did not exist in the brains of animals killed by bleeding, that the quantity of blood in the cerebral vessels was not affected by posture or gravitation, that congestion of these vessels was not found in those conditions in which it might be well expected (hanging, etc.) and that compensatory readjustments between the different sets of cerebral vessels always maintained a constant vascular volume. Subsequently Kellie wrote

that in the ordinary state of these parts we can not lessen, to any extent, the quantity of blood within the cranium, by arteriotomy or venesection; whereas if the skull of an animal be trephined then hemorrhage will leave very little blood in the brain.

Within the next two decades following the publication of the results of Kellie's experiments, many clinical observations were reported in substantiation of this conception—that the vascular content of the brain was at all times practically constant. This Monro-Kellie doctrine received wide publicity through its acceptance by Abercrombie (4). This eminent surgeon, in discussing apoplexy, thus summed up his views on the subject (p. 300):

In this investigation it is unnecessary to introduce the question, whether the brain is compressible, because we may safely assert that it is not compressible by any such force as may be conveyed to it from the heart through the carotid and vertebral arteries. Upon the whole, then, I think we may assume the position as being in the highest degree probable, that, in the ordinary state of the parts, no material change can take place in the absolute quantity of blood circulating in the vessels of the brain.

Burrows in 1843 (5) was probably the first to question the absolute accuracy of this doctrine which so firmly considered the brain as of fixed incompressible bulk. He emphasized strongly the importance of the cerebro-spinal fluid, as the means of replacing the loss of blood during hemorrhage, for he felt that the amount of intracranial blood was obviously diminished by systemic bleeding.

"Whether the vacated space is replaced by serum, or resiliency of the cerebral substance under diminished pressure, is another question" was Burrows' summary of the possible readjustment for variations in the volume of the cerebral blood. As far as can be ascertained, this is the first statement of the view that the volume of the brain may be altered in accord with pathological or physiological conditions within the cranium. Burrows presents one of the most satisfactory conceptions of the whole process of fluid changes within the cranium (p. 32):

Those who have maintained this doctrine of the constant quantity of blood within the cranium, have not, I believe, taken into due consideration that large proportion of the contents of the cranium which consists of extra-vascular serum. Regarding this serum as an important element of the contents of the cranium, I admit that the whole contents of the cranium, that is, the brain, the blood, and this serum together, must be at all times nearly a constant quantity.

It was only when the subject of a constant blood volume in the cranium was subjected to experimental test that reliable data were obtained. Kussmaul and Tenner (6) demonstrated the unreliability of post-mortem observations and came to the conclusion, advanced by Burrows and supported by the experimental work of Donders (7), that variations in the total volume of blood in the cranium occurred. These early experiments, as pointed out by Leonard Hill (8) in 1896, are not conclusive as variation in the blood volume in one part of the cerebral vascular system might well be compensated by readjustments in another. Following many other investigators who used various methods of experimental attack, Leonard Hill concluded that (p. 77): "The volume of blood in the brain is in all physiological conditions but slightly variable."

More recently (1914) Dixon and Halliburton (9), in the course of an extensive study of the cerebro-spinal fluid, have come to the conclusion "that the cranial contents cannot any longer be regarded as a fixed quantity without the power of expanding or contracting in volume."

It must be assumed, however, that with certain reservations, the data favor the idea of a relatively fixed total volume of the cranial contents but with the capacity for change in any one of the three chief elements concerned.

The conception of a more or less constant cranial content is closely related to the questions which are naturally called forth by the experimental modification of brain bulk, detailed in foregoing sections of this paper. For within the closed cavity the alteration in volume of any element must be at the expense of the other elements. First of the possible explanations of the experimental alteration in brain bulk is that relating to the blood volume of the cranium. Are the vascular readjustments following the intravenous injection of hypotonic and hypertonic solutions sufficient to account for the definite change in brain bulk? In one of his original experiments, in which the cranium of a dog had been trephined, Kellie observed a recession of the brain away from the skull during exsanguination. Ecker (9) also observed in a trephined animal a remarkable shrinkage of the brain when the loss of blood from division of the carotids became excessive. The converse of this vascular diminution of the brain volume was recorded also by Ecker, who found that pressure on the thorax of a trephined dog caused protrusion of the brain into the cranial opening. Burrows also comments on this possibility of hernia through the trephine opening occurring in those cases in which the blood supply to the brain was markedly increased. These early observations on the relation of the cranial vascular supply to the volume of the brain during life have been confirmed and substantiated by many other workers on the cerebral circulation and cerebro-spinal (intracranial) pressure.

In our own experiments the modification of brain bulk has been produced both in the opened and in the intact skull. Observations on venous and arterial pressures under such experimental conditions have been made; these will be reported at another time. But that these alterations in brain bulk are independent of changes in volume of the blood in the vascular bed, may be deduced from other findings. The fact that similar changes occur in both the trephined and the unopened skull is strong evidence against the view that these changes in brain bulk depend on alterations in vascular volume and the persistence of the anatomical change after formalin fixation makes such a view untenable. For it must be assumed that with death of the animal, opening of the chest, introduction of a cannula in the aorta, injection of formalin through this vessel and release of the pressure by incising the right auricle, any vascular alterations existing in life are no longer maintained; so that the persistence, after such fixation, of a given brain bulk, if due simply to the amount of blood in the capillary bed and other vessels of the brain, would be impossible. That changes in bulk do persist after fixation as above, is ample evidence that such changes are maintained by some fundamental and comparatively stable alterations in the substance of the brain itself. A further fact, which shows that the changes in volume of the brain as produced in these experiments are fundamentally independent of vascular alterations, is that brains fixed by immersion in formalin, as well as those preserved by arterial injection of the fixing agent, retain in part the changes in bulk produced by intravenous injection. Following several experiments in which, after opening of the skull the brain bulk was changed by intravenous injection, the heads of the animals were cut from the body and immersed in formalin. That the skull and dura were freely open during experimentation in these cases and that all the vessels of the neck were severed before fixation by immersion and not by injection and that after such treatment the brain still maintained the vol-

ume change brought about by the intravenous injection, are further evidence that the changes in bulk are independent of vascular alterations. While, as has been emphasized, the method of preservation does not accurately maintain the condition existing in life, it nevertheless makes possible the recognition of undeniable evidence of change in brain bulk. Vascular alterations may account for some changes in brain bulk which occur in the living animal, but the changes persisting in death and after the technical procedures employed in this investigation are quite evidently due to some other cause.

The other variable factor which may operate within the cranium in producing changes in brain bulk involves the cerebro-spinal fluid. We have already noted the lasting rise in the pressure of the cerebro-spinal fluid following the intravenous injection of a hypotonic solution, and the production of swollen brains by such injections. Conversely, a definite decrease in the size of the brain has been found in those cases in which the pressure of the cerebro-spinal fluid has been markedly lowered by intravenous injection of hypertonic solutions. In considering these results it becomes rather difficult to determine with absolute accuracy the primary factor involved in producing these alterations. Does the modification of the bulk of the brain determine the pressure-change in the cerebro-spinal fluid or are both dependent individually on some more fundamental cause? That change in brain volume in our experiments is not caused alone by changes in the pressure of the cerebro-spinal fluid is demonstrated by its occurrence in the opened skull, for with the trephine opening and the dura incised, the fluid pressure becomes minimal, and any rise in pressure is within certain limits relieved. That fundamental osmotic changes in the blood are responsible for the changes in the pressure of the cerebro-spinal fluid, following intravenous injections of solutions of various tonicity, seems a reasonable conclusion. Although it is probable that change in the volume of the brain may affect the pressure of the cerebro-spinal fluid, and possible that changes in the pressure of the fluid may alter the bulk of the brain, in these experiments there is evidence that primary alterations in brain bulk and cerebro-spinal fluid pressure, both, are caused by fundamental osmotic changes in the blood supplied to the brain.

Such considerations force one to conclude that the alteration in the volume of the brain following intravenous injections of hypotonic or hypertonic solutions is quite independent of change in either the volume of the blood supply to the brain or of the pressure of the cerebro-spinal fluid. With the diminution in bulk the pressure of the cerebro-spinal fluid falls—a partial compensation for the evacuated space formerly occupied by the brain of normal size. Conversely, an increased bulk of the brain may cause dislocation of a certain volume of the cerebro-spinal fluid, thus raising its pressure as determined in a manometer.

Relating this experimental modification of the brain bulk to the restricted Monro-Kellie doctrine it becomes evident that another variable factor must be introduced. The brain should no longer be considered as incompressible and of fixed volume as the early writers assumed it to be, but as subject to variation in size under experimental conditions. Monro, of course, qualified his theory by consideration of matter "effused or secreted from the blood vessels," and Burrows suggested that the brain possessed "resiliency of the cerebral substance under diminished pressure." Pathologically the increase in bulk of the brain is well known in the cerebral edemas of trauma, acute infections and certain other conditions. Similarly, pathological states characterized by diminished volume of the brain are also quite common. The Monro-Kellie doctrine then requires marked modification; the view so well advanced by Burrows is probably the more correct. This leads one to assume that the cranial cavity is relatively fixed in volume and is completely filled by brain, cerebro-spinal fluid and blood; variations in any one of the three elements may occur, compensation being afforded by alteration in the volume of one or both of the remaining elements.

The underlying processes involved in the modification of brain bulk by the intravenous injection of hypertonic and hypotonic solutions seem concerned then with osmotic changes in the blood. That the osmotic pressure of the blood is an essential factor in such experimental changes in brain bulk is shown by the fact that no alteration in the volume of the brain follows relatively large doses of Ringer's solution (100 cc. in a cat) but occurs promptly on intravenous injection of far smaller amounts of distilled water or concentrated salines. Just how this change in osmotic value of the blood affects the brain tissue and alters its volume can only be speculated upon at the present time. The change is limited apparently by the potential distensibility or contractility of the brain in the particular animal used. Thus, in old cats, the alterations in brain volume have not been so marked as in younger animals, though the contractility seems to persist longer than the distensibility. On the other hand, in young animals the change in cerebral volume is of far easier accomplishment. Capacity for osmotic changes in these animals must be about the same; the resultant modification of the brain bulk then is limited by anatomical factors. Finally, in the closed skull certain changes take place, limited by the potential powers of change in the brain itself and by the intradural capacity; in the trephined skull, the only limitation to change is the intrinsic capability for contraction or expansion of the brain itself.

SUMMARY

1. Intravenous injection of a hypertonic solution (30 per cent NaCl or saturated $NaHCO_3$) is followed by a marked decrease in size of the brain; when the skull is opened the brain may be seen to fall away several millimeters from the inner surface of the skull after such injection.

2. Intravenous injection of a hypotonic solution (water) causes a marked swelling of the brain; when openings are made in the skull the brain will rise, forming tense herniae protruding several millimeters through the trephine openings.

3. These changes are independent of the volume of the fluid injected and are probably due to fundamental osmotic effects of the hypotonic and hypertonic solutions.

4. The brains of old cats fail to respond readily to intravenous injection, particularly to the intravenous injection of hypotonic solutions.

5. Internal changes, recognizable histologically, have been found quite constantly in the brains of animals which have been given intravenous injections of hypertonic or hypotonic solutions and which have not been trephined. On the contrary, in animals in which the skull is opened and the brain thus allowed to change its volume freely, these histological changes have not been demonstrated.

BIBLIOGRAPHY

(1) Weed and McKibben: This Journal, 1919, xlviii, 512.

(2) Monro: Observations on the structure and function of the nervous system, Edinburgh, 1783.

(3) Kellie: On death from cold and congestion of the brain, Edinburgh, 1824. Reprint from Trans. Med. Chir. Soc.

(4) Abercrombie: Pathological and practical researches on diseases of the brain, etc., Edinburgh, 1828.

(5) Burrows: On disorders of the cerebral circulation, etc., (London, 1846); Philadelphia, 1848.

(6) Kussmaul and Tenner: On the nature and origin of epileptiform convulsions, etc. Trans. by Bronner, New Sydenham Society, London, 1859.

(7) Donders: Schmidt's Jahrbuch, 1851, lxix, 16.

(8) Hill: The physiology and pathology of the cerebral circulation, London, 1896.

(9) Dixon and Halliburton: Journ. Physiol., 1914, xlviii, 128.

(10) Ecker: Physiol. Untersuch. über die Bewegungen des Gehirns, etc., Stuttgart, 1843.

I N 1926, Percival Bailey, in association with Harvey Cushing, introduced a system of classifying gliomas which has been of considerable value to neurosurgeons since that time.[11] The classification of intracranial neoplasms has always been a difficult task.[20] However, the intensive studies of Cushing, Bailey, and their colleagues established order in this confusing area, and, for the first time, an accurate evaluation of the clinical behavior and prognosis of these tumors could be made.[1—12,14,20]

In the early days of modern neurosurgery, pathology

" . . . seemed far ahead of surgery, since the meningeal tumors had already been described in masterly fashion by Louis and Cruveilhier; Johannes Müller and Cruveilhier had published a beautiful study of the pearly tumors; the chordomas had been described by Müller and the real age of discovery in the pathology of intracerebral tumors had been opened by Virchow's detection of the glia in 1835 and 1846 and a little later he had even been able to describe various types of gliomas. He already knew the soft and hard types, the myxoid and medullary, as well as the telangiectatic and hemorrhagic ones. He described the ependymal tumors and the neuromas of the eighth nerve and succeeded in separating the psammomas and fibromas from the sarcomas of the dura mater. If we study this period of rapidly developing knowledge of the nervous system, it is most striking to see how each discovery of a normal element is rapidly followed by the description of a corresponding tumor. . . .

" . . . We already find at this time a very characteristic subgrouping of the gliomas into spider cell gliomas and so on. But this was not generally accepted and Virchow's influence was so great that his system, as modified by Borst,[13] was the rigid framework of pathological teaching in all countries until the beginning of the twenties of this century.

"The new development was already foreshadowed at the beginning of this century with the occurrence of two events outside the Virchow tradition of pathology. These were examples of the use of finer methods in the analysis of the origin of brain tumors. In 1902, shortly after Weigert had demonstrated blepharoplasts in ependymal

cells, Mallory[15] was able to show these structures in certain 'sacral' tumors, making the origin of these tumors from ependymal cells highly probable. Again in 1903, Muthmann and Sauerbeck,[17] studying a fourth ventricle tumor by serial sections, were able to demonstrate its origin from the velum posterius.

" . . . In 1911, Pick and Bielschowsky,[18] to whom we owe much brilliant work in neuroanatomy and neuropathology, were occupied in studying the neuronal tumors. They began to classify them, not only according to their resemblance to normal ganglion cells, but also to the various stages of maturation. . . . A few years later in 1918, Ribbert,[19] in his classical study of the gliomas, created a similar genealogical tree for these tumors. . . .

"To reach the decisive period in the development of classification, two conditions were necessary, 1) the accumulation of pathological material to an extent previously unknown, i.e., this was dependent upon the development of neurosurgery as a specialty, and 2) a new mode of working on a scientific problem i.e., a 'team' studying the same problem from various aspects."[20]

These conditions were met at the Peter Bent Brigham Hospital in Boston. Beginning in 1922, Percival Bailey, stimulated by the discoveries of Cajal and Hortega in the normal structure of the interstitial tissues of the brain, attempted to formulate a classification of gliomas that would be of practical value to the neurosurgeon. After his early attempts to identify microglia and oligodendroglia had proved unsuccessful, Bailey began to group Cushing's collection of tumors on an empirical basis according to frequently recurring types of structure. From this experience, Bailey gradually formulated his scheme of the histogenesis of the brain and his classification of the gliomas. He submitted this material to Dr. Cushing in the spring of 1925. Cushing added a thorough clinical evaluation of the classification, and the entire work was published in 1926.[5,7,11]

Following the publication of this over-all scheme, Bailey then published individual accounts of several of the major types of glioma.[9,10,12] The most outstanding of these was his thorough study of the oligodendrogliomas in association with Paul Bucy.[7,9]

Since Bailey's pioneering work, more advanced techniques for studying neuropathological material have been developed,[16] and many other classifications of brain tumors have been introduced.[14,20] None, however, has been as influential as the original classification. Its essential features have remained of practical value to the neurosurgeon since 1926.

References

1. BAILEY, P. Further remarks concerning tumors of the glioma group. *Johns Hopk. Hosp. Bull.*, 1927, *40:* 354–389.
2. BAILEY, P. Histologic atlas of gliomas. *Arch. Path. Lab. Med.*, 1927, *4:* 871–921.
3. BAILEY, P. Histologic diagnosis of tumors of the brain. *Arch. Neurol. Psychiat.*, Chicago, 1932, *27:* 1290–1297.
4. BAILEY, P. Cellular types in primary tumors of the brain. In: *Cytology & cellular pathology of the nervous system.* W. Penfield, Ed. New York: P. B. Hoeber, 1932, *3:* 905–951.
5. BAILEY, P. A review of modern conceptions of the structure and classification of tumors derived from the medullary epithelium. *J. belge Neurol.*, 1938, *38:* 759–782.
6. BAILEY, P. Intracranial tumors. *Springfield, Ill.: Charles C Thomas*, 1948, 2nd ed., xxiv, 478 pp..
7. BAILEY, P. Personal communication.
8. BAILEY, P., BUCHANAN, D. N., and BUCY, P. C. Intracranial tumors of infancy and childhood. *Chicago: Univ. of Chicago Press*, 1939, xiii, 598 pp.
9. BAILEY, P., and BUCY, P. C. Oligodendrogliomas of the brain. *J. Path. Bact.*, 1929, *32:* 735–751.
10. BAILEY, P., and BUCY, P. C. Astroblastomas of the brain. *Acta psychiat., Kbn.*, 1930, *5:* 439–461.
11. BAILEY, P., and CUSHING, H. A classification of the tumors of the glioma group on a histogenetic basis with a correlated study of prognosis. *Philadelphia: J. B. Lippincott Co.*, 1926, 175 pp.
12. BAILEY, P., and EISENHARDT, L. Spongioblastomas of the brain. *J. comp. Neurol.*, 1932, *56:* 391–430.
13. BORST, M. Ein Sacraltumor von hirnartigem Bau. *Beitr. path. Anat.*, 1902, *31:* 419–439.
14. COSTERO, I. Pathology of glial neoplasms. In: *The biology and treatment of intracranial tumors.* W. S. Fields, and P. C. Sharkey, Ed. Springfield, Ill.: Charles C Thomas, 1962, xi, 505 pp. (see pp. 178–211).
15. MALLORY, F. B. Three gliomata of ependymal origin: two in the fourth ventricle, one subcutaneous over the coccyx. *J. med. Res.*, 1902, *8:* 1–10.
16. MEYER, A. Some recent trends in neuropathology. *J. ment. Sci.*, 1960, *106:* 1181–1194.
17. MUTHMANN, A., and SAUERBECK, E. Ueber eine Gliageschwulst des IV. Ventrikels (Neuroepitheli-

oma gliomatosum columnocellulare veli medullaris posterioris) nebst allgemeinen Bemerkungen über die Gliome überhaupt. *Beitr. path. Anat.*, 1903, *34:* 445–488.
18. PICK, L., and BIELSCHOWSKY, M. Über das System der Neurome und Beobachtungen an einem Ganglioneurom des Gehirns (nebst Untersuchungen über die Genese der Nervenfasern in "Neurinomen"). *Z. ges. Neurol. Psychiat.*, 1911, *6:* 391–437.
19. RIBBERT, H. Über das Spongioblastom und das Gliom. *Virchows Arch.*, 1918, *225:* 195–213.
20. ZÜLCH, K. J. The present state of the classification of intracranial tumors and its value for the neurosurgeon. In: *The biology and treatment of intracranial tumors.* W. S. Fields, and P. C. Sharkey, Ed. Springfield, Ill.: Charles C Thomas, 1962, xi, 505 pp. (see pp. 157–177).

OLIGODENDROGLIOMAS OF THE BRAIN.*

PERCIVAL BAILEY AND PAUL C. BUCY.

From the Surgical Clinic of Dr Harvey Cushing, Peter Bent Brigham Hospital, Boston, Massachusetts, and from the Surgical Laboratories of the Albert Merritt Billings Hospital, University of Chicago.

IN 1922 one of us, while in charge of Dr Cushing's laboratory at the Brigham Hospital, began a series of attempts to determine whether the microglia and oligodendroglia, newly distinguished by del Río-Hortega (15), participated in the formation of tumors of the brain. For many years all efforts were fruitless. Both microglia and oligodendroglia could readily be found in the cortex adjacent to the tumor but never within the tumor itself. In 1925 Penfield (19) reported the discovery of microglia within a brain-tumor, but playing the role of phagocytes, not as constituent cells of the neoplasm. Since with technique for microglia it is possible to impregnate phagocytes of any kind we have never felt Penfield's demonstration to be conclusive, as he has himself admitted (21).

Nevertheless several tumors were discovered which we thought must be composed of oligodendroglia and this belief was first expressed in an article by Bailey and Hiller (6). The neoplastic cells of these tumors were small, with scanty cytoplasm and round nuclei containing abundant chromatin. Mitotic figures were very rare. Between the nuclei was a delicate fibrillary material which could not be impregnated nor stained differentially by any method then at our disposal. When degenerated it formed a honeycomb around the nuclei so that the cross-section had much the appearance of a section of woody plant. Scattered

* Reprinted from *The Journal of Pathology and Bacteriology*, 1929, *32:* 735–751, with the kind permission of the Editor.

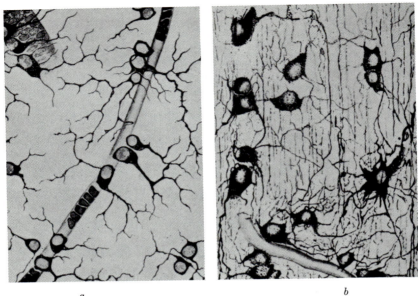

a   *b*

FIG. 1.—(*a*) Copied after Hortega. Normal oligodendroglia. Note especially those with a single process. (*b*) Copied after Penfield. Normal oligodendroglia. Note the large cell which resembles somewhat an astrocyte.

astrocytes were usually present. These tumors were described by Bailey and Cushing (5) under the name of oligodendrogliomas.

In looking back over previously described gliomas we were able to identify but three cases possibly of the same type, namely, those of Landau (16), of Ziveri (26), and of Roussy, Lhermitte and Cornil (24) the last said (without proof) to be composed of microglia. Since the appearance of the monograph of Bailey and Cushing reports of similar tumors have been published by Carnegie Dickson (10), by Schaffer (25) and by André-Thomas and Jumentié (1). Definite proof of the presence of oligodendroglia was however still lacking. It was not until February and March of 1928 that fresh operative material was obtained from four tumors in which the presence of oligodendroglia was proven beyond doubt. Since that time by the use of the Globus-Penfield modification of the method of del Río-Hortega we have positively identified nine other such tumors in Dr Cushing's series.

It is scarcely necessary to give detailed accounts of all these various tumors. The four recent tumors will be completely described and a table will serve to summarise the salient points concerning the other cases, followed by a general description covering all the gliomas of this type with which we are familiar. But before turning our attention to these tumors it might be well to pause a moment to refresh our minds concerning the structure of the oligodendroglia and the changes it undergoes in pathological conditions.

STRUCTURE OF THE OLIGODENDROGLIA.

The original description of the oligodendroglia (if one excepts the fragmentary notes of Robertson (23)) was published in Spanish by del Río-Hortega (15). Satisfactory accounts in English may be found in the articles of Bailey and Hiller (6) and of Penfield (20).

An oligodendroglial cell contains a spherical nucleus which is smaller than the nucleus of a neuroglial cell and has a denser chromatinic network. The cytoplasm forms a finely granular mass which may be rounded but is often polygonal and lies usually excentrically to the nucleus. It contains a centrosome, a Golgi-apparatus, a few mitochondria, and is heavily impregnated by the silver-carbonate method of Hortega (fig. 1). From the body of the cell arise one or more delicate processes which taper rapidly to an even calibre throughout their course; they may even be of the same calibre right up to their point of origin. Small swellings at irregular intervals along the course of the processes contain granules known as gliosomes. The processes are delicate, usually short, and sometimes branch dichotomously.

The oligodendroglia is found in most abundance along the long fibre-tracts but is to be found also in the cortex especially as satellites of the neural cells.

In acute degenerative lesions the oligodendroglia undergoes a change called by Penfield and Cone (22) "acute swelling"; the cell-body enlarges, the cytoplasm is rarified except at the extreme periphery and the nucleus becomes pyknotic. A more chronic degenerative change results in the formation of mucocytes (Pélissier (17), Bailey and Schaltenbrand (7)) but it is not certain that the acute swelling always results in the transformation of the cytoplasm into a substance giving the reactions of mucus (Ferraro (11)).

Progressive changes on the part of the oligodendroglia are unknown. It is uncertain whether they take part in the process of gliosis.

It will be evident from the descriptions that the tumors in the following cases are composed of cells having the structure of oligodendroglial cells and undergoing the same degenerative changes.

CASE REPORTS.

Case 5, *P.B.B.H., Surg. No. 13924. Calcified tumor of the left central region. Osteoplastic exploration with evacuation of cyst and partial extirpation. Secondary operation. Third operation. Fourth operation. Oligodendroglioma. (Reported previously by Bailey, Sosman, and van Dessel* (8)).

P.E.M., aged 43, was admitted 27th January 1921, complaining of headaches and convulsive attacks, having been referred by Dr C. J. Durham of Muskegon, Mich.

He had been well until 1904, when he had a generalised convulsion with unconsciousness. After that he had several other convulsive attacks at intervals of from three weeks to a year. In 1915 his memory began progressively to fail. Since September 1920, his attacks were more frequent, and he began to have minor attacks during which he would for a few minutes lose the ability to speak. After the attacks he would have headaches for a day or so.

On admission to the hospital he had a right facial paresis, some impairment of memory, haziness of the upper margins of both discs, with slight dysarthria and some hesitation at times in speaking. A roentgen examination of the head showed a definite area of calcification in the left hemisphere in about the region of the central fissure. On 2nd February 1921, Dr Cushing turned down a left bone-flap disclosing a large tumor, about 4.5 cm. in diameter, lying just in front of the fissure of Rolando. This tumor contained a cystic cavity from which 30 c.c. of fluid were evacuated. A portion of the tumor was removed and the wound closed.

Following the operation his difficulty of speech was slightly increased, but this later improved. Roentgen-ray treatment was begun before he was discharged, 24th February, with the facial paresis somewhat improved, optic discs unchanged and his speech defect somewhat better. Roentgen-ray treatments were continued by Dr Hollis Potter of Chicago. He continued to have epileptic attacks about every three weeks until 1st May 1924, when he began again to have difficulty of speech and impairment of motion of his right arm and leg. Since that time he had felt weak and miserable. His speech had grown worse and worse. He began to drag his right leg in walking. He didn't understand very well what he read.

He was re-admitted to the hospital on 26th August 1924, with some slight haziness of the left optic disc. He had a very slight right hemiparesis especially of the face. The right side of the body was colder and perspired more easily than the left. He had a very pronounced aphasia,

both motor and sensory. On 29th August 1924, a roentgen treatment was given without benefit. On 4th September 1924, Dr Cushing re-elevated the old bone-flap, evacuated a cystic cavity containing about 30 c.c. of fluid and removed a great deal of the mass of the tumor which was not definitely circumscribed. Following the operation, his aphasia improved gradually and on 18th September 1924 he was given another roentgen treatment, and discharged. At that time he was feeling well; the decompression was soft; he had a slight right facial paresis; and there had been some improvement in his ability to talk and read. On 6th February 1925, he wrote that he was feeling well, had had no epileptic attacks since 30th May 1924, scarcely ever had headaches, and was back at work in his office. Further roentgen treatments were given by Dr Vernon Moore of Grand Rapids, Mich.

On 23rd March 1925 he was examined by Dr V. G. J. Stuart of Grand Rapids, who could find no paresis or sensory disturbances or, in fact, any defect of his nervous system or his mentality, but in September 1926 he began to have twitching attacks of the right side of the face, accompanied by numbness of the right hand, and on two occasions (October 1925 and May 1926) there were convulsions with loss of consciousness. Lately there was increased difficulty in speaking. He was readmitted on 6th December 1926, when the old operative incision was reopened disclosing a reddish-gray tumor about 4 cm. in diameter in the supra-marginal region, which was shelled out apparently completely.

There was an increased paresis of the right arm which persisted, but his speech was slightly improved. He was discharged on 26th December 1926. His speech improved and he went back to work, being troubled only by occasional attacks of twitching in the right side of his face. Beginning in September 1927, his difficulty of speech increased and he began to have headaches and weakness of the right hand. Severe convulsions with loss of consciousness induced him to seek admission again on 13th February 1928.

He had then a very pronounced anomia and considerable mental confusion. The optic discs were choked 1–2 diopters. There was also a right hemiparesis and astereognosis in the right hand. On 21st February 1928 the old wound was reopened and a large mass of soft grayish tumor removed. In the midst of this mass was a cyst containing 15 c.cm. of fluid.

He was discharged on 18th March 1928 with a right hemiplegia predominating in the arm and aphasia about as on admission. He had some convulsive attacks which were fairly well controlled by luminal. When last heard from in February 1929, he seemed to be developing an extracranial extension in the neck.

Microscopical description. Microscopically the material removed at the first operation shows a very cellular tumor of fairly uniform appearance. It is composed of cells whose nuclei contain abundant chromatin. The nuclei, for the most part, are round and of a uniform size, but many ovoid and irregular forms are seen. The cytoplasm is finely granular and eosinophilic; it is small in amount and very indistinct. A few mitotic figures are seen. The intercellular material is of a homogeneous eosinophilic character (fig. 2a) staining a rusty red with phosphotungstic acid hematoxylin and bright-red with mucicarmine. In some areas the nuclei are closely packed together, the intercellular material is missing and some of the cells are arranged in typical pseudo-rosettes (fig.

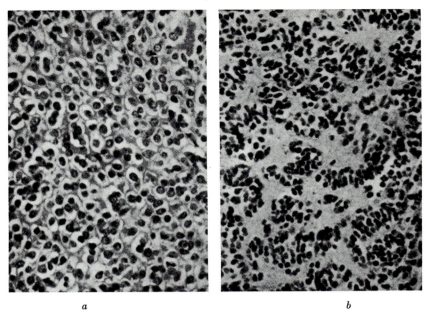

a   b

Fig. 2.—Case 5. Tumor removed at first operation. Methylene blue-eosin. ×300. (a) Extensive hyaline transformation of the intercellular tissue. (b) Arrangement of nuclei resembling that of medulloblastomas.

2b); these nuclei are more or less ovoid in shape and in
these areas mitotic figures can be seen, and here the
tissue cannot be differentiated from that of a medulloblastoma. However, such areas occupy only a very
minor part of the tumor, the remainder presenting the
typical picture of spherical nuclei uniformly arranged
and separated by definite intercellular material.

The tissue is moderately vascular and occasionally
separated into large bundles by wide connective-tissue
septa. The gold-sublimate method shows very few
astrocytes. In the sections prepared according to Penfield's modification the cells take the stain very well,
except in the medulloblastoma-like areas. In the well-
stained portions all of the cells have a moderate amount
of cytoplasm about a clear, usually round, vesicular
nucleus. There are many bipolar and unipolar cells, the
processes of which are thick and wavy. They appear to
be spongioblasts. However, most of the cells have three
or four processes which are narrow and usually short and
a moderate amount of cytoplasm from which the processes arise abruptly.

The tissue removed in December 1926 is moderately
vascular, extremely cellular and of marked uniformity
both of cellular distribution and nuclear size and shape
(fig. 3b). In the gold-sublimate preparations few astrocytes are seen but more than in the tissue from the first
operation. The tissue was improperly fixed for the silver-
methods and as a result imperfectly impregnated. However, by substituting lithium carbonate for sodium
carbonate in the preparation of the silver for Penfield's
method we were able to obtain fair impregnations. These
show many typical small oligodendroglia (fig. 4b) and a
few unipolar and bipolar cells. No astrocyte-like forms
are seen. There are, however, many oval nuclei, the
cytoplasm of which does not stain.

The tissue removed in 1928 has changed considerably
in appearance from that of 1921. The cells now all have

spherical nuclei of uniform size and distribution (fig. 3a).
There is also considerable perivascular calcification to
be seen. Staining with scarlet red reveals a little fat in
the tumor, all of which is intracellular, and occasionally
extends away from the cell in a row of granules presumably in a cytoplasmic process. In this manner the
cytoplasm and processes of many cells, typical oligodendroglia, are well seen. The gold-sublimate preparations show many astrocytes, many of which are very
large and have numerous processes; others are of small
size.

In the silver-carbonate preparations are seen many
more astrocyte-like cells than in the gold-sublimate
preparations. A very few bipolar and unipolar cells are
also present. These sections show many typical oligodendroglia with spherical nuclei, a narrow zone of cytoplasm and three or four short processes which arise
abruptly from the cell-body and are of constant size.
Many very large cells, evidently gigantic oligodendroglia,
are also seen. These cells have the same general characteristics as the small cells differing only in the fact that
they are much larger and have relatively more cytoplasm. There are also a few cells which show acute
swelling (fig. 4a).

Comment. The X-ray plate taken previous to
operation has unfortunately been lost, but fragments of tumor from the first operation were preserved and radiation reveals irregular areas of calcification. The long postoperative survival can in
part be explained by roentgen treatment and repeated operations, but not entirely so. The longest postoperative survival of a medulloblastoma
under similar treatment in our experience has
been 63.5 months (J. H., P.B.B.H., Surg. No.
13981) and of a glioblastoma multiforme 42

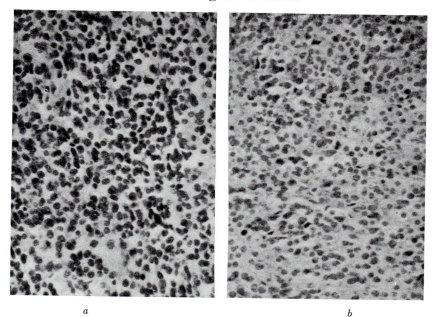

a   *b*

FIG. 3.—Case 5. (*a*) From third operation. Nuclei more numerous and irregular. HE, ×300. (*b*) From second operation. Showing typical appearance of oligodendroglioma. Methylene blue-eosin. ×300.

months (C. A. P., P.B.B.H., Surg. No. 17165). It is too early to make any remarks concerning a possible extracranial extension. Gliomas do not metastasise outside the leptomeninx (retinal gliomas excepted) and rarely spread by direct extension into the extracranial tissues. We have

seen only one other similar extracranial proliferation. We will return later to the question of the origin of the astrocytes, so numerous in the later specimens. In all the material oligodendroglial cells were very numerous, clearly dominating the microscopical appearance.

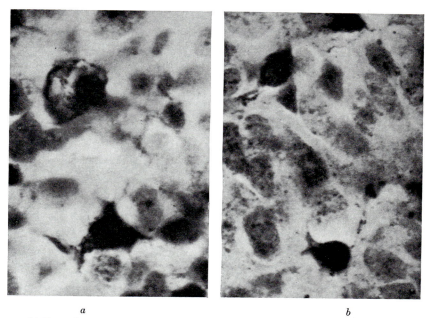

a   *b*

FIG. 4.—Case 5. (*a*) From the third operation. Oligodendroglial cells; one acutely swollen. Silver carbonate. ×1200. (*b*) From the second operation. Lithium carbonate. ×1200.

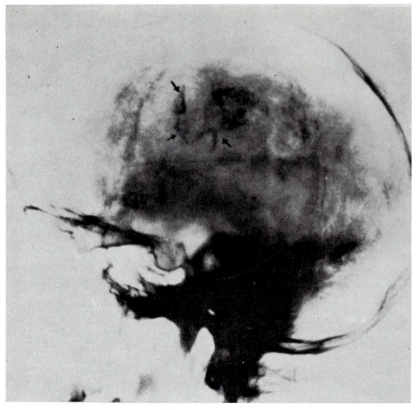

Fig. 5.—Case 11. Calcification visible in roentgenogram.

Case 11, P.B.B.H., Surg. No. 30778. Calcified tumor of left precentral region. Epilepsy. Extirpation of tumor. Oligodendroglioma.

On 21st February 1928, there was admitted Henry C.G., age 45, referred by Dr E. N. Libby of Boston and complaining of epilepsy.

In May 1922 he had his first attack, beginning with a burning sensation in the right side of the tongue. There was twitching of the right arm and finally unconsciousness and incontinence. A second similar attack occurred on 22nd September and a third in November of the same year. Since then he had only minor seizures with sometimes clouding of consciousness for a few seconds and twitching of right face and neck. These minor attacks increased in frequency until they lately had occurred two or three times daily. Since 1925 the right face drooped. In the last six months there had been some weakness of the right hand and also some difficulty in speech just before the convulsions. There had never been any headache.

Examination disclosed a right lower facial paresis and slight haziness of the nasal margins of both optic discs. Auditory acuity was lowered in both ears since an attack of malaria 22 years previously.

Roentgen examination revealed multiple streaks of calcification close to the surface in the left parietal region just behind the coronal suture, involving an area roughly circular in outline and about 4 cm. in diameter (fig. 5).

On 6th March 1928 an osteoplastic operation (Horrax-Cushing) disclosed a firm tumor in the precentral region, 4 cm. in diameter, extending upward from about 1 cm. above the Sylvian fissure. It involved also the frontal convolutions, particularly the second. It was covered by a large number of fine blood-vessels. A mass of the tumor was removed to a depth of about 2 cm.

Immediately following the operation there was an increase of aphasia. On 7th March and again on the following day there were attacks of twitching in the right face. Speech became reduced to "yes" and "no." On the afternoon of 8th March the wound was reopened and a large extradural clot was evacuated. Recovery was then rapid although minor epileptic seizures continued until 13th March. There was a notable increase in vocabulary, especially for French and German which before operation he had entirely lost.

He was discharged 24th March 1928. When last examined on 4th February 1929 he was much improved, spoke more freely, and his decompression was quite soft.

Microscopical description. The tissue is very cellular (fig. 6a). The nuclei are round, of a constant size and uniformly distributed. They have a heavy diffuse chromatinic network with one or two dense accumulations at or near the center. No mitotic figures are seen. The cytoplasm is very indefinite, finely granular and eosinophilic. The intercellular network is also rather indistinct. There are many small blood-vessels and considerable perivascular proliferation of connective tissue. Some calcium is deposited about the vessels in the exten-

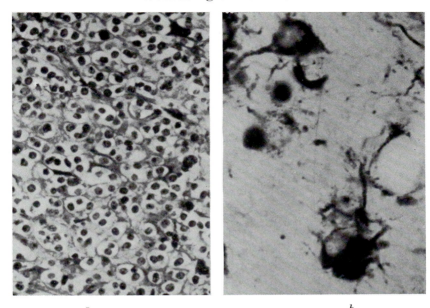

Fig. 6.—Case 11. (a) Oligodendroglioma showing several nuclei in the compartments. Phosphotungstic acid-hematoxylin. ×300. (b) Typical oligodendroglial cells. Silver carbonate. ×1200.

sive degenerated areas and there is occasionally proliferation and swelling of the endothelial lining of the vessels.

The sections stained with scarlet red show a great deal of fat in the tumor both intercellular and intracellular, and by no means limited to the necrotic areas. The Cajal technic for nerve-fibres reveals a considerable number running through the tumor. No connection between the neoplastic cells and these fibres can be found; they undoubtedly have their origin in the neighbouring cerebral tissue. The gold-sublimate preparations demonstrate many myelinated fibres which could not possibly have arisen from the tumor itself. In the sections prepared according to Globus's modification of Cajal's gold-sublimate method many astrocytes scattered throughout the tumor are seen, very poorly impregnated. Many of them have thick wavy processes.

In the silver-carbonate preparations a few nuclei seem to have no cytoplasm but about most of them can be seen a narrow zone of cytoplasm from which two or three processes arise rather abruptly (fig. 6b) to pass for varying distances into the surrounding tissue. These processes remain of practically the same calibre throughout their course. There are also many gigantic cells with a large amount of cytoplasm and usually three or four large processes, very similar in shape to the smaller ones. They have never been observed to have "sucker feet." There are also a few large cells with a large number of processes, many of which are quite short and end on the wall of a vessel. These cells are unquestionably astrocytes. All stages of transition between the true astrocytes and the gigantic oligodendroglia can be seen. Many of these large cells cannot therefore be definitely classified.

Comment. Again in this case there was development of symptoms over a period of many years before operative interference was necessary. The tumor was moreover calcified and the absence of mitotic figures speaks also in favor of the benign nature of the lesion, which, as in the previous case, had extended to the surface of the brain.

Case 12, P.B.B.H., Surg. No. 30880. Calcified tumor of left occipital region. Headaches, impairment of vision and hemianopsia. Extirpation. Oligodendroglioma.

On 9th March 1928 there was admitted Hans G., aged 39, referred by Dr Carl A. Schillander of Springfield, Mass., and complaining of headaches and loss of vision.

About a year and a half before admission he began to have diplopia and recurring attacks of blurred vision. Severe headaches in the frontal region occurred about the same time and occasional vomiting. About six months after the onset he noticed that he was unable to see to the right side and became unable to read, the print looking as he said like "a jumbled-up mess." Lately his memory had failed.

Examination disclosed a right homonymous hemianopsia, a paresis of the left sixth nerve and bilateral choked discs of 5 diopters elevation. The roentgen rays moreover revealed an irregular streaky calcification in the left occipital lobe (fig. 7).

On 13th March 1928 a left occipital operation (Horrax-Cushing) revealed bulging and flattened convolutions over the left occipital lobe. A transcortical incision came down on soft tumor at a depth of 1 cm. A large mass of soft reddish-gray tumor containing a few small cystic cavities was removed, and a decompression made in the temporal region.

The next day he had a sensation of flickering lights off to the right side and remarked that he had occasionally had such attacks for the previous ten years but only re-

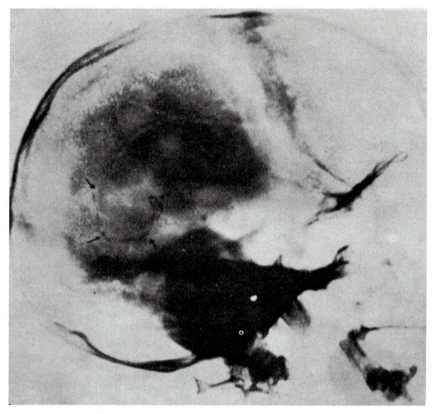

FIG. 7.—Case 12. Calcification as shown by X-rays.

membered them when they returned after the operation. He was discharged on 3rd April 1928. His visual acuity had slightly improved. The decompression was slightly bulging. When last heard from on 5th February 1929, he was well but very irritable and unable to work.

Microscopical description. The tissue removed presents an unusually uniform appearance (fig. 8a) of closely packed cells with a moderate number of blood-vessels and intervascular connective-tissue strands. The cells have a very indistinct, faintly eosinophilic granular cytoplasm. The nuclei are all practically round and of an almost constant size, varying from about 10 to 15 μ in diameter. They contain a moderate amount of chromatin scattered throughout the nucleus but accumulated particularly in a small round or irregular mass at the center. Rarely a mitotic figure can be found. There are to be seen a few cells with darkly staining cytoplasm and a few short processes. These are apparently abnormal astrocytes.

The sections stained with scarlet red show a considerable quantity of fat throughout the tumor-tissue, accumulated in large and small globules. In some instances it closely invests the individual nuclei and seems to lie within the cell itself; elsewhere it is definitely intercellular. The brain-tissue about the tumor contains a much greater quantity of fat than the tumor itself.

The gold-sublimate preparations are very granular. Scattered astrocytes with typical bodies, several processes and "sucker-feet" can be seen. There are also innumerable cells which are very poorly seen in these preparations; their nuclei are spherical and about them can be seen in a few cases a narrow zone of cytoplasm from which arise abruptly from one to four fine short feebly-impregnated processes; these are morphologically oligodendroglia.

In the sections prepared according to Penfield's modification of Hortega's silver-carbonate method only the nuclei of many of the cells can be seen. In others a faint ring of finely granular lightly-staining cytoplasm is also visible. Still others show a well-stained zone of cytoplasm about a spherical nucleus, identical with those nuclei which are bare. The cytoplasm in these cases may be a very narrow zone or a large rectangular or triangular area from which arise abruptly short narrow processes of even calibre from their origin (fig. 8b). Many typical swollen oligodendroglia are seen. These have a nucleus at the center surrounded by a wide zone of slightly granular lightly-staining material which is encompassed by a dark ring.

The method of Perdrau demonstrates an abundant network permeating the tissue in every direction. On superficial examination it appears to be formed by the connective-tissue but careful scrutiny and comparison with sections stained by phosphotungstic acid hematoxylin make it certain that much of this network is a homogeneous material in which no trace of fibrillae can be found. The fibrils are sharply impregnated around the blood-vessels.

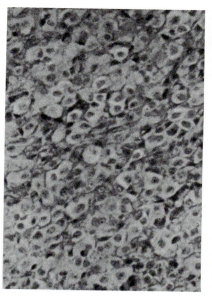 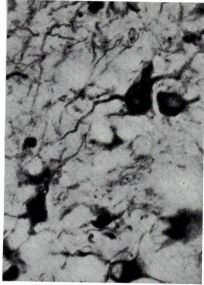

a b

Fig. 8.—Case 12. (a) Oligodendroglioma with very slight degenerative change. Methylene blue-eosin. ×300.
(b) Numerous oligodendroglial cells. Silver carbonate. ×780.

The endothelial cells of the small blood-vessels are swollen and proliferated. In some areas they have undergone a hyaline transformation in which calcium-salts have been deposited.

Comment. The flickering hallucinations of light which the patient remembered to have had for many years often occur with occipital tumors, and again in this case give evidence of the chronicity of the lesion.

Case 13, P.B.B.H., Surg. No. 31054. Calcified tumor in right parietal region. Headache, untidiness, and weakness of left foot. Extirpation. Oligodendroglioma.

On 31st March 1928 there was admitted Mary D'A., age 56, referred by Dr F. C. MacDonald of Roxbury, Mass., complaining of headaches, vomiting and weakness of the left foot.

It was noted by her family that as early as June 1927 she was listless and neglectful of her household. In September she complained of headache. In October she became untidy and careless of her personal appearance. In November she occasionally vomited. She complained also of a sensation of pins and needles in the left hand and began to drag the left foot. She had repeated stuporous attacks and finally on 28th March became frankly comatose and was brought to the hospital.

When admitted she was unable to stand; the tendon-reflexes were greatly exaggerated on the left side; there was a left hemihypesthesia to pain; the disc-margins were hazy but there was no measurable elevation. Roentgen examination disclosed an irregular mass of calcification about 3×5 cm. in extent in the right parieto-occipital region close to the surface of the brain (fig. 9).

On 12th April a right osteoplastic operation (Horrax-Cushing) revealed a soft spreading vascular glioma in lower parietal region. A large mass about 5 cm. in diam-

eter was removed. A subtemporal decompression was made.

The patient recovered promptly, became talkative and happy and was walking well when discharged on 3rd May 1928. The decompression was bulging slightly. When last examined on 26th March 1929 she was quite free from symptoms. The decompression was soft.

Microscopical description. The tissue removed is quite cellular and of very uniform appearance (fig. 10a). It is permeated by numerous small capillaries. The nuclei are round and contain a moderate amount of chromatin which is scattered diffusely throughout the nucleus. The nuclei are almost of a constant size: but there are a few very large ones. The cytoplasm is very indefinite and is finely granular. There is a large amount of intercellular material of a finely granular or homogeneous appearance in which few fibrils can be distinguished. There are many large areas of necrosis. No increase in perivascular connective tissue of any moment is seen, although there are many areas containing perivascular calcification. No mitotic figures can be found.

The scarlet-red preparations reveal practically no fat in the tumor-tissue except in the necrotic areas. The gold-sublimate method shows a moderate number of astrocytes. They vary greatly in size. The larger ones have a multitude of processes, some of which are rather short.

In the silver-carbonate preparations the majority of the nuclei have no surrounding cytoplasm; however many of them have two or three short processes which arise abruptly from a narrow zone of cytoplasm (fig. 10b). There are some giant-cells of this same type which are undoubtedly hypertrophic oligodendroglia. A few typical swollen oligodendroglia are also seen. There are many large cells with numerous processes, probably transitions to astrocytes.

Comment. The clinical course was shorter in this

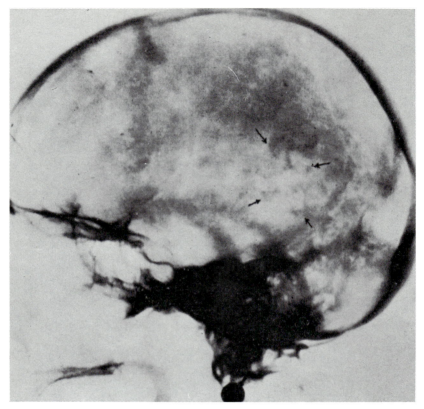

Fig. 9.—Case 13. Calcification in parieto-occipital region.

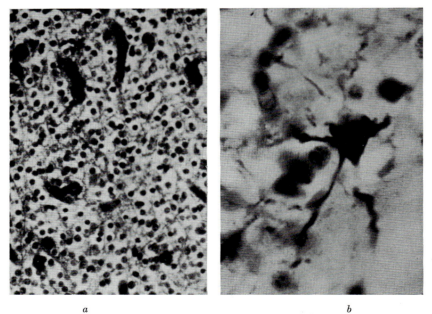

a　　　　　　　　　　　　　　　　　　　　　　　　　　*b*

Fig. 10.—Case 13. (*a*) Typical nuclei and arrangement of an oligodendroglioma. Phosphotungstic acid-hematoxylin. ×300. (*b*) Typical oligodendroglial cell. Silver carbonate. ×1200.

case, probably because of the location of the lesion in the relatively silent parietal area. The calcification and absence of mitotic figures are indications of a benign slowly advancing lesion.

From these four cases, therefore, we have the impression that tumors of this type are chronic and slowly growing in spite of the occasional presence of mitotic figures. This impression is confirmed by the study of the entire group as given in the table. . . .

DISCUSSION.

Clinical description. From the foregoing records it is at once apparent that the oligodendroglioma is predominantly a tumor of the cerebral hemispheres of adults, although we have seen one possible case at the age of five. Carnegie Dickson's patient also was only six years old. The tumor in his case, moreover, was in the third ventricle and we see no reason why such tumors should not occur also in the cerebellum and spinal cord. There is no marked predominance in either sex. It is evident also that these are slowly growing tumors, the average being 57.5 months of symptoms before the operation and the postoperative survival being 39.2+ months. The average total survival is 96.7+ months. The microscopic findings agree with the clinical course in that there are few mitotic figures to be found. Moreover, the tumors are almost invariably calcified. Since the introduction of the Potter-Bucky diaphragm calcification has been visible in the X-ray films of every patient but one.

Roentgen description. The calcification seen in the X-ray films is not typical of this type of glioma and does not serve to distinguish it from the other types in which calcification occurs. van Dessel (9) has shown that it may occur in any slowly-growing glioma. The deposits of calcium usually appear as blotchy or wavy irregular shadows (*cf.* figs. 5, 7, 9).

Microscopical description. The tissues were all fixed in 10 per cent. formalin. This naturally precluded the use of the original gold- and silver-methods of the Spanish school. However, when Globus (13) and Penfield (18) published their modifications of these methods for formalin-fixed tissues we immediately tried them on this particular tumor-series and found them to be very satisfactory. Throughout all of this work, in every case, companion-sections of normal human cerebral tissue were always simultaneously impregnated in the same baths. Thus the silver-stains, which are notoriously subject to slight variations, were always controlled and unspecific preparations were always discarded. All of the tissues were first stained with either hematoxylin and eosin, or methylene blue and eosin. All tissues were also stained with Mallory's phosphotungstic acid-hematoxylin. In many cases blocks from the tumor had originally been refixed in Zenker's fluid and stained in the laboratories of the Peter Bent Brigham Hospital. In those cases in which such preparations were not avail-

able blocks were prepared according to the technic of Davidoff and then stained. This method gave beautiful preparations. In most of the cases frozen sections were stained with scarlet red and counterstained with hematoxylin.

Frozen sections were always prepared according to Penfield's modification of Hortega's silver-carbonate method for staining the oligodendroglia and microglia; and according to Globus's modification of Cajal's gold-sublimate technic for the major glia. Where it seemed indicated frozen sections were prepared according to Cajal's silver-pyridine methods for myelinated and unmyelinated nerve-fibres. Perdrau's modification of Bielschowsky's silver-method for impregnating the connective tissue was also used in most cases.

In addition we perfected two modifications of Penfield's technic which proved very advantageous for some tumors. Our first modification was the one which proved of the greatest value although it altered the method but little. Instead of using the weak solution of ammonium hydroxide as Penfield suggests we substituted 10 per cent. ammonia as was suggested by Globus in his modifications. This improved the preparations very much. It may have been due to the fact that all of the tissues had been in formalin for at least a few months and some of them for many years. The second modification was of much less value. We substituted Hortega's silver-carbonate solution prepared with lithium carbonate for the silver-solution prepared with sodium carbonate as used by Penfield. This resulted in a much darker impregnation but the preparations lost in specificity. Astrocytes were stained particularly well in the tumor and poorly in the normal brain as compared with the original method of Penfield, which did not stain them at all in the normal brain and only poorly in the tumor. The lithium-prepared solution also stained fewer oligodendroglia than the true method of Penfield but those which were impregnated were very clear (fig. 11). In one case, on tissue fixed in Zenker's fluid, the original method was of no value while the lithium-modification gave beautiful preparations (*cf.* fig. 4b).

In some of the tumors so many oligodendroglia were impregnated that individual cells could not be clearly distinguished (fig. 12a). In these and other cases various measures, such as varying the time in the silver-bath and increasing the time of toning in the gold-chloride bath, had to be taken to reduce the number of cells impregnated in order that microphotographs showing the contour of the individual cells could be obtained (fig. 12b). In most instances a definite effort had to be made to find areas in which isolated cells stood out sufficiently clearly from the mass of cells to be illustrative. After observing the extreme cellularity of these tumors in ordinary preparations it can be easily understood that complete impregnation of all of the cells and their processes is not satisfactory for careful study and demonstration.

Microscopically this group of tumors presents characteristics which are sufficiently clear to permit of no confusion with any other members of the glioma-group. Preparations stained with hematoxylin and eosin or methylene blue and eosin are

Oligodendrogliomas

Case	Name	Hospital Surg. No. B = Brigham H = Hopkins	Sex	Age at admission	1st symptom	Length of pre-operative symptoms	Operative procedure	Post-operative survival after 1st operation	Location of tumor	Calcification in X-ray	Remarks
						Months		Months			
1	Marion M.	B 4636	F	45	Headache	36	Osteoplastic exploration, May 4, 1916 Partial extirpation, June 11, 1925	148+	Left central	+	Unusually large number of astrocytes. Calcification seen only in X-rays taken in 1925.
2	Delia K.	B 5490	F	48	Epilepsy (sensory attacks)	72	Partial extirpation, Oct. 14, 1916	24	Right post-central	0	Died of increasing growth of tumor.
3	Edwin M.	B 13185	M	25	Headache	3	Subtemporal decompression, May 8, 1922 Osteoplastic exploration, Sept. 12, 1923 Re-exploration, June 12, 1924	23	Septum lucidum.	0	Died of blockage of cerebrospinal fluid circulation.
4	Dabney L.	B 13583	M	40	Lassitude	11	Partial extirpation, Nov. 30, 1920	51	Left central	0	Died of increased growth of tumor.
5	Paul M.	B 13924	M	43	Epilepsy	204	Partial extirpation, Feb. 2, 1921; Sept. 4, 1924; Dec. 6, 1926; Feb. 21, 1928	95+	Left central	+	Has developed what seems to be an extra-cranial extension in neck.
6	Ellen C.	B 20125	F	33	Headache	60	Osteoplastic exploration, Nov. 28, 1923	24	Right frontal	+	Died of status epilepticus.
7	Dennis M.	B 20535	M	43	Headache	8	Partial extirpation, Jan. 24, 1924	42	Right frontal	+	Died of intraventricular extension.
8	Light C.	B 26448	F	52	Headache	8	Partial extirpation, June 9, 1926	29+	Right frontal	+	Living and well.
9	Ethel McR.	B 28534	F	45	Lassitude	16	Partial extirpation, April 12, 1927	21	Left frontal	+	Sudden death: apoplexy(?)
10	Ferdinand H.	B 29140	M	47	Epilepsy	132	Partial extirpation, Dec. 27, 1927 (Spurling)	24+	Left temporal	+	Many spongioblasts in tumor. Living and well.
11	Henry G. G.	B 30778	M	45	Epilepsy	68	Partial extirpation, March 6, 1928	10+	Left precentral	+	Living and well.
12	Hans G.	B 30880	M	39	Hallucinations of light	120	Partial extirpation, March 13, 1928	10+	Left occipital	+	Living and well.
13	Mary D'A.	B 31054	F	56	Negligence	10	Partial extirpation, April 12, 1928	9+	Right parietal	+	Living and well.

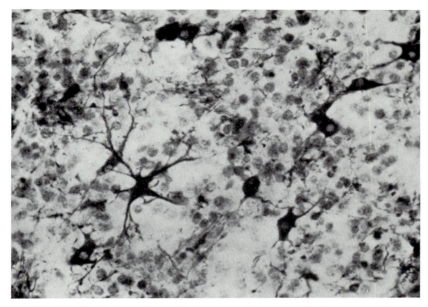

FIG. 11.—Typical oligodendroglia in a tumor impregnated by the non-specific
lithium-modification. One astrocyte is also seen. ×380.

usually sufficient for a positive diagnosis of any tumor of this type. Of the nine tumors originally placed in this group, on the basis of such stains, in the monograph of Bailey and Cushing (5), six have subsequently been proven by specific impregnation to be composed essentially of oligodendroglia and the three others were tumors which had been imperfectly fixed so that we were unable to secure satisfactory impregnations. It is only for the proof of the true nature of the cells in the tumor that detailed histologic studies such as this are necessary.

As we have stated the picture presented by sections stained with the methods commonly used in

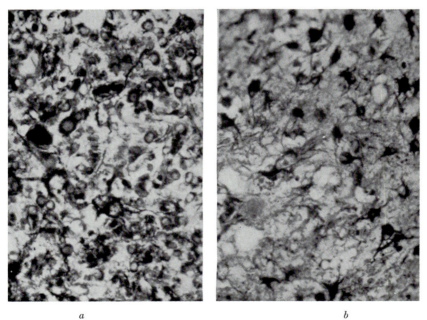

a

b

FIG. 12.—Oligodendrogliomas. (a) Practically every cell is impregnated. Silver carbonate. ×300. (b) From another tumor with looser structure. Silver carbonate. ×320.

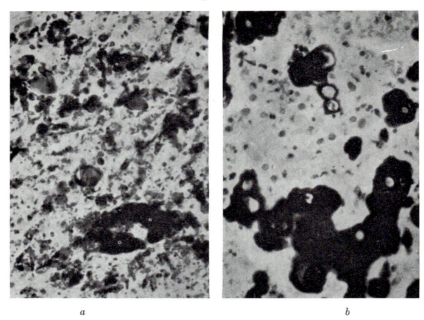

a   *b*

Fig. 13.—(*a*) Extensive fatty degeneration in an oligodendroglioma. Scarlet red. ×300. (*b*) Calcification occurring
   in the walls of blood-vessels. Methylene blue-eosin. ×300.

any pathological laboratory is typical. The tissue
is exceedingly cellular and presents a remarkable
uniformity. The nuclei, which in these stains are
the only distinct part of the cells, are almost all
perfectly round and of a fairly constant size. They
are distributed thickly but uniformly over the
field. They range from about 10 to 20 μ in diameter in the various tumors and contain a moderate
amount of chromatin which is scattered diffusely
throughout except for one or two small darkly
staining accumulations near the center resembling
nucleoli. There are rarely any mitotic figures to be
seen. The cytoplasm is very indistinct, is finely
granular and eosinophilic. The individual cells are
separated from each other by a fibrillary intercellular material which serves to "box-in" each
individual cell. Occasionally two or three nuclei
may be found in one such "box" (*cf.* fig. 6*a*). This
intercellular material varies in appearance. A
large part of it has often undergone a homogeneous transformation (*cf.* fig. 2*a*). The remainder is
made up of a mixture of intervascular connective-
tissue fibres, protoplasmic processes of astrocytes
and the delicate processes of the oligodendroglia.

The vascularity of the tissue varies considerably. In most of the cases it is moderate in amount
but in a few an extensive thick network of fine
capillaries is present. In many we see an increase
in the perivascular connective tissue which is frequently associated with a deposition of calcium-
or iron-salts about the vessels (fig. 13*b*). These
areas of calcification are most prevalent in the
necrotic or semi-necrotic portions of the tumor al-

though they are found elsewhere as well. The
microscopic centers of calcification are undoubtedly the forerunners of the large masses of calcium
which characterise so many of the tumors in the
roentgenograms.

Many of the specimens show in addition to the
perivascular changes a marked proliferation of the
endothelial lining of the blood-vessels (fig. 14*a*).
Carnegie Dickson reported this same finding in
what appeared to be a typical example of an
oligodendroglioma. In his case he saw proliferation so extensive as to occlude completely some of
the vessels. Such marked hyperplasia was rarely
observed in our tumors.

Necrotic areas are relatively common and vary
from quite extensive ones of two or three centimeters in diameter to those which are microscopic
in size. They contain only fat and an eosinophilic
granular material surrounded by tumor-tissue.
Occasionally they have broken down to form
small cysts. Stains for fat reveal varying amounts
in the different tumors. In some it lies abundantly
between the cells and within the cells themselves
(fig. 13*a*); others show none at all or very little.
The fat may lie in the processes as well as in the
cytoplasm of the cell-body and thus very clearly
outline the contour of typical oligodendroglial
cells (fig. 15*b*).

In several cases nerve-fibres, both myelinated
and unmyelinated, can be found running through
the tumor in large numbers (fig. 15*a*). These have
no connection with the tumor-cells and are evidently the remnants of the invaded cerebral tis-

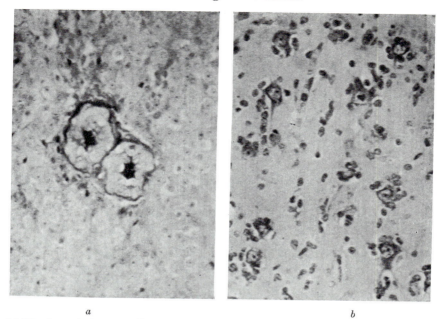

a   *b*

Fig. 14.—(*a*) Blood-vessels from an oligodendroglioma. Note the proliferation of the endothelium. Methylene blue-eosin. ×300. (*b*) Increase in oligodendroglial cells around neurones of cortex near an oligodendroglioma. Methylene blue-eosin. ×300.

sue. In studying the neighboring neural tissue in two cases a marked satellitosis was found (fig. 14*b*). This extended several millimeters from the tumor. About the neurocytes were as many as 15 or 20 small round nuclei. As one approached the tumor their number greatly increased until finally

the tissue had the appearance of tumor-tissue containing many neurocytes, as in the case of Landau (16). This layer soon gave way to tissue containing no neurocytes and only typical small round oligo-nuclei. In all cases the line of junction between the tumor and the cerebral tissue is not

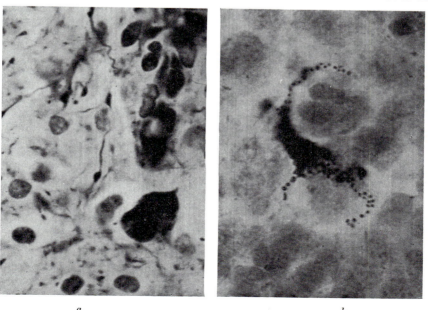

a   *b*

Fig. 15.—(*a*) Unmyelinated neural fibres passing through an oligodendroglioma. Reduced silver. ×1000. (*b*) Oligodendroglial cell with droplets of fat in the processes (retouched). Scarlet red. ×1200.

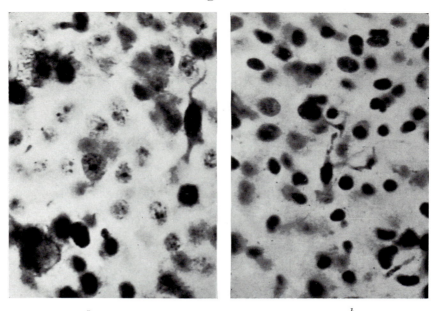

a   b

FIG. 16.—(a) Microglial cell in the margin of an oligodendroglioma.
Hortega-Penfield. ×1000. (b) Similar cell. ×700.

clean-cut. In one tumor a few microglia were found (fig. 16) at the periphery where it joined the cerebral tissue. These undoubtedly are from the invaded tissue as they cannot be found elsewhere in this tumor and are not seen in any of the other cases.

On the other hand the various staining methods reveal numerous astrocytes scattered throughout these tumors. They are not more plentiful at the periphery and with a few rare exceptions they all appear to be perfectly healthy normal or hypertrophied cells. Many of them have the cell-body applied to the vessel-wall after the manner of the perivascular cells of Andriezen (2). In one instance in which specimens were secured at a secondary operation from the same individual after an interval of seven years we find a marked increase in the number of astrocytes. In one tumor (case 1) a large area is found which is very loose in texture, contains very few cells and is quite avascular. These cells are not oligodendroglia but are typical astrocytes. It would seem therefore that here we have the possibility of a mixed oligodendroglioma and astrocytoma. In one other tumor (case 10) a large number of spongioblasts are present.

For our present purposes, that is for demonstrating the true nature of these extremely cellular yet paradoxically slowly growing, calcifying tumors, the silver preparations are the most interesting. These preparations demonstrate that the small round nuclei which compose almost all of the tissue are surrounded by cytoplasm which gives rise to a few short processes. The cytoplasm varies somewhat in amount between two types of cells: the small cell and the giant-cell. Except for their size there is no essential difference between the two. In the small cells the cytoplasm is a narrow zone immediately surrounding the nucleus and arising abruptly from it are a few, usually three or four, short processes which, differing from those of the astrocytes, do not taper but remain of a constant size throughout their length. In the giant-cells there is more cytoplasm which usually assumes a rectangular or polyhedral shape (figs. 17b and 19b), the processes of which are longer and proportionately thicker than in the small cells and arise abruptly from the cell-body. Typical cells of this type do not have "sucker feet" which connect with the blood-vessels as do the astrocytes.

There are also many cells which appear to be transitions between the gigantic oligodendroglia and astrocytes. It is impossible definitely to classify them as belonging in either group. Some of them have a nucleus and cell-body similar to the oligodendroglia but with several long tapering processes. Many of the cells which we have previously taken to be protoplasmic astrocytes are doubtless of this nature (cf. Bailey (3), plate XXIII). Some of them have poorly developed "sucker feet" (fig. 17a). Practically every stage of gradual transition from typical oligodendroglia to typical astrocytes can be found (fig. 19a). These

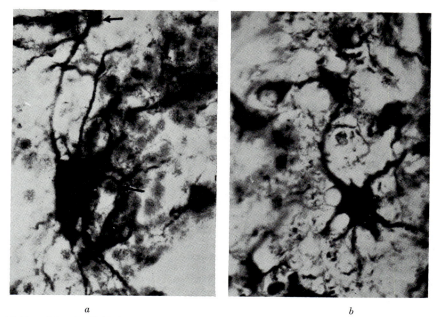

a   b

Fig. 17.—(a) Transitional cell. Body resembling that of an oligodendroglial cell but with "sucker feet" (arrows).
Gold-sublimate. ×700. (b) Gigantic oligodendroglial cell. Silver carbonate. ×780.

transitional cells are usually impregnated poorly with both methods and are often fuzzy with numerous delicate processes (fig. 18).

In every tumor typical swollen oligodendroglia can be demonstrated. These cells have a small pyknotic nucleus at the centre of a fairly wide layer which is either clear or slightly granular and

is surrounded by a definite heavily-impregnated membrane (fig. 20). Frequently a few fine bands running between the outer membrane and the nucleus can be seen. The number of such swollen cells varies in the different cases. Those specimens which were obtained many hours post mortem contain many swollen and few typical oligoden-

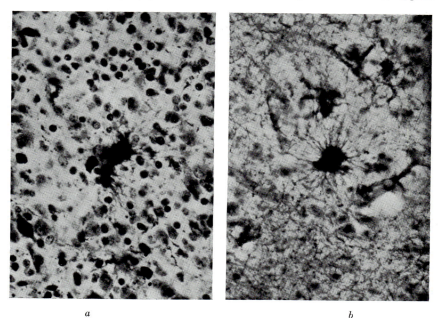

a   b

Fig. 18.—Transitional cells stained: (a) with silver carbonate and (b) with gold-sublimate. ×380.

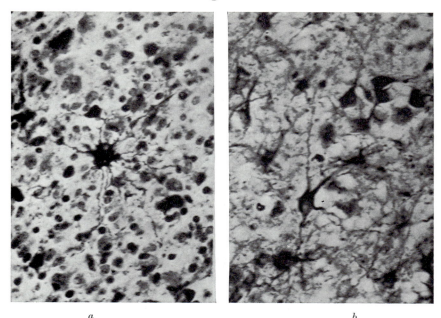

a   b

FIG. 19.—(a) Oligodendroglial cell of transitional type. Silver carbonate. ×380.
(b) Gigantic oligodendroglial cell. Silver carbonate. ×420.

droglia, while those specimens which were obtained at operation and fixed immediately have as
a rule fewer swollen cells and more cells with
typical cytoplasm and processes.

In addition the Penfield technic impregnates
feebly many unipolar and bipolar cells. These can
also be seen poorly in the gold-sublimate preparations. They are thick and have heavy wavy processes (fig. 21b). They appear to be spongioblasts.
There are also many unipolar cells with typical
oligo-bodies and one process arising abruptly from
the cytoplasm (fig. 21a). These are morphologi-

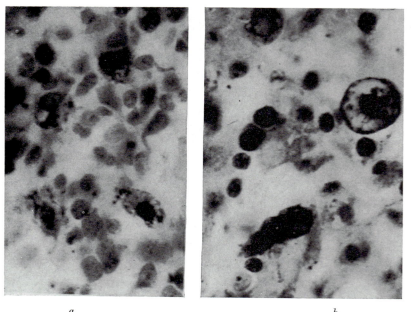

a   b

FIG. 20.—Swollen oligodendroglial cells. Silver carbonate. (a) ×780. (b) ×1000.

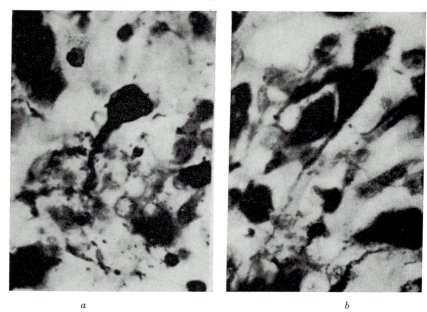

a   *b*

Fig. 21.—(*a*) An oligodendroglial cell with a single process. Compare with Fig. 1.
(*a*) Silver carbonate. ×850. (*b*) Unipolar spongioblasts. Gold-sublimate. ×850.

cally oligodendroglia with one process. Such cells are depicted in Hortega's original description (15) of the oligodendroglia (*cf.* fig. 1).

The degenerative changes which occur in these tumors result not only in acute swelling of the neoplastic cells but also in the deposition in their cytoplasm of numerous globules of fat, so that they resemble the scavenger cells of the central nervous system (fig. 22). In addition there occurs a finely granular or homogeneous transformation of the cytoplasm of other cells (fig. 23*b*) and of the intercellular fibrillary material. The resultant degen-

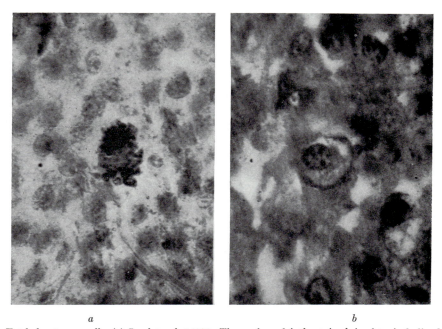

a   *b*

Fig. 22.—Fat-laden tumor-cells. (*a*) Scarlet red. ×850. The nucleus, faintly stained, is of typical oligodendroglial type. (*b*) Hematoxylin-metanil yellow ×1000. Vacuolated cytoplasm after removal of fat.

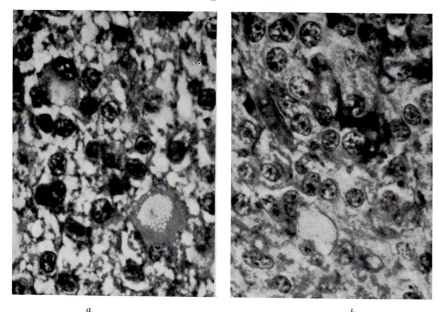

a   *b*

Fig. 23.—Oligodendroglioma. Hematoxylin-mucicarmine-metanil yellow. × 850. (*a*) Cells resembling those found in
Schilder's encephalitis (astrocytes?), one of which contained droplets of fat. (*b*) One mucocyte above; below
is a neoplastic cell with the typical cytoplasm of a so-called "Gitter cell."

erative product stains faintly with eosin and with anilin blue but often very deeply with mucicarmine. The mucicarmine-stain can also be found in the peripheral cytoplasm of swollen cells, but at times the entire body of the cell is deeply stained (fig. 23). In other cells the center of the body is filled with fat-globules (fig. 23*a*) and the periphery takes a deep-red stain with mucicarmine. These cells resemble those found often in Schilder's encephalitis. At other times the mucinoid material seems to be entirely intercellular. In these cases typical mucocytes can be found in the surrounding cerebral tissue, while in the tumor the red stain is so diffuse and general as to obscure the individual cells.

Theoretical considerations. From the conditions present in these tumors we may derive some suggestions concerning the oligodendroglia and its relation to the other interstitial cells of the central nervous system. It is evident that the foregoing descriptions confirm the opinion of Hortega, which has been supported by Penfield, that the oligodendroglia and the classical neuroglia are closely allied. There are numerous cells in all these tumors which it is practically impossible to classify. They have characteristics of both oligodendroglia and of astrocytes. Moreover there are numerous other cells which are equally difficult to classify; they might be either unipolar spongioblasts or unipolar oligodendroglia such as Hor-

tega has depicted. The presence of all these transitional cells indicates clearly the close kinship of the oligodendroglia and the astrocytes. On the other hand the conditions in those tumors are just as clearly opposed to the attempt of Ferraro and Davidoff (12) to bring together the oligodendroglia and the microglia. No cells were seen in these neoplasms which resembled microglia except in the border near the brain-tissue. It is true that many cells were found resembling the "Gitter-cells" described by Ferraro and Davidoff (12), but we have elsewhere insisted (3*a*) that the term "Gitter-cell" is a morphological one, meaning simply that the cell is full of fat-granules and gives no indication of any phagocytic activity.

SUMMARY

1. Proof has been obtained, by specific impregnations, of the existence of brain-tumors composed essentially of oligodendroglia.

2. These tumors are predominantly situated in the cerebral hemispheres of adults.

3. They almost invariably contain sufficient deposits of the salts of calcium or iron to be visible in X-ray films.

4. Oligodendrogliomas are slowly growing gliomas with a relatively good prognosis.

5. The records of four such tumors are given in detail as well as data concerning nine other proven and four presumptive cases.

BIBLIOGRAPHY

1. ANDRÉ-THOMAS AND JUMENTIÉ, J.   Un cas de tumeur du ventricule latéral, *Revue neurol.*, 1928, ii. 202–206.

2. ANDRIEZEN, W. L. . . . . .   On a system of fibre-cells surrounding the blood-vessels of the brain of man and mammals and its physiological significance, *Intern. Monatschr. f. Anat. u. Physiol.*, 1893, x. 532–540.

3. BAILEY, P. . . . .   Histologic Atlas of Gliomas, *Arch. Path. and Lab. Med.*, 1927, iv. 871–921.

3a. BAILEY, P. . . . .   Discussion of symposium on interstitial tissues, *Trans. Am. Neurol. Assoc.*, 1927, 53rd Session, p. 162.

4. BAILEY, P., AND BUCY, P. C. . .   Oligodendrogliomas of the brain; preliminary note, *Proc. Chicago Path. Soc.*, 1929.

5. BAILEY, P., AND CUSHING, H. .   Tumors of the glioma group, Lippincott, 1926.

6. BAILEY, P., AND HILLER, G. . .   The interstitial tissues of central nervous system, a review, *Jour. Nerv. and Ment. Dis..*, 1924, lix. 337–361.

7. BAILEY, P., AND SCHALTEN-   Die muköse Degeneration der Oligodendroglia, *Deuts. Zts. f. Nervenh.*, BRAND, G.   1927, xcvii. 231–237.

8. BAILEY, P., SOSMAN, M. C., .   Roentgen therapy of gliomas of the brain, *Am. Jour. of Roentg. and Ra-* AND VAN DESSEL, A.   *dium Therapy*, 1928, xix. 203–264.

9. DESSEL, A. VAN . . . .   L'incidence et le processus de calcification dans les gliomes du cerveau, *Arch. franco-belges de chirurgie*, 1925, xxviii. 845–874.

10. DICKSON, W. E. C.. . . . .   Oligodendroglioma of floor of third ventricle, *Brain*, 1926, xlix. 578–580.

11. FERRARO, A. . . . . . .   Acute swelling of the oligodendroglia and grape-like areas of disintegration, *Arch. of Neurol. and Psych.*, 1928, xx. 1065–1079.

12. FERRARO, A., AND DAVID-.   The reaction of the oligodendroglia to injury of the brain, *Arch. of Path.* OFF, L.M.   *and Lab. Med.*, 1928, vi. 1030–1053.

13. GLOBUS, J. H. . . . . . .   Cajal and Hortega glia-staining methods, *Arch. of Neurol. and Psych.*, 1927, xviii. 263–271.

14. HORTEGA, DEL RÍO . . . .   Algunos observaciónes acerca de la neuroglia perivascular, *Bol. de la Soc. española de Hist. Nat.*, April 1925, 1–21.

15. HORTEGA, DEL RÍO . . . .   La glia de escasas radiaciones (oligodendroglia), *Boletín de la Real. Soc. española de Hist. Nat.*, 1921, xxi. 63–92.

16. LANDAU, M.. . . . . . .   Das diffuse Gliom des Gehirns, *Frank. Zts. f. Path.*, 1910, v. 469–514.

17. PÉLISSIER, G. . . . . . .   Syndrome Wilsonien consécutif à la névraxite épidémique, *Thèse de Montpellier*, 1924.

18. PENFIELD, W. . . . . . .   Method of staining oligodendroglia and microglia (combined method), *Am. Jour. of Path.*, 1928, iv. 153–157.

19. PENFIELD, W. . . . . . .   Microglia and the process of phagocytosis in gliomas, *Am. Jour. of Path.*, 1925, i. 77–89.

20. PENFIELD, W. . . . . . .   Oligodendroglia and its relation to classical neuroglia, *Brain*, 1924, xlvii. 430–452.

21. PENFIELD, W. . . . . . .   Phagocytic activity of microglia in the central nervous system, *Proc. N.Y. Path. Soc.*, 1925, xxv. 71–77.

22. PENFIELD, W., AND CONE,   Acute swelling of oligodendroglia, *Arch. of Neurol. and Psych.*, 1926, xvi. W. . . . .   131–153.

23. ROBERTSON, W. F. . . . .   A microscopic demonstration of the normal and pathological histology of mesoglia cells, *Jour. of Ment. Science*, 1900, xlvi. 724.

24. ROUSSY, G., LHERMITTE, J., .   Essai de classification des tumeurs cérébrales, *Ann. d'anat. Path. mèd-chir.*, AND CORNIL, L.   1924, i. 333–382.

25. SCHAFFER, K. . . . . . .   Bemerkungen zur Histopathologie des Hirnglioms, *Monatsschr. f. Psych. und Neurol.*, 1927, lxv. 208–229.

26. ZIVERI, A. . . . .   Sopra un caso di tumore dei lobi frontale e temporale destri con alcune considerazioni sui gliomi, *Revista di pat. nerv. e mentale*, 1918, xxiii. 286–310.

Neurosurgical Classic—14

Eᴀʀʟʏ in the course of his extensive clinical studies of cortical function and of epilepsy,[28,31,32,35,36] Dr. Wilder Penfield made a chance observation that has led to a major contribution to the understanding of cerebral function.

In the nineteenth century, neurosurgeons first began to employ the experimental techniques of Fritsch and Hitzig, Ferrier, Sherrington, and others, to study the cortical localization of motor functions in man.[1,41—43] Frequently these techniques were used to map out the area of the brain to be removed in patients with focal epilepsy.[5]

"More exciting were the two cases published in 1909 by Harvey Cushing on sensations resulting from stimulations of the post-Rolandic area in man. Operating under local anaesthesia he established the sensory function of the human postcentral strip. Penfield, since that day . . . , has greatly extended these observations on both the motor and sensory and other responsive areas of the brain. . . .

"Ferrier many years ago said that all parts of the cortex would prove to be excitable, but he could not demonstrate excitability himself except from restricted areas of the brain: the greater part was unresponsive. Ferrier's prophecy was long unfulfilled, and only recently has come closer to confirmation. Thus we now know that responses must be looked for not only in movements of the limbs or in sensations or in flashes of light or sounds or odours but in two other directions. The first is in the autonomic or visceral changes that may be the replies to stimulation of some areas. . . . This work has mainly been done on animals. The second and much the more exciting, discovery was made by Penfield—that stimulations of the temporal lobe in human beings may evoke experiences, pictures in the mind. . . . "[5]

The following is Dr. Penfield's account of his first experiences with this phenomenon:

" . . . I was operating upon a woman under local anaesthesia in the Royal Victoria Hospital and was applying to different points on the temporal lobe of her brain a stimulating electrode. She (E.W.) told me suddenly that she seemed to be living over again a previous experience: she seemed to see herself giving birth to her baby girl. That had happened years before, and meanwhile the girl had grown up. The mother was now lying on the operating table in my operating room, hoping that I could cure her attacks of focal epilepsy.

"This, I thought, was a strange moment for her to talk of that previous experience, but then, I reflected, women were unpredictable and it was never intended that men should understand them completely. Nevertheless, I noted the fact that it was while my stimulating electrode was applied to the left temporal lobe that this woman had had this unrelated and vivid recollection. That was in 1931.

"It was more than five years later when a somewhat similar psychical state made its appearance during electrical stimulation. This time, however, it seemed certain that the stimulus had somehow summoned a past experience.

"The Montreal Neurological Institute was opened in 1934, and a patient, J.V., a girl of 14 years, was admitted in June 1936. . . . She was complaining of seizures during which she sometimes fell unconscious to the ground in an epileptic convulsion. But, immediately preceding such an episode, she was aware of what seemed to be a hallucination. It was always the same: an experience came to her from childhood. . . .

"At operation, under local anaesthesia, I mapped out the somatic sensory and motor areas for purposes of orientation, and I applied the stimulator to the temporal cortex. 'Wait a minute,' she said, 'and I will tell you.' I removed the electrode from the cortex. After a pause, she said: 'I saw someone coming toward me, as though he was going to hit me.' It was obvious also that she was suddenly frightened.

"Stimulation at a point farther forward caused her to say, 'I imagine I hear a lot of people shouting at me.' Three times, at intervals and without her knowledge, this second point was stimulated again. Each time she broke off our conversation, hearing the voices of her brothers and her mother. And on each occasion she was frightened. She did not remember hearing these voices in any of her epileptic attacks.

"Thus the stimulating electrode had recalled the familiar experience that ushered in each of her habitual attacks. But stimulation at other points had recalled to her other experiences of the past, and it had also produced the emotion of fear.

Our astonishment was great, for we had produced phenomena that were neither motor nor sensory, and yet the responses seemed to be physiological, not epileptic. . . . "[25]

Dr. Penfield's subsequent experiences with similiar patients has led to two important neurophysiological concepts: the definition of the centrencephalic system and its importance to consciousness, and the role of the temporal lobe in memory and in psychomotor epilepsy.[2-27,29,30,33,34,37-40] Reproduced below is Penfield's initial account of these ideas, as given in the Harvey Lecture delivered October 15, 1936.

References

1. BRAZIER, M. A. B. The historical development of neurophysiology. In: *Handbook of physiology. A critical, comprehensive presentation of physiological knowledge and concepts.* J. Field, Ed. Washington, D.C.: American Physiological Society, 1959, Sect. 1, *1:* 1–58.
2. FEINDEL, W., and PENFIELD, W. Localization of discharge in temporal lobe automatism. *Arch. Neurol. Psychiat., Chicago,* 1954, *72:* 605–630.
3. FEINDEL, W., PENFIELD, W., and JASPER, H. Localization of epileptic discharge in temporal lobe automatism. *Trans. Amer. neurol. Ass.,* 1952, 14–17.
4. JASPER, H. H. Implications for the neurological sciences. In: *Electrical stimulation of the brain. An interdisciplinary survey of neurobehavioral integrative systems.* D. E. Sheer, Ed., Austin: Univ. of Texas Press, 1961, xiv, 641 pp. (see pp. 557–562).
5. JEFFERSON, G. Man as an experimental animal. *Lancet,* 1955, *1:* 59–61.
6. MILNER, B., and PENFIELD, W. The effect of hippocampal lesions on recent memory. *Trans. Amer. neurol. Ass.,* (1955), 1956, 42–43.
7. MULLAN, S., and PENFIELD, W. Illusions of comparative interpretation and emotion. Production by epileptic discharge and by electrical stimulation in the temporal cortex. *Arch. Neurol. Psychiat., Chicago,* 1959, *81:* 269–284.
8. PENFIELD, W. The cerebral cortex and consciousness. *Harvey Lect.,* 1937, 35–69.
9. PENFIELD, W. The cerebral cortex in man. I. The cerebral cortex and consciousness. *Arch. Neurol. Psychiat., Chicago,* 1938, *40:* 417–442.
10. PENFIELD, W. Psychical seizures. In: *Psychiatric research. Papers read at the dedication of the laboratory for biochemical research, McLean Hospital, Waverly, Massachusetts, May 17, 1946.* Cambridge, Mass.: Harvard Univ. Press, 1947, 113 pp. (see pp. 81–99).
11. PENFIELD, W. Observations on the anatomy of memory. *Folia psychiat. neerl.,* 1950, *53:* 349–351.
12. PENFIELD, W. Epileptic automatism and the centrencephalic integrating system. *Res. Publ. Ass. nerv. ment. Dis.,* 1952, *30:* 513–528.
13. PENFIELD, W. Memory mechanisms. *Arch. Neurol. Psychiat., Chicago,* 1952, *67:* 178–191.
14. PENFIELD, W. Temporal lobe epilepsy. *Brit. J· Surg.,* 1954, *41:* 337–343.
15. PENFIELD, W. Studies of the cerebral cortex of man. A review and an interpretation. In: *Brain mechanisms and consciousness.* E. D. Adrian, F. Bremer, H. H. Jasper, and J. F. Delafresnaye, Ed. Oxford: Blackwell Scientific Publications, Ltd., 1954, xv, 556 pp. (see pp. 284–304).
16. PENFIELD, W. The permanent record of the stream of consciousness. In: *Proceedings XIV international congress of psychology (Montreal, 1954).* Amsterdam: North-Holland Publishing Co., 1955, 256 pp. (see pp. 47–69).
17. PENFIELD, W. The twenty-ninth Maudsley lecture: The role of the temporal cortex in certain psychical phenomena. *J. ment. Sci.,* 1955, *101:* 451–465.
18. PENFIELD, W. Thoughts on the function of the temporal cortex. *Clin. Neurosurg.,* 1957, *4:* 21–31.
19. PENFIELD, W. Functional localization in temporal and deep sylvian areas. *Res. Publ. Ass. nerv. ment. Dis.,* 1958, *36:* 210–226.
20. PENFIELD, W. Some mechanisms of consciousness discovered during electrical stimulation of the brain. *Proc. nat. Acad. Sci., Wash.,* 1958, *44:* 51–66.
21. PENFIELD, W. The excitable cortex in conscious man. *Liverpool: University Press,* 1958, ix, 42 pp.
22. PENFIELD, W. The rôle of the temporal cortex in recall of past experience and interpretation of the present. In: *Ciba Foundation symposium on the neurological basis of behaviour, in commemoration of Sir Charles Sherrington, 1857–1952.* G. E. W. Wolstenholme, and C. M. O'Connor, Ed. Boston: Little, Brown & Co., 1958, xii, 400 pp. (see pp. 149–174).
23. PENFIELD, W. Centrencephalic integrating system. *Brain,* 1958, *81:* 231–234.
24. PENFIELD, W. The interpretive cortex: the stream of consciousness in the human brain can be electrically reactivated. *Science,* 1959, *129:* 1719–1725.
25. PENFIELD, W. A surgeon's chance encounters with mechanisms related to consciousness. *J. roy. Coll. Surg. Edinb.,* 1960, *5:* 173–190.
26. PENFIELD, W. Neurophysiological basis of the higher functions of the nervous system—introduction. In: *Handbook of physiology. A critical, comprehensive presentation of physiological knowledge and concepts.* J. Field, Ed. Washington, D. C.: American Physiological Society, 1960, Sect. 1, *3:* 1441–1445.
27. PENFIELD, W., and BALDWIN, M. Temporal lobe seizures and the technic of subtotal temporal lobectomy. *Ann. Surg.,* 1952, *136:* 625–634.
28. PENFIELD, W., and ERICKSON, T. C. Epilepsy and cerebral localization. A study of the mechanism, treatment and prevention of epileptic seizures. *Springfield, Ill.: Charles C Thomas,* 1941, x, 623 pp.
29. PENFIELD, W., and FLANIGIN, H. Surgical therapy of temporal lobe seizures. *Arch. Neurol. Psychiat., Chicago,* 1950, *64:* 491–500.
30. PENFIELD, W., and JASPER, H. Highest level seizures. *Res. Publ. Ass. nerv. ment. Dis.,* 1947, *26:* 252–271.
31. PENFIELD, W., and JASPER, H. Epilepsy and the functional anatomy of the human brain. *Boston: Little, Brown & Co.,* 1954, xv, 896 pp.

32. PENFIELD, W., and KRISTIANSEN, K. Epileptic seizure patterns. A study of the localizing value of initial phenomena in focal cortical seizures. *Springfield, Ill.: Charles C Thomas*, 1951, viii, 104 pp.

33. PENFIELD, W., and MILNER, B. Memory deficit produced by bilateral lesions in the hippocampal zone. *Arch. Neurol. Psychiat., Chicago.*, 1958, *79:* 475–497.

34. PENFIELD, W., and MULLAN, S. Illusions of perception and the temporal cortex. *Trans. Amer. neurol. Ass.* (1957), 1958, 6–8.

35. PENFIELD, W., and RASMUSSEN, T. The cerebral cortex of man. A clinical study of localization of function. *New York: Macmillan Co.*, 1950, xv, 248 pp.

36. PENFIELD, W., and ROBERTS, L. Speech and brain-mechanisms. *Princeton, N. J.: Princeton Univ. Press*, 1959, xiii, 286 pp.

37. PEROT, P., and PENFIELD, W. Hallucinations of past experience and experiential responses to stimulation of temporal cortex. *Trans. Amer. neurol. Ass.*, 1960, 80–82.

38. SCARFF, J. E. Fifty years of neurosurgery, 1905–1955. *Int. Abstr. Surg.*, 1955, *101:* 417–513 (see p. 484).

39. WALSHE, F. M. R. Some reflections upon the opening phase of the physiology of the cerebral cortex, 1850–1900. In: *The history and philosophy of knowledge of the brain and its functions. An Anglo-American symposium*, London, July 15th–17th, 1957. F. N. L. Poynter, Ed. Springfield, Ill.: Charles C Thomas, 1958, x, 272 pp. (see pp. 223–234).

40. WALTER, W. G. The neurophysiological aspects of hallucinations and illusory experience. *London: Society for Psychical Research*, 1960, 24 pp.

41. WILKINS, R. H. Neurosurgical classic—XII. J. Neurosurg., 1963, *20:* 904–916.

42. WILKINS, R. H. Neurosurgical classics—XIX. J. Neurosurg., 1964, *21:* 424–431.

43. WILKINS, R. H. Neurosurgical classic—XXII. J. Neurosurg., 1964, *21:* 724–733.

THE CEREBRAL CORTEX AND CONSCIOUSNESS*[1]

WILDER PENFIELD

*Professor of Neurology and Neurosurgery,
McGill University, Montreal*

A NEUROSURGEON has a unique opportunity for psychological study when he exposes the brain of a conscious patient, and no doubt it is his duty to give account of such observations upon the brain to those more familiar with the mind. He may find it difficult to speak the language of psychology, but it is hoped that material of value to psychologists may be presented, the application being left to them. It seems to me quite proper that neurologists should

* Reprinted from *The Harvey Lectures*, 1937, 35–69, with the kind permission of The Williams & Wilkins Company.
[1] Lecture delivered October 15, 1936

push their investigations into the neurological mechanism associated with consciousness and inquire closely into the localization of that mechanism without apology and without undertaking responsibility for the theory of consciousness.

To make such an inquiry is to ask a very old question, as is shown by the following quotation from Zophar, the Naamathite, in the Book of Job:

> "Surely there is a vein for the silver
> And a place for gold where they fine it;
>
> . . . .
>
> But where shall wisdom be found?
> And where is the place of understanding?"

REVIEW OF RELEVANT LITERATURE

The cerebral cortex has apparently acquired an increased functional specialization as the mammalian scale is ascended, ending in a very remarkable increase in man. Lashley (1929) concluded from his work on rats that the capacity of these animals to learn (maze habits) was reduced, depending upon whether more or less cerebral tissue was destroyed. This decrease was not influenced by the nature of the cytoarchitectural fields removed. This function therefore depended, in his opinion, only upon the amount of cortical tissue present and not upon its anatomical specialization.

Pavlov (1927), working upon dogs, concluded that the special function of the cerebral cortex is to establish new nervous connections and so to ensure a perfect functional correlation between the organism and its environment. It is, he said, the essential organ for the maintenance and establishment of conditioned reflexes. In contrast to Lashley's findings in the rat, Pavlov admitted that removal of the posterior portions of the cerebral cortex destroyed the activity of the special analyzers for acoustic and visual reflexes, while tactile reflexes were disturbed very little indeed. On the other hand, bilateral removal of the anterior one-half of the cerebral cortex destroyed the tactile analyzer and interfered little with learning and retention of visual and auditory reflexes. He found that bilateral removal of the temporal lobes in dogs damaged the auditory analyzer most. Babkin, working in Pavlov's laboratory, showed that after such an operation the dog learned to respond to single tone auditory stimuli but he never reacted to the calling of his name, never appreciated successive compound auditory stimuli.

Fulton (1934) and his associates, working upon monkeys and chimpanzees, have accurately demonstrated a considerable amount of specialization of function in the pyramidal and "extra-pyramidal" portions of the cerebral cortex, a specialization which to a large extent is exclusive.

In man the increase of specialization of certain areas of the cerebral cortex is as striking as the enormous increase in the total quantity of the cerebral cortex. Capacity for replacement, described by Lashley as almost universal in the rat, is still present in man to a very considerable extent, especially in infancy. But in the adult man, one occipital lobe is essential to useful vision of any sort in the opposite field; lesions of the motor cortex on one side result in irrecoverable crossed hemiplegia, and the cortical sensory areas are irreplaceable for certain forms of sensation in the opposite limbs. Furthermore, the appearance of speech has resulted in the development of a unilateral highly specialized localization within the cortex. The aphasia which becomes permanent following destruction of certain areas of the human brain, still so poorly defined, indicates an enormous increase in specialization as compared with the disturbance of the understanding of a dog for compound auditory stimuli after removal of both temporal lobes.

The cerebral cortex of man has been divided into separate cytoarchitectural areas by the histological studies of Vogt (1926), von Economo (1929), Campbell (1905), Brodmann (1925) and others, as shown by figure 1. It would seem reasonable, a priori, that the differences that exist in the cell arrangement of these regions should correspond with a difference in function. This certainly is the case in the motor and visual areas and must be so to some extent in the others. The fact that marked substitution is possible in infancy and that some substitution is possible later does not alter the fact that under normal conditions there is specialization of use of the cortex for special purposes in focal areas.

Foerster (1936) has made an effort to delimit function in the human cerebral cortex according to the cytoarchitectural fields of Vogt and Brodmann. This attempt has been successful to some extent at least. After a study[2] of well over one hundred cases of electrical exploration of the human cortex in conjunction with Dr. Edwin Boldrey, I have been unable as yet to outline functional representation within the same sharp limits, with the exception of the precentral and postcentral gyri and perhaps the calcarine cortex.

Hughlings Jackson (1931) pointed out years ago that recoverability from clinical lesions of the nervous system is chiefly a matter of quantity of nervous tissue involved, a conclusion startlingly like that of Lashley and Pavlov. Jackson, however, described, or rather predicted, three levels of functional differentiation in the central nervous system. The lowest level was in the spinal cord, medulla and pons, where the individual units of the body, such as muscles, had individual representation. At the middle level, which he suggested would be found in the sensori-motor portion of

[2] To be published presently.

the cerebral cortex, there was re-representation, not of the individual parts, but of peripheral function, such as co-ordinated movements and elaborations of sensations.

Pavlov, after exhaustive physiological analysis, arrived at a similar conclusion in regard to the cerebral cortex which he did not limit to sensorimotor cortex as Jackson had done. He stated that probably the entire cortex represented a complex system of analyzers of internal as well as external environment of the organism. He suggested that all tissues of the body would eventually be found to be included in this representation.

Jackson went one step further, inferring that there must also be a still higher level of integration, a final sensory and motor arrangement which might form the neural substratum of consciousness, and he suggested that this might be found in the frontal and prefrontal regions.

STIMULATION OF THE CEREBRAL CORTEX IN CONSCIOUS PATIENTS

The patients referred to below were operated upon without any anesthetic and without receiving a pre-operative sedative. Local anesthesia was used to avoid pain and the brain exposed widely by means of osteoplastic craniotomy. The operative wound was carefully ringed about and a sheet arranged perpendicularly so that the patient's face and body were fully exposed below the operative field. Thus he could be observed by those who sat beyond the sterile barrier and could converse with them.

Response is obtained from the human cortex most easily from the vicinity of the central fissure of Rolando, that is, from Brodmann's areas 4 and 6 anteriorly, and 1, 2 and 3 posteriorly (Fig. 1). These responses are not obtained from exactly fixed areas like the keys of a piano, but they vary considerably from case to case. During a specific operation they remain constant in position but can be influenced by facilitation and inhibition. Outside of the motor cortex the same area in different brains may give marked differences of response depending apparently upon the frequency of some previous experience, such as the aura of an epileptic seizure. These unusual responses may well be explained by the process which Pavlov has termed conditioning.

VOCALIZATION

The discussion may be best opened by a description of vocalization which has been produced by us only recently since we have begun to use a thyratron stimulator. It has not previously been described as an isolated phenomenon in man, and Leyton and Sherrington (1917) observed that they could not produce it in anthropoids with faradic stimulation. Gibbs and Gibbs (1936) pro-

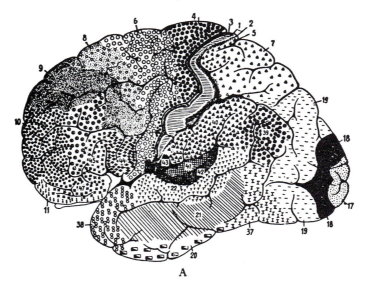

A

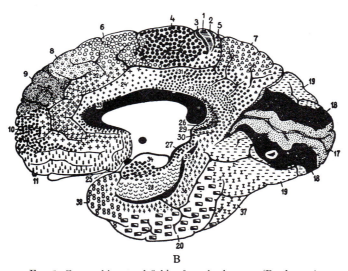

B

Fig. 1. Cytoarchitectural fields of cerebral cortex (Brodmann).

duced purring in cats by stimulation in the vicinity of the infundibulum.

(1) The patient, H. My., was an intelligent man of 32 who worked as a railroad fireman. He had complained of epileptic seizures for three years before admission. The cause of these seizures was found to be a small glioma of benign type deep in the frontal lobe near the midline and anterior to the motor gyrus (Fig. 2, T). In April 1935 the right hemisphere was exposed by osteoplastic craniotomy and careful stimulation experiments were carried out. Reference to figure 2 shows a photograph of the cerebral cortex of this patient during operation. The patient was quiet

and co-operative and talked freely with the operator and with the specially trained observer, Miss Mary Roach. The numbers on the small paper squares which may be seen on the surface of the brain indicate the order in which stimulation with positive result was carried out; number one representing the first stimulation and number two the second, and so forth. The rest of the exposed brain was explored completely with the electrode without result. The results of the positive stimulations were as follows:

When point 13 was touched with the electrode the patient reported sensation in the left little finger and extension of the little finger was observed. This was repeated twice without warning to the patient and with the same result. At 1 a feeling of "electricity" was produced in the left middle finger. There was no movement associated with the sensation. At 2 a feeling of "electricity" was produced in the left index finger; at 11 flexion of the left arm and forearm and extension of the fingers. This last was repeated once with the same result.

Stimulation at 10 produced closure of the left hand. The patient reported feeling a strong sensation "like hold on to electricity," meaning that his hand tingled while it closed. At 3 there was sensation over the lower lip on the left side. At 4 a sensation was produced like electricity in the left side of the tongue. Stimulation at 6 produced violent swallowing and after a short interval of silence the patient stated he had felt "electricity" in the mouth. Stimulation at 7 produced a feeling in the mouth.

These numbers are therefore seen to lie on either side of the central fissure of Rolando. There is no way of determining the central fissure in a living patient except by stimulation because of the great variability in cortical pattern, especially in pathological cases. Number 7 lies just below the fissure of Sylvius; number 6 just above it. On the precentral gyrus at the point 5 which lies between areas from which movement of the upper extremity and of the face were produced, stimulation resulted in vocalization. Because of the fact that this was the first example of such vocalization,

stimulation of this point was repeated thirty-one times, but without undue fatigue.

At the first response the patient emitted a somewhat groaning "Oh." After stimulation stopped he said, "I do not know why I made that noise." This was repeated four times with the same result. The intensity of thyratron stimulation was 28, the frequency of the stimulus being between 60 and 70 per second. When asked why he continued to make this noise the patient said "I don't know. Something made me speak and I felt something touch up there." This last may have been due to some pressure upon the unanesthetized scalp. The next time he was stimulated he said, "You must have made me do that." The same strength of stimulus produced numerous sensory results in the other areas of the cortex but no other motor response.

At the seventh stimulation Dr. Colin Russel observed the patient carefully during his vocalization. He remarked that the mouth opened widely without any expression of fear or emotion while crying. At the eighth stimulation he vocalized loudly and when asked afterwards whether he felt anything he said, "Felt anything—sure it felt as though you were pulling the voice out of me." The longer the stimulation was continued the louder the tone seemed to become and the higher the pitch. The fourteenth stimulation was therefore prolonged to see the effect. In this instance vocalization continued for a period of six seconds and ended in a tremolo (probably when his

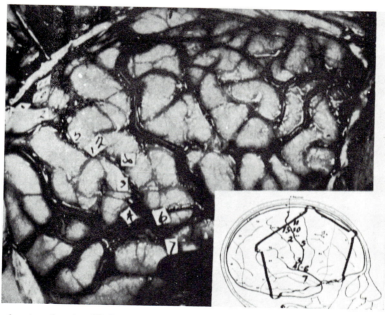

Fig. 2. Cerebral cortex of patient H. My. photographed during operation. The numbers placed upon the brain indicate points from which motor or sensory responses were obtained by stimulation. T indicates position of oligodendroglioma. Inset shows position of craniotomy exposure.

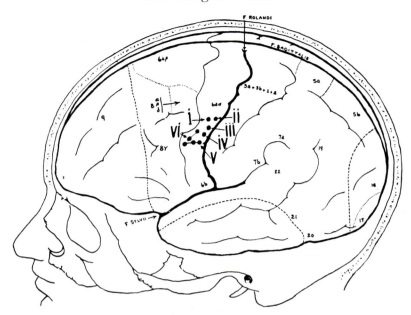

Fig. 3. Chart to show localization of points from which vocalization was obtained in six different cases. The Roman numerals indicate the number of each case as it appears in the text.

breath gave out). On one occasion he vocalized, then drew a deep breath and continued to cry.

At the eighteenth trial area 12, about 6 mm. below 5, was stimulated, using a somewhat stronger stimulus. This was repeated at both areas on the twentieth trial and it was noted that the tone of the voice was higher at 5 than it was at 12, but it was true that the effect seemed greater when 5 was stimulated, which may perhaps account for the higher tone.

On the twenty-second stimulation the patient was informed that he was to try not to call out when stimulated. He said he would try. I warned him when I was going to stimulate but the vocalization began almost immediately after stimulation and continued until the electrode was withdrawn. I then said to the patient, "I win," and he replied, "You did," and laughed. But he added, "I guess I would have won if I had been on that side of my head."

In general, the patient was unable to stop the cry or to influence it in any way. He was as surprised at the first sound of his own voice as we were and he dissociated himself at once from this artificial employment of his own cortex. He knew he had not willed it.

At a distance of 1 mm. from a circumscribed area, using a monopolar electrode, no result was obtained but on moving the electrode 1 mm. nearer, the vocalization would regularly occur in typical fashion. With the same intensity of stimulus used to produce this vocalization no motor movements could be obtained anywhere. A

stronger stimulation had to be used to produce flexion of the hand on the same convolution above this point, and below the same, stronger stimulation produced violent swallowing. On returning to the vocalization area even the strong stimulation did not produce any additional associated motor movements but only the sound of his voice in the vowel "O" or "A." There was nothing at any time to suggest words.

At ward rounds nine days later the following note was made on the patient's history: "On discussing with the patient his sensation at the time when vocalization was produced on the operating table, he states that it did not sound as though he were saying anything he wanted to say, but as though his voice came with a rush, as something beyond his control. There was no sensation of the mouth, tongue or face at the time of vocalization.

"He says he felt no sensation anywhere but 'just as though something drawed it out of my mouth.'

"He dreamed next day after operation that someone was making him speak but he did not seem to be on the operating table. There is at present no speech disturbance nor has there been since operation."

In five subsequent cases vocalization has been produced by stimulation of the cortex in a roughly corresponding area upon the precentral gyrus of the left side in two and of the right in three cases. The location of the vocalization point in all six

breath gave out). On one occasion he vocalized, then drew a deep breath and continued to cry.

At the eighteenth trial area 12, about 6 mm. below 5, was stimulated, using a somewhat stronger stimulus. This was repeated at both areas on the twentieth trial and it was noted that the tone of the voice was higher at 5 than it was at 12, but it was true that the effect seemed greater when 5 was stimulated, which may perhaps account for the higher tone.

On the twenty-second stimulation the patient was informed that he was to try not to call out when I stimulated. He said he would try. I warned him when I was going to stimulate but the vocalization began almost immediately after stimulation and continued until the electrode was withdrawn. I then said to the patient, "I win," and he replied, "You did," and laughed. But he added, "I guess I would have won if I had been on that side of my head."

In general, the patient was unable to stop the cry or to influence it in any way. He was as surprised at the first sound of his own voice as we were and he dissociated himself at once from this artificial employment of his own cortex. He knew he had not willed it.

At a distance of 1 mm. from a circumscribed area, using a monopolar electrode, no result was obtained but on moving the electrode 1 mm. nearer, the vocalization would regularly occur in typical fashion. With the same intensity of stimulus used to produce this vocalization no motor movements could be obtained anywhere. A

stronger stimulation had to be used to produce flexion of the hand on the same convolution above this point, and below the same, stronger stimulation produced violent swallowing. On returning to the vocalization area even the strong stimulation did not produce any additional associated motor movements but only the sound of his voice in the vowel "O" or "A." There was nothing at any time to suggest words.

At ward rounds nine days later the following note was made on the patient's history: "On discussing with the patient his sensation at the time when vocalization was produced on the operating table, he states that it did not sound as though he were saying anything he wanted to say, but as though his voice came with a rush, as something beyond his control. There was no sensation of the mouth, tongue or face at the time of vocalization.

"He says he felt no sensation anywhere but 'just as though something drawed it out of my mouth.'

"He dreamed next day after operation that someone was making him speak but he did not seem to be on the operating table. There is at present no speech disturbance nor has there been since operation."

In five subsequent cases vocalization has been produced by stimulation of the cortex in a roughly corresponding area upon the precentral gyrus of the left side in two and of the right in three cases. The location of the vocalization point in all six

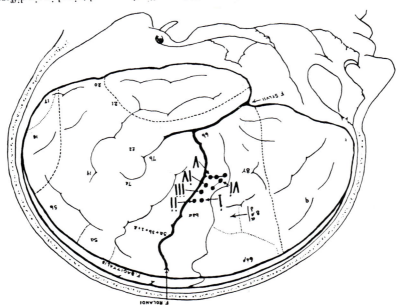

Fig. 3. Chart to show localization of points from which vocalization was obtained in six different cases. The Roman numerals indicate the number of each case as it appears in the text.

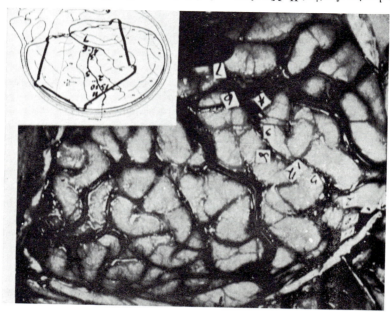

FIG. 2. Cerebral cortex of patient H. M., photographed during operation. The numbers placed upon the brain indicate points from which motor or sensory responses were obtained by stimulation. T indicates position of oligodendroglioma. Inset shows position of craniotomy exposure.

served. This was repeated twice without warning to the patient and with the same result. At 1 a feeling of "electricity" was produced in the left middle finger. There was no movement associated with the sensation. At 2 a feeling of "electricity" was produced in the left index finger; at 11 flexion of the left arm and forearm and extension of the fingers. This last was repeated once with the same result.

Stimulation at 10 produced closure of the left hand. The patient reported feeling a strong sensation "like hold on to electricity," meaning that his hand tingled while it closed. At 3 there was sensation over the lower lip on the left side. At 4 a sensation was produced like electricity in the left side of the tongue. Stimulation at 6 produced violent swallowing and after a short interval of silence the patient stated he had felt "electricity" in the mouth. Stimulation at 7 produced a feeling in the mouth.

These numbers are therefore seen to lie on either side of the central fissure of Rolando. There is no way of determining the central fissure in a living patient except by stimulation because of the great variability in cortical pattern, especially in pathological cases. Number 7 lies just below the fissure of Sylvius; number 6 just above it. On the precentral gyrus at the point 5 which lies between areas from which movement of the upper extremity and of the face were produced, stimulation resulted in vocalization. Because of the fact that this was the first example of such vocalization,

stimulation of this point was repeated thirty-one times, but without undue fatigue.

At the first response the patient emitted a somewhat groaning "Oh." After stimulation stopped he said, "I do not know why I made that noise." This was repeated four times with the same result. The intensity of thyratron stimulation was 28, the frequency of the stimulus being between 60 and 70 per second. When asked why he continued to make this noise the patient said "I don't know. Something made me speak and I felt something touch up there." This last may have been due to some pressure upon the unanesthetized scalp. The next time he was stimulated he said, "You must have made me do that." The same strength of stimulus produced numerous sensory results in the other areas of the cortex but no other motor response.

At the seventh stimulation Dr. Colin Russel observed the patient carefully during his vocalization. He remarked that the mouth opened widely without any expression of fear or emotion while crying. At the eighth stimulation he vocalized loudly and when asked afterwards whether he felt anything he said, "Felt anything—sure it felt as though you were pulling the voice out of me." The longer the stimulation was continued the louder the tone seemed to become and the higher the pitch. The fourteenth stimulation was therefore prolonged to see the effect. In this instance vocalization continued for a period of six seconds and ended in a tremolo (probably when his

duced purring in cats by stimulation in the vicinity of the infundibulum.

(1) The patient, H. M'y., was an intelligent man of 32 who worked as a railroad fireman. He had complained of epileptic seizures for three years before admission. The cause of these seizures was found to be a small glioma of benign type deep in the frontal lobe near the midline and anterior to the motor gyrus (Fig. 2, T.). In April 1935 the right hemisphere was exposed by osteoplastic craniotomy and careful stimulation experiments were carried out. Reference to figure 2 shows a photograph of the cerebral cortex of this patient during operation. The patient was quiet

and co-operative and talked freely with the operator and with the specially trained observer, Miss Mary Roach. The numbers on the small paper squares which may be seen on the surface of the brain indicate the order in which stimulation was carried out; number one representing the first stimulation and number two the second, and so forth. The rest of the exposed brain was explored completely with the electrode without result. The results of the positive stimulations were as follows:

When point 13 was touched with the electrode the patient reported sensation in the left little finger and extension of the little finger was ob-

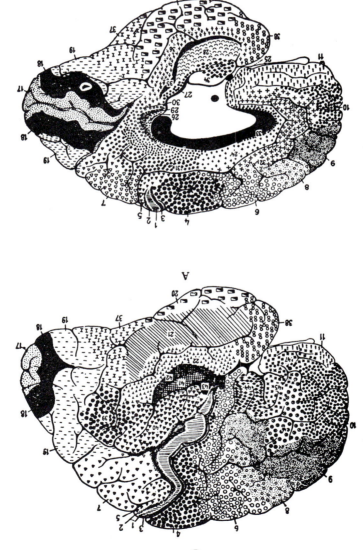

Fig. 1. Cytoarchitectural fields of cerebral cortex (Brodmann).

enormous increase in the total quantity of cerebral cortex. Capacity for replacement, described by Lashley as almost universal in the rat, is still present in man to a very considerable extent, especially in infancy. But in the adult man, one occipital lobe is essential to useful vision of any sort in the opposite field; lesions of the motor cortex on one side result in irrecoverable crossed hemiplegia, and the cortical sensory areas are irreplaceable for certain forms of sensation in the opposite limbs. Furthermore, the appearance of speech has resulted from the development of a unilateral highly specialized localization within the cortex. The aphasia which becomes permanent following destruction of certain areas of the human brain, still so poorly defined, indicates an enormous increase in specialization as compared with the disturbance of the understanding of a dog for compound auditory stimuli after removal of both temporal lobes.

The cerebral cortex of man has been divided into separate cytoarchitectural areas by the histological studies of Vogt (1926), von Economo (1929), Campbell (1905), Brodmann (1925) and others, as shown by figure 1. It would seem reasonable, a priori, that the differences that exist in the cell arrangement of these regions should correspond with a difference in function. This certainly is the case in the motor and visual areas and must be so to some extent in the others. The fact that marked substitution is possible in infancy and that some substitution is possible later does not alter the fact that under normal conditions there is specialization of use of the cortex for special purposes in focal areas.

Foerster (1936) has made an effort to delimit function in the human cerebral cortex according to the cytoarchitectural fields of Vogt and Brodmann. This attempt has been successful to some extent at least. After a study[2] of well over one hundred cases of electrical exploration of the human cortex in conjunction with Dr. Edwin Boldrey, I have been unable as yet to outline functional representation within the same sharp limits, with the exception of the precentral and postcentral gyri and perhaps the calcarine cortex. Hughlings Jackson (1931) pointed out years ago that recoverability from clinical lesions of the nervous system is chiefly a matter of quantity of nervous tissue involved, a conclusion startlingly like that of Lashley and Pavlov. Jackson, however, described, or rather predicted, three levels of functional differentiation in the central nervous system. The lowest level was in the spinal cord, medulla and pons, where the individual units of the body, such as muscles, had individual representation. At the middle level, which he suggested would be found in the sensori-motor portion of

the cerebral cortex, there was re-representation, not of the individual parts, but of peripheral function, such as co-ordinated movements and elaborations of sensations.

Pavlov, after exhaustive physiological analysis, arrived at a similar conclusion in regard to the cerebral cortex which he did not limit to sensori-motor cortex as Jackson had done. He stated that probably the entire cortex represented a complex system of analyzers of internal as well as external environment of the organism. He suggested that all tissues of the body would eventually be found to be included in this representation.

Jackson went one step further, inferring that there must also be a still higher level of integration, a final sensory and motor arrangement which might form the neural substratum of consciousness, and he suggested that this might be found in the frontal and prefrontal regions.

STIMULATION OF THE CEREBRAL CORTEX IN CONSCIOUS PATIENTS

The patients referred to below were operated upon without any anesthetic and without receiving a pre-operative sedative. Local anesthesia was used to avoid pain and the brain exposed widely by means of osteoplastic craniotomy. The operative wound was carefully ringed about and a sheet arranged perpendicularly so that the patient's face and body were fully exposed below the operative field. Thus he could be observed by those who sat beyond the sterile barrier and could converse with them.

Response is obtained from the human cortex most easily from the vicinity of the central fissure of Rolando, that is, from Brodmann's areas 4 and 6 anteriorly, and 1, 2 and 3 posteriorly (Fig. 1). These responses are not obtained from exactly fixed areas like the keys of a piano, but they vary considerably from case to case. During a specific operation they remain constant in position but can be influenced by facilitation and inhibition. Outside of the motor cortex the same area in different brains may give marked differences of response depending apparently upon the frequency of some previous experience, such as the aura of an epileptic seizure. These unusual responses may well be explained by the process which Pavlov has termed conditioning.

VOCALIZATION

The discussion may be best opened by a description of vocalization which has been produced by us only recently since we have begun to use a thyratron stimulator. It has not previously been described as an isolated phenomenon in man, and Leyton and Sherrington (1917) observed that they could not produce it in anthropoids with faradic stimulation. Gibbs and Gibbs (1936) pro-

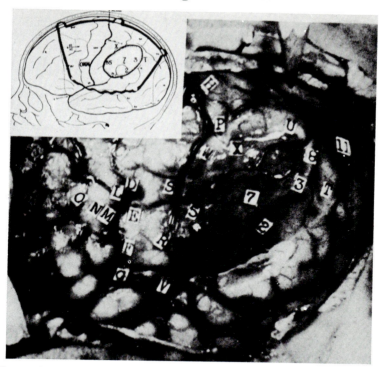

Fig. 4. E. L. Woman of 39 years who had had occlusion of a cerebral artery six years previously leaving deep cyst roofed by translucent membrane and floored by the ependyma of the underlying ventricle. Photographed during operation. Inset indicates localization of cyst.

cases is transposed to the left hemisphere in figure 3.

(2) H. Mi. was an intelligent young man of 27 years. Stimulation in the precentral gyrus produced vocalization (II, Fig. 3). On the same gyrus above the area, elevation of both brows symmetrically was produced; below the area, swallowing.

(3) Patient F. R. gave vocalization after stimulation of a similar point (III, Fig. 3) which lay just anterior to points in which mouth and tongue sensation could be produced. It was below the locus for movements of the right eye but it was not so discrete an area as in the first case mentioned above, and it was associated with drawing of the face to the right and a feeling of nausea. This spread was doubtless due to epileptic habit, as stimulation 2 cm. anterior and below produced an epileptic seizure which resembled those from which he habitually suffered and in which there was an epileptic cry at the beginning.

(4) E. M. was a young woman of 22. Vocalization was produced from the left precentral gyrus (I, Fig. 3) in an area no greater in diameter than 3–4 mm. The cry was somewhat quavering and was produced three times. Above it flexion of the wrist was obtained. Below it twitching of the lower lip and jaw resulted, more on the right side.

(5) F. W. was a boy of 17 years. Vocalization was produced from the left hemisphere at IV in figure 3, just below an area from which closure of both eyes was produced. When he had closed them both, the patient remarked that he could not help closing the right eye. The vocalization point was just anterior to the source of numbness in the right side of the tongue.

(6) E. L. was a housewife of 39 years who had suffered from epileptic seizures for six years following a vascular accident. This vascular lesion had produced the cyst seen in figure 4, situated in the left parietal lobe. There was no aphasia but the patient was a little childish.

The central fissure was mapped out by thyratron stimulation as may be seen by reference to figure 4. The inset in that figure indicates the cerebral localization.

A—pricking sensation right fingers; B—shaking of whole right hand; C—sensation in right fingers; D—sensation in nose; E—sensation in right thumb and closure of jaw; F—sensation in right side of chin; G—sensation in tongue and chin; I—flexion of elbow; K—flexion of fingers; L—slight tremor in right side of face with sensation in that cheek and chin.

M—vocalization "Umgh." Patient then said "What is that?" Without replying I repeated the stimulation. Vocalization was repeated and her mouth pulled to the right. I then asked her why she made that noise. She replied that it hurt her in the chin. N—vocalization in same tone but clonic as though regularly interrupted. O—vocalization in definite tremolo. Patient was saying "I can't do—" and carried the "do" over into the sound of vocalization as the area was stimulated. When asked again why she made that noise she replied "I don't know."

The stimulation of O was repeated for longer duration. Vocalization resulted until the patient's breath seemed to be exhausted, whereupon a small epileptiform attack was reported, consisting of pulling of nose, mouth and face to the right, and inward rotation of the right arm.

The size of the area (M, N, O in figure 4, or V in figure 3) from which vocalization was obtained was not greater than from 6–7 mm. in diameter. It was observed that stimulation at O produced a sound different from that at M. It was discontinuous so that it sounded like speech but one could make out no words.

When the patient was told to count to twenty stimulation at a little distance did not influence the counting. When the electrode was brought nearer she seemed to continue the "eleven" sound. Stimulation below M during the counting caused her to stop on two trials. When asked why she stopped she replied, "I tremble so."

The electrical exploration was continued and it is interesting that sensation in the chin and right face which was found to accompany vocalization when M and O had been stimulated, was produced by stimulation at a distance over the surface of the cyst at T, 5 and 7 with no vocalization. Stimulation at 2 and 3 produced sensation in both sides of the face, in chin and tongue, and slight closure of mouth in clonic manner. These stimulations just mentioned were upon the translucent covering of a fluid-filled cyst. After removal of the cyst this translucent material was found still to contain nerve fibres. This is an example of the spread of excitability that so often is found in cases of epilepsy. It may be called epileptic facilitation perhaps. In this case it seems evident that it is produced by activation of superficial nerve fibres which cross the surface of the cyst to the postcentral convolution at F and G, as there was no grey matter present and no other fibre layers.

GENERAL OBSERVATIONS ON CORTICAL STIMULATION

Simple movements, when they are produced, appear to the patient to be quite involuntary. In our whole series of patients we have found none who was under the impression that he was carrying out these movements of his own volition. A public school teacher remarked about the movement that had been produced in her face, "It seems involuntary." And another intelligent young woman observed, "My leg moved itself."

Likewise, sensation when produced electrically is referred at once to the periphery as an unexplained sensation.

I have often asked a patient to make an effort not to move the hand, face or foot and followed this by stimulation of the motor area for this part. The result is usually a movement over which he has no control and he is never at any time in doubt about this. With or without warning restimulation of that area will ordinarily reproduce the same movement.

On the other hand, a patient is sometimes able to prevent a movement by an act of will power. In the case of F. W., stimulation of area 6a beta of Brodmann (Fig. 3), which Vogt has named the frontal adversive field, produced closure of the right hand and a hot feeling down the right side of the body. The patient was instructed to make an effort to keep his right hand still if he could do so. The stimulation was repeated without warning the patient. He reported the same feeling of a flush in the right side of his trunk and he held his hand quite still. A somewhat more complicated example of a patient's effort to oppose the effect of cortical stimulation is the following.

The cortex of an intelligent young girl, H. T., was stimulated anterior to the lower end of the right precentral gyrus while she was counting from one to forty. At the time of stimulation the patient hesitated slightly and the observer reported that there was pulling of the mouth to the left. She continued to count, however. When her task was finished the patient stated to me that, "It was hard to continue." She was able, therefore, to continue to count although the left side of her mouth had been forced to go into involuntary movement by stimulation of the right cortex.

Patients sometimes state that they have a strong desire to move which they are able to control, or at all events do control. F. S., an Italian who found some difficulty in expressing himself in English, after stimulation at nearby points in area 6a beta (Fig. 3), made the following observations: (1) "My nerves shook all over; wanted to pull me to the left." (He showed agitation probably because he thought he was about to have one of his habitual epileptic fits.) (2) "Wanted to fall to the left side." (3) "Head feels like it wants to move down to left leg and left leg up to head."

After the patient, R. M., had been subjected to stimulation in the same area, Vogt's frontal adversive field, he said that he had felt as though his "eyes were going to turn to the left." There was, however, no turning of his eyes at that time. Another patient, H. T., when stimulated in the same field on the right side, said she felt as though she wanted to turn her head to the left. She made no obvious movement.

The patient J. H. tried to resist movements produced by stimulation of areas 4 and 6 of Brodmann without success. However, stimulation at a distance produced downward plantar flexion of the opposite foot together with an aura of an habitual attack. This was repeated without warning. The patient explained that he had a desire to move the foot down at that time. He was asked to resist it and stimulation of the same point was repeated. The patient's foot moved upward in the opposite direction and the whole leg was drawn up in an exaggeration of opposition.

On the other hand, at times a patient may have the feeling of movement without there being any observable change of position of the part. F. W. stated that at the time of stimulation of the left postcentral lobule he had sensation of movement in the right thumb. No movement in the thumb could be seen, however. Stimulation at this point was repeated at a later time without warning to the patient and he reported the same sensation.

Stimulation may sometimes produce a feeling of paralysis in a part without any objective change in the appearance of that part. For example, H. Mi., when stimulated in the left postcentral lobule reported that he felt a tremor in the upper lip on the right side, and that he lost control of the lip. There was no obvious movement. When the right precentral lobule was stimulated, H. T. reported that she was unable to speak and unable to open her eyes. This stimulation was at a point just below an area where marked closure of both eyes had been produced. This sort of response may possibly indicate the production of an inhibitory discharge.

When a sensation is produced from stimulation of the cerebral cortex it is usually described as numbness or electricity. Quite exceptionally the patient uses an adjective which suggests a feeling of cold or warmth. For example, when the cortex of the patient D. R., an intelligent young boy, was stimulated in the left postcentral region, he reported at 2 "electricity" in the thumb and first two fingers of his right hand. At 4 he said he felt something cold at the right side of his mouth, both inside and out. At 5 he reported a feeling of electricity in the thumb and first finger. At 7 he stated there was a feeling inside of his mouth in the lower jaw, which he described as a "sticking" sensation. The feeling of heat down the side has been reported above under the patient F. W.

Pain has been produced by stimulation of the cerebral cortex, particularly in the frontal adversive field, but this has been in relation to the aura of an epileptic seizure which perhaps it would be better not to discuss at this time. Stimulation of the olfactory lobe causes the patient to exclaim with some surprise that he smells something. Patient E. M. said the odor resembled "oxygen." Patient F. R. said that it smelt like "something burning."

More complicated sensations may also be produced. For example, the patient J. C. said that she felt afraid and that she had a sensation in her abdomen, when the anterior end of her second temporal convolution was stimulated. The next stimulation at an adjacent point produced a train of phenomena which must be considered epileptiform but which illustrates a number of points made above. The patient had first a feeling in the abdomen, next the feeling of fear and then a desire to move the left hand. There was a plucking movement with her left hand. When she was asked, "Why do you move your left hand and not your right?" she replied, "That one wants to." She added that the movement was "involuntary." This stimulation was repeated several times without warning but with the same result. On one occasion she was warned that the stimulation was coming and was urged to keep her left hand still, if she could. On this occasion she reported the same sensation but kept her hand quite still. During this stimulation she cried a little; afterwards she said she wanted to move her hand but prevented herself from doing so. It should be added here that the feeling in the abdomen and the feeling of fear were phenomena which sometimes appeared in the epileptic seizures to which this patient was subject.

What do these observations indicate as far as the relationship of consciousness to the cortex is concerned? Crude motor movements are made by stimulation of the pyramidal and parapyramidal cortical motor areas but the individual is fully conscious that he has not done it—he has not willed it. He says rather, that it was involuntary, or the hand moved itself. If a bit of sensory cortex is activated the patient feels a crude sensation in the hand but it never occurs to him that he has imagined it. He hears his own voice crying as the result of stimulation and when he has finished he exclaims in surprise that his voice was drawn out of him, and next day he may live over the experience in a dream that someone is making him speak.

As far as introspection is able to go the patient concludes that the activity of his own stimulated cerebral cortex is on a plane quite distinct from his own conscious thinking. The electrode of the surgeon may provide him with a new sensory experience or it may initiate a motor movement against which he is able to struggle by means of such other cortical mechanisms as are still at his disposal.

But before generalizing any further a brief consideration of certain aspects of epilepsy may be interposed.

EPILEPSY

"Epilepsy," Hughlings Jackson said, "is the name for occasional sudden, excessive, rapid and local discharges of grey matter." As this discharge may take place in different areas of the nervous system, so the character of the discharge may vary greatly from movement to sensation and from dream to mental lapse. But in general the movements are violent and purposeless, the sensations crude and the dreams simple.

Jackson conceived that during a seizure there was a discharge in the grey matter of the brain which began at some local point and spread from that point, producing a march of outward phenomena. This conception had two results. Firstly it provided an hypothesis for the understanding of epilepsy. Secondly, it provided him with a key to the localization of function in the brain. By the study of epileptics he concluded that cerebral convolutions represented the function of certain peripheral parts, ten years before Hitzig and Ferrier demonstrated this to be a fact by electrical stimulation of the convolutions of animals.

Consider as an example the "Jacksonian" seizure which begins by localized movement of the great toe and spreads in succession to the leg, arm, hand and face of the same side. The discharge of the pyramidal cells in the toe area of the precentral gyrus progressively spreads downward through the length of the gyrus. In so doing it maps out the contiguity of cortical representation of these parts. The spread is from one area of grey matter to another, rather than along internal association pathways to more distant centres.

Another example may be cited. An epileptogenic focus in the posterior part of one temporal lobe (Penfield 1935) produced in a patient the following habitual chain of phenomena: (1) the hearing of a roaring noise, (2) a sense of dizziness, (3) salivation and (4) micropsia or the hallucination that everything looked small. Of these phenomena two are sensory, one motor and one hallucinatory. Discharge of certain areas of the brain has produced each. But the spread has taken place in this manner not because special association pathways exist between these areas. The spread has followed the pattern described because of contiguity of representation.

Epileptogenic discharge of ganglion cells is sudden, overwhelming and undiscriminating, as though they were for the moment affected by a miniature hurricane. The result of this focal hurricane indicates that there exists focal representation in the brain and indicates which areas are neighbors. The site of the initial discharge must be sought by the clinician. The cerebral cortex apparently is not the only region where epileptic discharge may take place. It may involve the grey matter at other levels in the central nervous system including the diencephalon and midbrain, and even on rare occasions the spinal cord.

An epileptic seizure is in some ways the direct opposite of paralysis. A unilateral seizure is on some occasions followed by unilateral paralysis which usually affects the part that was earliest and most severely involved in the seizure. Such a post-seizure paralysis may consist in a monoplegia, a hemiplegia, an aphasia, a mental stupor or even complete coma and diplegia.

The cause of these post-seizure paralyses was thought by Jackson to be fatigue of the discharging cells. It was suggested by Kinnier Wilson to be a phenomenon of after-discharge inhibition. The present evidence suggests that these paralyses are due to post-convulsive spasm of the cerebral arteries or at least to the focal cerebral anemia which frequently follows epileptic seizures of whatever variety (Penfield 1933).

The important point to be borne in mind is that, except during the duration of complete coma and diplegia, these paralyses are due to focal or local inactivity of nerve cells just as the epileptic discharge is due to regional activation of the same. Thus the post-epileptic negative state may have for our present purpose a localizing value similar to that of the positive local discharge of a focal epileptic seizure.

It should be remembered, further, that there is paralysis of voluntary function in any part of the brain during epileptic discharge in that part. If it be an area which is too complex to express itself during the discharge there will be no evidence of the fit other than absence of function. A discharge occurring within the speech area signalizes its occurrence only by silence, by the inability to speak. This has the same outward effect as post-epileptic paralysis although the cause is quite different.

Epileptic disturbances of consciousness will be taken up under the headings of dream state and automatism. Further discussion of loss of consciousness in epilepsy will appear in the final section on generalities.

DREAM STATES

Hughlings Jackson applied this term to alterations of consciousness which appear in epileptic states, alterations without loss of consciousness. In a dream state a patient may have a sudden feeling of strangeness, of unexplained familiarity, but some capacity is retained for conscious insight, and he may know that this is another fit. He may suddenly see a complicated scene which in fact comes from some past experience, but he can still reason and is aware of the unreality of the condition. Jackson called this double awareness mental diplopia.

An example of such a dream state may be given somewhat in detail: J. V., a young girl of 14 years, had suffered from epileptiform seizures from the age of 11, characterized by sudden fright and screaming when she would hold on to people for protection. This was followed by falling and occasionally a major convulsion. In infancy, at the close of an anesthetic, she had had a single convulsion followed by coma and transient left hemiplegia.

Following a typical but severe seizure which was induced after her admission to the hospital she had transient weakness of the left side and a positive Babinski sign on the left side. On careful questioning it was learned that during the preliminary period of fright she invariably saw herself in a scene that she remembered at the age of 7 years.

The scene was as follows: A little girl was walking through a field where the grass was high. It was a lovely day and her brothers were walking ahead of her. A man came up behind and said, "How would you like to get into this bag with the snakes?" She was very frightened, screamed to her brothers and they all ran home, where she told her mother about the event. Her mother remembers the fright and the story and the brothers still remember the occasion and remember seeing the man.

Following that she occasionally had nightmares in which the scene was re-enacted. Three or four years later, at the age of 11, she was recognized as having attacks by day and in the attacks she habitually saw the scene of her fright. She saw a little girl whom she identified with herself in the now-familiar surroundings. She was conscious of her environment at the time of the attack and would call those present by name and yet she saw herself as a little girl with such distinctness that she was filled with terror lest she should be struck or smothered from behind.

At operation under local anesthesia adhesions between dura and arachnoidea were found indicating an old subdural hemorrhage and cortical atrophy most marked in area 19 of the occipital lobe, the area from which her curious complicated aura could be reproduced. This change was probably due to a hemorrhage in infancy at the time of the anesthesia.

The central fissure was mapped out as seen in figure 5, from Y to M. At point 13 and also 17 stimulation caused her to state that she saw stars on the opposite side. At 16 and 14 the aura of an attack was produced. After stimulation at 16 she said, "Wait a minute and I will tell you." Then a little later she said, "I held on to the bar" (as she had been asked to do) "and the bar seemed to be walking away from me. I saw someone coming toward me as though he were going to hit me." In a moment she called, "Don't leave me." The point 14 was stimulated without the patient's knowledge. She suddenly said, "Say something,"—then a little later, "I had the funny feeling. It was like an attack."

At another point nearby, but from which the mark was accidentally displaced before the photograph was taken, stimulation had previously produced her first aura. She stared suddenly and then cried, "Oh, I can see something coming at me. Don't let them come at me." She remained staring and fearful for 30 seconds, although the stimulation was of much shorter duration. A little later she said, "It didn't feel like an attack at first but right after it felt like an attack coming on; it sort of started and then passed off. First time it has

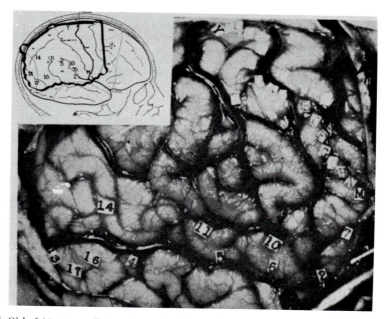

Fig. 5. J. V. Girl of 14 years suffering from epileptiform seizures ushered in by a complicated aura which could be initiated by electrical stimulation at points 14 and 16. Brain photographed during operation.

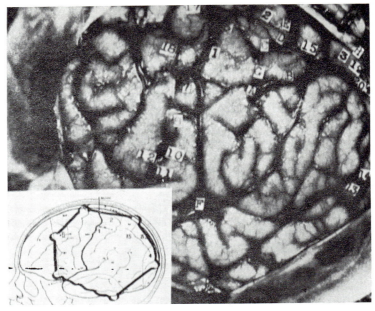

Fig. 6. M. B. Woman of 30 years. Complicated habitual aura could be initated by stimulation at point 4. Photographed during operation.

felt like an attack since last Wednesday." Wednesday had been the day when several seizures were induced.

Stimulation was carried out at a number of points from the first temporal convolution backward through cortical area 22 to the site of the origin of her aura in area 19 (Fig. 1). These stimulations caused the patient to cry out that she heard a large number of people shouting. Once she said, "They are yelling at me for doing something wrong; everybody is yelling." On enquiry she said she could hear her mother and brothers. Stimulation at 2 (Fig. 5) caused her to say, "I imagine I hear a lot of people shouting at me." The stimulation was repeated twice without warning and for not over 2 seconds. Each time the voices were heard again, the duration of the voices being 8 and 7 seconds respectively. A third time the stimulation was repeated without warning and she said, "I hear them again." At 10, "Oh, there it goes, everybody is yelling," and after an interval, "Something dreadful is going to happen." At 11, "There they go, yelling at me, stop them!"

If her epileptogenic discharge began at 16 or 14 and passed forward over points 11, 10 and 2, she would have had her typical hallucination, felt the dread and eventually heard accusing voices before any convulsive phenomena were observed. As she did not remember the voices in an ordinary seizure it seems likely that she had an amnesia for this part of the march, not an infrequent occurrence in this region.

This is an example of the reproduction of a complicated memory of an event which actually occurred between the time of receiving an injury to the brain and the onset of the seizures. This is not without precedent. I have studied a patient whose attacks were originating somewhat farther forward in one temporal lobe as proven by stimulation and who saw herself giving birth to a child during the aura. The picture she saw reproduced the surroundings of that event as it had actually happened.

A somewhat different type of complicated aura may be mentioned briefly. M. B., an intelligent young woman of 30 years, suffered from epileptiform attacks characterized by (1) an hallucination of being far away or of seeing things small, (2) dizziness or sensation of turning, (3) tinnitus, (4) numbness in right hand, all followed at times by loss of consciousness and a generalized convulsive seizure. At operation, in area 5b, a somewhat yellowish soft convolution was found and from this convolution and its vicinity her aura could be reproduced. In figure 6 the numbers 3 and 4 are laid upon it.

Stimulation of the post-central convolution at 1 produced numbness in the thumb and at 2 numbness in the right side from axilla to umbilicus; 4— "Felt like I was going far away; sometimes like that before an attack. Like when things look far away." 3—Dizziness "like before an attack." 15— "Felt as though I was falling out of bed." The stimulation was repeated without warning. She said suddenly, "Yes, the same thing—felt as though I was falling."[3]

If the epileptogenic disturbance began at 4 and moved to 3, then 15 and finally 2 and 1, she might well have complained first of an hallucination of being far away, next of dizziness, then of falling, and finally numbness in the right hand. If the disturbance had spread still further forward there would have been convulsive movements.

In such cases it may be said that there is an alteration in consciousness but actually there is a new phenomenon being presented to the conscious individual. In the case of J. V., this phenomenon arises from a discharge which is occurring within the cortex of cytoarchitectural area 19. At the same time that patient, because she retained consciousness, differentiated between the spurious phenomenon which might be called synthetic and the actual existence of the outside world as presented to her by the unoccupied regions of the cerebral cortex. In the case of M. B. a disturbance originating in area 5b gave her the hallucination of being far away and yet she retained an understanding of her surroundings.

AUTOMATISM

Quite different from the above dream state is the post-epileptic automatic state. The subject is in full control of his body but does not know what he is doing. He may respond if spoken to. He may obey a command or may resent violently and dangerously any interference.

You may prefer to call this an alteration in consciousness but it seems to me a loss of consciousness on an exceedingly high level, if the expression is permissible. He has no present responsibility nor will he have future memory of what he does.

A brief example may be cited. An intelligent and sensitive young patient gave a history of major seizures sometimes followed by violent behavior which distressed him as well as his parents. While in bed on the public ward of the Royal Victoria Hospital he had a seizure during his sleep, characterized by convulsive movements of both sides and frothing at the mouth. He then got out of bed and without putting on his slippers or bathrobe he began to look for something under his bed—possibly his slippers. He walked about and then got into bed with another patient. When nurse, doctor and prospective bed-fellow opposed him he fought them violently. On coming to himself he had no recollection of the incident and was chagrined to learn of it.

Jackson considered such a state to be invariably

[3] Foerster (1936) has described a similar case of a woman who had an epileptogenic scar in the left parietal lobe near the midline. Stimulation here caused the patient to feel as though she were rolling off the table to the right.

due to post-epileptic paralysis, paralysis of the highest level of neural activity, the substratum of consciousness. He therefore considered the state to be a phenomenon of release from higher control. If it is in truth post-convulsive paralysis I would suggest, on the basis of what we now know, that there remains an effective anemia in the region wherein consciousness is represented. Sometimes the preceding seizure is very slight indeed. At other times there is no evidence of any such seizure. But the same is true in other spheres. A hand may become suddenly paralyzed without sign of convulsion, doubtless due to a spontaneous anemia without preceding epileptogenic reflex.

It is quite possible, however, that it is not always post-epileptic. If an epileptic fit may take place in the same level or area of the brain as the post-epileptic paralysis, then automatism must be possible during a fit caused by discharge in this highest level as well as in the post-discharge period. Some petit mal seizures must be of this nature.

GENERALITIES

For the purposes of this discussion it seems to be unnecessary to inquire into the mechanism by which a conscious decision receives its initial activation in neuronal conduction or even to inquire as to whether such decisions are reflex. It is enough to be able to recognize when an individual is conscious and when he loses consciousness, to be able to describe what portions of the central nervous system may be paralyzed without abolishing consciousness and what portions may be still active when consciousness is gone. Finally one may hope to indicate those areas which are necessarily inactive when consciousness is abolished by a paralyzing lesion.

In the epileptic's dream state as described above, an hallucination is presented to him by discharge within one portion of the cerebral cortex but the patient retains insight into his real environment due, no doubt, to normal function in other parts of his cerebral cortex. He may even be able to say to an observer (as J. V. did) "Wait a minute," and after the dream is over to recount it in detail. This may be in a sense a doubling of consciousness but it is not a loss. In the post-epileptic automatic state the patient still has cortical mechanism intact, and furthermore he still has co-ordinating control of those mechanisms. He is a perfect machine but he has either lost consciousness exclusively or there has been a temporary removal of one element of consciousness. By analogy, this must either be produced by paralysis of a small area of the brain or by paralysis of scattered mechanisms with a unit blood supply.

Most often consciousness is lost by such patients in association with certain epileptic phenomena and as one part in the habitual pattern. In general, an epileptic disturbance may spread a considerable distance over the cortex, especially the post-central cortex before consciousness is lost. On the other hand, the loss of consciousness during a true seizure may be primary without any manifestation other than a blank expression and arrest of speech (petit mal). The return of consciousness in such a patient may be without sign and he may continue his train of thought without knowledge of the gap. The neurological mechanism, temporarily inactive, must be the same or similar to that which is paralyzed in automatism.

In a more severe petit mal seizure there are usually, as pointed out by Jackson, certain associated phenomena such as "deep pallor and a slight wave of universal movement." Such a lapse is sometimes regularly associated with loss of the mechanism for maintaining erect posture and the patient suddenly falls to the ground. If there is an aura preceding simple loss of consciousness it is most often an epigastric or a visceral one.

Let us consider for the moment that consciousness has a localizable representation in the brain: like movement, vision, hearing and speech. From the nature of the associated phenomena just described, one might suggest that that representation finds its topographical localization near to the representation of autonomic function in the hypothalamus and close to the third ventricle from which region facial blanching might be produced and where visceral sense may be represented and adjacent to the upper end of the nerve circuits in the midbrain which maintain standing. This topographical localization does not signify a belief in a punctate centre but rather a general region. The exact position may be wrong but the reasons to search for such localization are valid.

We may make another observation about consciousness and epilepsy. It is invariably lost at the beginning of those attacks in which the convulsion is generalized from the start. Now if there is an as yet uncharted area of the brain where all sensory and motor processes are re-represented epileptogenic discharge here would result in involvement of all somatic and visceral functions simultaneously and would obliterate consciousness from the beginning.

Hughlings Jackson found this problem a favourite one. He often quoted from Herbert Spencer these words: "The seat of consciousness is that nervous centre to which mediately or immediately the *most heterogeneous* impressions are brought."

On a lower functional level vision has its nervous mechanism in the occipital lobes and hearing in the temporal lobes. That is, a sound produces a neural activity in the temporal lobes which forms the basis of hearing. In the motor region the neural activity forms the basis for voluntary movement. If we had no other evidence, knew no

anatomy of tracts, had never used an experimental animal, the study of human epilepsy would have shown us these facts concerning voluntary movement, hearing and seeing.

In an analogous manner the evidence from the study of epilepsy suggests that there is such a region where those neural activities converge, which are the indispensable substratum of consciousness. The elements are there both for sensation and for the initiation of movement.

But perhaps it would be well, before yielding to the temptation of anatomical localization, to reconsider the physiological and psychological results of cortical stimulation independent of epilepsy.

The phenomena produced by cortical stimulation are crude. The movements involve many different muscles that depend on a very wide innervation in the brain stem and spinal cord, and yet the result is simple flexion or extension of a part or a turning movement which accomplishes nothing purposive. If stimulation of a cortical motor area is carried out during the execution of some voluntary act by the subject, the motor mechanism in question is snatched away from his control, but he may continue to carry out the act if there are other mechanisms available not so stimulated. Thus the girl (H. T.) continued to count aloud even though one side of her mouth was caused to contract in the useless manner of a motor discharge. She said she found it hard work but she succeeded, no doubt due to the fact that she was using the other side of her mouth appropriately by means of the mouth motor mechanism from the opposite hemisphere.

If, however, vocalization is being produced by stimulation of one hemisphere, the larynx, diaphragm and all the accessory muscles of phonation are pre-empted by this discharge. The individual cannot speak or alter the vocalization however hard he may try. A homologous vocalization mechanism exists in the opposite hemisphere but the final common path of this discharge has already been pre-empted by an electrode.

The demand of an electrode is not always irresistible. Although stimulation of Brodmann's area 4 or 6 produces a movement which the patient cannot inhibit, nevertheless in the epileptic brain stimulation at a distance from the motor cortex sometimes produces what the patient describes as a desire to move a certain part. By making a conscious effort he can prevent such movement and in his effort to do so he may, at the time of stimulation, make the opposite movement (J. H.). On the other hand, if the fingers of one hand are caused to close by an irresistible electrical stimulus the patient can quite easily use the other hand in an efficient manner to try to force the fingers open.

An electrode can produce no more evidence of a

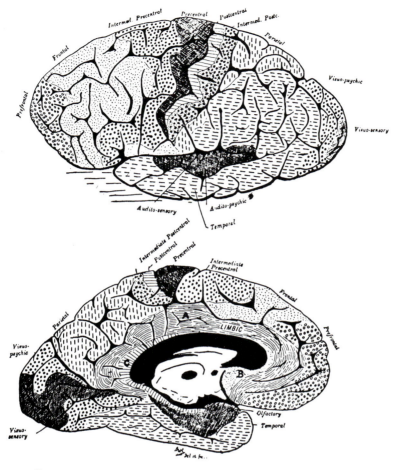

FIG. 7. Cytoarchitectural fields of cerebral cortex (Campbell, 1905).

directed, purposeful, skilful movement than is to be found on the mockery of action produced by an epileptic cortical discharge.

Sensory and hallucinatory phenomena of a more complicated nature may be produced in the posterior two-thirds of the hemispheres, but only when those phenomena have previously formed a part of a recurring epileptic fit which seems to prepare that portion of the cortex for local conditioned reflexes. The stimulation seems to reproduce a familiar chord the harmony of which has become the characteristic expression of that area of cortex when stimulated.

The above discussion applies to the sensorimotor cortex. No mention has yet been made of the frontal lobes anterior to areas 4, 6a alpha and 6a beta of Brodmann. This is what Campbell (1905) called the frontal and prefrontal cortex (Fig. 7). It is dangerous to give this area a name because of the confusion of terminology that already exists, as pointed out by Walshe (1935), but for convenience of discussion it may be called the extra-motor frontal cortex.

In regard to this portion of the frontal lobe Pavlov wrote that it should (probably) be included with the rest of the cerebral cortex. But a clearer impression of his eventual opinion may be gathered from the letter of his pupil, Professor Boris P. Babkin, who wrote to me as follows: "Many of the experimental data obtained by you on man point in the same direction as the facts obtained by us in Pavlov's laboratory, namely that the cortex is primarily a representation of the receptors scattered over the external and internal surfaces of the body. However, in the last years of his life Pavlov came to the conclusion that the frontal region of man serves for higher neural activities than the formation of conditioned reflexes. Thus, if a conditioned stimulus is regarded as a signal, there also may be formed 'signals of signals,' e.g. words. The 'centre' for the formation of these signals of signals would be the frontal region. Pavlov never touched the problem of consciousness. At any rate in the dog it is not located in the frontal lobes, as I know from my own experiments involving extirpation of this part of the hemispheres."

Hughlings Jackson suggested that in the "prefrontal" area was to be found the highest level of re-representation. But he suggested this in the same tentative manner that he once suggested, in the days before Hitzig, that motor and sensory representation would be found in the corpus striatum.

In my own experience no convulsive phenomena have been produced by electrical stimulation of the extra-motor frontal cortex as yet, and no responses of any sort have been produced other than what may be called autonomic alterations, but these so rarely as to make conclusion premature. Possibly other forms of electrical current may give a different result. But, so far, no alteration and no arrest in consciousness have been produced here even by strong stimulation, and neither has been reported by others.

Fits which originate from focal lesions in the frontal pole are characterized, it is true, by initial loss of consciousness followed by adversive movements before the appearance of generalized convulsions. Radical extirpation of the whole of one frontal lobe, including all of the extra-motor cortex and back into area 6a beta, may be carried out in a conscious patient without his losing conscious insight during the procedure or memory of the details of the event afterward. After immediate recovery the most important detectable sequel, in my opinion, is "impairment of those mental processes which are prerequisite to planned initiative" (Penfield and Evans, 1935).

If this large area of cortex in both frontal lobes were necessary for the existence of consciousness it seems likely that there would be at least a temporary loss of consciousness during the removal of one lobe and until the remaining lobe could take over the function of both. And yet one occipital lobe may be removed without the patient being aware of any interference with vision or of the reduction of his visual field. Furthermore, the fact that epileptiform discharge in the extra-motor frontal cortex obliterates consciousness may be likened to the fact that such discharge, if it be a strong one, in one occipital lobe may produce complete temporary blindness, a blindness that applies to the whole visual field and the patient says everything is dark.

All of this would suggest that the frontal lobes anterior to recognized motor areas are utilized in conscious processes but that they are not indispensable to the existence of consciousness. It is conceivable that these lobes represent an elaborative field for a more essential concentration of nerve tracts which lie posteriorly and more centrally in the brain. But it should be pointed out that stimulation of this area of the brain in man has cast no light upon its function as yet and I should like to exclude the extra-motor frontal cortex from any conclusions reached here in regard to the remainder of the cerebral cortex.

Long-continued unconsciousness appears clinically in patients who have a lesion of an area somewhere above but not far removed from the midbrain and in the vicinity of it. Details will be omitted here, but twice, after posterior fossa operations, patients of mine have gone into a condition eventually resembling sleep, in which they lived several months with stomach-tube feeding. In another case a similar state followed operative removal of a tumour which extended into the pulvinar and which was followed by unconsciousness from which the patient began to rouse after six weeks of artificial feedings. Such localization as has been achieved for sleep, normal and pathological, also implicates this general region (Hess, 1932).

It is, of course, impossible to state that in such unconscious states as those just described all sense perception is gone. One may conclude no more than that volitional aspects of consciousness are non-existent and that no later memory of the state persists. In a discussion of this general field with Professor Charles Hendel he has pointed out to me that in one sense I cannot escape the formulation of some definition of consciousness, at least by implication, and that my argument applies particularly to volitional consciousness or the motor element of consciousness. It is true that if there is such a thing as sense perception or pure sensory consciousness in the absence of all volitional capacity the evidence produced in this study seldom applies to it, and patients have no memory of such a state. Nevertheless, after an epileptic seizure a patient may say he heard and saw what was happening during the seizure but could give no outward sign. The physiological explanation that seems evident for this state is that the necessary cortical motor mechanisms were taken away from him by the epileptic disturbance while certain sensory cortical mechanisms were not so pre-empted. At such a time the patient could hardly be called unconscious.

The common published conception of the cerebral cortex seems to be that it represents the highest level in the scale of nervous activity. The objective evidence derived from a study of epilepsy and from the study of conscious patients during brain operations supports the view of Hughlings Jackson that the sensori-motor cerebral cortex represents only a middle level of integration.

Man is one of a million species of animals, some of which at least would seem to be conscious. Parker (1934) pointed out the conservatism of nature in regard to changes of the central nervous system as compared with the radical variety of outward form. The human cerebral cortex has developed coincidentally with man's acquisition of new skills and new adjustments to his environment. *A priori*, there seems to be no reason why the neural mechanism essential to consciousness should migrate outward into the newly exfoliated hemisphere.

In a conscious individual it must be from somewhere that neuronal impulses pass to the motor areas of the hemispheres producing complicated behaviour which cannot be simulated by electrical stimulation anywhere over the cortex. Hallucinations involving elaborate memory of visual and auditory pictures can be produced by such stimulation but the patient retains conscious insight into the unreality of the experience. The same epileptic and post-epileptic processes which paralyze discrete areas of the cerebral cortex also may abolish consciousness. Therefore it seems reasonable to assume that there is a discrete area of the brain the integrity of which is essential to the existence of conscious activity.

Finally, there is much evidence of a higher level of integration within the central nervous system that is to be found in the cerebral cortex, evidence of a regional localization of the neuronal mechanism involved in this integration. I would suggest that this region lies, not in the new brain, but in the old, and that it lies below the cerebral cortex and above the midbrain.

Such localization does not signify that other parts of the brain play no rôle in this mechanism. All parts of the brain may well be involved in normal conscious processes but the indispensable substratum of consciousness lies outside of the cerebral cortex, probably in the diencephalon.

This discussion has avoided the subject of the nature of consciousness. That is a psychological problem. It has been concerned with the localization of the "place of understanding" and by place is meant the localization of those neuronal circuits most intimately associated with the initiation of voluntary activity and with the sensory summation prerequisite to it.

REFERENCES

BRODMANN, K. Vergleichende Lokalizationslehre der Grosshirnrinde, Leipzig, 1925.

CAMPBELL, A. Histological studies on the localization of cerebral function, Cambridge, 1905.

FOERSTER, O. The motor cortex in man in the light of Hughlings Jackson's doctrines. Brain, 59: 135, 1936.

FULTON, J. Paralyses of cortical origin. Proc. Calif. Acad. Med., 1, 1934.

GIBBS, E. AND GIBBS, F. A purring center in the cat's brain. J. Comp. Neurol., 64: 209, 1936.

HESS, W. The autonomic nervous system. Lancet, Dec. 3, 1199, 1932.

JACKSON, H. Selected writings of John Hughlings Jackson, London, 1931.

LASHLEY, K. Brain mechanisms and intelligence. Chicago Univ. Press, Chicago, 1929.

LEYTON, A. AND SHERRINGTON, C. Observations on the excitable cortex of the chimpanzee, orang utan and gorilla. Quart. J. Exp. Physiol., 11: 135, 1917.

PARKER, G. The origin, plan and operational modes of the nervous system. New York, 1934.

PAVLOV, I. Conditioned reflexes. Translated by Anrep, Oxford Univ. Press, London, 1927.

PENFIELD, W. The evidence for a cerebral vascular mechanism in epilepsy. Annals of Int. Med., 7: No. 3, 1933.

PENFIELD, W. Focal epileptic discharge in a case of tumour of the posterior temporal region. Can. Med. Assn. J., 33: 32, 1935.

PENFIELD, W. AND EVANS, J. The frontal lobe in man: a clinical study of maximum removals. Brain, 58: 115, 1935.

VOGT, C. AND VOGT, O. Die vergleichend-arkitektonische und die vergleichend-reizphysiologische Felderung der Grosshirnrinde unter besonderer Berücksichtigung der menschlichen. Die Naturwissenschaften, 14: 1191, 1926.

VON ECONOMO, C. The cytoarchitectonics of the human cerebral cortex. Oxford Univ. Press, London, 1929.

WALSHE, F. On the "Syndrome of the premotor cortex" (Fulton) and the definition of the terms "premotor" and "motor." Brain, 59: 49, 1935.

Since their introduction by Dr. Walter Dandy in 1918 and 1919,[7–10] pneumoventriculography and pneumoencephalography have become routine techniques for the diagnosis of various neurological diseases. The importance of these innovations has been stressed frequently, and many consider them to be the most important of Dandy's various outstanding contributions to neurosurgery.[1,4–6,13,14,16,18–21]

Prior to the introduction of these techniques, a few isolated cases of craniocerebral trauma had been described in which intracranial and intraventricular air was visualized by roentgen ray.[5,12] The best known of these cases was reported in 1913:[17]

On November 24, 1912, ". . . a middle-aged man was admitted with a head injury to a New York hospital under the care of Dr. W. H. Luckett. He was x-rayed by Dr. W. H. Stewart, who detected a fracture in the posterior wall of the frontal sinus. The patient was treated conservatively and discharged from hospital, but returned some three weeks later having suffered a relapse. On December 14 a further radiographic examination of the skull was undertaken by Dr. Stewart. He reported that these x-rays showed the ventricles enormously dilated by what was probably air or gas. As a result of these findings Dr. Luckett operated and during the course of the operation tapped one of the ventricles and noticed that air or gas was released. The patient died three days later and at autopsy the fracture in the posterior wall of the frontal sinus was confirmed and part of the bone was found to be depressed about one centimeter. The brain was removed in toto and placed under water. Bubbles emerged through a laceration in the base of the frontal lobe and this laceration was shown to communicate with the anterior horn of the ventricle. The fluid in the ventricle at the time of the operation was examined bacteriologically and found to be sterile. It was therefore assumed that air, not gas, was present."[5]

However, despite this accidental visualization of the ventricular system, the diagnostic potentials of this phenomenon were not appreciated until about 5 years later. On January 3, 1917, a patient of Dr. Dandy's, ". . . . whose abdomen he was about to explore for intestinal perforation chanced to have a chest x-ray taken on the way to the operating room . . . Air was clearly visible under the diaphragm. Operation confirmed the presence of intraperitoneal air, as well as the perforated typhoid ulcer through which it had escaped. The usefulness of this discovery has been amply confirmed on hundreds of subsequent occasions.

"It is of interest that this was the very roentgenogram that originally suggested to Dandy the use of air to outline the cerebral ventricles!"[6]

"Because brain tumors were so infrequently revealed by roentgenograms of the skull Dandy searched for a technique by which he might visualize the cerebral ventricles, for the latter were usually displaced or distorted by an intracranial neoplasm."[20] After unsuccessful attempts with the various media used in pyelography, ". . . Dandy substituted air for ventricular fluid and obtained a clear outline of the ventricular system. Thus ventriculography was born in 1918."[20]

In 1919, Dandy ". . . demonstrated that the cerebral structures might be visualized if the air were injected into the lumbar subarachnoid space. Within two years Bingel[2] in Germany, Jacobaeus[15] and Widerøe[22] in Norway, unaware of Dandy's work, independently injected air into the lumbar subarachnoid space to demonstrate roentgenologically, tumors of the spinal cord. Bingel[3] gave the procedure the name of pneumoencephalography or encephalography."[20]

"Dandy favored ventriculography and most of his studies were with that technique, whereas in Europe, especially Germany, encephalography became popular. The procedures were not uncritically received by the medical profession. In America, a few early fatalities, which occurred before surgeons realized that, in the case of brain tumors, the air study must be followed by craniotomy, led to a reserved skepticism of the new practice for several years . . ."[20]

"It seems obvious that ventriculography was not always an innocuous procedure, for Dandy advised, in comatose patients, ventricular estimation, a procedure he devised in 1923 and one which he considered better tolerated than ventriculography.[11] The usual occipital perforations were made. The upper ventricle was tapped, the fluid aspirated and measured. The lower one was similarly treated. A disparity in the amounts of fluid removed was thought to indicate a tumor on the side having less fluid. If a ventricle contained more than 25 cc. of fluid, it was considered obstructed. If communication between the ventricles was questioned 1 cc. of a neutral suspension of indigo carmine was injected into one ventricle and the other aspirated in search of the dye. To differentiate between a tumor obstructing the aqueduct and pseudotumor, a spinal puncture was advocated twenty minutes after the dye had been injected in the ventricle.

"Ventricular estimation never gained popularity but the dye test, originally used to determine whether a hydrocephalus was obstructive or communicating, became a routine procedure."[20]

Since their introduction, ventriculography and encephalography have been modified frequently by changes in positions, contrast media, and roentgen-ray techniques.[20] The basic ideas, however, have remained unchanged for almost half a century, a fitting tribute to their inherent worth. Dandy's classical 1918 paper on ventriculography is reprinted below and his 1919 paper on encephalography will be reprinted in a forthcoming issue of the *Journal of Neurosurgery*.

References

1. BAGLEY, C. Obituary. Walter E. Dandy. *J. nerv. ment. Dis.*, 1946, *104:* 456–457.

2. BINGEL, [A.] Braunschweig. Ärztlicher Kreisverein. *Med. Klin.*, 1921, *17:* 608.

3. BINGEL, A. Encephalographie, eine Methode zur röntgenographischen Darstellung des Gehirns. *Fortschr. Röntgenstr.*, 1921, *28:* 205–217.

4. BLALOCK, A. Dr. Walter E. Dandy. Birthday number. *Surgery*, 1946, *19:* 577–579.

5. BULL, J. W. D. History of neuroradiology. *Brit. J. Radiol.*, 1961, *34:* 69–84.

6. CAMPBELL, E. Walter E. Dandy—surgeon, 1886–1946. *J. Neurosurg.*, 1951, *8:* 249–262.

7. DANDY, W. E. Ventriculography following the injection of air into the cerebral ventricles. *Ann. Surg.*, 1918, *68:* 5–11.

8. DANDY, W. E. Ventriculography following the injection of air into the cerebral ventricles. *Amer. J. Roentgenol.*, 1919, *6:* 26–36.

9. DANDY, W. E. Röntgenography of the brain after the injection of air into the spinal canal. *Ann. Surg.*, 1919, *70:* 397–403.

10. DANDY, W. E. Localization of brain tumors by cerebral pneumography. *Amer. J. Roentgenol.*, 1923, *10:* 610–612.

11. DANDY, W. E. A method for the localization of brain tumors in comatose patients. The determination of communication between the cerebral ventricles and the estimation of their position and size without the injection of air (ventricular estimation). *Surg. Gynec. Obstet.*, 1923, *36:* 641–656.

12. DANDY, W. E. Pheumocephalus (intracranial pneumatocele or aerocele). *Arch. Surg., Chicago*, 1926, *12:* 949–982.

13. FIROR, W. M. Memoir. Walter E. Dandy. 1886–1946. *Ann. Surg.*, 1947, *126:* 113–115.

14. HORRAX, G. Neurosurgery. An historical sketch. *Springfield, Ill.: Charles C Thomas*, 1952, xi, 135 pp. (see pp. 92–95).

15. JACOBAEUS, H. C. On insufflation of air into the spinal canal for diagnostic purposes in cases of tumors in the spinal canal. *Acta med. scand.*, 1921, *55:* 555–564.

16. JEFFERSON, G. Obituary. Walter Dandy. *Brit. med. J.*, 1946, *1:* 852–853.

17. LUCKETT, W. H. Air in the ventricles of the brain, following a fracture of the skull. Report of a case. *Surg. Gynec. Obstet.*, 1913, *17:* 237–240.

18. SACHS, E. The history and development of neurological surgery. *New York: P. B. Hoeber, Inc.*, 1952, 158 pp. (see pp. 79–81).

19. SCARFF, J. E. Fifty years of neurosurgery, 1905–1955. *Int. Abstr. Surg.*, 1955, *101:* 417–513.

20. WALKER, A. E. Diagnostic procedures. In: *A history of neurological surgery*. A. E. Walker, Ed. Baltimore: Williams & Wilkins Co., 1951, xii, 583 pp. (see pp. 23–39).

21. WALKER, A. E. Walter Edward Dandy (1886–1946). In: *The founders of neurology*. W. Haymaker, Ed. Springfield, Ill.: Charles C Thomas, 1953, xxvii, 479 pp. (see pp. 417–420).

22. WIDERØE, S. Om intraspinal luftinjektion og om dens diagnostiske betydning ved rygmarvslidelser, saerlig ved svulster. *Norsk. Mag. Laegevidensk.*, 1921, *82:* 491–495.

VENTRICULOGRAPHY FOLLOWING THE INJECTION OF AIR INTO THE CEREBRAL VENTRICLES*

By Walter E. Dandy, M.D.
of Baltimore, Md.

(From the Department of Surgery, the Johns Hopkins Hospital and University)

The value of röntgenography in the diagnosis and localization of intracranial tumors is mainly restricted to the cases in which the neoplasm has affected the skull. In an analysis of the X-ray findings in one hundred cases of brain tumor from Doctor Halsted's Clinic, Heuer and I[1] have shown that in only 6 per cent. of the cases did the tumor cast a shadow, and in these it was only the calcified areas that were differentiated by the X-rays from the normal cerebral tissues.

In those instances (9 per cent. of our cases) in which a tumor has encroached upon the sphenoid, ethmoid or frontal sinus, the invading portion casts a shadow in the röntgenogram. Such shadows are due to the displacement of the normally contained air by tissues which are less pervious to the X-ray. This group of shadows is of minor practical importance because the growth can be recognized by the destruction of the walls or bony septa of the sinuses.

Since the X-rays penetrate normal brain tissues, blood, cerebrospinal fluid and non-calcified tumor tissue almost equally, any changes in the brain produced by altered proportions of these components will not materially alter the röntgenogram.

Although skull changes are shown by the X-ray in 45 per cent. of our cases and are frequently pathognomonic, on the whole they represent late stages of the disease. As intracranial tumors come to be diagnosed and localized earlier, the value of the X-ray will be correspondingly diminished.

For some time I have considered the possibility of filling the cerebral ventricles with a medium that will produce a shadow in the radiogram. If this could be done, an accurate outline of the cerebral ventricles could be photographed with X-rays, and since most neoplasms either directly or indirectly modify the size or shape of the ventricles, we should then possess an early and accurate aid to the localization of intracranial affections. In addition to its radiographic properties, any substance injected into the ventricles must satisfy two very rigid exactions: (1) It must be absolutely non-irritating and non-toxic; and (2) it must be readily absorbed and excreted.

The various solutions and suspensions used in pyelography—thorium, potassium, iodide, collargol, argyrol, bismuth subnitrate and subcarbonate, all in various concentrations—were injected into the ventricles of dogs, but always with fatal results, owing to the injurious effects on the brain. Marked œdema, serosanguineous exudate, and petechial hemorrhages resulted. The severe reactions that are sometimes encountered after the intraspinous injection of most therapeutic remedies indicate the dangers even from carefully prepared solutions. A slight acidity or alkalinity may result even in death. It seems unlikely that any solution of radiographic value will be found which is sufficiently harmless to justify its injection into the central nervous system. Suspensions are precluded because they are not absorbed.

Ventriculography, therefore, seems possible only by the substitution of gas for cerebrospinal fluid. It is largely due to the frequent comment by Doctor Halsted on the remarkable power of intestinal gases "to perforate bone" that my attention was drawn to its practical possibilities in the brain. Striking gas shadows are present in all abdominal and thoracic radiograms. The stomach and intestines are often outlined by the contained air, even more sharply than when filled with bismuth. A small collection of gas in the intestines often obliterates the kidney outlines. A perforation of the intestines may be diagnosed by the shadow of the air that has accumulated under the diaphragm. Gas gangrene may be diagnosed by the air blebs (of B. welchii) in the tissues. Pneumothorax is sharply outlined because the normal lung tissues are eliminated. The paranasal sinuses and mastoid air cells show up in a thick skull by virtue of the air, and pathological conditions of the sinuses are evident because inflammatory or tumor tissue replaces the air. From these and many other normal and pathological clinical demonstrations of the radiographic properties of air it is but a step to the injection of gas into the cerebral ventricles—pneumoventriculography.

Methods.—Several gases are inert and readily absorbable, and in these respects satisfy the requirements for injection into the cerebrospinal system. Although it is possible other gases give even better results, we have used only air in the injections here described. The merits of other gases are now being studied.

In order to obtain a skiagram of the lateral cerebral ventricles filled with air, it is necessary to remove at least more cerebrospinal fluid than the contents of one ventricle and to replace this fluid with an equal quantity of air. Before closure of the fontanelles, one can readily make a ventricular puncture through the interosseous defect. After union of the sutures, it is necessary to make a small opening in the bone.

Air and water in a ventricle behave exactly as they would in a closed flask. Following any change in position the fluid gravitates to the most dependent part and the air rises to the top. Owing to the free communication between the third, the right and the left lateral ventricles through the foramina of Monro, fluid and air will readily pass from one ventricle to the other. Because of the curves in the ventricular system, however, it is obvious that in any given position, only part of the ventricular fluid can gravitate to the point of the needle, so that this amount only can be aspirated. If desired, fluid can be removed from the remaining recesses by tilting the head, just as one manipulates a curved tube to replace the fluid with air. Theoretically, it should be possible to remove nearly all the ventricular fluid by suitable manipulations of the head, but for practical purposes enough fluid can be obtained from one correct position. Visualization of the ventricular system will

* Reprinted from *Annals of Surgery*, 1918, *68:* 5–11, with the kind permission of the Chairman of the Editorial and Advisory Board.

[1] Röntgenography in the Localization of Brain Tumor, Based Upon a Series of One Hundred Consecutive Cases. The Johns Hopkins Hosp. Bull., 1916, xxvii, 311. Also: A Report of Seventy Cases of Brain Tumor. The Johns Hopkins Hosp. Bull., 1916, xxvii, 224.

best indicate the most appropriate location for ventricular puncture and the proper position of the head. It will then be seen that the most fluid can be obtained from a puncture in the anterior part of either lateral ventricle (Fig. 2). The head should be placed with the face down and partially rotated so that the ventricle to be aspirated is beneath and the needle enters at the most dependent point possible. This position permits the maximal drainage of fluid from the opposite lateral and the third ventricles. Aspiration through a puncture in the posterior or descending horn permits a fairly complete removal of the fluid from one ventricle and from that portion of the other lateral ventricle which is anterior to the foramen of Monro. In the aspiration of fluid from the posterior horn of the lateral ventricle, the patient must lie with the face directed upward and backward and the head rotated from 30 to 40 degrees toward the side of the needle.

The exchange of air for cerebrospinal fluid must be made accurately. If the air injected is greater in volume than the fluid withdrawn, acute pressure symptoms will result. To attain accuracy we have used a Record syringe with a two-way valve attachment (Fig. 1). A small amount of fluid (20 c.c.) is aspirated and an equal quantity of air injected. This is repeated until all the fluid has been removed. By aspirating and injecting in small quantities, injury to the brain from negative pressure is prevented. Not knowing the size of the ventricles beforehand, we have no way of estimating the amount of air necessary to fill one ventricle. For this

reason we have preferred the removal of all the fluid that can be readily obtained. This has been found to be but little greater than the contents of one ventricle.

Needless to say, owing to the lighter weight of air, the ventriculogram represents the ventricle farthest from the X-ray plate. To insure the best results the sagittal plane of the head should be parallel with the plate. Valuable assitance can also be obtained from anteroposterior X-rays. The head should then be placed so that the sagittal plane is vertical, preferably with the occiput resting on the plate. With the latter precaution a more even distribution of air on the two sides is obtained and the ventriculogram represents the anterior portions of both lateral ventricles. For special points in diagnosis additional anteroposterior views may be taken of the posterior and descending horns of the ventricle by placing the forehead on the plate.

Results Following Injection.—We have injected air into the cerebral ventricles at least twenty times. In some instances the injection has been repeated. The amount of air injected has varied from 40 to 300 c.c., the larger quantities in cases of internal hydrocephalus. Only once has there been any reaction, and in this case the injection (300 c.c.) was made forty-eight hours after the first stage of an operation for cerebellar tumor (Fig. 3). The reaction was characterized by a rise of temperature, nausea, vomiting, and increased headache, all of which were quickly relieved after release of the air by a ventricular puncture. Ten days later, a large cerebellar tumor was removed, the patient making an uneventful

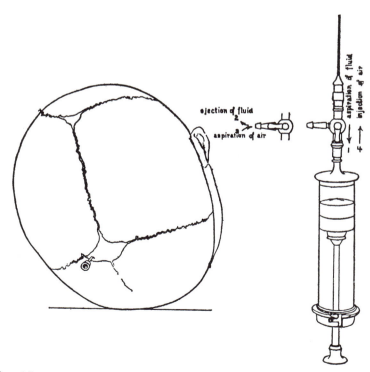

Fig. 1.—Showing oblique position of head for aspiration of fluid and injection of air. The forehead is resting on plate. Note point of entrance of the needle into anterior fontanelle on dependent side. Figure on right shows record syringe and two-way valve attachment used for this purpose.

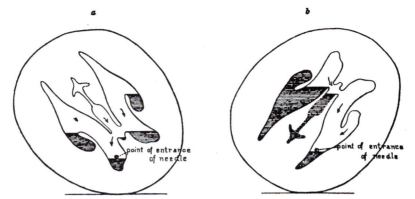

Fig. 2.—Diagrams showing relative amounts of cerebrospinal fluid that can be removed from a single ventricular puncture: (1) when forehead is down (a) and (2) when occiput is down (b). Shaded area represents the fluid which remain in the ventricular system after the greatest possible quantity has been removed. Unshaded area represents maximum quantity of air which can be injected to replace the fluid withdrawn. It is evident that more fluid can be removed when the puncture is made anteriorly and the forehead is dependent.

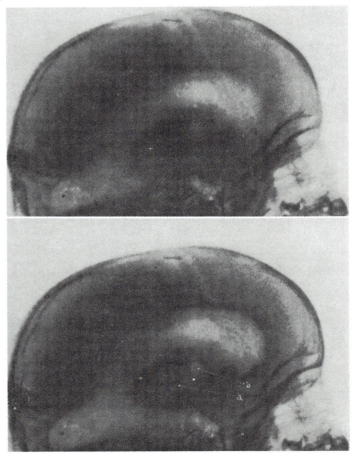

Fig. 3.—Ventriculogram in a child three year sold, with tuberculous meningitis. The ventricle is slightly dilated an early obstructive hydrocephalus having resulted from closure of the foramina of Magendie and Luschka by exudate. The separation of the frontoparietal sutures also indicates intracranial pressure. a, third ventricle; probably the foramen of Monro. The body, the posterior horn, and the descending horn of the lateral ventricle are obvious.

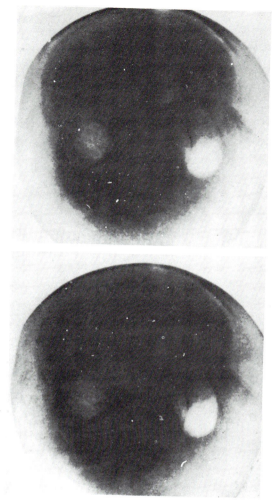

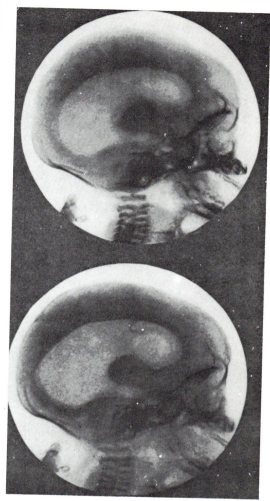

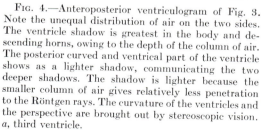

Fig. 4.—Anteroposterior ventriculogram of Fig. 3. Note the unequal distribution of air on the two sides. The ventricle shadow is greatest in the body and descending horns, owing to the depth of the column of air. The posterior curved and ventral part of the ventricle shows as a lighter shadow, communicating the two deeper shadows. The shadow is lighter because the smaller column of air gives relatively less penetration to the Röntgen rays. The curvature of the ventricles and the perspective are brought out by stereoscopic vision. a, third ventricle.

Fig. 5.—Ventriculogram of moderately distended ventricle in a case of communicating hydrocephalus. The size of the head is normal. Note the obliteration of the more normal ventricular contour shown in Fig. 3. The posterior horn is supplanted by a diffuse posterior bulging. The deeper shadow in the anterior part of the ventricle is due to air in the opposite ventricle.

recovery. All of the injections have been made in children varying from six months to twelve years of age. Invariably the lateral ventricle has been sharply outlined in the radiogram. In two instances the third ventricle and the foramen of Monro were visible (Figs. 3 and 8). In none, however, have we observed the fourth ventricle or the aqueduct of Sylvius. The practical value from pneumoventriculography is expected principally from the shadows of the lateral ventricles.

Day by day the air shadow diminishes and eventually disappears. In a case of internal hydrocephalus it re-

quired two weeks. Possibly in more normal cases the time may be less, as air in other body tissues vanishes much more rapidly. In all probability absorption of air injected into the ventricles takes place by the same channels as in the case of the ventricular cerebrospinal fluid. In a previous communication[2] it has been shown that cerebrospinal fluid is almost entirely absorbed from the subarachnoid space; that only a very slight absorption takes place from the ventricles. Phenolsulphonephthalein in a closed ventricular system disappears in from ten to twelve days, whereas it is absorbed

[2] Dandy and Blackfan: Am. J. Dis. Child., 1914, viii, 406; 1917, xiv, 424. Also J. Am. M. Assoc., 1913, lxi, 2216.

in from ten to twelve hours when the ventricles communicate with the subarachnoid space, where the absorption of cerebrospinal fluid normally takes place.

Air introduced into the ventricles acts in no way differently from the air included at every intracranial operation. Following tumor extirpation especially, the resulting defect fills with air which, unless displaced by salt solution, is shut in when the dura and scalp are sutured. For a few days pending its absorption from tumor defects the patient may be conscious of the

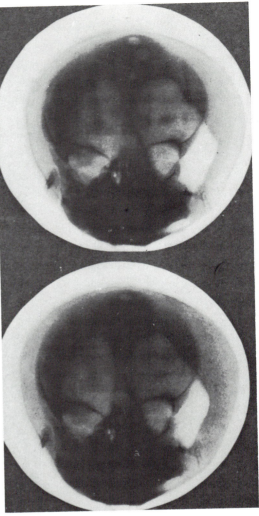

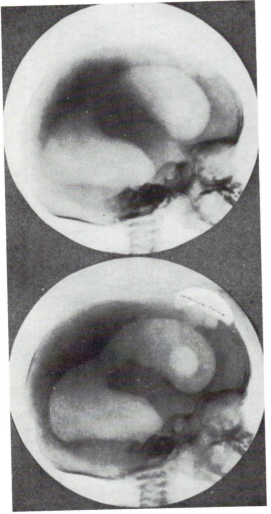

Fig. 7.—Anteroposterior view of Fig. 6. Note the fairly equal distribution of the air in the two ventricles. This is probably due to the more extensive communication due to the enlarged foramina of Monro. *a*, third ventricle.

movement of the air when the head is turned, but its presence is without any other effects.

The Value of Ventriculography.—Even in the few cases here reported ventriculography has proven of great practical value. For the first time we have a means of diagnosing internal hydrocephalus in the early stages. Internal hydrocephalus is one of the most insidious diseases of the brain and is rarely diagnosed before a considerable amount of cortical destruction has resulted. This is true of adults as well as of children. With exact visualization of the ventricles the findings are pathognomonic. Not only the existence of hydrocephalus but its degree and the amount of brain destruction are at once evident from the ventriculogram.

In one case (in an infant six months old) an internal

Fig. 6.—Ventriculogram (lateral view) of a more distended ventricle in a fairly advanced case of communicating internal hydrocephalus. Note the ventricular hernia and its neck communicating with the anterosuperior part of the lateral ventricle. It was necessary to draw the hernia in the lower picture because the X-ray shadow of the hernia on the X-ray plate was so slight as to be visible only by an oblique or reflected light. The constriction in the centre of the ventricle is due to the fact that air does not fill the ventricle.

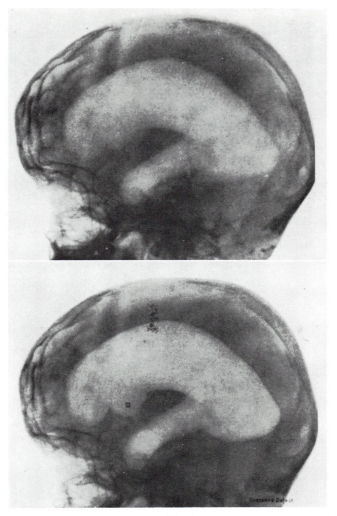

Fig. 8.—Ventriculogram (lateral view) in a large head with closed sutures. The convolutional atrophy of the skull, indicative of internal hydrocephalus, is evident in the occipital and frontal regions. The markings are intensified by the air in the ventricles. III is third ventricle. The downward projection from the third ventricle is probably the infundibulum. The patient was twelve years old. A large cerebellar tumor had been removed.

hydrocephalus was suspected from a bulging fontanelle, but the ventriculogram showed no enlargement of the ventricles. Another child (three years old) remained drowsy for several days after apparent recovery from an attack of epidemic cerebrospinal meningitis. The spinal fluid was clear and contained no organisms. The ventricular fluid was turbid and organisms were present; the ventriculogram demonstrated a greatly enlarged ventricle. The diagnosis of obstructive internal hydrocephalus, clinically unsuspected, was made with absolute certainty from the ventriculogram.

In two other children measurements of the head were normal but hydrocephalus was suspected because of abnormally large fontanelles. In each case the ventriculogram demonstrated ventricles which nearly filled the cranial chamber (Fig. 5).

One of the most interesting diagnoses, made possible only through the ventriculogram, was in a colored child eight months old. The head was definitely larger than normal, indicating the probability of an internal hydrocephalus. Over the anterior fontanelle, but slightly to one side, was a portruding tumor suggesting a meningocele, and this diagnosis had been made. Air injected into the lateral ventricle passed directly into the tumor. In the lateral ventriculogram the tumor was seen to arise from the greatly distended ventricle by a narrow neck (Fig. 6). An anteroposterior ventriculogram showed this communication to be unilateral. The diagnosis of a ruptured cortex with a (false) ventricular hernia was established, and subsequently verified at necropsy.

In another case a large cerebellar tumor was removed from a boy twelve years old. The large head, the marked convolutional atrophy of the skull, blindness, and the location of the tumor, made the diagnosis of internal hydrocephalus certain, but only the ventriculogram gave an accurate estimation of its advanced degree and the amount of brain destruction (Fig. 8).

Without a ventriculogram the diagnosis of internal hydrocephalus in children is frequently guess-work; with the ventriculogram the diagnosis is absolute.

We have as yet not obtained a normal ventriculogram. In one of these cases the ventricle was small but not known to be normal. It is possible that one of the earliest signs of internal hydrocephalus may be alteration in the shape of the ventricle due to the pressure effects on parts of the wall which are least resistant. The obliteration of the angle between body and posterior horn in Fig. 5 (contrasted to Fig. 3) suggests this probability, but ventriculograms of the intervening stages and the normal are lacking.

We have not yet applied ventriculography to adults, but expect to do so in all cases in which the diagnosis is obscure. In a boy of twelve years the ventriculogram was even sharper than in younger children. In adults we should expect the ventriculogram to be at least as sharp or possibly even more so because of the greater contrast between the density of air and bone. Several possibilities are anticipated from ventriculograms in adults: (1) The enlarged ventricles in internal hydro-cephalus should be absolutely defined. (2) Tumors in either cerebral hemisphere may dislocate or compress the ventricle and in this way localize the neoplasm. (3) Tumors growing into the ventricles may show a corresponding defect in the ventricular shadow. (4) A unilateral hydrocephalus may be demonstrable if the air cannot be made to enter the opposite ventricle.

CONCLUSIONS

1. The outlines of the lateral cerebral ventricles can be sharply outlined by the X-ray if air is substituted for cerebrospinal fluid.

2. The injection of air into the ventricles has had no deleterious effects in twenty cases.

3. Ventriculography has already proved of great practical value in the diagnosis and localization of many intracranial conditions. It is invaluable in internal hydrocephalus.

NOTE.—*Explanation of Figures.*—Two pictures are shown in each figure number. The upper one is the untouched photographic reproduction of the X-ray plate; the lower is the same photograph retouched by Miss Norris in order to overcome photographic loss of detail, and especially to emphasize the lines and special points which would otherwise be lost to the reader.

Neurosurgical Classic—16

T HE May 1963 issue of the *Journal of Neurosurgery* contained a reprint of Dr. Walter Dandy's classical 1918 paper on ventriculography. His companion work on encephalography is reproduced below.

RÖNTGENOGRAPHY OF THE BRAIN AFTER THE INJECTION OF AIR INTO THE SPINAL CANAL

By Walter E. Dandy, M.D.*
of Baltimore, Md.

(From the Department of Surgery, The Johns Hopkins Hospital and University)

As was shown in a recent publication,[1] one or more of the cerebral ventricles can be sharply outlined in a röntgenogram if the ventricular fluid be withdrawn and replaced by an equal quantity of air. In the course of this work it was soon noted that in many cases some of the air had passed out of the ventricular system and could be seen in filaments on the surface of the brain, that is, in the sulci. In order to reach the sulci from the point of injection in a lateral ventricle, the air must have followed the normal pathways by which cerebrospinal fluid circulates. It must have passed through the foramen of Monro into the third ventricles, thence into the fourth ventricles, through the aqueduct of Sylvius, and then, having left the ventricular system, it must have entered the cisterna magna by way of the foramen of Magendie and the paired foramina of Luschka. Finally, from the cisterna magna it must have passed along the various cisternæ under the base of the brain and then by numerous branches have reached the termination of the subarachnoid space—the sulci. Not infrequently, the entire subarachnoid space was graphically defined by the air shadows.

These observations at once gave promise of new possibilities in intracranial diagnostic study. Many lesions of the brain affect part of the subarachnoid space directly or indirectly. In hydro-

* Reprinted from *Annals of Surgery*, 1919, *70:* 397–403, with the kind permission of the Chairman of the Editorial and Advisory Board.

[1] Dandy, W. E.: Ventriculography Following the Injection of Air Into the Cerebral Ventricles. *Ann. Surg.*, July, 1918. Fluoroscopy of the Cerebral Ventricles. The Johns Hopkins Hosp. Bull., February, 1919.

cephalus of the communicating type, adhesions at the base of the brain obliterate the cisternæ and the cerebrospinal fluid cannot reach the sulci over the cerebral hemispheres; a local area of subarachnoid space may be obliterated by a tumor situated on or near the surface of the brain; a defect in the brain due to atrophy must necessarily be filled with cerebrospinal fluid, which may maintain communication with the subarachnoid space. These, and no doubt many other conditions, should be demonstrable by the absence or by the presence of air over the cerebral hemispheres.

After the injection of air into a cerebral ventricle a certain amount will soon appear on the external surface of the brain if the head is carefully manipulated so that the air is guided to the small aqueduct of Sylvius and the fourth ventricle. But the time of escape of air from the ventricles and of its appearance in the cerebral sulci are variable. The more completely the ventricles are filled with air the greater the probability that it will appear externally; and the more dilated the iter and the foramina of Luschka and Magendie (as in hydrocephalus) the more readily will air appear externally. Nevertheless, it was evident that at best the amount of air that will reach the cerebral sulci must vary greatly, according to the conditions existing in each individual case.

The problem therefore before us was: How can we in every case be sure of obtaining a complete injection of the subarachnoid space? The solution lies in the direct injection of air into the spinal canal. By this method the influence of the ventricular system is entirely eliminated; the air passes directly into the cisterna magna and thence into the ultimate ramifications of the subarachnoid space.

The technic is essentially similar to that described elsewhere for intraventricular injections. A small quantity of spinal fluid is withdrawn and an equal amount of air injected into the spinal canal. This process of substitution is repeated until the fluid ceases to appear on aspiration. There is no need to sterilize the air, because it is always free from pathogenic organisms.

Undoubtedly this procedure is not devoid of danger. Medullary distress, even fatal results, might well follow from increased intracranial pressure if the amount of air injected were even slightly in excess of the fluid withdrawn. The danger would certainly appear to be much greater in intraspinous than in intraventricular injec-

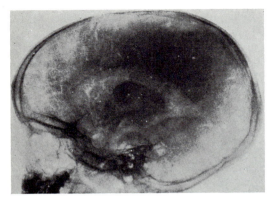

Fig. 1. Photograph of a roentgenogram of the head after injection of air into a lateral ventricle. The air has passed out of the ventricular system and filled the cerebral sulci, which appears as a network of lines. The cisterna interpeduncularis and the major branches passing to the cerebral sulci are fairly distinct just above the sella turcica. The lateral ventricle is normal.

tions, because in the latter direct pressure on the medulla in large measure is inhibited by the tentorium cerebri. In my own cases no bad effects have followed and the results have led me to believe that with proper care and judgment the procedure is entirely harmless. I have always left the open needle in the spinal canal for two or three minutes after the injection has been finished, thus rendering the intraspinous pressure directly under control. If the needle is left open, the intraspinous becomes equal to the atmospheric pressure, which is less than the normal intraspinous pressure. This reduced pressure is an additional safeguard against any possible development of a "reactive" intracranial pressure.

The position of the body is all-important in intraspinous injections—in fact, in all air injections, because the air rises as the fluid gravitates. The head must be at least twenty degrees higher than the needle. With each injection the air will then rush to the brain and a new supply of fluid will fall to the point of the needle. No doubt the sitting posture would be more satisfactory, because it would allow a more complete and uniform injection of the subarachnoid spaces over both cerebral hemispheres. In the recumbent position, which I have used exclusively, mainly for the comfort of the patient, it is possible that the injection may be more complete over the surface of the higher hemisphere than over the lower hemisphere, and that on turning the patient from one side to the other (in order to take both right and left lateral views of the head) important changes in the distribution of the air may be induced by the effects of gravity. In the sitting posture, rotation of the head would not alter the position of the air in the spaces, because gravity would not be

brought into play, and a more accurate photograph of the "air mantel" on each hemisphere would be obtained. If, however, the intracranial subarachnoid space is thoroughly injected, there should be but little change due to gravity and the recumbent posture should prove practically as effective as the sitting posture. Additional experience will probably indicate the position of choice.

I have injected air intraspinously into eight patients—four children and four adults—from Professor Halsted's service, without any bad effect. The amount of air has varied from 20 to 120 c.c. In one patient a mild headache followed but disappeared in three hours; vomiting but no headache occurred in another case; in the others no complaints were made. In reality, the effects should be much the same as those following the usual lumbar puncture.

One difficulty in the injection procedure should be mentioned. The aspiration must be gentle because the needle may plug at times, presumably with fibres of the cauda equina. If the suction is very gentle this may be obviated. In no case was there pain from injury to the nerves.

It must always be remembered that spinal punctures are very dangerous in all patients with intracranial tumors. A spinal puncture should never be made (if a tumor is present) unless the intracranial pressure has been previously relieved by a ventricular puncture or by some other procedure.

What becomes of the air? Air disappears from the subarachnoid space quite rapidly. It is absorbed as from other tissue spaces and undoubtedly passes directly into the blood. Usually no air is demonstrable in the röntgenogram twenty-four hours after the injection. Absorption from the subarachnoid space is many times faster than from the ventricles.

Practically all cerebrospinal fluid is absorbed from the subarachnoid space; very little from the ventricles, and the absorption of ventricular fluid occurs only after it has passed into the subarachnoid space.[2] When air is injected into a lateral ventricle, its rate of absorption seems to depend upon the freedom of access to the subarachnoid space. If the ventricles are normal the air will disappear in the course of a few days. If an internal hydrocephalus is present, the absorption time is greatly increased because an obstruction prevents the air from reaching the subarachnoid space. In cases of ventricular dilatation it may require two to three weeks for the air to disappear. The rate of absorption of air from the ventricles and the subarachnoid space appears to be relatively the same

[2] Dandy, W. E., and Blackfan, K. D.: Internal Hydrocephalus. Am. J. Dis. Child., 1914, viii, 406. Second paper: Am. J. Dis. Child., 1917, xiv, 424. Also: J. Am. M. Ass., 1913, lxi, 2216.

as that for the absorption of fluids from these cavities, although the absolute time required is greater for the absorption of air.

Röntgenography of the Normal Subarachnoid Space.—If the spinal and intracranial subarachnoid spaces are normal, the air which has been injected intraspinously will fill all the intracranial spaces (Figs. 1–3). The cisterna magna shows as an air-filled space of varying size, anterior to the squamous part of the occipital bone. The cisterna chiasmatica, which is the anterior terminus of the cisternæ, usually shows quite distinctly, and from it several branches may be seen passing upward into the cerebral sulci. The intensity of the shadow of the cisternæ under the medulla, pons, and midbrain is greatly modified by the dense bone at the base of the skull, notably the petrous part of both temporal bones. The continuity of the shadow of all the cisternæ can, however, nearly always be traced if the X-ray is good and the injection has been complete. The sulci appear as a network of lines over all the surfaces of the cerebral hemispheres. In general appearance the injected sulci suggest very closely the shadows of the vessels in the diploe, although the arrangement is different. In the earlier ventriculograms, in which only a few sulci contained air, the shadows were erroneously looked upon as markings of the diploëtic veins. Sulci have not been observed around the cerebellum, but frequently an envelope of air can be seen completely surrounding it. This envelope of cerebellar air is continuous with the cisterna magna. In one plate in which the upper part of the spinal canal was included, the spinal subarachnoid space was full of air, and in this column of air the shadow of the spinal cord was very distinct (Fig. 5).

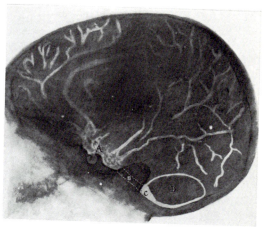

Fig. 3. A retouched photograph of a roentgenogram of the head after an intraspinous injection of air. The subarachnoid space is probably normal. The lines of the component parts of the subarachnoid space have been intensified because of the loss of detail through photographic reproduction. *A*, cisterna interpeduncularis; from it many large branches can be seen establishing direct communication with the cerebral sulci. *B*, cisterna shadow subdued by the dense temporal bones. This part of the cisterna can be seen in many X-rays. *C*, cisterna magna; from it the cerebellar subarachnoid space completely encircles the cerebellum (*D*). The large horizontal sulcus shown directly connecting with the cisterna, in all probability, is on the mesial aspect of the brain and passes around the corpus callosum. It is impossible to tell which of the other sulci are median and which are external.

The cerebellum frequently appears as an island (Fig. 3). Since the tentorium cerebelli is in apposition with part of the pericerebellar subarachnoid space, the shadow of this space marks the under surface of the tentorium. In cases in which the lateral ventricles are enormously dilated, a ventriculogram will delimit the upper margin of the tentorium. By combining the upper and lower shadows in such a case, the outlines of the tentorium are quite sharply seen. Mention of this is made merely to show how sharply the X-rays will differentiate tissues in a medium of air.

Localization of Intracranial Lesions by Intraspinous Injections of Air.[3]—The cisternæ may be regarded as the vital part of the subarachnoid space. Inasmuch as they form the trunk of the subarachnoid tree, all cerebrospinal fluid must traverse them in order to reach the cerebral sulci. The sulci are important because in them practically all cerebrospinal fluid is absorbed. Any obstruction in the cisternæ, therefore, leads to hydrocephalus because of a diminished absorption of cerebrospinal fluid. Hence it becomes of

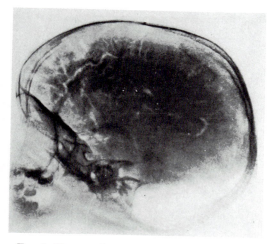

Fig. 2. Photograph of a roentgenogram of the head after an intraspinous injection of air. The sulci and cisterna are more distinct than after the intraventricular injection as shown in Fig. 1.

[3] The röntgenographic detail in these plates we owe to the skill of Miss Mary Stuart Smith, in the X-ray service of Doctor Baetjer.

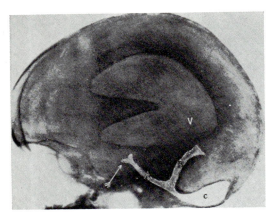

FIG. 4. Retouched photograph of a roentgenogram of the head after an intraspinous injection of air. The patient had internal hydrocephalus. It will be noticed that none of the sulci are injected as in Figs. 1, 2, and 3. At the arrow, an obstruction due to adhesion has blocked the cisterna. *A*, cisterna pontis and medullaris. *B*, cerebellar subarachnoid space, also only partly open. *C*, cisterna magna, considerably enlarged. *D*, lateral ventricle, which partially filled with air after the intraspinous injection.

the utmost importance to determine whether the cisternæ are patent or whether they have been obliterated. Intraspinous air will always reach the sulci if the cisternæ are patent; and conversely, if the air does not reach the sulci, the cisternæ must be obstructed at some point. Furthermore, with a good X-ray one can see just where the obstruction is situated.

In this series of eight cases, the location of the lesion has been accurately determined in three. In the remaining five, the subarachnoid space was normal. In the three patients in whom the lesion was located by means of intraspinous air, other methods had entirely failed. The findings in these cases will be briefly stated.

In a case of hydrocephalus, 110 cc. of air were injected intraspinously. It filled the cisterna magna, extended along the cisterna medullaris, and was stopped at the point of obstruction in the cisterna pontis (Fig. 4). This obstruction, due to adhesions from meningitis, had prevented the air reaching the sulci and thereby caused hydrocephalus. Necropsies have shown that communicating hydrocephalus is usually caused by adhesions in the cisternae.[4] I have since produced this disease in animals by occluding the cisterna with a perimesencephalic band of gauze.[5]

The injection of air gave still further information. Although it could not reach the cerebral subarachnoid space, which is normally the path of least resistance, it

[4] Dandy, W. E., and Blackfan, K. D.: Internal Hydrocephalus (second paper). *Am. J. Dis. Child.*,1917, xiv, 424.
[5] Dandy, W. E.: Experimental Hydrocephalus. To appear in *Annals of Surgery*.

passed through the basal foramina of Luschka and Magendie, the fourth ventricle, the aqueduct of Sylvius, the third ventricle, the foramen of Monro, and partially filled a lateral ventricle (Fig. 4). The fact that the air passed into the ventricle showed that the hydrocephalus was of the communicating type. It should be noted that air has not been observed to enter the ventricle except in hydrocephalus. Normally, the cerebellum is in such close apposition to the floor of the fourth ventricle that, despite the absence of valves, the retrograde flow of air into the fourth ventricle is prevented. It is conceivable that the precise localization of the obstruction by the air method may render operative relief for the obstruction possible.[6]

Our second case presents an even more interesting pathology. The patient was a child three years of age. She had passed through an attack of acute cerebrospinal meningitis, but instead of complete recovery, lethargy and vomiting had ensued. Internal hydrocephalus was suspected by Doctor Blackfan, and confirmed by ventriculogram. A month later a second ventriculogram showed a measurable increase in the size of the lateral ventricle, but the rate of growth was mark-

[6] In the December number of the *Annals of Surgery*, 1918, I presented a form of treatment for communicating hydrocephalus. If it should be possible, in a certain number of cases, to restore the channel of the cisternae, this treatment would be superior to a bilateral choroid plexectomy.

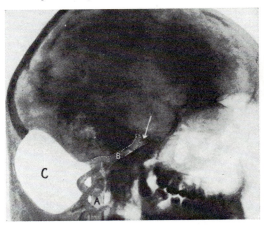

FIG. 5. Retouched photograph of a roentgenogram of the head, after an intraspinous injection of air. The patient was suffering from the effects of an intracranial tumor which was localized only by the aid of the air injection and after a cerebellar exploration had revealed no growth. The operative defect in the occipital bone can be seen. In this region an enormous collection (*C*) of cerebrospinal fluid has accumulated. This corresponds to a greatly enlarged cisterna magna. Even the upper part of the spinal cord is visible because the spinal canal is filled with air. *B*, cisterna medullaris and pontis. The arrow points to the block in the cisterna. Here a midbrain tumor was found and partially removed through a transcerebellar incision. It had closed both the aqueduct of Sylvius and the cisterna. The large collection of fluid (*C*) is due to the occlusion of the cisterna. It will be seen that none of the cerebral sulci contain air.

edly less than in the typical form of this disease. The air passed freely along the cisternæ and into the sulci over a very restricted area of the cerebral cortex (Fig. 6), not more than one-fourth of all the sulci showing the injection. Nor could it be determined whether the injected area was bilateral or unilateral. Exactly the same röntgenographic findings were present in the two X-rays taken a month apart; in fact the same convolutions could be traced in both. The sulci could be followed into the cisterna chiasmatica.

These data supply a new conception of the pathology of hydrocephalus. The inflammatory process has sealed off all the main branches which radiate from the cisternæ, with the exception of one or possibly more which supply the anterior fourth of the cerebral cortex on one or possibly both sides. Absorption of cerebrospinal fluid from this restricted area has been sufficient to retard to a great extent, though not to prevent, the development of hydrocephalus. Should more branches from the cisternæ subsequently open, it is quite probable that, owing to the increased absorption which would follow, the accumulation of fluid will be entirely arrested. Such a development could easily explain many spontaneous cures in hydrocephalus. It is very doubtful if these pathological changes in the brain would be detected at necropsy.

A third case was in a boy of nineteen, who was suffering from intracranial pressure. An internal hydrocephalus was discovered. But what had caused the hydrocephalus? From his symptoms a tentative diagnosis of a cerebellar tumor was made, and since the signs and symptoms pointed to both sides equally, a vermis tumor seemed most likely. After a thorough cerebellar exploration I was unable to find any trace of the tumor. The foramen of Magendie was normal. Three weeks after this operation, the phenolsulphonephthalein test showed that a complete obstruction was present at some point between the third ventricle and the foramen of Magendie. Air (120 c.c.), injected intraspinously, was stopped in the anterior end of the cisterna pontis; none reached the cerebral sulci (Fig. 5). These findings could admit of only one interpretation—the pressure of a tumor in the region of the aqueduct of Sylvius, which had occluded it and the cisterna pontis. At operation a tumor as large as a hickory nut was found in the midbrain, and partially removed after bisection of the vermis of the cerebellum. The iter had been completely obliterated by the tumor.

Another interesting radiographic finding in the case was the enormous amount of fluid which had collected at the base of the brain after the first operation. We have frequently noticed after cerebellar operations in which a tumor was not found that such an accumulation of fluid followed, but the explanation had never been clear. The X-ray picture seems to indicate that the closure of the cisternæ causes the fluid to accumulate, or, in other words, bring about a localized hydrocephalus; the fluid forms in the fourth ventricle (the iter being closed). Another point of interest in this röntgenogram is the sharp outline of the spinal cord (Fig. 5).

A fourth case was that of a boy of eighteen. Hydrocephalus of a year's standing had followed an acute illness which had been diagnosed as measles. At operation the hydrocephalus was found to be due to closure of the foramina of Luschka and Magendie by dense adhesions. I made a new foramen of Magendie and wanted to be

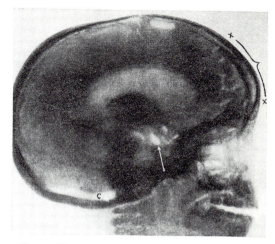

Fig. 6. Photograph of roentgenogram of head after injection of air into ventricle (not retouched). This patient had an early hydrocephalus following acute cerebrospinal meningitis. Only a small area of the cerebral sulci contain air (cf. brackets between X and X on surface). The obstruction which caused the hydrocephalus was not in the cisternæ but in the main branches which radiate to the sulci. The arrow points to the cisternæ which appear as a series of "blotches"; part of this appearance is probably due to the dilated trunks (obstructed above) which pass from the cisternæ to the cerebral sulci. The partial filling of the cerebral sulci (X to X) explains the slow development of the hydrocephalus. C, cisterna magna.

sure that it was functioning before allowing the patient to go home. Six weeks after the operation, air injected into the ventricles passed through the new foramen of Magendie and filled the cisterna magna and many of the cerebral sulci. We now could feel certain not only that the foramen of Magendie was patent, but also that all the subarachnoid space was receiving cerebrospinal fluid for absorption. The boy has since resumed his studies in college.

It also seems probable that we shall be able to localize spinal cord tumors by means of intraspinous injections of air. In one of our cases (Fig. 5) the spinal cord and the surrounding air-filled space are sharply outlined. Should the spinal canal be obliterated, either by a tumor or possibly by an inflammatory process, it is conceivable that the air shadow will extend up to the level of the lesion. Its intensity will naturally be greatly reduced by the great density of the spine, and particularly of the bodies of the vertebræ. A lateral view of the spine, by eliminating the maximum amount of bone, will probably give the best results. If the spinal canal is not obliterated by the tumor, the injected air will pass freely into the intracranial subarachnoid space, none being left in the spinal canal. This happened in one of our cases in which a spinal cord tumor was sus-

pected. The passage of air into the brain was difficult to explain at the time of the injection, as the
symptoms had been present for four years and a
tumor of such duration would certainly have
blocked the spinal canal. At operation a chronic
transverse myelitis was found. Instead of an enlargement of the spinal cord, there was a constriction, which readily explained the failure of air to
stop at the suspected zone.

As yet we have not had an opportunity of studying the radiographic findings in tumors of the
cerebral hemispheres. It is conceivable that local
effects may be noted in the sulci, or possibly even
the direct or indirect effects of pressure on the
cisternæ may be discovered.

The practical value of intraspinous injections
has been thoroughly established by the results in
the few cases here reported. As a matter of fact,
we shall often be able to localize a tumor from
either a ventriculogram or from an X-ray of the
subarachnoid space alone, an analysis of the signs
and symptoms of the individual case enabling us
to determine which should be tried first. From the
data obtainable from the combination of intraventricular and intraspinous injections it is difficult to see how intracranial tumors can escape
localization.

CONCLUSIONS

1. By substituting air for cerebrospinal fluid
through a lumbar puncture, all parts of the subarachnoid space can be clearly seen in a röntgenogram.

2. Not infrequently, an air shadow will completely surround the cerebellum, showing clearly
its size and shape.

3. The spinal cord can be seen surrounded by a
column of air.

4. The cisternæ appear as large collections of
air at the base of the brain; the cerebral sulci as a
network of tortuous filaments of air.

5. After an intraspinous injection, provided
that the subarachnoid space is intact, the air will
always fill the cerebral sulci.

6. But if the cisternæ are blocked at any point
by a tumor or adhesions, the air will not be able to
reach the cerebral sulci.

7. The exact position of the obstruction in the
cisternæ can often be seen in the radiogram. In
one of our cases of communicating hydrocephalus,
the obstruction was in the cisterna pontis. In a
second case of communicating hydrocephalus the
cisternæ were patent but all except one or two of
the main branches were occluded. In a third case
a tumor was located in the midbrain solely by
means of the radiogram.

8. In a case of hydrocephalus, air passed from
the spinal canal into the lateral ventricle, demonstrating the patency (and dilatation) of the
foramina of Magendie and Luschka, the aqueduct
of Sylvius, and the foramen of Monro. The
hydrocephalus was, therefore, of the communicating type.

9. A case of hydrocephalus was cured by con-
structing a new foramen of Magendie. Six weeks
later, air injected into the ventricles passed
through the new foramen, showing that it was
still functioning. The air also filled the cerebral
sulci, an indication that the entire arachnoid space
was patent.

EXPLANATION OF FIGURES

Much detail is lost in photographing and re-
producing the figures. Figs. 1, 2 and 6 have not
been retouched. Figs. 3, 4 and 5 have been retouched (even to the extent of being almost
diagrammatic) in order to show clearly the essential details which otherwise would have been lost
to the reader.

Neurosurgical Classics—17 and 18

Shortly after the introduction of air myelography for the demonstration of spinal tumors[1,2,5,6,13,14] Sicard and Forestier described positive contrast myelography employing an iodized poppy-seed oil (Lipiodol).[3,7–10,12] Because this procedure provided sharper contrast and easier interpretation, it initially received widespread interest. However, it was soon found to be associated frequently with meningeal irritation. In addition, the viscidity of Lipiodol led to occasional false filling-defects, and made its complete removal difficult. Because of these problems, the interest in Lipiodol myelography waned, and it was not often performed after 1930.

During the following ten years, neurosurgeons became aware of the disease process of protrusion of the intervertebral discs, and interest in myelography was again stimulated. A number of new contrast media were proposed, but most were discarded because of unpleasant side effects.[12] In 1941, the relatively nonirritating iodine-containing oil, Pantopaque, was introduced.[4,11,12] This oil, less viscid than Lipiodol, was found to outline better the finer structure of the spinal canal, and proved easier to remove. Since that time, no better contrast medium for myelography has been introduced.[4]

The two papers reproduced below represent the two major steps in the development of present-day myelography.

References

1. Arnell, S. Myelography with water-soluble contrast, with special regard to the normal roentgenpicture. *Acta radiol., Stockh.,* 1948, suppl. 75, 85 pp.
2. Bingel, A. Intralumbale Lufteinblasung zur Höhendiagnose intraduraler extramedullärer Prozesse und zur Differentialdiagnose gegenüber intramedullären Prozessen. *Dtsch. Z. Nervenheilk.,* 1921, *72:* 359–370.
3. Bucy, P. C. Jean Athanase Sicard (1872–1929). In: *The founders of neurology.* W. Haymaker, Ed. Springfield, Ill.: Charles C Thomas, 1953, xxvii, 479 pp. (see pp. 382–385).
4. Bull, J. W. D. History of neuroradiology. *Brit. J. Radiol.,* 1961, *34:* 69–84.
5. Dandy, W. E. The diagnosis and localization of spinal cord tumors. *Ann. Surg.,* 1925, *81:* 223–254.
6. Jacobaeus, H. C. On insufflation of air into the spinal canal for diagnostic purposes in cases of tumors in the spinal canal. *Acta med. scand.,* 1921, *55:* 555–564.
7. Sicard, J.-A., and Forestier, J. Méthode radiographique d'exploration de la cavité épidurale par le Lipiodol. *Rev. neurol.,* 1921, *37:* 1264–1266.
8. Sicard, [J.-A.], and Forestier, [J.] Méthode générale d'exploration radiologique par l'huile iodée (lipiodol). *Bull. Soc. méd. Hôp. Paris,* 1922, 3 s. *46:* 463–468.
9. Sicard, J.-A., and Forestier, J. Diagnostic et thérapeutique par le Lipiodol. Clinique et radiologie. *Paris: Masson & Cie.,* 1928, 370 pp. (see pp. 51–140).
10. Sicard, J. A., and Forestier, J. The use of lipiodol in diagnosis and treatment. A clinical and radiological survey. *London: Oxford University Press,* 1932, ix, 235 pp.
11. Steinhausen, T. B., Dungan, C. E., Furst, J. B., Plati, J. T., Smith, S. W., Darling, A. P., Wolcott, E. C., Jr., Warren, S. L., and Strain, W. H. Iodinated organic compounds as contrast media for radiographic diagnoses. III. Experimental and clinical myelography with ethyl iodophenylundecylate (Pantopaque). *Radiology,* 1944, *43:* 230–234.
12. Walker, A. E. Diagnostic procedures. In: *A history of neurological surgery.* A. E. Walker, Ed. Baltimore: Williams & Wilkins Co., 1951, xii, 583 pp. (see pp. 23–39).
13. Widerøe, S. Om intraspinal luftinjektion og om dens diagnostiske betydning ved rygmarvslidelser, saerlig ved svulster. *Norsk. Mag. Laegevidensk.,* 1921, *82:* 491–495.
14. Widerøe, S. Über die diagnostische Bedeutung der intraspinalen Luftinjektionen bei Rückenmarksleiden, besonders bei Geschwülsten. *Zbl. Chir.,* 1921, *48:* 394–397.

GENERAL METHOD OF RADIOLOGICAL EXPLORATION BY IODIZED OIL (LIPIODOL)*

By Messrs. Sicard and Forestier

For a long time it has been recognized that the preparation of iodized oil, the so-called Lipiodol,

---

* Translation of Méthode générale d'exploration radiologique par l'huile iodée (lipiodol), by MM. Sicard and Forestier, *Bull. Soc. méd Hôp. Paris,* 1922, 3 s. *46:* 463–468, printed with the kind permission of La Societé Médicale des Hôpitaux de Paris.

has the capacity to stop X-rays. However, radiologists have pointed out this fact only as a matter of simple curiosity.

We have thought that this particular quality of Lipiodol could be applied usefully to the radiological study of the cavities of the body. The results obtained have confirmed our hypothesis.

Lipiodol results from the complete and total combination of iodine and poppy-seed oil (Lafay). (We owe Mr. Lafay thanks for the liberality with which he has made Lipiodol available to us, as well as for the determinations of iodine which he has been kind enough to make in patients subjected to this medication.) Iodine is found concealed in this combination. The product is transparent, keeps the coloring of the original oil, but appears of a great density, not supernatant, but falling to the bottom of the water. Under the influence of a long stay in the open air, it becomes blackish, "and in this case it is preferable not to inject it" (Lafay). One cc. of iodized oil contains about 0.54 gm. of iodine. This oleo-iodine is tolerated remarkably by the tissues. We have sometimes injected it in a dose of 10–12 cc. in a single lumbar-muscle hypodermic injection without provoking more than a local reaction of a transitory type. It causes no redness of the skin, it leaves no hardened tissue, and out of several hundred injections we have noted neither abscess nor general or local incident, and no appreciable tendency to encystment or to *vaselinome*. The injections can be repeated with impunity, even daily, into muscular or cellular tissues, up to an aggregate amount of 80–100 cc. (we have not yet exceeded this figure) without provoking the least sign of intolerance. It can be injected intravenously (Rathery).

Furthermore, because of its heavy density, Lipiodol responds to gravity and passes readily into cavities or muscular interstices. It gives, either with impregnations at some distance removed from the original site of injection (fluid cavities and cerebrospinal fluid, for example) or with uninterrupted passages through tissues (muscles, epidural cellular tissue, etc.), movements of iodized oil of great interest to follow under radiological control. It remains visible radiologically for a long time in the tissues.

Thus, it is proved that Lipiodol combines all requisite conditions for exploring the cavities of the body without danger: great opacity to X-rays, absence of causticity and of toxicity, absolute tolerance, capacity for passage and prolonged visibility.

We first studied in a therapeutic and diagnostic respect the action of Lipiodol injected into the epidural cavity in patients with lumbar hyperesthesia, lumbar arthritis, or in those with lumbo-ischialgia (see Sicard and Forestier. Exploration de la cavité épidurale par le lipiodol. Societé de Neurologie, December 1921). We have, thus, obtained most convincing radiological illustrations.

The epidural cavity can be approached by the sacrococcygeal hiatus, as we have already demonstrated, or through the yellow ligaments all along the vertebral segments.

Sacrococcygeal injection of 2 cc. of Lipiodol permits, as soon as the day following injection, recognizing radiographically the epidural upward extension of the oleo-iodine to about the 5th lumbar vertebra. Tracks and spaces of iodized oil appear at the level of the sacral canals.

Epidural injection of Lipiodol made higher up by the lumbar method in the way of ordinary spinal puncture—rachicentesis—(but with a special trocar needle designed to avoid the opening of the dura mater and the egress of cerebrospinal fluid) permits seeing as early as a few hours after injection the lower extension of the oleo-iodine to the coccyx. If by a mechanical contrivance, such as placing blocks of wood under the feet of the bed, a kind of so-called static Trendelenburg position maintained for some ten hours is realized in the patient so injected, radiography will permit revealing, after this lapse of time, the high epidural localization of the iodized oil to the vicinity sometimes of the upper dorsal vertebrae, and that is realized by the tracks of iodized oil uninterrupted from the point of original departure of the injection.

It is understood that, according to the amount of Lipiodol injected, 2–6 cc. for example, and according to the point-of-reference epidural stages, the epidural cavity can be consulted methodically in its different segments when there is investigation, for instance, of a neoplastic diagnosis or one of Pott's disease, indicated by pressure.

The epidural injections of iodized oil are painless and remain painless. The radiographic pictures become fixed almost definitely twenty-four hours after injection. The extension is halted from that time on and the resorption of the Lipiodol is so slowly produced that radiologic pictures taken in case of need, even several months later, are hardly altered. Patients with lumbar hyperesthesia, lumbar arthritis, and lumbo-ischialgia benefit remarkably from the direct epidural therapy.

Injection of Lipiodol made no longer into the epidural cavity *but into the cerebrospinal fluid* after lumbar puncture is well tolerated, with this reservation, however, that the habituation of the subarachnoid sac to the foreign substance of iodized oil is accomplished only after a painful period of 2–3 days. It is necessary to warn about the appearance during this initial stage, 6–7 hours after injection, of symptoms of pain in the legs; namely, various paresthesias and formications, transitory reactions which are lessened markedly by the classic injection of morphine. Furthermore, these reactions are a function of the injected dose of iodized oil. They are at least reduced when the amount of the injection into the cerebrospinal fluid does not exceed 0.5 cc., but even in higher doses of 5–6 cc. the action of the sphincter has never been disturbed.

The Lipiodol in the subarachnoid sac obeys the effect of gravity. It collects, in the standing position, entirely at the bottom of the terminal sacral space, which it delineates as tapering into a point. In the dorsal or lateral decubitus, the Lipiodol extends into the stratum that spreads out along the posterior or lateral spinal tracts. It then forms a sheath around these tracts which detaches itself and is blackish, at radiography, over an extent of several centimeters. The Lipiodol in the cerebrospinal fluid persists for months without a tendency toward resorption. After this initial period of adaptation of 2–3 days, it is tolerated remarkably without provoking any trouble.

Injection of Lipiodol made into the lumbar subarachnoid space has given us very encouraging therapeutic results during tabes with shooting pains of the lower limbs and, likewise, during certain forms of syphilitic paraplegia.

We pass quickly over other more or less isolated attempts at injection of iodized oil into the cerebral arachnoid mater in general paralysis or into fistulous passages, articular collections of fluid, and urethral strictures. Our medical practice in this respect is still too limited.

On the other hand, we have pursued the study of this procedure applied to exploration of the broncho-pulmonary tree. . . . Thus, iodized oil in organic combination of high concentration appears to us tolerated perfectly by the lung. One should be able to use it as a potent therapeutic agent because of its content in active principle and in the non-injurious form in which it is found. However, again, because of its opacity for X-rays, it permits carrying out on the living a radiological exploration of certain portions of the trachea and of the bronchi in a manner such as that used for the digestive passages.

It has seemed to us that, in its entirety, this method of new investigation by Lipiodol with respect to the cavities that up to now have remained unexplored radiologically, such as the epidural and the subarachnoid cavities, or the tracheobronchial-pulmonary tree, would be interesting to call to your attention and productive of practical deductions.

IODINATED ORGANIC COMPOUNDS AS CONTRAST MEDIA FOR RADIOGRAPHIC DIAGNOSES

III. Experimental and Clinical Myelography with Ethyl Iodophenylundecylate (Pantopaque)[*][1]

THEODORE B. STEINHAUSEN, M.D., CLARENCE E. DUNGAN, M.D., JOSEPH B. FURST, M.D., JOHN T. PLATI, PH.D., S. WILLARD SMITH, M.D., A. PERRY DARLING, M.D., and E. CLINTON WOLCOTT, JR.,

with

STAFFORD L. WARREN, M.D. AND WILLIAM H. STRAIN, PH.D.

Department of Radiology, School of Medicine and Dentistry, The University of Rochester, Rochester, N. Y.

Ethyl iodophenylundecylate is one of a number of iodinated organic liquids that has been studied as a contrast medium for myelography. This new medium is a mixture of isomeric esters of which the principal constituent is probably that shown in the accompanying formula. It contains 30.5 per cent iodine and has a density of 1.263 at 20°C. The name Pantopaque[2] was coined for this mixture to provide radiologists and clinicians with a convenient designation. The chemistry of this and of related diagnostic aids is discussed elsewhere (1, 2).

$$I-\langle\!\!\langle\rangle\!\!\rangle-\overset{\displaystyle CH_3}{\underset{\displaystyle |}{CH}}-(CH_2)_8COOC_2H_5$$

Ethyl iodophenylundecylate (provisional)

Prior to its clinical use, ethyl iodophenylundecylate was tested intrathecally in dogs in a series of comparative experiments against iodized poppy-seed oil. In these tests the new medium proved to be much easier to handle, produced discomfort of shorter duration, and in most of the animals was almost completely absorbed within a year. The clinical results have paralleled those obtained in animal experimentation.

As is shown in Table I, iodized poppy-seed oil is

TABLE I

Coefficients of Viscosity of Myelographic Media

Medium	$\eta^{25°C.}$	$\eta^{37.5°C.}$
Ethyl iodophenylundecylate	0.372	0.217
Iodized poppy-seed oil	8.06	3.76
Ratio	1:22	1:17

* Reprinted from *Radiology*, 1944, *43:* 230–234, with the kind permission of The Radiological Society of North America, Inc.

[1] These studies were aided by a grant from the Research Laboratories of the Eastman Kodak Company. They were presented before the Radiological Society of North America, at its Twenty-eighth Annual Meeting, Chicago, Ill., Nov. 30–Dec. 4, 1942, and submitted for publication in June 1944.

[2] Pantopaque is a registered trade-mark.

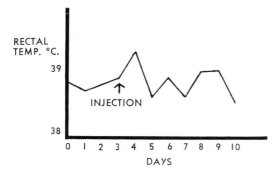

CHART 1. Typical transient fever following intrathecal injection of ethyl iodophenylundecylate in dogs.

twenty-two times as viscous as ethyl iodophenylundecylate at 25°C., and seventeen times as viscous at 37.5°C. Because the new medium is so
fluid, it is easily injected or removed with an 18- or
20-gauge needle and flows freely in the spinal
canal immediately after injection. In dogs, however, where lumbar punctures are nearly impossible, and where the space relations of the canal
are such that both media flow very slowly, practically none of the injected material can be removed.

Following intrathecal injection of 3 to 5 cc. of
ethyl iodophenylundecylate in dogs, there is a
period of slight fever, lasting one or two days, as is
shown in Chart I. During this time. the dogs are
clinically well, but a fair proportion may exhibit
mild distress when the head is bent. After two or
three days, however, this symptom disappears.
With iodized poppy-seed oil, on the other hand,
there is no fever, but the period of distress when
the head is bent may persist for ten to fourteen
days. Sections taken from the spinal cords of dogs
sacrificed at varying intervals show that both
media are encysted after a lapse of about six
weeks. The encystment is particularly noticeable
in the cauda equina area and is not found generally throughout the cord. Typical sections showing the type of encystment that occurs are reproduced in Figure 1. As is evident from these photo-
micrographs, the size of the cysts with ethyl
iodophenylundecylate is considerably less than
that of those produced by iodized poppy-seed oil;
this is probably referable to the greater viscosity
of the poppy-seed oil. Cord sections taken at
intervals from dogs injected intrathecally with
ethyl iodophenylundecylate show that the physiological response about the cysts is essentially a
foreign body reaction.

Acute toxicities for ethyl iodophenylundecylate
were determined by intraperitoneal and intravenous injections. The LD 50 for intraperitoneal
injections was found to be 4.6 gm./kilogram for
mice and 19 gm./kilogram for rats. Control experiments with iodized poppy-seed oil showed no

toxic effects with rats even when the medium was
injected intraperitoneally at a level of 25 gm./
kilogram. The injected ethyl iodophenylundecylate was completely absorbed in six weeks, however, while the iodized poppy-seed oil was not
absorbed during the life of the experimental
animal. The more rapid rate of absorption of the
new medium may well be the sole cause of its
relatively greater toxicity. Intravenous injections
in dogs showed that ethyl iodophenylundecylate
was without effect at a level of 0.5 gm./kilogram
but was lethal at a level of 1.0 gm./kilogram.
Emulsification with water containing small
amounts of Igepon T (sodium olelylmethyl-
taurine) or of methyl cellulose reduced the toxicity
considerably, and doses of 1.0 gm./kilogram were
given intravenously to dogs with safety.

With the assurance from these experimental
studies that the new medium was safe, it was first
tested clinically on Nov. 23, 1940, by Drs. Paul
Garvey and Nathaniel Jones in Case I, reported
below. The absence of untoward developments

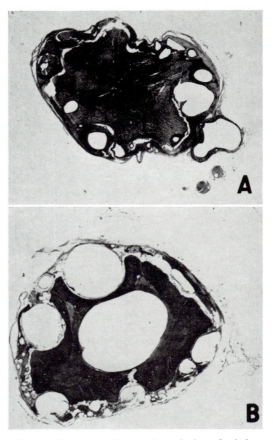

FIG. 1. Cyst formation in the spinal cord of dogs
following intrathecal injection of (A) ethyl iodophenylundecylate and (B) of iodized poppy-seed oil. The
sections represent extremes in pathology.

led to its use in 4 additional patients. The satisfactory outcome in these first few cases was followed by a wider use, until now the new medium has been tested in numerous clinics. The most extensive series of cases[3] have been compiled by Dr. William P. Van Wagenen (Rochester, N.Y.), Dr. R. Glen Spurling (Louisville, Ky.), and Dr. William V. Cone (Montreal, Canada). From their experience it is evident that the best results are obtained if 3 to 5 c.c. of ethyl iodophenylundecylate are injected and later removed by the general procedure of Kubik and Hampton (3). In this way up to 90 per cent of the injected medium is easily removed and the small amount of residuum is completely absorbed within a few weeks.

[3] As of November 1942.

Case Histories

CASE I (Unit No. 171887): A 53-year-old male with complete paralysis from the waist down as the result of pressure on the dorsal cord from a dissecting aortic aneurysm was injected on Nov. 23, 1940, with 5 c.c. of ethyl iodophenylundecylate at L4 after removal of 8 c.c. of crystal-clear spinal fluid. Fluoroscopy showed a persistent constriction at L3 and L4, and also between L4 and L5. The patient experienced no reaction from the injection. Death occurred from a rupture of the aneurysm seventeen days later. A postmortem examination showed that the contrast medium was still mobile. Sections (Fig. 3) of the spinal cord showed a few polymorphonuclear cells around the nerve roots. There was no evidence of encystment in any portion of the cord.

CASE II (Unit No. 173025): A 28-year-old white male with embryoma of the left testicle with bone and pul-

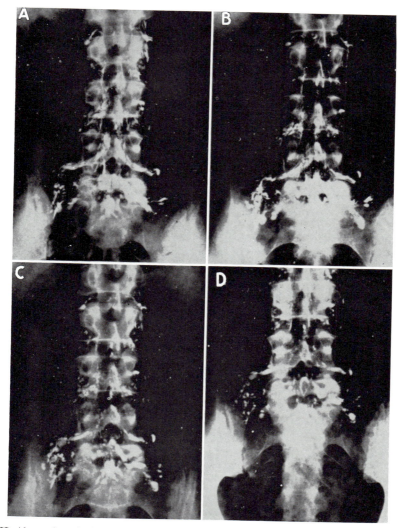

FIG. 2. Case II: Absorption of ethyl iodophenylundecylate in unusual case in which the nerve sheaths are filled with the medium. A. Immediately after injection. B. After three days. C. After forty days. D. After five months.

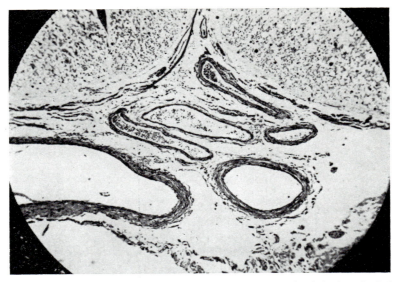

FIG. 3. Case I: Section from the spinal cord seventeen days after injection of ethyl
iodophenylundecylate. A few polymorphonuclear cells are seen.

monary metastases was injected with 5 c.c. of ethyl
iodophenylundecylate on Jan. 7, 1941. Films (Fig. 2)
taken at intervals up to May 29, 1941, show a gradual
absorption of over half of the injected contrast medium.
Immediately after injection the Pantopaque became
immobile as a result of filling the nerve sheaths, particularly the sheaths of the sciatic nerves. During the week
immediately following the injection, the patient had a
slight paresthesia in the lower leg. Otherwise there were
no clinical symptoms. Death occurred at home and an
autopsy was not obtained.

CASE III (Unit No. 183121): A 29-year-old female

with clinical symptoms of a ruptured nucleus pulposus
was injected on Sept. 9, 1942, with 3 c.c. of ethyl iodophenylundecylate. A diagnosis of extra-medullary compression between L4 and L5 was somewhat equivocal.
The contrast medium was removed and the patient was
placed on fracture boards. On Sept. 21, 1942, 3 c.c. of
Pantopaque was again injected, but fluoroscopy showed
that some of it was extradural. For several days the
patient experienced increased leg pain, especially after
manipulation. Finally, on Sept. 28, 1942, a third examination was made with 3 c.c. of ethyl iodophenylundecylate and a positive diagnosis of a lesion at the disk space

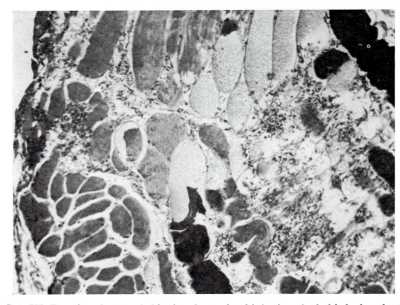

FIG. 4. Case III: Reaction about probable site of extradural injection of ethyl iodophenylundecylate.

of L4 on the left side was obtained. A laminectomy was performed on Sept. 30. A section taken at the probable site of the extradural injection showed striated muscle and fibrous tissue. In the section reproduced in Figure 4 dense fibrous connective tissue is seen having a structure consistent with that of ligamentum flavum. In this tissue there is no evidence of any inflammatory reaction. Other portions of the section show striated muscle and areas of fairly loose connective tissue. Some of the striated muscle bundles appear to contain more than their normal number of nuclei, while others show considerable degenerative change. Instead of normal striated myofibrils the muscle sheaths contain a granular débris. This degeneration could be due to some local irritant, but similar changes are often seen without any known foreign matter in the vicinity. Several areas of the less dense connective tissue show infiltration by polymorphonuclear leukocytes in addition to many small round cells and a few larger monocytes. No definite droplets of contrast medium are seen, and there is no localized focal necrosis or abscess formation.

Summary

Ethyl iodophenylundecylate (Pantopaque), a new contrast medium for myelography, is more fluid and is therefore more easily injected and removed than previously described oil-type contrast media. In addition to these physical advantages, the medium is absorbed from the subarachnoid space with relative rapidity.

260 Crittenden Blvd.
Rochester 7, N. Y.

References

1. STRAIN, W. H., PLATI, J. T., AND WARREN, S. L. J. Am. Chem. Soc. 64: 1436, 1942.
2. PLATI, J. T., WITH STRAIN, W. H., and WARREN, S. L. J. Am. Chem. Soc. 65: 1273, 1943.
3. KUBIK, C. S. and HAMPTON, A. O. New England J. Med. 224: 455, 1941.

Neurosurgical Classic—19

CAROTID arteriography is used widely as a diagnostic procedure in modern neurosurgery. The development of this important technique primarily was the result of the efforts of one man—Antonio Caetano de Abreu Freire Egas Moniz.

Egas Moniz led an unusually varied and productive life.[3,16,18] His nonmedical achievements alone were impressive. As a politician, Egas Moniz created and directed the Centrist Party. He was a political prisoner at one point in his career, and at another he was almost killed by a schizophrenic assassin. During the first World War, Egas Moniz was the Portuguese Ambassador in Madrid, and later Minister of Foreign Affairs. He was also president of the Portuguese delegation to the Paris Peace Conference in 1918. In 1951 he was asked to be President of Portugal, but he refused. Egas Moniz also was active in other fields. He wrote an operetta, taught mathematics, fought a duel, became a gourmet, and still found time to write on the history of playing cards and to publish a biography of Pope John XXI.

Even more outstanding were the medical achievements of Egas Moniz. After distinguishing himself as a student at the University of Coimbra, he studied neurology at La Salpêtrière with Raymond, Pierre Marie and Dejerine, and at L'Hôpital de la Pitié with Babinski. Egas Moniz became a professor of medicine at the age of 28, the first occupant of the chair of neurology at the University of Lisbon, and the author of over 300 medical publications. Partly in collaboration with the neurosurgeon Pedro Manuel de Almeida Lima, he developed two major neurosurgical techniques—carotid arteriography and prefrontal leucotomy. The latter work brought Egas Moniz the 1949 Nobel Prize for physiology and medicine.

In developing carotid arteriography Egas Moniz persevered in the face of numerous difficulties.[3,16] Prior to his investigations, contrast radiography for neurological diagnosis had become known in the forms of ventriculography, encephalography, and myelography.[5,20–22] Techniques of carotid injection had been described, and radiographic studies of the anatomy of various organs had been performed in cadavers by arterial injections of radiopaque materials.[6,15,19] Egas Moniz applied these ideas and techniques to his project, but the applications were not easy.[3,5] Even after a number of contrast media had been screened carefully in animals, those thought safe for human experimentation were shown to cause irritation of tissue and pain. The percutaneous injection of the internal carotid artery was tried in four patients. This proved so difficult that it was supplanted by direct injection after surgical exposure of the artery. Other problems were posed by the intravascular dilution of the contrast medium, and the inadequacies of the available radiological equipment. While a successful technique was being developed, nine patients were given intracarotid injections. Of these, six subsequently had transient neurological symptoms and one died. To the credit of Egas Moniz, he persevered and gained eventual success.

Numerous papers on carotid arteriography were published by Egas Moniz and his collaborators in 1927[5–9] and the ensuing years. In 1931 Egas Moniz presented his studies at the First International Neurological Congress in Bern,[10,17] and published a book describing his first 180 arteriograms.[11] Other volumes by Egas Moniz and by Almeida Lima followed.[1,2,12–14] With later improvements in contrast material, techniques of injection, and radiological equipment, carotid arteriography became employed widely.[19] It has fulfilled the expectations of Egas Moniz in the diagnosis of intracranial neoplasms. But more important, carotid arteriography has permitted the modern neurosurgical attack on carotid and cerebral vascular lesions.[4,16]

The initial report by Egas Moniz, which was presented to the Société de Neurologie in Paris on July 7, 1927, is reproduced below.

References

1. ALMEIDA LIMA, P. Contribuição para o estudo da circulação dos tumores intracranianos. Lisbon, 1938. Cited by Almeida Lima[2] (p. 95).
2. ALMEIDA LIMA, P. Cerebral angiography. London: Oxford University Press, 1950, xiii, 221 pp.
3. BULL, J. W. D. History of neuroradiology. Brit. J. Radiol., 1961, 34: 69–84.
4. BULL, J. W. D. A short history of intracranial aneurysms. Lond. clin. med. J., 1962, 3: 47–61.
5. EGAS MONIZ. L'encéphalographie artérielle, son importance dans la localisation des tumeurs cérébrales. Rev. neurol., 1927, 2: 72–89.
6. EGAS MONIZ. A prova da encefalografia arterial. Lisboa méd., 1927, 4: 297–344.
7. EGAS MONIZ. Injections intracarotidiennes et substances injectables opaques aux rayons X. Pr. méd., 1927, 35: 969–971.
8. EGAS MONIZ. La radioartériographie cérébrale. Bull. Acad. Méd., Paris, 1927, 98: 40–45.
9. EGAS MONIZ. Radiografia das artérias cerebrais. J. Soc. Sci. med. Lisboa, 1927, 91: 323–335.
10. EGAS MONIZ. La localisation des tumeurs cérébrales par l'encéphalographie artérielle. Proc. first int. neurol. Congr. (Bern, 1931), 1931, xxv, 440 pp. (see pp. 61–66).
11. EGAS MONIZ. Diagnostic des tumeurs cérébrales et épreuve de l'encéphalographie artérielle. Paris: Masson & Cie, 1931, iii, 512 pp.
12. EGAS MONIZ. L'angiographie cérébrale. Ses applications et résultats en anatomie, physiologie et clinique. Paris: Masson & Cie, 1934, 327 pp.
13. EGAS MONIZ. Clinica della angiografia cerebrale. Torino: I.T.E.R., 1938, 142 pp.
14. EGAS MONIZ. Die cerebrale Arteriographie und Phlebographie. Berlin: J, Springer, 1940, viii, 413 pp.
15. KNAUER, A. Ueber die Behandlung der Paralyse und der Hirnsyphilis mit Salvarsaninjektionen in die Karotiden. Münch. med. Wschr., 1919, 66: 609–611.
16. PERINO, F. R. Egas Moniz. Founder of psychosurgery, creator of angiography. Nobel Prize winner, 1874–1958. J. int. Coll. Surg., 1961, 36: 261–271.
17. SACHS, E. The history and development of neurological surgery. New York: P. B. Hoeber, Inc., 1952, 158 pp. (see p. 81).
18. STEVENSON, L. G. Nobel prize winners in medicine and physiology, 1901–1950. New York: H. Schuman, Inc., 1953, ix, 291 pp. (see pp. 264–271).
19. WALKER, A. E. Diagnostic procedures. In: A history of neurological surgery. A. E. Walker, Ed. Baltimore: Williams & Wilkins Co., 1951, xii, 583 pp. (see pp. 23–39).
20. WILKINS, R. H. Neurosurgical classic—VII. J. Neurosurg., 1963, 20: 450–458.
21. WILKINS, R. H. Neurosurgical classic—VIII. J. Neurosurg., 1963, 20: 531–536.
22. WILKINS, R. H. Neurosurgical classic—X. J. Neurosurg., 1963, 20: 721–727.

ARTERIAL ENCEPHALOGRAPHY, ITS IMPORTANCE IN THE LOCALIZATION OF CEREBRAL TUMORS*

By EGAS MONIZ

(Institut d'Investigations scientifiques Rocha Cabral et de la Clinique neurologique de Lisbonne)

THE Sicard test of intraspinal injections of Lipiodol has rendered important services in the localization of medullary compression. At the same time it has constituted a big step forward in semeiology, for the principle of putting into relief the radiographic opacity of the Lipiodol introduced into the cavities of the body has overtaken neurology and has become a general method which has progressed daily.

Recently the pathology of the gall bladder has been clarified considerably by the method of Graham, Cole and Copher. They have founded their experiments upon the action of certain preparations of phthalein and their selective elimination by bile, which was demonstrated by Abel and Rowestre for the study of the functional capacity of the liver. Graham, Cole and Copher started their work in 1923. They sought a compound with a phenolphthalein base with a fairly high atomic weight, such as, for instance, bromine or iodine, which, eliminated by the biliary channels, would show up the bladder as opaque to x-rays. They selected intravenous sodium tetraiodophenolphthalein and demonstrated the possibility of obtaining good pictures of the bladder in the dog. The American authors recognized at the beginning that the substance used was fairly toxic and replaced it with sodium tetrabromophenolphthalein. With bromine and iodine they obtained the desired results, except that the radiographic effects of iodine were more clearly visible than those of bromine.

After prolonged experimentation the authors decided upon phenoltetraiodophthalein as the most-to-be-recommended product, if it is pure. The undesirable effects on the animals, in some cases fatal, which were observed at the beginning with sodium tetraiodophenolphthalein were caused by impurities of the products. This was why they preferred the brominated compounds, which are less toxic but had to be used in larger quantities.

Having discovered the substance, it was now

---

* Translation of: L'encéphalographie artérielle, son importance dans la localisation des tumeurs cérébrales. Revue neurologique, 1927, 2: 72–89. Printed with the kind permission of Masson & Cie, Paris, France,

necessary to study the means of entry. The gastric route, the intestinal, either by the introduction of coated substances or by using an Einhorn duodenal tube, and the rectal route have been practically abandoned.

Graham, Cole and Copher preferred the intravenous route, as being the most practical and the simplest, but taking special precautions with the manner of introducing the substance.

Phenolphthalein generally is used in a dose of 4 grams per 35 cc. of recently distilled water. The intravenous injection is pushed in very slowly, because the fall in arterial pressure is troublesome with rapid injections.

The method of the American authors shows the advantages of using opaque substances in the study of cavities normally not shown up by x-rays.

We used another route in the hope of obtaining visualization of the brain through the opacity of its vessels, particularly the arteries. This is the direction taken by our work.

Ventriculography has already been carried out to define the position of cerebral tumors. We believed that if we succeeded in visualizing the cerebral arterial network, it would also be possible to localize tumors on the basis of the alterations shown in the contexture of the arterial framework.

Before summarizing our experiments and our results in animals and humans, we should glance at the ventriculographic data obtained, as being an element in the diagnosis of cerebral tumors.

We are indebted to Dandy for the method of radiographic visualization of the lateral ventricles. His first note is dated 1918.[1] Since then, Dandy and his associates have published other works and British and German neurologists have taken up this direction to obtain the localization of cerebral tumors by the study of the differences in appearance of the normal ventricles and those in brains with neoplasms.

The most commonly used substance for obtaining radiographic contrast was air. Oxygen or CO_2 has also been injected. Dandy has used thorium, potassium iodide, collargol, Argyrol and bismuth substrate, but the results were poor. Sicard used rising Lipiodol, that is iodinated oil with a lower percentage of iodine than the descending Lipiodol. Jacobaeus and Schuster also used Lipiodol. But air still remains the preferred substance. Resorption varies from a few hours to a few weeks. It is introduced into the ventricles either directly, or in cisternal or lumbar injections (Purves Stewart).

Most authors prefer direct puncture. This is performed by means of a cranial trepanation, either, for the anterior horn, 2 cm. from the median line, somewhat forward from the frontoparietal suture, or for the posterior horn at a point situated 3 cm. behind and 3 cm. above the external auditory orifice (Kocher). Other authors have given different points (Grant, Sicard, etc.).

In general 5 to 10 cc. of cerebrospinal fluid is drawn from the ventricle, and an equal quantity of air is injected, after which we wait for 2 to 3 minutes. Pressure becomes roughly equal to atmospheric pressure. Next we inject 20 to 120 cc. of air.

However, the methods are fairly variable (Dandy, Bingel, etc.). The radiographs are made with a Potter-Buckey diaphragm.

Ventriculography has often provided valuable information for the localization of tumors; but there are radiographs that show a deformation of the ventricles and it is still rather difficult to define the precise point at which the neoplasm is situated.

Recently, A. Elsberg and S. Sittler[2] have made studies on cadavers of subjects who died of cerebral tumors, and upon making comparisons between ventriculographs and moulages they arrived at the following conclusions:

1. In the case of a tumor of the right posterior fossa, one sees a displacement outside the posterior horn of the right ventricle, with a reduction in the capacity of the right ventricle.

2. In the case of a tumor of the frontal and right temporal lobes, radiography shows a considerable lengthening of the distance between the anterior and posterior horns on the side of the tumor, while on the opposite side they come closer to one another. In the case of an occipital tumor there is a distention of the two horns showing roughly the same appearance.

In his book Jüngling[3] has shown a series of figures with fairly informative diagnosis. But interpretation often remains extremely difficult, and, at least in a large number of cases, does not provide an indisputable localization.

In a discussion of the *Section of Neurology of the Royal Society of Medicine*[4] the question was presented by Sargent, who considered that ventriculography was a clinical aid in the diagnosis of tumors. But he warned against the method being used more than in doubtful cases or cases impossible to diagnose by neurological means. Two questions arise in connection with ventriculography: the danger of air injection and

[1] W. E. Dandy. Ventriculography following the injection of air into the cerebral ventricles. *Annals of Surg.*, July 1918, p. 5.

——— Roentgenography of the brain after the injection of air into the spinal canal. *Annals of Surg.*, October 1919, p. 397.

[2] *Arch. of Neur. and Psych.*, October 1925.

[3] O. Jüngling and H. Peiper. *Ventrikulographie und Myelographie in der Diagnostik des Zentral-nervensystems*, Leipzig, 1926.

[4] Meeting held, April 10, 1924, *Brain*, 1924, p. 380.

the difficulty of a definite diagnosis even in cases with ventricular deformation.

Sargent makes ventriculographic interpretations dependent upon radiographic progress and upon generalization and perfectioning of radiological stereoscopy and the Potter-Buckey diaphragm.

The principal objection against ventriculography is the danger of air injections into the ventricles replacing cerebrospinal fluid. However, Sargent believes that this drawback could be modified with practice and experience. He even believes that such neurological exploration should be made by neurosurgeons, who, knowing the intracranial physiology, would, with their experience, be able to avoid surprises occasioned by such interventions.

At the end of 1924 he had made 13 injections in ten cases. One blind child with hydrocephalus died three days following the injection but the death could have been the result of natural causes.

Another patient, a woman with an unlocalized tumor who had undergone double puncturing of the posterior horns without yielding any cerebrospinal fluid, died seven days later. An autopsy was refused.

These two deaths made it clear to Sargent that the method should be used with caution.

McConnell has made ventriculographs in fifteen cases of cerebral tumors and in ten cases obtained the desired localization, which represents a fairly considerable percentage. He had two deaths, one eight hours, the other fourteen hours following the injection of air. In the two patients the tumor was situated in the posterior fossa of the cranium. In many cases he observed considerable reactions, which he attributed to the increased intracranial pressure. McConnell believes that the danger could be diminished by replacing the liquid with air in small quantities, 2 to 5 cc.

He recognizes that there are great difficulties in interpreting radiographs. For example, the posterior horn is often absent or cannot be distended. The absence of air does not signify that there is pressure at this point.

Wilfred Harris believes that ventriculography is so dangerous that it should only be used in very special cases. Jefferson is of roughly the same opinion. As to the method of injecting the air, most use direct introduction by cranial trepanation. McConnell always performs this at the Keen point; Sargent performs a double puncture of the posterior horns. James Stewart prefers the introduction of air by lumbar puncture. In his opinion this method is less severe and the results are the same. McConnell claims that this method is not preferable, since there is no assurance of filling the ventricles full of air.

From this discussion it may be deduced that there are two points upon which we must pause: 1.

the danger of the method, and 2. the difficulty in interpreting the radiographs, for, as was stated by Purves Stewart, even in the most successful cases one does not invariably obtain an indication of the position of the tumor.

As to the danger of ventriculography opinions of surgeons and neurologists are not in complete accord. Dandy regards it as very slightly dangerous. In his first 100 cases of ventriculography he had 3 deaths. Burgel, out of 200 or more, had only 2 deaths. Weigeldt, Schott and Eitel, Wartenberg, did not have any deaths out of a large number of cases. On the other hand other authors had a higher percentage. Adson, Ott and Crawford had 6 out of 72 cases; Grant, 5 out of 40; Denk, 7 out of 67; Jüngling, 8 out of 60.

Regarding the localization of tumors by ventriculography, the authors once again are not entirely in accord. Out of 97 ventriculographies (1922–23) Dandy was able to make a diagnosis in 32 cases. Grant, out of 40 cases, was able to confirm the diagnosis in 15 cases, etc.

In other words ventriculography is a method to be utilized in the localization of cerebral tumors, but one which must be undertaken with care and carried out with prudence. There are certain dangers that must be avoided and reduced. The diagnosis is not always definite and in some cases it cannot be made; but in those cases in which there is no other means of clarifying the diagnosis, and since we are dealing with gravely ill subjects, ventriculography, with all its dangers and uncertainties, is a method to be used and perfected.

De Martel does not believe the injection of air into the ventricles to be harmless. He lost two patients and prefers the injection of a colored substance, also suggested by Dandy. These have been very useful to him without in any way harming any of the patients undergoing this procedure. De Martel punctures the posterior horns of the two lateral ventricles. He extracts from one of the two ventricles a certain amount of cerebrospinal fluid (a few cubic centimeters). This liquid is replaced by the same amount of methylene blue. After a quarter of an hour of waiting a few cubic centimeters of cerebrospinal fluid are drawn from the other ventricle. If this liquid is blue in color, one may conclude that the two lateral ventricles and the third ventricle communicate to a large extent with one another. After another quarter of an hour the inferior cerebellar cistern is punctured; if this liquid is not colored, one may suspect the existence of a tumor of the lower part of the cranium, which by compressing the walls of the fourth ventricle, obstructs the aqueduct of Sylvius and prevents the passage of the colored liquid outside the third ventricle, or even of a tumor in the region of the third ventricle. Sometimes one cannot puncture one of the two lateral ventricles, and the dye injected into the other ventricle passes freely across the third and fourth ventricles. In this case one must consider the existence of a tumor situated on the side of the lateral ventricle which has not been punctured and the cavity of which is probably obliterated by pressure from the tumor.

This method, according to De Martel, who is far from being infallible, has made it possible for him on several occasions to diagnose "roughly" the site of the tumor on one of the hemispheres. Such a localization, even though approximate, could be very useful for the surgeon.

All the above descriptions justify some further investigations, although these seem even more hazardous. While ventriculography and intraventricular injections of dye, which are fairly dangerous, only provide information regarding localization of cerebral tumors in certain cases, the method of arterial encephalography which we are about to propose might help in resolving certain problems of localization. We do not regard this problem as having been completely solved, but the knowledge acquired is the first step on a road which appears to promise good results.

Patients with cranial hypertension, as a rule, reach the neurologist very late, either through the fault of the general practitioner who does not interpret the headaches and vomiting correctly and postpones examination of the fundus of the eye, or because the patients reach the ophthalmologist voluntarily only when vision is lost or practically lost. Often patients come and ask for our care when they are blind. Clinical interest is much reduced in these cases, particularly when other symptoms of hypertension (headaches, vomiting, etc.) are attenuated. Surgical intervention could never restore the patients' vision and in view of the uncertainty in the diagnosis of localization, most prefer not to be operated on in these circumstances. We do not advise this intervention even if localization has been made, once the headaches have disappeared or only occur very rarely. Such cases are generally lost to any kind of intervention.

In the case of patients who come for consultation in the first phase of papillary edema, even if we do not have a diagnosis of probable localization, immediate cranial decompression is indicated. But if we were able to diagnose the site of the tumor, it would probably be possible to achieve a radical cure, and towards this end everything should be risked.

Ventriculography, intraventricular injections of dye, arterial encephalography on which we are pinning our hopes, are methods which should be used with the object of obtaining a localization which might guide the surgeon in a radical operation.

To achieve visualization of the arteries of the brain one needs an opaque, non-oily substance which can easily pass through the capillaries in such a way as to avoid any kind of embolism, and one which is harmless. This was our first task.

But since the substance had to be introduced through the internal carotid, it was necessary to know if this artery would allow its introduction without adverse effect and if the brain would accept the opaque substances selected without severe reactions.

Another question to be resolved was the avoidance of immediate dilution of the aqueous solution in the mass of the blood, which would cause a loss of visualization if it could not be introduced at the first attempt, in all probability by substituting blood. Each systole should spurt 160 cc. of blood into the organism. We have calculated that this quantity for each internal carotid should amount to between 3 and 4 cc. of blood. Thus, in a period of 5 cardiac rotations, the intracarotid injection made within this period (4 seconds) would be dissolved in 20 cc. of blood, which would eliminate the visibility of the liquid introduced.

At the same time it was necessary to have access to a very good x-ray installation— which we did not —to obtain photographs at the precise moment, so as to avoid dilution taking place too rapidly. In addition, temporary binding of the carotid would be indispensable for this operation.

Once a visualization of the arterial network has been obtained, one should have a fairly constant normal picture. If there is a cerebral neoplasm the network should present fairly appreciable modifications, at least in certain regions sufficient to allow a definition if not of the entire extent of the tumor, at least one point or another where it gives rise to a displacement of the arterial network. If we are dealing with a highly vascularized tumor, one could very probably obtain a visible spot by penetration of the opaque liquid by x-rays.

The outline presented above shows the course taken in our experimentation.

One cannot determine the size of tumors according to the intensity of the general symptoms of hypertension. All neurologists have encountered some surprises on this score. Large tumors, for instance tumors of the corpus callosum,[5] may grow and develop without causing any appreciable disturbance.

On the other hand there are small tumors which give rise to a very remarkable hypertensive symptomatology. Sometimes they arise rapidly and give the impression of inflammatory processes. In other cases they appear slow and progressive. In other words it is impossible to correlate the symptoms observed with the volume of the tumor.

It would be very helpful if the radiographic methods of investigation of the brain could give

[5] Egas Moniz. Tumeurs du corps calleux, a work which will appear in a future number of L'Encéphale.

us all the information necessary for localization, spread, etc. of the intracranial neoplasm. But in solving this grave diagnostic problem the principal objective is the localization of at least a part of the tumor.

For example, in the case of a tumor of the corpus callosum, to which we referred earlier, the arteries, the callosal and the marginal callosal, should be changed. In the left hemisphere, in which the anterior horn of the much dilated lateral ventricle was invaded by neoplasm, the arterial circulation should also show considerable modifications.

We thought exclusively of the internal carotid and the arterial network derived from it because the internal carotid gives rise to the anterior cerebral and the sylvian, two strong arteries which irrigate the greatest part of the brain and particularly the silent part of the brain, that is the zone where the neoplastic invasion did not produce appreciable symptoms of localization.

The vertebral arteries nourish the diencephalon and the cerebellum where localization is relatively easy because it is manifested by disturbances which are well known to neurologists. Furthermore, they are not easy of access, and since they irrigate the bulb, the introduction of substances could give rise to grave and immediate consequences.

The internal carotid is localized in its own hemisphere. The anterior communicants between the two anterior cerebral arteries and the posterior communicants, which are branches of the basilary trunk, are the only possible passages to the opposite hemisphere. The injected substances will thus remain in the circulation of the internal carotid involved. Constant irrigation of the communicants by the blood of the internal carotid of the other side and the two vertebrals will prevent not only the entry of the opaque substance but will send blood to the carotid which is tied temporarily.

Of the opaque substances we preferred strontium bromide at the beginning. In another paper[6] we have presented our conclusions on this subject.

Among bromides those of strontium and lithium are the most opaque. Sodium and potassium bromide also provide satisfactory opacity. Strontium bromide is somewhat less toxic than lithium bromide, but the latter is useful from this standpoint, since large quantities of it can be injected into veins without disturbance. However, lithium bromide is somewhat more irritating than strontium bromide. Their intravenous injection in a high concentration produces a painful sensation in the channel of the vein, but this is transient.

Strontium bromide, preferred by us, never

gives rise to this phenomenon, but concentrated solutions from 30% and above cause a sensation of heat, at first localized in the head and later generalized throughout the body, which is transient but fairly uncomfortable. It is comparable to that produced by the intravenous injection of calcium chloride. Lithium bromide also produces these phenomena, but with a lesser intensity. These sensations of heat can be avoided if the injections are given slowly.

Strontium bromide in high doses gives rise to hardening of the veins which we corrected by adding 10% glucose.

Under these conditions we have been able to inject, without adverse effect, solutions containing up to 80% of strontium bromide and in very high quantities (10 to 15 cc.) without any discomfort on the part of the patients.

Parkinsonian postencephalitic patients have derived much profit from these injections. Despite the disagreeable sensation, they asked for them.

We have established that 70% solutions of strontium bromide were entirely harmless. At 80% we observed faintness in one patient, which led us to stop short of this amount.

We determined the opacities of the various bromides, notably 10 to 80% strontium bromide by placing a box of small rubber tubes full of progressive solutions of this salt into the cranium. We observed that the opacity starting from 30% is fairly considerable, but even the 10% solution is visible across the cranium (fig. 1). We experimented with this salt in animals and then in humans. We shall deal with the results obtained shortly.

After an accident had occurred, we took another direction. It seemed to us that bromides were less toxic, and particularly less irritating than iodides; we had selected them for this reason. However, we knew that iodides were more opaque than bromides, because opacity to x-rays is a consequence of the much higher atomic weight of iodine (127) than of bromine (80). One must also take into account the atomic weight of the associated metal; but the iodides, generally speaking, are much more opaque than the bromides. We repeated the experiments we made with bromides using iodides, and decided upon sodium iodide, which incidentally was already in clinical use, in intravenous injections. By injecting the cerebral arteries of cadavers with 30%, 20% and 10% and even 7.5% solutions it was observed that they were still visible across the cranium. We believe that this observation is so important that we are publishing four of the radioarteriographs obtained with these injections (figs. 2, 3, 4 and 5). In figure 2 (head preserved in formol) the penetration of the 30% solution of sodium iodide is not satisfactory. In figure 3 the arterial network ob-

---

[6] Egas Moniz. Les injections carotidiennes et les substances opaques. *Presse médicale*, 1927.

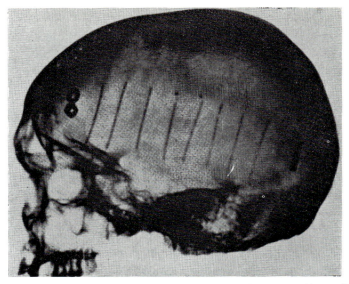

FIG. 1. Opacity of strontium bromide in solutions ranging from 10% to 80%.

tained with a 20% solution is fairly well visible. In figure 4, with a 10% solution, the arteries are still visible. The 7.5% solution, within the limits of visibility, shows some of the more important arteries. This fact, which was entirely unexpected, could be used in other clinical investigations outside neurology.

We have injected into the veins of humans 10–50% solutions of sodium iodide. It was observed that up to 30%, the injections, even when carried out at a certain speed, are not painful. At 30% some patients complained of pains along the course of the vein. These are intensified and become constant when this percentage is exceeded. The addition of other substances (glucose, bromide, etc.) does not modify the painful reaction. We stopped at 25%, which still provides a very good opacity and does not give rise to any pain upon intravenous injection.

Iodides are less well tolerated by the tissues than bromides. Particular care must be taken in making the injections, to avoid their extravasa-

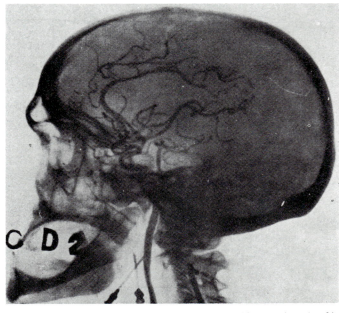

FIG. 2. Arterial network derived from the internal carotid. Injection of 30% NaI.

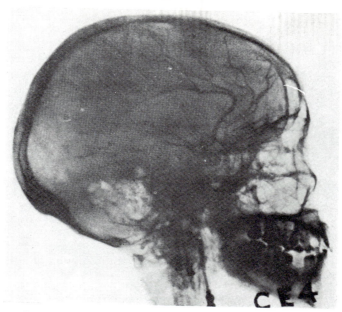

FIG. 3. Internal carotid injected with 20% NaI and vertebral with 10% NaI.

tion outside the vessels. However, iodides are harmless to arteries. Brooks, who injected them in cases of arteritis obliterans in 100% dosages, observed after the amputation of one of the limbs that the arteries did not present any macroscopic or microscopic lesions.

We have studied other iodides which we did not use. Most make up unstable solutions. Strontium and lithium iodide liberate iodine, even in low concentrations. Rubidium iodide, which is very opaque, is not toxic, but produces pains even at fairly low dosages.

Sodium iodide is not very stable either. Above 30% the liberation of iodine is almost constant, particularly if one keeps the ampules for some time and if they are exposed to light. As a precaution we use recent solutions, if possible sterilized on the day of application. When the ampules

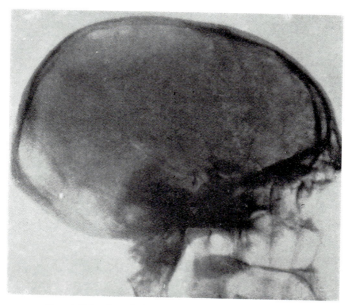

FIG. 4. Injection of the internal carotid with 10% NaI.

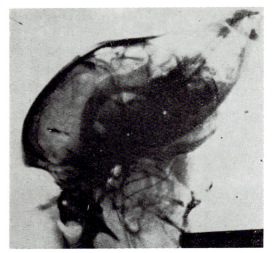

FIG. 5. In a live dog, visualization of some cerebral arteries. The internal carotid is visible, very thin, also the internal jugular and the vertebral veins.

appeared slightly yellow, we did not use them. One must also consider the chemical purity of the salts to be used.

The experiments performed by us on animals were numerous, and were made either to determine the toxicity of the drugs selected, or to establish the effects of the substances used on the brain, using intracarotid injections, or to detect the injected cerebral arteries in radiographs.

For the determination of toxicity we injected

rabbits and dogs. The results for strontium bromide and lithium bromide and for sodium iodide were entirely reassuring in the doses to be administered to humans. Experiments made with intravenous and subcutaneous injections have shown their harmlessness at even high percentages.[7] We obtained a confirmation of these results with intravenous injections in humans.

With intracarotid injections it was observed that dogs maintain a greater resistance to the substances introduced. We have two dogs alive, one weighing 8 kg. in which we injected 3 cc. of a solution of 100% strontium bromide into the carotid and a female dog in which we injected 1.5 cc. of a 25% solution of sodium iodide into the carotid.

The carotids of the dog are fairly resistant to the injections, although they behave variously. Sometimes they form hematomas, in others, blood spurts out after the injection, and in some the arteries showed no reaction. We never had any unfavorable complications here, nor were there any such in humans.

The dog was the animal selected for radiographic experiments. It was not a good subject for this, since the cranium presents lines in radiography caused by the bony rugosity of the muscular insertions which are very numerous and extensive in the head of the dog.

The internal carotid of the dog is very thin and cannot be reached directly. For this purpose we

[7] Egas Moniz. Injections intracarotidiennes et substances opaques. *Presse médicale*, 1927.

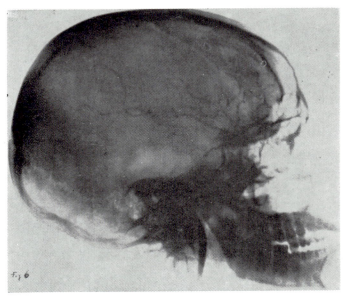

FIG. 6. Arterial encephalography of the cerebral carotid network in a live human. Case of a large hypophysial tumor. The carotid is pulled forward, and the origin of the sylvian is also higher. The anterior cerebral, much reduced in volume, is deformed in its direction.

tied the common carotid above its point of origin, at the same time pressing the occipital artery which is as thick in the dog as the internal carotid and which originates above it and very close to it. But this was not sufficient to obtain a radiograph of the arteries of the dog brain. It was necessary to prevent the passage of blood from the common carotid, to avoid dilution of the opaque substance used. This lower ligature was therefore carried out and the opaque liquid was injected into the isolated segment, which forced the entry of the liquid into the internal carotid, without mixture of the carotid blood.

The first radiographs were negative. They were made with a Potter-Buckey and with a fairly long exposure. Thus we noticed that a condition which is indispensable for success is the radiophotograph to capture the progress of the substance across the arteries, now maintained by the blood of the collateral vessels. The photographs which we were able to obtain with the machine belonging to our hospital were very long—a quarter of a second—but we nevertheless succeeded in obtaining positive results. This radiological inadequacy was the most serious difficulty to be overcome in all our experiments. It was even the indirect cause of other obstacles which we encountered and of the fact that we did not reach definite results rapidly. I hope that this situation will be improved shortly but do not know whether, solely with a more powerful instrument, we would obtain what is indispensable for us. We will return to this subject later.

In the dog we injected sometimes strontium bromide, sometimes lithium bromide in a 100% concentration into the carotid. We discovered the outlines of some cerebral arteries and veins of the neck in three cases. Figure 5 shows an injected head. The cerebral arteries are visible in the hemisphere and at the base (with some veins?). These results encouraged us to pursue the experiments on humans.

Before going further studies were made on cadavers in order to establish thoroughly the arterial tree of the brain and to confirm certain anatomical concepts by means of radioarteriographs. In fact we also used this work, which was carried out in collaboration with Almeida Dias and Almeida Lima,[8] to present certain radioanatomical concepts and new ideas on the cranioencephalic topography. By means of stereoscopic radiography we were able to separate the two carotid systems of the brain: the internal, or anterior cerebral, and the external or sylvian.

These experiments were very informative. One can see very good networks by simultaneously

injecting through the internal carotid and the vertebral artery on the same side, a 100% solution of sodium iodide under pressure.

We made a large number of radiographs on cadavers in order to obtain the normal picture of the distribution of the arteries seen with x-rays. We did everything possible to obtain cadavers of persons having died of cerebral tumors. These, with alterations in the arterial network, would provide a partial demonstration of the hypothesis suggested by us; but within six months of experimentation we were only able to obtain one cadaver which was of use from this standpoint.

The experiments underwent considerable changes according to the development of our work. There was always one great difficulty to overcome: the entry of the blood at the moment of injection of the opaque solution, which immediately lowered the concentration, in other words, the possibility of obtaining visualization of the vessels.

We had this difficulty with the dog and overcame it by tying the carotid. It should be noted that in the dog the communicating arteries are not comparable to those in humans. The problems appeared to be much more difficult to solve. But the opacities were well defined, well observable and consequently, in order to obtain the picture of the arteries, we had to have: 1. a solution which, when mixed with the existing blood, should still be opaque; 2. an apparatus which could give photographs rapid enough to capture the progress of the liquid in the vessels.

Our experiments can be divided into two stages, that of the injection of strontium bromide and the other the administration of sodium iodide. We began by attempting to inject the covered internal carotid in humans. The attempt was made in four cases. Before this we sought to reach the internal carotid at the point of entry into the carotid orifice, without result. It is possible that we did not succeed because we used very fine 0.5 and 0.6 mm. needles. The blood never spurted out because of their small diameter and length (5 cm.). Having abandoned this approach we were guided by the edge of the sternomastoid in the triangle formed by its border, the anterior surface of the digastric and the omohyoid.

In our *first case* we had the impression that we had reached the carotid, in a case of general paralysis. We had injected 7 cc. of a solution of 70% strontium bromide without consequences. It is probable that the injection was made into the internal jugular, since the patient did not experience any pain.

In the *second case* the injection was made into the internal carotid and since the patient was in a condition to allow the making of the first radiograph, the common carotid was compressed to prevent the entry of blood into the internal

[8] Egas Moniz, Almeida Dias et Almeida Lima. La radiartériographie et la topographie cranio-encéphalique. *Journal de Radiologie*, 1927.

carotid during injection of the opaque liquid. The painful reaction was fairly violent following the introduction of 5 to 6 cc. of the solution. The patient rose suddenly and it was impossible to make the radiograph.

In the *third case*, that of a parkinsonian patient, who had greatly profited from the intravenous injection of strontium bromide, the sensation felt was again disagreeable but we decided to continue. This patient subsequently had a Claude Bernard-Horner syndrome which has since gone completely.

The *fourth patient* had a rather disagreeable surprise in store for us. The needle emerged from the artery and the greater part of the liquid (more than 10 cc.) was extravasated into the surrounding cellular tissue. There were no grave consequences. The patient had a temperature of around 38° for a few days, slow resorption, no abscess. The patient continued to have a Claude Bernard-Horner syndrome, from which he improved gradually. After this accident we decided to make the intervention on an exposed artery. The surgeon, Mr. Antonio Martins, was kind enough to undertake to expose and inject the internal carotid.

Fifth case. This was a female patient aged 20 years with an unlocalized cerebral neoplasm. She was blind. Once the right internal carotid was exposed the ligature was made and a 70% solution of strontium bromide was injected. The artery was punctured twice and approximately 4 cc. of the liquid were injected. At the beginning of the injection the patient complained. She had a neuropathic background and became highly agitated. Later she suffered from a type of anesthesia: disturbance in speech, and after one minute, cessation of speech. There were no other consequences. The radiographs were negative. They were taken somewhat late. The results of the injection were without adverse effect on the patient. She had some fever the following day (39°) and transient dysphagia. On the third day she was restored once more.

The *sixth case* was a progressive postencephalitic parkinsonian patient, very severe, aged 48 years. He had considerable muscular rigidity, trembling, transient diplopia, retropulsion with repeated falls, blepharospasms, great difficulty in talking. Scopolamine was not beneficial. Intravenous injections of large quantities of strontium solution brought some improvement. We selected this patient with the double object of obtaining an arterial radiograph and to see the result of the direct action of strontium bromide on the brain. The carotid having been exposed, we injected 13 to 14 cc. of a solution of strontium bromide after tying the artery. The patient complained of severe pain. In order to obtain four radiographs we kept the ligature on for 2 minutes. The first radiograph, which is blurred, nevertheless shows the arterial penetration of the opaque fluid. Another radiograph, made immediately afterwards, shows only the internal carotid injected, and a small amount of opacity in the upper part of the anterior cerebral, which demonstrates that a thrombus immediately formed in this artery. Another radiograph made at the moment of removing the ligature of the carotid shows the sylvian and particularly the posterior cerebral, which showed us that the pressure of the carotid blood overcame the current originating from the vertebral. Since the blood was not able to pass through the anterior cerebral, pressure was exercised on one side, on an area of the vertebral, and on the other, on the ophthalmic. Then the patient exhibited a syndrome of thrombophlebitis and died eight hours after the injection. The state of this patient's arteries probably contributed to this accident;[9] but we made a technical error by keeping the ligature of the internal carotid on for a prolonged period, and after the injection. The high dose of the drug may also have been the cause of trouble; but we are unable to explain the immediate formation of the anterior cerebral thrombus which we never observed in animals. Could the development of the vascular and perivascular lesions of severe encephalitides be explained by the action of bromides?

This accident led us to abandon bromide solutions and turned our attention to iodides in such a way as to obtain sufficient opacity with doses lower than those used with bromides.

At this point we began a study of the opacity of iodides and their action upon tissues and vessels. As has been stated, solutions of sodium iodide are visible across the cranium, even in very low doses, such as 10% and even 7.5%, and we were able to inject into the veins, without harmful effects, solutions of sodium iodide up to 50%. These injections are not painful up to 30%.

Under these conditions we took 22 to 25% solutions for intracarotid injections. We had to determine the dose to be injected without injury to the patient and sufficient to give the necessary opacity. For this we believe that large quantities of liquid are not necessary, for when they enter the arterial circulation of the communicants (the internal carotid being tied) the greater part of the substance will disappear. The quantity to be introduced had to be such that, mixed with the blood contained in the part of the carotid above the ligature, it should give a solution of about 20%, which is still fairly opaque. For this 3 to 5 cc. of a 25% solution of sodium iodide had to be

---

[9] Histopathological examination of the brain, under the direction of Professor Parreira, is not yet complete.

injected. Since the x-ray apparatus of our hospital makes $\frac{1}{4}$ sec. pictures we were able to introduce up to 5 cc. of substance.

This liquid with a probable concentration of 20% comes into contact with the blood proceeding either from the anterior communicant or the posterior communicant. We do not know the amount brought in by the arteries into the hemispheric circulation as substitute for blood from the internal carotid. But we have calculated that for each cardiac revolution they would bring in the blood corresponding to the entry of the liquid injected in one second, that is, roughly one cubic centimeter. Even under these conditions—and the substances are not immediately dissolved, the two liquids, blood and iodide running side by side—we would obtain an opacity of 10%, which is sufficient to visualize at least a part of the largest arteries of the brain. However, it was necessary to capture the progress of the liquid with very rapid pictures.

We have tried intracarotid injections of 22% sodium iodide (first case) and 25%, without harm to the patient. These were carried out in 4 cases, one of which does not count because we were puncturing a bad artery and the experiment was abandoned without making radiographs. In the other three cases the injections were made without adverse effect into the internal carotid with solutions of sodium iodide in the dosages mentioned.

The *first case*, a patient with a cerebral neoplasm, with a suspected right frontoparietal localization because of a slight opacity detected by radiography, and since he was blind in the right eye and saw very little with his left eye, received an injection of 3 cc. of 22% solution of sodium iodide. He received a local novocain anesthetic and also, in advance, an injection of morphine chlorhydrate with $\frac{1}{2}$ mg. of atropine sulfate. At the instant of making the radiograph the ligature was removed from the internal carotid, hoping thus to profit from the entry into the cerebral circulation of the opaque mass which was stagnating in the carotid cisterna. The result should have been positive had we had very fast, instantaneous photographs at our disposal; but with $\frac{1}{4}$ second and with the speed of the blood coming from the carotid the picture was taken without leaving even vestiges of opacity.

In the sixth case of the bromide series we obtained the outlines of the sylvian and posterior cerebral arteries by this method. Visualization was more pronounced in the posterior cerebral, possibly because opposition from the blood current coming from the basilary trunk briefly held up the current coming from the internal carotid, giving it an appreciable degree of visualization.

Radiography in the first case of the iodide series

was entirely negative. There was no trace of any opacity in the arteries.

When the internal carotid was punctured the pulse slowed down from 90 to 56. The patient merely complained of a slight pain in the ear. The following day he revealed a certain degree of dysphasia and his temperature rose to 38°. On the third day he was up and has been in good health since.

The *second case*, a blind patient who has been in our service for some years because of cranial hypertension, did not show any obvious symptoms of localization. There were no cerebellar symptoms, but on the other hand, there was very pronounced nystagmus, even in the intermediate position of the eyeballs. The patient suffers from generalized epileptic attacks, which are more pronounced towards the left, which led us to make the sodium iodide test on the right. He has recently gained a fair amount of weight. No other symptoms. This being so, it appears to us impossible to determine any localization. Local anesthesia was with novocain and the carotid was exposed and injected before tying. Entry of blood into the syringe was very violent and to the 5 cc. of 25% solution, 3 cc. of blood were added, which lowered the concentration to about 15%. In other words if the solution finds 1 cc. in the communicating arteries, even if radiography was made between two cardiac revolutions, which did not in fact occur, the concentration would be reduced to 7.5%, which is the limit of visibility in cadavers.

However, in radiography the internal carotid is fairly well visible as far as the upper curve. It did not appear to us to be normal. We even suspected that it had assumed this shape because of pressure from a neoplasm but since the other arteries are not visible nothing can be claimed for certain.

Passage of blood from the communicating arteries dragged the contents along. The wave of blood probably pressed at the moment of making the radiograph, and the sodium iodide shadow, already much delayed, was lost during the time required to obtain the picture.

The patient complained during the injection of transient pain, not very intense, in the temples, to some extent in the eyes and in the right ear. The pulse fell from 95 to 60 during the injection. Slight dysphasia the following day. On the third day he was up and took his meals without difficulty.

Third case in the iodide series. Boy of 20 years with a hypophysial tumor. A typical Fröhlich-Babinski syndrome. He was blind and had recently had severe attacks of vomiting and pronounced headaches. Grave condition.

In this patient for the first time a satisfactory method was followed: the internal carotid was exposed and injected before tying, because once ligated it is very difficult to reach. The blood was not allowed to enter the syringe[10] and the artery was tied rapidly. Five cc. of a 25% solution of sodium iodide was injected. Then the artery was untied immediately. The patient experienced no pain. There was no fall in his pulse rate. There was some dysphasia the following day. After the third day he was in good condition.

He received two injections of 1 centigram of morphine and atropine during the 45 minutes preceding the injection.

The radiograph (fig. 6) shows the carotid pulled forward and without the upper curvature. The sylvian, very well visible, is also pulled forward and upward. The anterior cerebral shows a different arrangement from that which is seen in normal networks and it is very thin and blurred.

The tumor is the cause of the changes in position of the internal carotid and of the sylvian and probably of the modifications in the anterior cerebral, but on this point we cannot say anything positive. All of this demonstrated by comparison of normal radiographs with these.

Our problem has now been presented. In live subjects one can obtain radioarteriographs of the brain and it can furnish elements for the localization of tumors. But the experiments must be continued if we are to obtain information which cannot be furnished by one case alone.

The method is very simple but quite possibly many modifications will yet be made. It will even be possible to give the injection with the artery covered, with compression of the common carotid, either with the fingers, or with compressors of the type described by Dupuytren. This depends upon the percentage of liquid to be introduced. Morphine anesthesia should be replaced by ethyl chloride or nitrogen protoxide if high concentrations are used.

The meningeal arteries, derived from the external carotid, can also be explored by injection. In making the injection into the common carotid it will be possible to obtain both networks (meningeal and cerebral), which are very easy to separate in radioarteriographs.

But the great problem to be resolved now is not that of the carotid injection and the percentages to be used, which have already been established, more or less. The radiological method is much more important. It could provide considerable simplifications and new aspects in vascular

encephalography, because we will be able to see not only the arterial network, but also the venous network and the sinuses.

A number of very quick photographs must be obtained, knowing that the progress of the blood is 10 meters per second. It is essential that these be successive pictures. It would be very interesting and very useful—since one would never lose the pictures—to make an actual cinematographic film of cerebral circulation with these opaque substances in motion. There is also another problem to be resolved: very rapid stereoscopic radiographs, so as not to lose the movement of the opaque liquids in the arteries. The solution of this problem appears somewhat more difficult, but stereoscopy would be a very valuable aid in showing the displacement of arteries caused by the pressure of tumors.

In summary, at the moment the problem has shifted to radiology which, we believe, will satisfy all our hopes before long. We will continue our experiments, but we will need a better x-ray apparatus. Without it no appreciable progress can be made.

For the time being, we advise the following method, which is harmless to the patients and able to provide a fairly satisfactory arterial encephalograph:

1. Preparing the patient with one or two injections of morphine and atropine.

2. Exposing the internal carotid.

3. Fixing the patient's head to the photographic frame by means of a bandage, to avoid movement of the head.

4. Making the injection into the carotid without allowing blood to enter the syringe.

5. Always taking good care to avoid the entry of air.

6. Immediately afterwards making the temporary ligature of the internal carotid with tweezers.

7. Immediately and rapidly injecting 5 to 6 cc. of a 25% solution of sodium iodide recently prepared and sterilized.

8. Making one or several radiographic pictures (as rapidly as possible), while continuing to inject the opaque fluid.

9. Immediately untying the temporary ligature of the internal carotid.

We have already cited some of our collaborators in our articles. We must also thank our friends: Assistant Eduardo Coelho, who was always beside us in the clinical experiments, Professor Cancela d'Abreu, Assistants R. Loff and L. Pacheco and Doctors A. Fernandes and M. Beirão, for the aid which they gave us in the course of this work.

---

[10] A device with a stopcock may be used with two syringes, one full of physiological serum, communicating with the needle at the moment of puncturing the artery, and the other with the substance to be injected. This device was used with the first injections we made with the carotid covered.

Neurosurgical Classics—20 and 21

THE invention of the ophthalmoscope and the early application of this instrument to the study of papilledema were largely the work of three young men— Hermann von Helmholtz, Albrecht von Graefe, and John Hughlings Jackson.

Von Helmholtz was born at Potsdam in 1821. He received his medical education at the Friedrich Wilhelm Institute in Berlin, and even as an undergraduate he demonstrated the genius that was apparent throughout his later career.[10,11] After graduation he was a surgeon in the Prussian Army for five years, and it was during this time that von Helmholtz performed his important studies on animal heat. These studies led to one of the most important contributions ever made in the field of physics—the theory of the conservation of energy.[10] During his subsequent career as Professor of Physiology at Königsberg, Bonn, and Heidelberg, von Helmholtz made several other outstanding contributions to medical physics.[9] He measured the velocity of the nervous impulse in motor and sensory nerves, he invented the ophthalmoscope, and he added many original observations on physiologic optics and acoustics.[10,15–17] In 1887 he became director of the Physico-Technical Institute at Charlottenburg, and he devoted the remainder of his life to basic studies in thermodynamics and electrodynamics.[10]

"The greatest discovery in the history of ophthalmology, not excepting the extraction of cataract, was the invention (1850) of the ophthalmoscope . . . , because by its use ophthalmology has been made an exact science. In the early years of the nineteenth century, *Prevost* (1790–1850) of Geneva demonstrated that the light from the eyes was from reflection and that it disappeared in the dark. *Jean Méry* (1645–1722) of Paris, a century earlier observed through the widely dilated pupils of a cat which by accident had been held under water, the highly colored fundus with its optic nerve. A short time later, *de la Hire* explained the cause by declaring that the water had

interfered with the refraction of light by the cornea and caused all the emergent rays to leave the eye in divergence. As the human eye began to be studied more closely, someone noticed that the eyes of an Ethiopian albino were luminous; and Scarpa (1752–1832) remarked that a reflection could be seen in certain deep-seated diseases, such as the 'amaurotic cat's eye.' Beer, in 1819, noted the red reflection in a case of absence of the iris; a few years later a normal eye, the pupil of which had been artificially dilated, permitted a similar observation. In these years the mystery of the blackness of the pupil was solved by the discovery that the fundus lies at the focus of the refractive powers of the cornea and lens, which powers keep the fundus invisible and the pupil dark.

"*Cumming*, a student in the London Hospital in 1846, by shading it from the light, was able to look directly into the eye of a fellow student and obtained both the 'retinal reflex' and the white light from the entrance of the optic nerve.

"In 1847, *Brücke* of Vienna by passing a tube through a candle flame was able to see the fundus, and reported that it was also possible to illuminate the pupil by the light reflected from an observer's spectacle lenses."[6]

" . . . The technical difficulty of placing the light and the observer's head in the same straight line was solved by the English mathematician, Charles Babbage[20] (1847), who held to his eye a mirror which served as the immediate source of light, in the centre of which a hole in the silvering acted as a window through which he looked . . .

" . . . To him should be credited the invention of the first ophthalmoscope, but his idea did not receive publication until seven years had passed (Wharton Jones, 1854[20]). In the meantime, von Helmholtz[15] (1851) had elaborated his ophthalmoscope and had elucidated the optical principles governing the path of the rays into and out of the eye, and since his discovery was . . . publicized and taken up intensively by von Graefe and the other leading ophthalmologists of the time, it is to von Helmholtz that the science of ophthalmoscopy must owe its inception. . . ."[9]

Von Helmholtz constructed his ophthalmoscope in 1850 and published his description of it in 1851.[15,25] It did not enjoy immediate popularity because of its crude construction and because few practitioners had enough background to comprehend the mathematics and physics involved.[25] However, during the following decade technical improvements allowed many original observations of intraocular pathology to be made, chiefly by ophthalmologists.[9] Among these original observations was the description by von Graefe of papilledema in association with intracranial tumor.

Friedrich Wilhelm Ernst Albrecht von Graefe was born in Berlin in 1828. As a young man he became interested in ophthalmology, and shortly became an exceptionally fine eye surgeon. As such he introduced iridectomy in the treatment of glaucoma and devised a special knife for his modified linear extraction of cataracts. In 1854, when von Graefe was 26 years old, he founded the Archiv für Ophthalmologie. During the subsequent years before his untimely death in 1870, von Graefe applied the newly-introduced ophthalmoscope to the study of glaucoma, embolism of the retinal artery, and various cerebral diseases.[6] In the course of these studies, von Graefe noted the occurrence of papilledema (called optic neuritis or choked disc until 1908[8]) in patients with brain tumors.[3,4,6,8,12,13] He advanced the explanation that this was due to mechanical hyperemia, and he correctly predicted that other causes of increased intracranial pressure would also be found to result in papilledema.[12,13]

Although von Graefe and others made many important observations with the ophthalmoscope, the value of this instrument in the study of affections of the nervous system was stressed most effectively by John Hughlings Jackson.[1–3,5,27,28] Jackson was born in 1834 in Yorkshire, England, and received his early medical training in York. After considering a career in philosophy, he was persuaded by Jonathan Hutchinson and Charles-Édouard Brown-Séquard to enter the field of neurology. Jackson's subsequent studies of focal epileptiform fits, involuntary movements, hemiplegia and speech disorders, as well as his philosophical interpretations of the functions of the nervous system, were of vital importance to the development of neurology and neurosurgery.[5,7,14,21–24,26–29]

In 1863, 1865 and 1866,[18,19] Jackson

" . . . published four papers on 'Defects of sight in diseases of the nervous system.' These papers are of surpassing interest in that they set forth the slow unravelling of the truth with regard to the nature and cause of optic neuritis of intracranial origin. He urged that routine ophthalmoscopic examination should be made in all cases of severe cerebral disease, whether the patient complained of defect of sight or not. He described the association of headache, vomiting and optic neuritis in cases of cerebral tumour, and laid great stress on the fact that the chief disease in a cerebral case, in which amaurosis is a symptom, rarely involves the optic nervous system. 'It is just as important,' he adds, 'to determine whether a patient's blindness depends on choroiditis, apoplexy of retina, or neuritis; as whether his bad talking depends on incoherence, defect of the faculty of language, or paralysis of the tongue.' "[3]

Today the ophthalmoscope is a virtually indispensable instrument for the evaluation of patients with intracranial disease. Its widespread use is due mainly to the pioneering efforts of von Helmholtz, who introduced the ophthalmoscope; von Graefe, who first used it to identify papilledema in association with brain tumors; and Jackson, who popularized its use in the diagnosis of neurological diseases.

References

1. ALPER, L. The history of neurology during the nineteenth century. *Bull. Univ. Miami Sch. Med.*, 1960, *14:* 75–81.
2. BALLANCE, C. Remarks and reminiscences. *Brit. med. J.*, 1927, *1:* 64–67.
3. BALLANCE, C. The dawn and epic of neurology and surgery. *Glasgow: Jackson, Wylie & Co.*, 1930, 40 pp. (see p. 26).
4. BERENS, C. The fundus changes and the blood pressure in the retinal arteries in increased intracranial pressure. Papilledema and optic atrophy. *Res. Publ. Ass. nerv. ment. Dis.*, 1929, *8:* 263–309.
5. BRAIN, R. The neurological tradition of the London Hospital or the importance of being thirty. *Lancet*, 1959, *2:* 575–581.
6. CHANCE, B. Ophthalmology. In: *Clio medica. A series of primers on the history of medicine.* E. B. Krumbhaar, Ed. New York: P. B. Hoeber, Inc., 1939, *20:* xvii, 240 pp. (see pp. 65–68; 76–80). Reprinted ed.: New York: Hafner Publishing Co., 1962.
7. CRITCHLEY, M. Hughlings Jackson, the man; and the early days of the National Hospital. *Proc. roy. Soc. Med.*, 1960, *53:* 613–618.
8. DUKE-ELDER, W. S. Text-book of ophthalmology. *St. Louis: C. V. Mosby Co.*, 1941, *3:* 2944–2965.
9. DUKE-ELDER, [W.] S., and SMITH, R. J. H. The

examination of the eye. In: *System of ophthalmology.* S. Duke-Elder, Ed. London: H. Kimpton, 1962, *7:* 233–365 (see pp. 286; 290–294).

10. EDITORIAL NOTE. Hermann Ludwig Ferdinand von Helmholtz. *Ann. med. Hist.,* 1921, *3:* 288–289.

11. GIBSON, W. C. The undergraduate activities of some contributors to neurological science. *Yale J. Biol. Med.,* 1955–1956, *28:* 273–284.

12. GLEW, W. B. The pathogenesis of papilledema in intracranial disease: a review of the literature. *Amer. J. med. Sci.,* 1960, n.s. *239:* 221–230.

13. v. GRÄFE, A. Ueber Complication von Sehnervenentzündung mit Gehirnkrankheiten. *v. Graefes Arch. Ophthal.,* 1860, *7,* Abt. 2: 58–71.

14. HEAD, H. Hughlings Jackson on aphasia and kindred affections of speech. *Brain,* 1915, *38:* 1–190.

15. [VON] HELMHOLTZ, H. Beschreibung eines AugenSpiegels zur Untersuchung der Netzhaut im lebenden Auge. *Berlin: A Förstner,* 1851, 43 pp.

16. [VON] HELMHOLTZ, H. Die Lehre von den Tonempfindungen als physiologische Grundlage für die Theorie der Musik. *Braunschweig: F. Vieweg & Sohn,* 1863, xi, 600 pp.

17. [VON] HELMHOLTZ, H. Handbuch der physiologischen Optik. *Leipzig: L. Voss,* 1867, xiv, 874 pp., with atlas.

18. JACKSON, J. H. Observations on defects of sight in brain disease. *Roy. Ophthal. Hosp. Rep.,* 1863, *4:* 10–19.

19. JACKSON, J. H. Observations on defects of sight in diseases of the nervous system. *Roy. Ophthal. Hosp. Rep.,* 1865, *4:* 389–446; 1865, *5:* 51–78; 1866, *5:* 251–306.

20. JONES, T. W. Report on the ophthalmoscope. *Brit. foreign med.-chir. Rev.,* 1854, *14:* 425–432.

21. KELLY, E. C., Compiler. John Hughlings Jackson. Introduction. *Med. Classics,* 1939, *3:* 915–917.

22. PENNYBACKER, J. The history of neurological surgery in the United Kingdom. *Oxf. med. Sch. Gaz.,* 1961, *13:* 152–162.

23. RIESE, W. The sources of Jacksonian neurology. *J. nerv. ment. Dis.,* 1956, *124:* 125–134.

24. RIESE, W. A history of neurology. *New York: MD Publications, Inc.,* 1959, 223 pp.

25. SHASTID, T. H. The description of an ophthalmoscope. Being an English translation of von Helmholtz's *"Beschreibung eines Augenspiegels"* (Berlin, 1851). *Chicago: Cleveland Press,* 1916, 33 pp.

26. SOMERS, J. A short history of neurology. *Univ. Mich. med. Bull.,* 1956, *22:* 467–481.

27. TAYLOR, J. The ophthalmological observations of Hughlings Jackson and their bearing on nervous and other diseases. *Brain,* 1915, *38:* 391–417.

28. TAYLOR, J., Ed. Selected writings of John Hughlings Jackson. *London: Hodder & Stoughton,* 1931, 2 vols. (see *1:* ix–xiv).

29. WALSHE, F. M. R. Contributions of John Hughlings Jackson to neurology. A brief introduction to his teachings. *Arch. Neurol., Chicago,* 1961, *5:* 119–131.

THE DESCRIPTION

OF AN

OPHTHALMOSCOPE*

BEING AN ENGLISH TRANSLATION OF

Von HELMHOLTZ'S
"Beschreibung eines Augenspiegels"
(BERLIN, 1851)

BY

Thomas Hall Shastid, A.B., A.M., M.D., LL.B., F.A.C.S.
SUPERIOR, WISCONSIN

And the first translation of this classic into any language

The present treatise contains the description of an optical instrument, by which it is possible in the living to see and recognize exactly the retina itself and the images of luminous objects which are cast upon it.[1] The instrument has, for this pur-

* Reprinted from *The Description of an Ophthalmoscope. Being an English Translation of Von Helmholtz's "Beschreibung eines Augenspiegels" (Berlin, 1851).* By Thomas Hall Shastid. *Chicago: Cleveland Press,* 1916, 33 pp.

[1] Even the ancients, as a matter of course, had noticed that the eyes of certain animals are brilliant in the dark. Thus Pliny (Book XI, Chap. 55): "The eyes of animals that see at night in the dark, cats for example, are shining and radiant, so much so that we cannot bear to gaze upon them; those of the shegoat, too, and the wolf are resplendent, and emit a light like fire." Pliny did not, however, attempt to explain the phenomenon.

In 1704, Jean Méry, of Paris, performed his famous experiment with a cat. Having immersed the animal in water, he first observed that the pupil dilated (as a result of suspended respiration) and then he beheld in all its glory the fundus of the animal's eye—the entrance of the optic nerve and all the colors and vessels of the choroid. Méry understood quite well enough that something more than mere pupillary dilatation was necessary to account for the possibility of observing the fundus of the eye when the eye was under water. His explanation, however, of the "something more" was wholly erroneous. He believed, that is to say, that the view of the fundus was rendered possible by the water's filling up a multitude of tiny "unevennesses" on the anterior surface of the cornea. Five years later, de la Hire stepped forward with the correct explanation. According to him, the water obviated the refraction of light by the cornea, so

pose, two different problems to solve. First, everything which we can see of the background of the uninjured eye appears to us absolutely dark. The cause of this lies, as I will show, in the light-refracting media of the eye, which, under ordinary circumstances, hinder us from seeing illuminated parts of the retina behind the pupil. Therefore, the first question is to discover a means of illumination whereby exactly that portion of the retina on which we gaze through the pupil may be adequately lighted. Secondly, we view the background of the eye only through the light-refracting media. These, however, cast images of the retinal objects, which, in general, do not lie for the observer within the limits of plain vision. We need, therefore, together with a proper procedure for illumination, also further optical expedients which will render possible for the observing eye a correct accommodation for the objects which it should see.

I. ILLUMINATION

In order to be able to find the essential conditions for the method of illumination, we must first

---

that all rays leaving a given point upon the fundus emerged from the eye not as parallel, but as divergent, rays. De la Hire also observed, incidentally, that the disturbing light-reflexes proceeding from a cornea *in aero* are done away with by the water.

In 1796 Fermin observed a certain luminosity in the pupils of an Ethiopian albino. In 1816 Scarpa remarked upon a similar phenomenon in a certain disease of the fundus, and, one year later, Beer described the same condition fully, inventing therefor the expression "amaurotic cat's eye"—a term which is still in use. In 1836 Hasenstein first produced a factitious luminosity by compressing the eyeball backward—making the eye, in fact, artificially hypermetropic. In 1847 Babbage, an English mathematician, exhibited to Wharton Jones, the distinguished London oculist, the model of an instrument invented by him for the purpose of examining the interior of the eye. It consisted of a small plane glass mirror, from which a portion of the silvering had been removed. This device, however, was first made kown to the world in 1854, by Wharton Jones (*Brit. and For. Medico-Chir. Review*, Oct., 1854). The services of Brücke (in 1845, published in 1847) and of Cumming (in 1846) are adverted to herein by Helmholtz.

The earliest reception of the ophthalmoscope is decidedly interesting. Thus, to quote from Koenigsberger, "*Hermann von Helmholtz*," (1906) p. 74: "The ophthalmoscope was, however, some time in making its way, on account of the mathematical and physical knowledge presupposed by the '*Description of an Ophthalmoscope for the Investigation of the Retina in the Living Eye*,' published in the autumn of 1851, and people were at first very shy of employing it. One distinguished surgical colleague told Helmholtz he should never use the instrument—it would be too dangerous to admit the naked light into a diseased eye; another was of opinion that the mirror might be of service to oculists with defective eyesight—he himself had good eyes and wanted none of it."—(T. H. S.)

of all make clear to ourselves why, as a rule, the ground of the eye behind the pupil appears to us to be of so deep a black.

The cause of this is not the condition of the pigment of the chorioidea; for, if the pigment layer absorbed the light which falls upon it even more completely than any other known black substance, still, there lie before the chorioidea parts which can reflect a quantity of light sufficient to render them visible. That is true, first of all, of the substance of the retina, which, to be sure, in the recent condition, is very transparent, and marks itself off but little against the dark pigmentary background; to a much higher degree, however, it is true of the blood-vessels of this membrane, whose tiny stems carry blood enough to exhibit a strongly red hue. Finally, there appears, even in the fundus of the eye, a shining white spot, namely, the place of entrance of the optic nerve, on which no pigment at all lies, and which, therefore, reflects all the light that falls upon it. And yet we observe, under ordinary circumstances, behind the pupil of the living eye, not the slightest trace of the red color of the blood, nor of the white color of the optic nerve.

It can be shown much better by a simple experiment, that not the color of the background, but only the refraction of the light in the ocular media, is the cause of the deep blackening of the pupil. Let one take any kind of small camera obscura well blackened within, and let him bring to the place where the picture is produced an opaque white card, for example one from thick white drawing-paper. Among other kinds of camera may be employed the ocular tubes of most microscopes, after the ocular glass has been removed therefrom, and the collective glass has been inserted. These tubes are, as a rule, precisely as long as the focal distance of the collective glass. If one sets them with the end which contains the ocular upward upon the white card, then they form a camera obscura of the kind we need. There are thrown, in this case, very bright images of the surrounding illuminated objects, on the white card, and still the interior of the instrument, when one looks into the lens in any desired direction, appears absolutely black. We have here a *fac simile* of the eye, where cornea and crystalline lens are substituted by the objective lens of the camera, and the retina by a clear white paper surface, but there occurs apparently the same complete darkness of the internal space as in the eye, as long as the paper surface lies precisely at the spot where the tiny images of external objects are produced. If one takes away the convex glass, or if one materially alters its distance from the paper surface, there appears to the beholder at once the clear white surface of the paper.

How, now, can the refraction of the light produce the phenomenon described? Let us consider the course which the rays of light must take, according to the physical laws of the refraction of light in the eye.

Let light fall from a luminous point upon a fittingly adapted eye, concerning which we assume that it is formed with absolute accuracy, that is, that all the incident rays from the point in question concentre upon a single point of the retina. Of the light which, by the ocular media, is caused to converge upon this membrane, the greater part is absorbed by the black pigment, while the smaller is reflected partly by the nerve elements and blood-vessels, partly by the layer of rod-shaped corpuscles. That which is thrown back by the latter structures, passes, as E. Brücke has shown, back out through the pupil, without becoming scattered to any other portion of the wall of the eye. In this way is avoided the spreading of perceptible quantities of dispersed light within the eye. The reflected rays, which, from the point of convergence on the retina, pass back out divergently to the refracting surfaces of the eye, follow then precisely the same path, in a reverse direction, by which the incident rays of the luminous point converged from the refracting surfaces of the eye until they reached the retina. From this it follows that the returning rays, even after they have passed clear through the refractive media and out of the eye, must coincide completely with the incident rays, must therefore finally all betake themselves to the original luminous point.

For, when two rays, which pass through several simply refracting media in a reverse direction, coincide in one of the same [media] they must do the same in all [the media]. On the limiting surfaces of the medium, that is to say, within which they coincide, the angle of incidence of the outcoming rays is identical with the angle of refraction of those which are entering. As, now, according to the laws of refraction, the proportion of the sine between the angle of incidence and the angle of refraction of the former, is precisely as large as that between the angle of refraction and the angle of incidence of the latter, so must also, on the other side of the refracting surface, the angle of refraction of the outcoming and the angle of incidence of the ingoing, rays, be equal. As, at the same time, all these rays lie in one plane, the plane of refraction, it follows that they also fall into one another [coincide] in the second medium. In like manner it follows further for the third, fourth medium, and so on.

Let us apply that to the case where any given system of refracting surfaces produces an exact image of the luminous point a at the point b, that is, where all the rays which proceed from a unite again in b, then follows the well known fact that in this case, always, a will be the image of b, if the latter sends out rays. Exactly upon the same paths, that is to say, on which rays from a proceed to b, they may also return from b to a. If now a is a luminous point outside the eye, and b its image, a point on the retina, then the ocular media will concentrate the returning light precisely at a into an image of b. The image of the illuminated retinal point will coincide exactly with the original point of luminosity. The same is still valid, also, when we have to do not with a luminous point, but with a luminous surface or a body, as soon as the eye is adapted for its outlines. All the incident light which is thrown back can always only return to its place of origin, and never can proceed in any other direction.

From this it follows that, without special expedients, we can see nothing of the illuminated portion of the retina, because we cannot bring our eye into the direction of the returning light without at the same time cutting off the incident light absolutely. To our pupil no light from the depths of the other's eye can return which has not proceeded from it [i.e., our pupil]. And as, in general, none at all has proceeded from our pupil, it sees in the darkness of the other's eye merely the reflection of its own blackness; only those portions of the retina become visible to it on which its own dark image is copied.

We have until now assumed that the observed eye furnishes absolutely accurate images. When that is not the case, the propositions heretofore laid down do not hold strictly true, the returning light will indeed proceed to the illuminating body, but it will also in part pass by that, and an observer who approximates himself to the line of direction of the incident light, will be able to perceive a part of the light which is coming out. On this fact are based the methods of Cumming (*Medic. Chirurg. Transactions*, Vol. 29, p. 284) and Brücke (*J. Müllers Archiv.* 1847, p. 225) for observing the illumination of human eyes. From what has been said it is manifest that, in this way, the illumination must be the greater, the less exactly the rays of a luminous point are concentrated on a point of the retina, therefore especially in faulty adaptation. Besides, I have convinced myself that one may observe a weak illumination, according to the method of E. Brücke, even in eyes with good acuity and under perfect adaptation for the luminous body, from which is to be concluded that, under all circumstances, a small quantity of incident light is scattered laterally. The cause thereof may be inexactness of the eye, incomplete transparency of its refracting parts, or diffraction at the border of the pupil.

In any case, the observer perceives, in this experiment, only a small part of the returning light, and indeed precisely that which is irregularly refracted and which cannot be used for the production of a regular image. Some other method is necessary for the attainment of our object, a method which makes it possible to look into the eye not merely somewhat, but exactly, in the direction of the incident light. The expedient for this has already been found in an accidental observation by E. Brücke. v. Erlach, who wore spectacles, saw, indeed, the eyes of an acquaintance shine, when the acquaintance saw reflected in the lenses of the spectacles a light which there was in the room. In this way, therefore, uncovered lenses were employed as illuminating mirrors, and through these very objects the observer looked toward the observed eye. Precisely the same expedient we shall employ for our purpose, replacing, however, the spectacle lenses to advantage by well ground plane glasses.

In a darkened room, where only a single source of light, a well burning lamp or an opening in the window shutter for the sunlight, is present, let one set a small, plane glass plate in such a way that the observed eye may perceive therein the mirrored image of the light, without, however, its necessarily gazing at this mirrored image directly. From out the anterior surface of the lens there falls, by this arrangement, light into the observed eye, and through the same glass at the same time the observer can view the eye, without, while so doing, being in the least aware of any light which is being reflected from its anterior surface. One sees that, in this way, it becomes possible to look into the subject's eye in precisely the same direction as that in which the light falls upon it. Under these circumstances the eye of the observer in fact receives light from out the depths of the other eye, and sees its pupil apparently grow luminous.

In Fig. 1, let A be the flame, C the glass plate, D the observed, G the observing eye. The light from A which falls upon the mirroring plate, is by that partly reflected, and the reflected part continues, according to the laws of catoptrics, as if it proceeded from the reflected image of the flame at B. For the observed eye this mirrored image represents the place of the luminous object, and upon its retina is thrown an inverted and minified image. Moreover, the axis of this eye can be turned in any direction, say toward the object H. According to the already developed rules, the refractive media of D cast the image of its retina and of its retinal images again at B. For B is the apparently present object for the eye D, and the rays returning from D must proceed again to their place of origin. On the way from D to B this light encounters once more the reflecting plate, a part is reflected and returns to the real flame A, another portion passes through the glass and strikes the eye of the observer G.

By this arrangement the pupil of the eye D appears to shine with a red light, and indeed as a rule more strongly than I have seen it do by Brücke's method. According to that method, there contributes to the illumination only the little light which, in the eye, is not completely and regularly refracted; according to the method just described, on the contrary, the entire light, with the exception of the part (to be sure not an inconsiderable part) which is lost by the passage through the reflecting glass. Moreover, the illumination is of very different strengths, when different portions of the retina receive the image of the flame. When the eye D turns in different directions, the clear retinal image must always remain in the prolongation of the line B D, and will therefore fall successively on various portions of the background. If it falls on the place of entrance of the optic nerve, then the most of the light is reflected, the pupil lights up with a strong yellowish white, almost as if the flame stood behind it. The retina proper, on the other hand, reflects less, and indeed red light. In general, the image of the flame upon it appears the brighter, the nearer; the darker, the farther, it lies from the place of entrance of the optic nerve. On the contrary, the place of direct vision, the yellow spot (which is struck when the observed eye D gazes directly at the mirrored image of the flame at B) reflects, by way of exception, very much less light than the parts which are nearest to it, and is therefore the most unfavorable spot for this experiment.

In order to fulfill the condition that the observer gaze into the eye exactly in the direction of the incident light, the glass plate may be directed either by the observed or by the observer. If the former is to do it, let him turn the plate first of all so that he sees therein the mirrored image of the light, then again so that this image appears to him exactly in the same direction as the observing eye, that, in other words, the latter and the mirrored flame cover each other. In this way the required condition is fulfilled. At the same time occurs this inconvenience, that the observed eye must look directly at the flame, the retinal image therefore falling precisely on the spot whence the light is the least reflected. If, however, the observed eye, after it has found the correct position, turns a little sidewise, in order to let the light shine more brightly, then the pupil becomes displaced and the correct position is disturbed. Still, one can then assist the matter by gentle turning of the mirror now this way and now that.

It is better, however, to perform the experiment in another way, whereby the observer holds the glass himself. One must, by this method, shade the face that is being observed, and make the reflecting plate so small that it is barely large enough to see through. The light reflected from it then produces on the shaded face of the observed a small, bright spot, which has about the form of the reflecting glass. This point should be so managed by the observer that its centre falls upon the observed eye, while he himself looks through the glass. In this way the glass may easily be placed

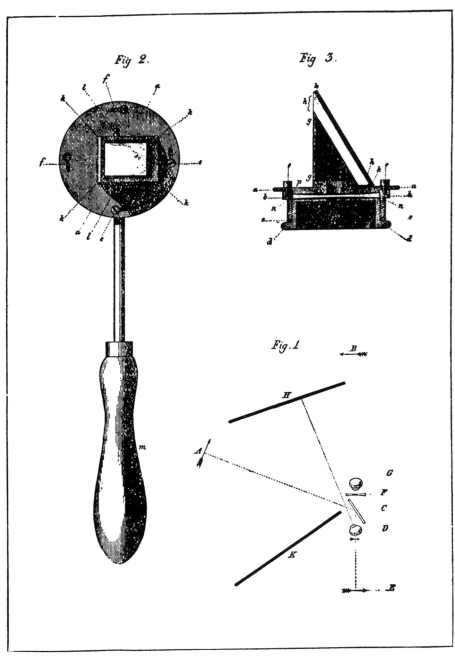

[Photographic Reproduction (Actual Size) of the Original Illustration in Helmholtz's ''Beschreibung eines Augenspiegels.'']

correctly, and the observed eye may, without the slightest difficulty, be turned toward all sides in order to cause the image of the flame to fall on different parts of the retina.

Every person can, furthermore, in similar fashion, by the aid of a bit of plane glass, see one of his own eyes grow luminous. He should step before a mirror, set up a lamp at one side, hold the glass before his right eye in such a way that he sees the flame reflected in the plate, and turn the glass so that the image of the flame coincides with the mirrored image of his left eye; then the left eye sees the mirrored image of his right pupil grow luminous, but of course only weakly so, because the retinal image falls on the outer side of the eye at a considerable distance from the optic nerve.

Moreover, the same simple expedient permits itself to be employed with advantage for illumination, in every instance when one wishes to look into a dark cavity with a narrow opening, for example, the auditory meatus, the nose, and so on. In order to view the drum membrane, one should seat the subject of the experiment with his back toward the window, preferably in sunshine, draw the auricle a little downward, and cast the reflected sunlight into the auditory meatus, while one gazes through the glass. In this way one may very easily and conveniently illuminate the tympanic membrane as strongly as he wishes, and so observe it.

In order to see the pupil become luminous, any simple plate of glass suffices for the mirror; one does not need in that case to pay particular attention to the intensity of the light. Should it be desired, however, by means of this light to recognize distinctly the structure of the retina and the character of the image of the flame, then one must endeavor to make the illumination as strong as possible. That can be done in two ways, namely, by a proper choice of the angle under which the incident light is reflected from the mirroring plane, and by an increase in the number of the reflecting plates. I will now unfold the principles which have guided me in this connection during the construction of my instrument, and which would also serve as a basis should oculists think it necessary to produce modifications of the instrument for practical purposes. For those of my readers to whom the physical conceptions involved are not familiar, I remark furthermore that this exposition is not necessary for an understanding of the sections to follow.

From every limiting surface of a glass plate, the more light is reflected the larger the angle of incidence, that is, the angle between the ray and a line which stands vertical to the plate. Since, in the case of reflection from the upper surfaces of transparent bodies, the light waves of different undulatory directions conduct themselves differently, we must think of the incident light as divided into two equal parts, of which the one is polarized parallelly to the reflecting surface, the other vertically thereto. The light-intensity of all the incident light we will call J, therefore that of each of the two divisions mentioned $\frac{1}{2}$ J, the angle of incidence (angle between the incident ray and the incident-perpendicular) a, the angle of refraction (between the refracted ray and the incident-perpendicular) a_1, the index of refraction n. If a is given, we find first of all a_1 by means of the equation

$$\text{sin. } a = n \text{ sin. } a_1$$

The intensity P of the light reflected from a limiting surface between air and glass and polarized vertically to the plane of incidence, is, according to the formula of Fresnel

$$P = \frac{J}{2} \cdot \frac{\tan^2 (a - a_1)}{\tan^2 (a + a_1)}$$

Likewise the intensity Q of the reflected light which is polarized parallelly to the plane of incidence

$$Q = \frac{J}{2} \cdot \frac{\sin^2 (a - a_1)}{\sin^2 (a + a_1)}$$

When several reflecting plates lie parallel, one behind another, and the illuminating surface is sufficiently large for its mirrored images, which are produced by the individual reflecting surfaces, to superimpose themselves, in greatest part, for the observed eye, then the individual images combine into one image of greater brightness. By computation of the quantities of light reflected to and fro between the different surfaces, one is able to determine for every system of parallel surfaces, how much light is, on the whole, reflected. For an indefinite number n of the reflecting surfaces one finds the sum II of the light polarized vertically upon the plane of incidence

$$\text{II} = \frac{nP}{J + 2(n - 1)P} J$$

and the sum Σ of that which is polarized parallelly to the plane of incidence

$$\Sigma = \frac{nQ}{J + 2(n - 1)Q} J$$

As I find these formulæ in no writing on physics I give their derivation briefly at the end of this essay.

The sum II+Σ gives us the entire quantity of light which is thrown back from the system of reflecting surfaces and which proceeds to the observed eye. We will set it down as equal to H, so that

$$H = \Pi + \Sigma$$

When the width of the pupil remains unchanged, the brightness of the retinal image is proportional to this quantity of light. The quantity of light returning from the eye we may therefore set down as equal to m H, where m designates a coefficient whose value is constant for different light-intensities, though dependent on the nature of the place on the retina from which the light proceeds. The returning light divides at the reflecting surfaces once more into a reflected and a transmitted portion, only the latter arriving in the observer's eye. The light which is reflected at the retina possesses, as is generally the case with diffuse reflected light, no longer any polarization, conducting itself in this respect, therefore, like the light from the light-source as it strikes upon the mirror. Inasmuch as, in addition, it falls upon the plates under the same angle, proportionately as much of it is reflected and transmitted as of the former [the light from the light-source]. If we designate the transmitted part by X, then we have the proportion

$$X : mH = (J - H) : J.$$

From this may be computed the quantity of light X, which passes into the eye of the observer. For H=0 and H=J; that is, when no light or all the light is reflected, X will=0. Between these extreme values of H exists a maximum of the value of X, which can be computed according to the known rules of the differential calculus. The maximum occurs when

$$H = \tfrac{1}{2}J.$$

Then will

$$X = \tfrac{1}{4}mJ.$$

By this condition is also determined for a given number of reflecting plates the angle under which the reflection must occur in order to give to the observer the brightest image. Unfortunately, the equation which expresses the dependence of the value H on the angle of incidence a, cannot be solved after a; we can therefore find the proper values of a only approximately by means of computational trials. Besides, it is of no use to drive the exactness of this computation very far, first, because the brightness for the observer is not materially altered, even when the position of the glasses is not that requisite for the maximum, and, secondly, because the alterations in the width of the pupil produced by different intensities of the incident light cannot be taken into account.

As the pupil of the observed eye becomes smaller under stronger incident light, the bright-ness of the retinal image will not increase entirely in the same proportion, when the values of H increase, as they should do according to the developed formulæ. It is therefore more advantageous to re-establish in the instrument the values of H as somewhat smaller than would be requisite for the maximum of H in the foregoing computation. One reaches, for example, the value, which slightly deviates from the foregoing maximum,

$$X = \tfrac{1}{5}mJ$$

when the light is reflected from one glass plate at an angle of about 70°, from three at an angle of 60°, of four at 55°, and these postions are therefore approximately the most advantageous.

The necessary brightness, therefore, can even be reached with a single glass plate for a mirror. The use of several plates at a smaller incidence-angle has, however, essential advantages if one would attain to distinct images of the retina. First of all, glass plates, even when they have well ground parallel surfaces, are not always internally of so homogeneous a structure as still to yield, by an oblique view, good, distinct images. Then, it is more difficult, by a very oblique view, to give to a reflecting plate the correct position toward the observed eye, and to hold the plate therein. Also, the observer, by the lateral parts of his head, cuts off more easily the rays of light which should fall upon the mirror; especially may this be avoided with difficulty when the angles of incidence are more than 70°. Finally, it remains to be especially considered that a small quantity of the light which falls into the observed eye is in fact reflected from its cornea and appears to the observer as a washed-out light spot in the visual field. This falls over the centre of the pupil, when the observed eye turns straight toward the mirror, therefore when it looks directly at the mirrored image of the flame; it falls more to one side when the observed eye gazes in any other direction, disturbing, however, the observation of the retina always more or less. It is therefore an essential advantage if one can weaken the corneal reflex for the observer to a considerable degree. Now, in fact, that image appears much weaker when 4 plates reflect at 56°, than when 3 reflect at 60° or one at 70°, while the retinal image, as already mentioned, holds to just about the same illumination. That is to say: the apparent brightness of the corneal reflex is not proportional to that of the retinal image, because the light which falls into the observed eye, and which is partly or wholly polarized by reflection, is depolarized by the diffuse reflection at the retina—something which does not occur from the specular reflection at the cornea. If the cornea, of the quantity of light A which falls upon it, reflects the portion μA, then the quantity of light which, in our experiments, passes from the cornea into the eye of the observer, equals, according to the same principles and the same designation as before,

$$\frac{\mu\Pi[J - 2\Pi] + \mu\Sigma[J - 2\Sigma]}{J}$$

Computation gives the result already stated. It is therefore from every point of view more advantageous to attain the necessary brightness by increasing the number of the plates, while they reflect the light at the polarization angle of 56°, than by increasing the angle of incidence, indeed the corneal reflex could be made to disappear entirely by increasing very much the number of the plates.

I have assumed, in the foregoing explanations, that the flame of a good oil-lamp with a double draught is employed as the light-source. When the experiment is properly conducted, the light of such a lamp is not so strongly reflected as very much to dazzle or fatigue the lateral parts of the retina of the observed eye. One can therefore easily continue the experiments as long as one likes. Only when the eye looks directly at the mirrored image of the flame, will this degree of brightness be found not long endurable. If one has at his disposal a more intense light, for example sunlight, which falls into a dark room through an opening in the window-shutter, then one can see the picture of the retina much brighter, if one, after proper weakening of the light, causes it to reflect from a mirroring-plate as vertically as possible, than when this takes place obliquely. The quantity of light which one may permit to enter into the eye is limited particularly by the sensitiveness of the latter. If, now, one has at his disposal excessively strong light, which by every kind of reflection, if it is not at the same time adequately weakened in another way, exceeds this limit, then the observer sees the retinal image, which has reached the limit of endurable intensity, at its brightest when as little as possible is lost at the second reflection. That is, however, the case when the light is thrown back from a plate almost vertically.

I have not had opportunity to institute such an investigation by means of sunlight; I do not believe, however, that, by that method, any considerable advantages are to be secured, because, in the case of vertical reflection, the apparent brightness of the disturbing corneal reflexes increases at a much higher rate than that of the retinal image.

There was expressed to me a number of times the supposition (at first blush a very plausible one) that, by a convex lens which should concentrate toward the observed eye all the light which falls upon it, the quantity of light falling into the eye and therefore also the brightness of the retinal image, could be considerably increased. I will therefore here direct attention to the fact that, in this way, not the brightness but only the size of the retinal image is increased. When we bring the eye to the point of union of the light-rays, which have passed through a lens, then the entire surface of the lens appears to us luminous with that light-intensity which belongs to the luminous point. Instead of the smaller retinal image of the luminous point, there forms itself for us therefore a larger one with the same intensity, that of the lens-surface. Moreover, by no complicated arrangement of lenses can the brightness be increased. In order to perceive this, we need only to remind ourselves of this fact from the theory of telescopes, that through no telescope or similar arrangement of lenses can an object of appreciable diameter appear brighter than with the naked eye. As, now, the inhabitant of the seeing eye subjectively perceives the surface no brighter through the lenses, so can, objectively, the image in his eye by the use of no sort of lenses be brighter than without them. For to an objectively brighter retinal image there must always correspond a stronger subjective light-perception.

2. Production of a Distinct Image of the Retina.

We now come to investigate how, by means of the light which, returning from the retina of the observed eye, falls into the eye of the observer, we may be able to receive distinct images of the retina itself, and of the picture of the light-source cast upon it. For this purpose let us take again our Fig. 1. According to the explanations just made, the ocular media will so refract the rays returning from points of the retina of the eye D, that they come together outside the eye and indeed in the corresponding points of the image B. The image which the ocular media cast of the retina and of the retinal image of the flame, coincides therefore in size and position with the first reflected image of the flame. An observer who (reckoning outward from the mirror) stands on the other side of B and at the distance of distinct vision from B, would therefore in fact be able to see that image of retinal objects distinctly. His visual field, however, limited by the pupil of the observed eye, would, at the comparatively considerable distance of the two eyes from one another, be so small that it would be impossible to combine the viewed details into a complete picture.

The regard which we must pay to the enlargement of the visual field, makes it much more necessary to approximate the two eyes as closely to each other as possible. Then, however, the image B falls in general behind the back of the observer, and can not be plainly seen by him. If, for example, in Fig. 1, the observing eye is at G, then it receives the light rays which proceed out of the eye D and which come together at the points of B. Now a normal eye can indeed unite upon its retina parallel rays, as these move from infinity, and divergent, as these come from nearer points, but not convergent rays. The simplest way to assist in this matter, and to make the convergent bundles of rays divergent, is a concave lens, which is inserted between the mirror and the eye of the beholder, as in Fig. 1 at F.

According to the known laws of refraction in concave lenses, the convergent rays which strike upon F will, after their exit from the lens, either be less convergent (when, that is to say, the focal distance is greater than FB) or they become parallel (when the focal distance equals FB) or, finally, divergent, as if they came from points of an image E behind the observed eye (when the focal distance is smaller than BF). In the latter case the concave lens acts precisely as it does in opera glasses, where it likewise converts the inverted imperfect image, which the objective lens should cast at its focus, and which lies on the side of the observer, into one which stands upright and which appears to the observer to be on the other side of the glasses. In our case, likewise, the ocular media form the objective glass of a microscope, which is constructed on the principle of a Gallileonian telescope, while the concave lens represents the ocular.

If the accommodation distance of the two eyes DB and GE are given, and in addition the mutual distances of the eyes and the concave lens are settled according to the principles above set forth, that is, made as small as the mirror permits, then is the focal distance which is to be given to the concave lens to be determined according to the known laws of refraction in lenses. This is found to equal

$$\frac{EF \quad BF}{EB}$$

or:

$$\frac{(EG - GF)(BD - DF)}{EG + BD - DG}$$

The greater are the accommodation distances EG and BD, the greater must also be the focal distance of F. The observer will, therefore, if one of the two eyes is short-sighted, employ stronger concave lenses, but, if one eye is far-sighted, weaker ones, than for two normal eyes. When the observing and the observed eye exchange their rôles, without altering the condition of their accommodation, there will generally become necessary a glass of a different focal distance, and, indeed, as GF < DF, a weaker one, when the more short-sighted eye observes, than when it is observed. Still, a closer consideration of the foregoing formula shows that this difference is extremely slight in the case of not too short-sighted eyes, so that, in the case of such, the same glass can serve for mutual observation.

The magnification is determined according to the known laws of optics in this way, that the image E, viewed from the center of the lens F, must appear under the same visual angle as B, its imaginary object. Since the eye G, the lens F and the eye D stand as closely together as possible, then will B appear from F only a little larger than from D. The eye G therefore sees the retinal image of the flame magnified, and indeed just as large, or, considered exactly, a trifle larger, than the eye D sees the original flame. The parts of the retina on which the image of the flame falls, appear likewise in the image E again, magnified of course in the same proportion as that.

According to what has just been said, the proportion of this enlargement is equal to that of the retinal image to its object. Let us take as the distance of the decussation-point of the refracted rays from the retina, according to Volkmann's measurings, 4 lines, for the distance of the object from the eye the normal visual distance of 8 inches, then the magnification is found to be 24 times.

We have compared the ocular media in our experiment with the objective of a microscope, the concave glass with the ocular. Now, in place of the latter, one should be able to produce a combination of two convex lenses, which stand at a distance from one another of less than the sum of their focal distances, as is the case in the ordinary compound microscope. The first of the lenses would, like the collective glass of this instrument, unite the weakly converging light-rays which proceed from the observed eye, more promptly to an image, which, situated between the lens and its focal distance, would exhibit the flame-image upright, the retina inverted. This image could then be seen magnified by the second convex lens. I have debated the results of such a combination, according to the known laws of optical instruments, with respect to magnification, illumination, visual field, etc. As the computation showed that in this way no essential advantages were to be secured, as compared with the simple concave lenses, it will here suffice to adduce those results very briefly. It is hereby presupposed that the first lens, so far as the mirror permits, is approximated to the observed eye, and that the observing eye lies close to the second lens.

First of all, as to the illumination, the maximum thereof is directly attained by a concave lens for the middle of the visual field. If the same thing is to occur by two convex lenses, then these must be so chosen and arranged that no other enlargement takes place than by the concave lens, that is, in such a way that the magnified retinal image of the flame appears to the observing eye under the same visual angle as the mirrored image of the flame does to the eye that is being observed.

If this enlargement is to occur, the image from the first lens must fall, as in the ordinary ocular tubes of the compound microscope, in the middle between both lenses. In the case of a weaker magnification, it is possible to cause a larger portion of the visual field to appear in the maximum of brightness; in the case of stronger, on the contrary, that can no longer occur even in the middle. As advantageous, therefore, as even a stronger magnification might be, still such a one is not practicable, because the illumination would thereby suffer too much, and a living eye would not well endure for a longer time without dazzling the incidence of still stronger light than that reflected from a good lamp. Then, too, is the fact that the living eye cannot be thoroughly fastened, as would be necessary for the fixation of individual parts of the image in the case of stronger magnification.

Next to be considered is the visual field. The part of the retina which one can survey is always the smaller the farther one removes oneself from the observed eye; the larger the nearer one comes to it. The limit of approximation is, however, set in this way: that the obliquely placed mirror-plates have to be inserted between the eye and the glass-lenses.

In order to compare by means of computation the effects of various lenses, we must therefore accept as equally great the distance of the concave glass and that of the first convex glass from the observed eye. If then at the same time the condition is observed, that the brightness in the middle of the visual field should reach its maximum, then are found definite focal distances of the convex lenses for every given distance from the eye, which make the visual field at its largest. If one choose the focal distances of both the convex lenses in accordance with these determinations, then it further appears that when the distance of the lens from the eye is smaller than the focal distance which one may give to the objective of a telescope from the aperture of the pupil without prejudicing the distinctness of the image, therefore in the case of achromatic lenses smaller than perhaps the tenfold pupillary diameter, the concave lens, if larger, the convex lenses can give a larger visual field.[2] Now, in the case of the closest possible approximation of the lenses to the observed eye, the distance between both will of course, on account of the mirror being placed in the interval between

the lenses, remain in general somewhat larger than the tenfold pupillary diameter, and one would therefore be able to secure by means of two convex lenses a slight advantage for the visual field. Inasmuch, however, as the lenses, in order to yield this advantage, must have focal distances of 36 to 40 lines, it may become very difficult to receive an image of the same distinctness as by a concave lens which may have a focal distance of 8 to 10 inches. I, at least, have not been successful in this matter, by the combination of such convex lenses as stood at my disposal. Moreover, it transpired, in the experiments with such lenses, that the correct location of the instrument for the perception of the retinal image is both found and kept with much greater difficulty. With a simple concave lens it is, to wit, not necessary that the axis of the lens be directed exactly upon the observed eye, if only the mirror casts light into it. This condition, however, must be observed in the case of two convex lenses.

Consequently it appears to be more advantageous to retain the simple concave lens as ocular, while one almost everywhere else in optics replaces it to decided advantage by convex lenses. A decided advantage of the latter occurs, to be sure, even in our case, which would make their employment desirable, to wit, the advantage that, by an altered distance of the lenses from each other, one can adjust the apparatus to all visual distances of the observed and the observing eye, while, for this purpose, one must exchange the concave lens for another. If one could completely make fast the head of the observed person and the instrument, convex lenses would in consequence be more convenient; without such arrangements, however, all their other advantages are outweighed by the disadvantage of the difficult placing of the instrument. I have therefore myself always employed only a simple concave lens.

3. DESCRIPTION OF THE OPHTHALMOSCOPE.

In order to institute observations of the kind described, it is convenient to unite the mirror-plates and the concave lens by means of a suitable frame. I propose for such a combination the name *Augenspiegel*, by analogy with similar instruments. The instrument is viewed in Fig. 2 from in front, in Fig. 3 exhibited in horizontal cross-section. The reflecting plates hh are fastened, by means of the brass piece gg, to the circular plate aa, at an angle which is equal to the chosen angle of incidence of the light rays—in the figure, 56°. The brass piece gg forms with the glass plates a hollow, right-angularly triangular prism. In Fig. 3 one sees into the inner cavity thereof, and has before him one of the right-angularly triangular basal surfaces. Of the three quadrangular lateral surfaces of the prism, that which corresponds to the hypothenuse of the basal surface, is formed by

---

[2] The sentence, in the original, is hopelessly obscure; it is, therefore, also obscure in the translation. The reader should recall the fact that Helmholtz, at the time when he wrote the "*Beschreibung*," was not yet master of a literary style, and I have deemed it far the fairer way not to force into the sentence a meaning of my own.—(T. H. S.)

the glass plates, that which corresponds to the longer cathetus stands free, that corresponding to the shorter cathetus lies on the disc aa, and carries a cylindrical process p, which, by means of a corresponding circular opening in the plate aa, so clasps through, that it holds the prism fast against the plate, but permits a turning on its axis. The glass plates are held against the prismatic brass piece by the frames kkkk, whose over-reaching lateral edges are secured to the brass piece gg by the screws ll. The disc aa rests on the cylinder bbcc without being permanently fastened to it. In the border of aa, namely, there are cut four openings of the form f, to which openings there correspond four screws ee with cylindrical heads and thin necks, inserted into the border of the cylindrical ring bb. In Fig. 2 are shown only two of these screws, in order to let the holes f be seen. The heads of the screws allow of their shoving through the broad circular portions of the openings, and if then the disc aa is turned about its center, the necks of the screws pass into the smaller, slit-shaped part of the same opening, while their heads lap over and fasten the disc to the ring bb. In that way it is possible to remove the disc very easily and quickly from the setting of the concave lens, and to exchange the lens for another. The concave lens nn lies between the plate aa and the floor of the cylindrical piece dd, which is screwed into bbcc and can be set back by screwing round, when it becomes necessary to lay two lenses one upon the other for very short-sighted eyes. The whole is fastened to the handle m. For a normal-eyed observer, the numbers 6 to 12 of the ordinary concave spectacle lenses, are sufficient for the adjustment to all adaptational conditions of the eyes to be invesigated. For the viewing of other normal eyes, I generally employed Nr. 10. For very short-sighted eyes, two lenses should be superimposed.

As to the reflecting plates, those of ordinary mirror-glass are not appropriate, because their two surfaces are as a rule not sufficiently parallel to cause the images which they cast of the lamp-flame to coincide in the way that they should. The glasses must therefore for our use be especially ground, in order to receive parallel surfaces, though this condition need not be fulfilled with such exactness as in the case of the plane-parallel glasses which one employs in the finer measuring instruments.

A good blackening of the non-reflecting surfaces is essential. Since, of the bright light which falls upon the instrument, only a proportionately small part returns from the retina of the observed eye, all the remaining remnants of the light, which might perhaps get into the eye of the observer, must be done away with. First of all, the inner surface of the ocular piece dd must be blackened, and the observer must place his eye as closely into it as possible, in order to cut off all the light which could fall from the flame upon this surface. Secondly, the outer surface of the disc aa and of the prismatic mirror-frame kkkk must be blackened, in order that blank metal surfaces, which are turned toward the observed eye, may not produce disturbing corneal reflexes. Thirdly, however, the inner surface of the mirror-frame is to be blackened with especial care. The light of the flame which falls on the reflecting plate, passes in greater part through, and strikes the plate gg. All that is not here absorbed, returns to the mirror, is reflected from this in the same direction to the observing eye, in which the weak light from the retina of the observed eye arrives, and mingles with the image of this membrane. I have found, in this matter, the general methods of procedure of mechanics for blackening brass-pieces to be inadequate, and the framework of the mirror must be tapestried internally with black velvet, which absorbs the light more completely.[3]

[3] The subsequent history of the ophthalmoscope "down to a time within the memory of men still living," is, very briefly, as follows: Ruete, in 1852, invented the "indirect method" (D. Augenspiegel u. d. Optometer, Göttingen, 1852). He employed a concave perforated mirror, held at a considerable distance from the observed eye, and between the mirror and the eye one (sometimes two) spherical convex lenses. Helmholtz, also, had made use of convex lenses, but these he had placed behind the mirror, finding them there, of course, of very little value (see herein).

Helmholtz, next, explained most thoroughly (Vierordt's Archiv, 1852, p. 827) the method which Ruete had invented. In the very same paper Helmholtz described what he called "the simplest method," by which an eye could be examined by means of only a candle, a screen and a convex spherical lens. He also mentioned (still in the same most memorable article) the so-called Rekoss discs—i. e., two rotatory discs, each containing four concave lenses inserted not far from the peripheries of the discs. One of the discs held lenses from 6 in. to 9 in. focus, the other those from 10 to 13 in. The Rekoss disc, or discs, with numerous modifications, is, as all are aware, in use at the present day. Rekoss was not an ophthalmologist, but an instrument-maker of Konigsberg (where Helmholtz at the time was living).

Coccius, in 1853, invented an instrument which found much favor for years. It consisted of a lens, set in a frame, in front of a plane mirror. The distance between the mirror and the lens could be altered very considerably.

Eduard Jaeger, in 1854, produced a combination of the Helmholtz and the Ruete instrument—that is to say, the plates of silvered glass in the Helmholtz instrument were made replaceable by a concave silvered mirror, such mirror to be used for the indirect method. To this affair of Jaeger's, Strawbridge, of Philadelphia, in 1871, added three interchangeable Rekoss discs.

The ophthalmoscope of Liebreich is too familiar to all to require the slightest description. So, almost, is that of Loring, with its single disc and double row of lenses, the disc being movable up and down for the purpose of bringing into action either the one row or the other.

When one desires to use the instrument, he sets the person to be examined in a dark room and next the corner of a table on which, at a level with the eye and sidewise from the face, stands a well-burning, double-draught lamp. It is convenient to set upon the table, at a fitting visual distance, some not too bright object, whereon one can point out to the observed eye certain points for fixation, for example a blackboard divided into squares, each of which is designated by a number, while one causes the eye to fix various points one after another. The image of the flame falls ever on different parts of the retina, which the observer, therefore, may investigate one after another in any order desired. Between the flame and the observed eye an opaque screen must be erected, in order to shade the eye, so that directly incident flame-light may not produce a very disturbing corneal reflex and a narrowing of the pupil. Still, the border of the shadow must pass very close before the observed eye, in order that the ophthalmoscope, which must itself remain in the light, may be carried toward that eye as closely as possible. The observer seats himself before the observed, brings the ophthalmoscope, without at first looking through it, into about the right position, when its reflecting surface casts a bright light upon the face. When one has so turned the mirror that the middle of its light falls upon the eye, and the axis of the instrument is directed precisely into it, one looks through. A person then has, as a rule, at once before him the bright image of the flame, or finds it after more or less moving about. Moreover, one can also, looking through the instrument, discern, to a certain extent, the eye and the clear light which must fall upon it, even if indistinctly and as if they were faded, and also, in that manner, with the help of these [the eye and the light upon it] discover the correct position. If, though the pupil appears luminous, one cannot see the various parts of the retina distinctly, then one must insert another concave lens. An observer who has accustomed himself to alter at will the adaptation of his eye, easily discovers whether he sees more plainly by a far-sighted or a near-sighted adaptation, and whether, accordingly, he must choose more or less strongly curved lenses. Moreover, many persons make the matter difficult, especially those who are not accustomed to looking through optical instruments, and short-sighted persons who see through them with diffi-

culty, insomuch as they involuntarily adapt the eye for great nearness, because they think of the object to be seen as being very close. In that way the eyes of the observer are greatly fatigued, and readily begin to be injected and to water. It is necessary here, as in the case of all optical instruments possessing an alterable adaptation, to adjust the eye for the distance, and then to adjust the instrument to the distance.

After a little practice it is not difficult to find the right lens and the correct position of the instrument. Also, one can easily, on his own eye, show these matters to anyone who has never yet seen them, in order first to render him familiar with the appearance of what he is going to look for. In that way it will be made much easier for him to discover independently the very same things in the eyes of others. Let the instructor, for this purpose, first of all discover the particular lens through which he can see the student's retina plainly, and then let him place this in the ophthalmoscope; then through the same glass the student can see distinctly into the eye of the teacher, if neither of the two is very short-sighted. In the latter case (as explained already) the more short-sighted person needs a somewhat weaker glass when he observes than when he is observed. Let the instructor, then, bring one of his own eyes into the position which has been described as that for the eye to be observed, and let him so hold the ophthalmoscope before him that he may be able, at the same time, to look through its central openings and glimpse the mirrored image of the flame in the mirror, hand over to the student the instrument in this position, and let him look through it. The student will then see in the eye the image of the flame. In order to teach him to recognize the appearance of the parts of the retina, let the teacher throw the image of the flame on the place of entrance of the optic nerve, because in that place the largest and most recognizable vascular trunks exhibit themselves. Let him, for this purpose, turn the eye gradually more and more to the inner side of the mirrored image of the flame, until this suddenly becomes smaller to him, or disappears. That happens, as is known, when the image falls upon the place of entrance of the optic nerve. Besides, most persons more easily succeed in seeing and recognizing the image of the flame than the tiny parts of the retina in the bright ground thereof.

4. VIEWING THE RETINA AND THE IMAGE OF THE FLAME.

Should one desire to investigate the retina completely, then it is convenient, as already mentioned, to set up a blackboard covered with numbers as a visual point for the eye to be investigated. As soon as this eye fixes one of the numbers, looking past the mirror a little to the inward

Wadsworth, of Boston, invented the "mirror obliquely set," which enables the observer today to look straight through the lenses instead of at an angle. Both the Loring and the Wadsworth instruments are especially valuable for refraction purposes.

The electric light ophthalmoscopes are in the hands of every practising ophthalmologist at the present day, and require no description.

side thereof, the observer will almost always recognize in the visual field one or two of the larger vessels. He causes the eye to turn to one of the near-lying figures, and notices whether he is brought nearer to the origin or to the branching of the vessels. While, in this way, he traces the vessels in the direction of their larger trunks, he comes at length to the place of entrance of the optic nerve. This distinguishes itself from the rest of the eye-ground by its white color, for it is not covered with pigment and a fine vascular network, but here the white cross-section of the nerve lies wholly free, at the very most shot through by tiny, isolated vessels. Mostly to the inner side, near by, the arteries and veins of the retina press forward from the depths. At times one sees a portion of the vessel still hiding in the substance of the nerve, and understands that, in the living, this substance is decidedly transparent. One distinguishes the two kinds of vessels from each other by the brighter color of the blood and the double contours of the walls in the arteries and in their first ramifications. I have not been able to recognize pulsations with certainty. The first main branches of the vessels border the optic nerve at its inner side, in order to spread out later, above and below, across the retinal field. The appearance of the sharply pencilled red vessels on the clear white ground is of surprising elegance. Somewhat farther to the inner side, close by the nerve, I have always remarked a small, sickle-shaped stripe of shadow, which appears to take its origin from a fold of the retina.

In the other parts, the ground of the eye looks reddish, and indeed first of all round about the optic nerve of a somewhat clear, light-red, the darker, on-the contrary, the farther you pass from that place. One sees here larger and smaller branching blood-red vessels, which stand out plainly from the back-ground. The ground itself appears to be not entirely homogeneous, but indistinctly reddish. This would seem to arise from the fact that the close capillary net is too fine, too weakly illuminated and too transparent to be distinguished plainly from the underlying weakly, light-gray substance of the retina. That the ground looks brighter in the vicinity of the optic nerve is no doubt owing to the fact that the retina here, on account of the superimposed fibres of the optic nerve, is thicker, while, toward its periphery, it becomes continually thinner. Moreover, the place of direct vision (the yellow spot) is essentially distinguished in appearance from the parts which lie immediately about it. In order to get this point before oneself, one causes the eye which is being observed to look directly at the mirrored image of the flame. The retina then appears much darker, grayish-yellow without intermixture of red; and one sees no traces of capillary vessels. Then, too, one is greatly an-

noyed while gazing on the yellow spot, by the tiny image from the cornea, which obtrudes itself precisely in the center of the visual field, while, during the observation of the lateral portions of the retina, it lies to one side.

After deciding what, in the healthy eye, can be made out concerning the nature of the retina, I have no doubt that one will be able to recognize all such disease conditions as permit of recognition by the sense of sight in other transparent parts— for example, the cornea. Increased repletion of the vessels and vascular varicosities must prove easy to make out. Exudates into the substance of the retina, or between that structure and the pigment membrane, must yield themselves to observation, very much as affections of the cornea do, by their brightness against a dark ground. If they lie in part before the retina, they will then enclose its vessels in a veil. I here recall that, according to Brücke, the recent retina is just about as transparent as the other ocular media, and that, apart from its vessels, it is only visible in our experiments because it is strongly illuminated on the deep-black ground of the pigment membrane. Fibrinous exudates, which are nearly always less transparent than the ocular media, must also for that reason, when they lie in the fundus of the eye, considerably strengthen the reflex. Then too I believe that opacities of the vitreous body will be much more easily and certainly recognizable, partly by the illumination of a reflecting glass-plate, partly by the ophthalmoscope. One will even be able to determine with ease, from the indistinctness of the image of the flame and of the retinal vessels, the degree of the opacity. If, in the case of such an opacity, scintillating particles have detached themselves, then too a person will be able to take note of these. In brief, I believe that I may hold the expectation not to be exaggerated, that all the alterations of the vitreous body and of the retina which, until now, have been found in cadavers, will also permit of recognition in the living eye—a possibility which appears to promise the most remarkable advances for the hitherto undeveloped pathology of this structure.[4]

Finally, it is of interest, for certain physiological purposes, to investigate the accuracy with which the eye forms images. It is best to employ for this purpose a thread, which one draws along hori-

[4] Probably the most significant sentence ever penned by an ophthalmologist. How gloriously the great man's prophecy has been fulfilled is known not merely to specialists and general practitioners, but even, in some degree, to first year medical students and the educated portion of the laity. In fact, there are just two kinds of ophthalmology, that which came before and that which followed after Helmholtz's "Beschreibung eines Augenspiegels."—(T. H. S.)

zontally before the flame. Its image remains single, while vertical threads are manifolded by the manifold reflections.

First of all one gets an opportunity to convince oneself, by the appearance of the image, that the different adaptations of the eye really depend upon alterations in the refractive media. One should cause to be fixed an object which is just about as far removed from the observed eye as the thread is from the flame. The observer then sees the elements of the retina and the image of the thread distinctly at the same time. Should the thread be carried nearer to or farther from the eye, then it becomes indistinct in the retinal image, or entirely disappears, while the parts of the retina remain sharp. One perceives from this that the retinal images of objects which stand at various distances from the eye, are in fact not equally distinct. Then again, one should so place the thread that it appears distinct in the retinal image at the same time with the vessels, and should cause the observed eye to fix a point which is either much farther or much nearer than that upon which it was formerly directed. Immediately one sees the retina and the image of the flame become gradually indistinct.

It should incidentally be remarked that, on the white surface of the optic nerve no image is cast, even when the image appears absolutely sharp on the immediately surrounding portions of the retina. Inasmuch as the observer, in the case of a person over whose optic nerve cross-section little vessels run, sees these quite as plainly as those of the retina adjacent, therefore that indistinctness of the image of the flame cannot proceed from the passage of the end of the optic nerve out of the level of the retina. I believe rather that one must regard the transparent condition of the optic nerve mass as the real cause.

Moreover, one is able, whenever it becomes necessary, to convince oneself readily in an objective manner of the presence and the degree of the short- or far-sightedness of the observed eye. Let the observer first investigate a normal eye, which he causes to fix objects at various distances, and notice what concave lenses he is obliged to use in the various stages of adaptation of the eye. In the investigation of any other eye, he then learns from the number of the concave glass through which he saw the retina distinctly the corresponding adaptational distance of the observed eye. The observer is, by this method, entirely independent of the assertions of the other person, for he himself sees, as it were with that other's eye, at least by means of its refractive media. In this way, for example, I was able to convince myself in a completely amaurotic eye, that that eye was simultaneously in a high degree short-sighted. In that way was decided in this case a question of great importance for the

anamnesis, whether, that is, certain earlier difficulties of sight recounted by the patient, should be referred to shortsightedness or to commencing amblyopia.

An important physiological conclusion thrust itself upon me in these investigations. The free-lying cross-section of the optic nerve is apparently so transparent that the light which falls upon it must penetrate deeply into the mass of the fibres, inasmuch as, now and then, one sees the bendings of the central artery and vein shimmering forward through the substance of the nerve. When the little image of the flame falls on the place of entrance of the nerve, then all its fibres, or at least a very large part of them, are struck by more or less intense light, and yet, obviously, they perceive no light. If they did perceive it, then that entire portion of the visual field which corresponds to them would have to appear illuminated. Not only, however, is that not the case, but there is even less light perceived than when the image falls upon some other portion of the retina. We must from this conclude that the fibres of the optic nerve are incapable of being affected by objective light (ethereal vibrations), while, nevertheless, they perceive every other kind of irritation as subjective light. This is a paradox, which, of course, has its ground in the ambiguity of the word "light," and is far removed from being an actual contradiction. The vibrations of the ether which we call light, produce, like every other mechanical or electrical irritation, when they strike the retina, the sensation which we call light. But from this, that the retina, protected from pressure and electrical currents and exposed to the action of ethereal vibrations, is much oftener struck and excited by the former than by the latter, it by no means follows that light must be regarded as an especially adequate irritant for the retina and the elements of the optic nerve and as standing in contrast to all the other kinds of irritation. There are no difficulties in supposing that all the irritations which are able to affect the optic nerve system produce sensations of light, that, however, the ethereal vibrations are able to act only on the retina. A similar state of affairs is found in the case of the nerves of touch, with respect to heat and cold. Here too the peripheral expansions behave differently from the trunks. For the latter, slight variations in temperature are no irritant at all, as it appears, and the greater variations, which are able to irritate, produce no temperatural sensations. Besides, one is able to conclude still further that, in the retina, not the fibres, which spread out in a radiating manner from the optic nerve, but the spherical elements, are sensitive to light. Were it the former, then must light which strikes on any place in the retina be perceived by all those fibres which in part end in this place, and in part pass across it on their way toward the retinal periphery. There would therefore extend, in the visual field, from every illuminated point, a bright shine toward the borders of the field, which is not the case. We may accordingly further conclude that even the continuations of the optic nerve fibres in the retina are insensitive to light. There remain only the ganglionic bodies and the nuclear-like structures of the retina, in which the ethereal oscillations are able to act as an irritant.

APPENDIX.

Derivation of the formula for the quantity of light which is reflected from several glass plates.

Whether this formula is correct for n reflecting surfaces is shown by the fact that it is also correct for (n+1). As it also proves right for n=1 and n=2, it must do the same for any desired value of n.

Let the quantity of light which at the given angle of incidence is thrown back by a reflecting surface, when the quantity 1 passes off of light polarized vertically against the plane of incidence, be p, that thrown back by n such surfaces $P_{(n)}$, that thrown back by (n+1), $P_{(n+1)}$. It is demonstrable that if

$$P_{(n)} = \frac{np}{1 + (n - 1p)} \quad \ldots\ldots\ldots\ldots 1)$$

then also that equation is correct which arises from this by the substitution of n+1 for n:

$$P_{(n+1)} = \frac{(n + 1)p}{1 + np} \quad \ldots\ldots\ldots\ldots 2)$$

For the sake of a better designation, let us assume that the system of n reflecting plates lies horizontal and that light falls on it from above. Let the (n+1)th surface be added to the system below. The quantity of light which passes downward from the lowermost nth surface of the compound system to the (n+1)th surface let us call x; that which, reflected from the (n+1)th surface, mounts to the system of the n surfaces, y. The quantity x is composed partly of the portion of the incident light which has passed through the system of n surfaces, partly of the portion of y which is reflected from this system. Therefore is

$$x = 1 - P_{(n)} + yP_{(n)} \quad \ldots\ldots\ldots\ldots 3)$$

The quantity y originates from that part of x which is reflected from the (n+1)th surface. It is therefore

$$y = xp \quad \ldots\ldots\ldots\ldots\ldots 4)$$

The quantity $P_{(n+1)}$ which passes upward from the uppermost surface, proceeds in part from that portion of the incident light which is reflected from the system of n surfaces, partly from that

portion of y which passes through this system. It is therefore

$$P_{(n+1)} = P_{(n)} + y(1 - P_{(n)}) \ldots\ldots\ldots 5)$$

If one eliminates x and y from equations 3, 4 and 5, one gets

$$P_{(n+1)} = P_{(n)} + \frac{p[1 - P_{(n)}]^2}{1 - pP_{(n)}} \quad \ldots\ldots\ldots 6)$$

If we place in this equation 6 the value of $P_{(n)}$ from the equation 1, we get in fact, after the necessary reductions, equation 2, whose correctness was to be proved.

For *one* reflecting surface is

$$P_{(1)} = p$$

Equation one (to be tested) gives the same value.

For *two* reflecting surfaces we get the value $P_{(2)}$ without employing equations 1 or 2, if, in the derivation of equation 6, we suppose that n=1 and $_{(n)}P=p$. Equation 6 then becomes

$$P_{(2)} = p + \frac{p(1 - p)^2}{1 - p^2}$$
$$= \frac{2p}{1 + p}$$

Equation 1 gives the same value.

As the latter accordingly is correct for n=1 and for n=2, then it follows from the proof adduced, that it is correct also for n=3, and if it is correct for n=3, that it also is correct for n=4, and so on to infinity.

In a precisely similar way the matter proceeds in the case of light polarized parallel to the surface of incidence.

If we assume the quantity of incident light to be equal to $\frac{1}{2}J$, and that $p = \dfrac{2P}{J}$, and designate that which we have here called P with II, we get the formula in question.

ABOUT THE COMPLICATION OF INFLAMMATION OF THE OPTIC NERVE WITH DISEASES OF THE BRAIN*

By
Prof. A. v. Gräfe.

One of the most instructive observations that examination with the ophthalmoscope has permitted is the frequent association of diseases of the optic nerve with extraocular diseases. About

_____
* Translation of: Ueber Complication von Sehnervenentzündung mit Gehirnkrankheiten, by A. v. Gräfe,

three years ago a patient came under my care who suffered from various cerebral symptoms, with left hemiplegia and paresis in the area of the facial nerve, intermittent epileptiform seizures, loss of memory, dulling of mental functions, and, in addition, progressive blindness. My first thought, while doing an external examination of the patient, was that the amaurosis was caused by paralysis of the optic nerve and, therefore, that no material changes in the eye, or possibly only signs in the papilla of secondary atrophy of the optic nerve would be evident. Contrary to this presumption, during examination with the opthalmoscope I found the papilla remarkably and irregularly swollen, it was markedly elevated on one side, but on the opposite side diminished gradually to the normal level. This normally transparent substance and the adjoining retina seemed gray and dense, with an unusual degree of redness, and for this reason the border of the choroid and the optic nerve was completely obscured. This opalescence was diffuse and in the upright image it had a striped appearance, seeming to follow the spread of the optic nerve fibers. The veins of the retina were widened, extremely tortuous, in certain parts very obscure, and were irregularly prominent in the opaque substance. The arteries were comparatively thin. The cloudiness of the retina diminished gradually from the border of the optic nerve and included a total zone of about 2 mm. in width, meaning a circle of about 5 mm. in diameter including the papilla. Without any doubt there was hyperemia and swelling of the optic nerve which, with the intense opacification of the substance, had to be considered inflammatory.[1] These intraocular findings, which were nearly the same in both eyes, could explain the almost complete blindness very well, but they were at least complicated by a disease of the brain, the diagnosis of which, after the consideration of all details which I don't want to mention here, fluctuated for a long time between a right-sided encephalitis and a cerebral tumor, but gradually was considered to be the latter. Because the rest of the cerebral symptoms existed long before the blindness, the inflam-

matory swelling of the optic nerves had to be considered subsequent to them, but what connection there was between the two diseases could not be determined. The patient expired, during an epileptiform seizure, after half a year of observation. The autopsy showed an expanding sarcomatous tumor in the right hemisphere. Unfortunately, examination of the eyes was not allowed. Incidentally, during the last month the optic nerves had changed their appearance considerably, the swelling had nearly completely disappeared, and the papillae had gained a more whitish appearance; the only difference between these findings and the ordinary findings of cerebral amaurosis with optic atrophy was the persistent tortuosity of the veins and the grayish opalescence of the part of the retina bordering on the papilla.

Again during the same year, a man in his thirties came to see me who had a similar complication of inflammatory swelling of the optic nerves, with amaurotic amblyopia and various cerebral symptoms. These latter symptoms never allowed, within the limits of my competence, a differential diagnosis between an encephalitis on the left side and a cerebral tumor. The degeneration of the papilla was exactly the same as in the other case, but the optic nerve was slightly redder and in the adjoining retina were some ecchymoses. It seemed to me remarkable that with the decrease of the swelling, the disturbance in function developed more and more into a hemianopic form similar to that associated with involvement of the left optic tract. His visual acuity increased somewhat but still remained very limited (Printing Sample No. 18). The optic nerve later nearly reached its normal level and was opaque and whitish, the veins remained partly tortuous, and the retina adjoining the optic nerve was only moderately opaque. After one and one-half years, the patient, who lived elsewhere, died from his cerebral disease and his physician was kind enough to send a short report on his autopsy. Also in this case, apparently there was a huge sarcoma in the left hemisphere.—Finally, in the years 1858 and 1859, two other similar patients were observed in my clinic. These two had the most distinct cerebral symptoms indicative of a central disease: One had a continuous roaring in his head, frequent vertigo with a tendency to fall to one side, recurrent epileptiform seizures followed each time by a very long stuporous state, weakness and sudden pains in the left arm, slow speech, disturbance in memory, apathy and somnolence; in the other, there were severe headaches, intermittent complete stupor, changes in smell and taste, difficulties in hearing, absence of sensation in the left part of the face, later a left hemiplegia, epileptiform seizures, and at greater intervals, disturbances in memory without other remark-

Albrecht v. Graefe's Archiv für Ophthalmologie, 1860, 7, Abt. 2: 58–71. Printed with the kind permission of Springer-Verlag, Berlin, Germany.

[1] The difference between this picture and that of primary retinitis of one or another form was primarily in the concentration of the swelling as well as of the opalescence in the papilla. The diminution of changes with the centrifugal flattening of the fibers, the striped appearance, the absence of all white points which usually appear as granular aggregates as an expression of disease of the middle layer of the retina, strengthened the opinion that just this layer of fibers was responsible for the conduction of the disease process from the optic nerve to the retina.

able disturbances in psychic functions. The pupils were remarkably dilated in both cases, the amaurosis did not start to develop until after most of the other cerebral symptoms had already developed. The optic nerve was affected in exactly the same way as previously described, and always on both sides. Again, the great degree of swelling and, in the first case, the excessively reddish discoloration were remarkable. The same characteristics were present as in the other patients, and especially in the first case there were a number of ecchymoses in the retina adjoining the papilla, which disappeared later. This patient died approximately one year after the first observation. The second died after a few months. The diagnosis of tumor of the cerebral hemisphere was decided upon because of the slow development of symptoms in both cases, the epileptiform seizures, the absence of all circumstances that would favor encephalitis or apoplectic encephalitis, and finally because of the changes in the optic nerve which had been found twice in association with tumors of the brain. Both diagnoses were confirmed by Professor Virchow. Again, we were dealing with sarcoma, and in both cases, in the right hemisphere.[2] The eyes of the latter patient, in whom the disease of the optic nerves had already reached its climax and the color of the swollen papillae had started to fade, were examined after they were hardened in chromic acid - potassium carbonate by Dr. Schweigger, who gave me the following report:

"It was not possible to preserve the eyes because they were already opened and had undergone examination, but the following changes could be found.

"The papillae are considerably swollen, and are protruding past the level of the choroid for a little more than 1 mm.[3]

"Immediately in the neighborhood of the

papilla, the retina is also thickened (up to 1 mm.). There is a hypertrophic development of the connective tissues in the nerve fiber layer; after picking this area for awhile, an arbitrary nucleus containing fiber cells and thickened neural fibers can be isolated. The latter show in their largest dimensions a diameter which exceeds the norm by about 4 to 6 times (0.012 to 0.016 mm.).

"At some distance from the papilla begins another peculiar change in the nerve fiber layer. The interspaces between the edges of the radiating fibers (more markedly refractive than usual) are filled with round, completely homogeneous structures (with an average size of 0.004 mm.) in which neither a nucleus nor a membrane can be recognized and which sometimes show a short ragged extension.

"On sections made from the papilla in the direction of the nerve fibers, one can recognize that these changes begin only at some distance from the papilla and always along the limiting surfaces, so that in the beginning they are always located between the existing nerve fibers and the limiting surfaces, while later they occupy the whole thickness of the nerve fiber layer. Probably these structures develop from a degeneration of the nerve fiber layer.

"Only small remnants of the ganglion cells can be found.

"The blood-vessels, especially in the vicinity of the papilla, have a considerably developed adventitia. Scattered in the retina (especially in the anterior part) a large amount of hemorrhage can be found."

In the other of the last-mentioned cases, which was at an even more advanced stage, Prof. Virchow found mainly a growth of the connective tissue elements, especially in the area of the periphery of the nerve. In both cases the changes were restricted to the papilla and the adjoining retina. The sections of the optic nerve outside the eye showed no remarkable anomalies.

According to these findings the previously-described disease probably consists of an inflammation of the optic nerve and the adjoining part of the retina (especially the inner layers) which leads to hypertrophy of the interstitial connective tissue and degeneration or destruction of the nervous elements. Although not the slightest elements could be found which showed evidence of a direct connection to the intracranial tumor, the coincidence between this inflammation of the optic nerve and the sarcomatous brain tumor which was observed four times seems to me to be reason enough to look for a common connection. For reasons which I will mention later, I came to the conclusion that the connection was probably only indirect and was caused by the effects of pressure which tumors of this kind have on the cavernous sinus. Necessarily, such pressure first

[2] I have mentioned the history of the disease and the findings at autopsy only briefly, partly because my notes are not complete in two of the four cases, partly because with this report I just wanted to fix the attention of the practicing doctor upon this matter, and partly because more distinct case histories will be published at another opportunity in connection with some similar considerations about complications of diseases of the eye and brain.

[3] In order to be certain of the micrometric height of the papilla on cuts which are made in the direction of the axis of the optic nerve, it is necessary to be sure that the cut goes through the middle of the papilla and really follows the direction of the optic nerve rather than oblique to the optic nerve because in oblique cuts the measurements are too large. Both requirements can be considered fulfilled if a sufficiently thin section contains central vessels in their entire length. The elevation of the normal papilla above the level of the choroid usually is a little more than 0.5 mm. under this condition (in the hardened eye).

leads to a congestion of blood in the retinal veins which can be seen by the widening and tortuosity of these veins; also tumefaction of the papilla caused by serous impregnation which slowly causes hypertrophy of the connective tissue could be related to such a mechanical hyperemia. It is more difficult if there are true inflammatory phenomena present, but even if these are not caused in a direct way from a mechanical hyperemia, an indirect cause certainly can be accepted. An organ that is affected by a mechanical hyperemia not only has less resistence to ordinary irritation, but the increase in volume itself and the extravasations of the blood could cause local irritation. In particular, the swelling of the optic nerve inside the resistant scleral ring could very well be the cause of irritation, and one even can think of a kind of incarceration of the papilla if this swelling has reached a certain level; also the relation of an inflammatory irritation to an extravasation of blood can be concluded to be similar to events in the brain. Such extravasations of blood could be demonstrated in nearly all cases, but can be missed in the ophthalmological examination, especially if they are present in smaller amounts because of their position behind the opaque inner retinal layers.

If this relationship between the nature of the disease and the mechanical hyperemia was to be considered true, it had to be demonstrated again in a similar way not only in brain tumors but also with other causes of pressure upon the base of the skull and the orbits. Experience has proved this theory right. However, I have to admit that such exquisite swellings of the papilla, as in these four cases, I have found again only three times in my practice, in one case in which a brain tumor was also found at autopsy (I did not mention this case because of the fragmentary observations of the other symptoms of the disease) and in two other cases in which the symptoms definitely pointed to a brain tumor, but in which there is no anatomical proof yet. In the following cases I observed a smaller degree of swelling but all the other characteristic changes:

1. In several cases of tumors of the orbits, the narrowing of the retinal artery was very distinct from the onset of the disease, which can be explained from the location of the cause of the pressure.

2. In one instance, where exophthalmos from inflammation of the fatty tissues of the orbits and amaurosis occurred after an abnormal case of erysipelas.

3. To a mild degree, in a case of inflammation of the tendon capsule. Here the conditions of the optic nerve and the retina returned completely to normal while in all the other cases it led to a partial or total atrophy. Probably in this case there was only a mechanical hyperemia with a serous impregnation.

4. In two patients on whom autopsy was not done, but whose symptoms pointed with great probability in the direction of an exudate at the base of the skull.

5. In several cases of subacute disturbances of the brain which were caused most probably by encephalitis or encephalomeningitis.

Still, I cannot consider the changes of the optic nerve that I have mentioned up to now as useless in the diagnosis of tumors of the brain, inasmuch as they, in their most marked form, especially tend to coincide with these tumors. But necessarily the conclusion has to be a careful one employing all the other signs at the same time. The continuation of observations, especially a series of autopsies, probably would prove that these changes in their most developed form not only occur in association with brain tumors, but also with other diseases in which the intracranial pressure is increased. But because this increase in pressure mainly occurs in tumors, there probably exists a relation which is not unimportant for diagnosis. I stress this opinion here especially because two discourses that I gave some time ago about this subject and whose protocols have been published in abbreviated form (Gazette hebdomadaire, 1859, and Berliner medicinische Centralzeitung, 1860) led to the misunderstanding that I implied complete pathognomonic relationships between these diseases of the optic nerve and brain tumors.

Certainly the relation of diseases of the retina to diseases of the brain is of great importance for the understanding of neurological diseases, especially in regard to the question of neuritis that was just discussed. This removes most of the basis for the conclusions that were reached in the time before the ophthalmoscope. If in the cerebral diseases that were causing several kinds of paralysis, amaurosis also occurred, in former times this was naturally explained by a paralysis of the optic nerve. And if conclusions were drawn from these cases about the crossing of the optic nerves, they resulted in errors. For instance in the literature several cases have been described in which unilateral disease of the brain caused complete amaurosis of the opposite eye; in my experience this never happens because of paralysis of the optic nerve. A unilateral disease in the hemisphere, if it is apoplexy, encephalitis or a tumor, always causes only hemianopic disturbances in one or two eyes if it has some effect on the centers of the optic nerve, but it never causes a complete amaurosis in the same or opposite eye. If this is the case, either the disease of the brain is not unilateral, but instead there are multiple foci, or at the same time there exist changes in the base of the skull which have a direct effect on the optic nerves, or there is a complication of the disease consisting of a peripheral disorder of the optic nerve or the retina. I have mentioned several times that I based these theories on the old knowledge of the semidecussation. Their influence on the prognosis of certain types of amaurosis related to cerebral disease is considerable. In a patient with apoplexy who remains with a hemianopic restriction of vision after the insult, total amaurosis never has to be feared as long as the characteristics of a unilateral disease, even with secondary encephalitis, are present.

Besides the above-mentioned form of neuroretinitis which is characterized by considerable swelling, redness, and cloudiness of the papilla, and in my opinion is caused by a mechanical hyperemia, another form occurs in association with encephalitic and encephalomeningitic processes which probably has the characteristics of a descending neuritis. In this form the papilla also swells and is obscure, the first, however, to a much less degree and without a steep rise at any place, and regarding the second, the color is more gray, perhaps reddish gray, but never as intensely hyperemic, and furthermore the changes develop much slower here than in the other cases, extend farther into the papilla and into all layers of the retina, in which most of the time white plaques and numerous apoplexies can be found. Anatomical examinations will have to decide if indeed, as I presume, the tract of the optic nerve is affected in continuity and if a direct conduction of the changes from the central focus exists, or if there is just an appearance of analogous processes in the nerve or in the retina. As an example of this type of disease, which doesn't seem to be very rare, I would like to present the following case:

A completely blind twenty-year-old girl was presented to me; some months before she developed a severe headache in the frontal and parietal areas without known cause, and in addition developed stupor, vomiting, delirium, and seizures in both upper extremities. For several days the patient remained in a nearly stuporous condition. Then slowly the symptoms of the disease decreased, but when the patient was in condition again to speak, she stated that she saw everything double and that she suffered occasionally from headaches. Her vision decreased within 14 days and at the end of this time there was a complete amaurosis. On examination was found: bilateral paresis of the abducens nerve (the cause of the former diplopia), incomplete anesthesia in the area of the left trigeminal nerve, paresis of several branches of the left oculomotor nerve and an absolute bilateral amaurosis with dilated and fixed pupils. What was more natural than to base the amaurosis also on a paralysis of the optic nerve; evidently there had been a meningitic process which could account for the

occurrence of all the paresis. However, the facts were different. By ophthalmoscopy there was bilateral inflammation of the optic nerve and of the retina, the optic nerves were reddish gray, cloudy, but only slightly swollen, the veins were wide, tortuous, the arteries small, the cloudiness of the retina in the area of the optic nerves was rather diffuse, only in some areas was there a slightly striped appearance visible at the greatest magnification, and the cloudiness extended widely in the area of the retina. Numerous little apoplexies, even at a distance of 4.5 mm. from the papilla, and little white stipples, points and plaques similar to those that appear in Bright's disease were visible. The area of the macula lutea on one side was degenerated in the usual star-like speckled manner. In short, in this case there was a neuritis and retinitis which were combined with meningitic or encephalomeningitic processes. Whether these or a coexisting paralysis of the optic nerve were the cause of the amaurosis is a different question. The picture of this disease, as mentioned above, in general was different from the other cases in the following ways: 1. because of the less marked swelling of the papilla, 2. because of the less marked widening of the papilla, 3. because of the expansion of the changes into the area around the optic nerve, 4. because of the participation of the middle and perhaps the posterior layers of the retina. This is shown (disregarding the expansion of the cloudiness outside of the area in which the fiber layer is large) by the appearance of small white points and groups of points and by the changes in the area around the macula lutea which is free from fibers.

A very similar case is even now under my treatment. A gentleman from Poland, some twenty years old, after a period of dull, intermittent, increasing, predominantly left-sided headaches, had fallen into a state of stupor, dullness of mental function, slow speech, and finally a semi-idiotic state. He slowly developed signs of right-sided paresis of the facial nerve, right hemiparesis, and bilateral amaurosis. A diagnosis was made of left-sided encephalitis or encephalomalacia with diffuse expansion and involvement of the cortex (possibly also multiple foci). The examination with the ophthalmoscope showed a neuroretinitis similar to that in the other patient except that up to now all the white points or plaques and the connected changes around the fovea centralis have been missing. If the peripheral disease could not have been proven, in order to explain the bilateral complete amaurosis I would have thought of multiple areas of softening, or possibly only right-sided softening, presuming that the absence of other paresis of cranial nerves, especially of the oculomotor nerves, indicated the absence of disease at the base of the skull (chronic meningitis).

Neurosurgical Classics—22 and 23

THE existence of cerebrospinal fluid has been known for centuries, but the study of this substance for diagnostic purposes was not possible until techniques were devised in the nineteenth century to permit its removal from the living patient with ease and safety.[4,5,11,15,16,29,31–33,37] Pearce Bailey wrote:

" . . . While it is probable that the Egyptian neurosurgeons encountered the fluid in their early surgical probings of the brain, which are described in Egyptian papyri of 3000 B.C., yet the first recorded evidence of its recognition is to be found in the writing of Hippocrates, who recognized it both in animals and in man. At that time, however, its true nature was not understood; its presence being attributed generally to pathological conditions, particularly hydrocephalus. Even later, such great physicians and scientists as Galen, Leonardo da Vinci and Vesalius were not aware that the fluid was normally present in the spaces within and around the central nervous system.

"The French surgeon, Ambroise Paré (1510–90), came closer to the root of the matter when he mentioned that some considered 'waterish moisture' was always present in the cerebral ventricles and he hinted at the function of the choroid plexuses. But it was not until the 18th and early 19th centuries, with the investigations of Cotugno, Haller, and most of all Magendie, that the cerebrospinal fluid was assigned a significant position in neurological anatomy, physiology, and chemistry.

"The Italian anatomist and clinician, Cotugno (1764), is generally credited as the first to positively demonstrate that a clear fluid filled the subarachnoid space and ventricular passages, but apparently his work at the time was largely overlooked, so that the potential significance of the cerebrospinal fluid to neurological research did not come into true perspective until François Magendie published his famous monograph in 1842. Herein Magendie described not only the appearance of the fluid, but demonstrated considerable knowledge of its physiological functions and its chemical composition. The latter, interestingly enough, was determined for Magendie by Lassaigne, who recorded both in animals and man, a water content over 98 percent, protein content less than 100 mg. percent, chlorides about 800 mg. percent, and the presence of bicarbonate, phosphate and calcium. Shortly thereafter Hoppe observed that the fluid reduced copper oxide, a reaction soon related to its sugar content.

"Magendie's monograph paved the way, during the middle and end of the 19th century, for broader studies on the physiology and formation of the cerebrospinal fluid, notably by Faivre (1854) and Retzius. Gustaf Retzius, versatile researcher in neuroanatomy at the Caroline Institute, with Axel Key, presented their view (1875–76) that the cerebrospinal fluid escapes from the subarachnoid space through the pacchionian bodies into the subdural space, then into the venous sinuses, and that some of it reaches the cervical lymphatics. It was much later when Weed (1914) advanced the opinion that most of the fluid is absorbed by the arachnoidal villi. But the theory of Retzius and Key that the fluid in the Virchow-Robin space flows into the subarachnoid space was accepted by Weed and forms the basis of his well known diagram which is still to be found in many textbooks on neuroanatomy today.

"While the work of Magendie and later of Retzius and Key opened a new vista of research on the cerebrospinal fluid, full-scale investigations on the fluid still could not advance rapidly due to lack of an easy portal of entry, by means of which ready access to the fluid could be gained. . . . "[3]

"The cerebral ventricles were tapped for hydrocephalus in ancient times, but the first puncture of the subarachnoid space appears to have been made by Corning[6] in 1885 for the purpose of injecting cocaine for anesthesia. However, Corning removed no fluid. Six years later Quincke[25] . . . and Morton[20] and Wynter[38] . . . independently tapped the lumbar subarachnoid space for the purpose of relieving intracranial pressure. Quincke reported his procedure and findings before an international congress and deservedly has been given the credit for introducing lumbar puncture to the medical profession. . . . "[33]

"Quincke would deserve a place in the history of medicine even if his only achievement had been the introduction of spinal puncture. No other single clinical method has done so much to clarify the understanding of diseases of the central nervous system. Quincke was born at Frankfurt-an-der-Oder, the son of a distinguished physician, who, with his family, later moved to Berlin. After studying medicine at Berlin, Würzburg and

298

Heidelberg under such celebrated men as Virchow, von Kölliker and Helmholtz, Quincke in 1867 became assistant to the great Frerichs. . . .

"Quincke's idea of spinal puncture for the withdrawal of fluid occurred neither by intuition nor by accident, and it is interesting to reconstruct the steps that led him to it. Searching for a simple and harmless way to relieve the increasing tension in hydrocephalus in children and thus save their lives, he reasoned that removal of the spinal fluid would break the vicious circle of the over-production and under-resorption of liquor caused by compression of the pacchionian granulations. As Frerichs' assistant, he had studied in 1872 the anatomy and physiology of the cerebrospinal fluid in dogs by injecting red sulphide of mercury into the spinal subarachnoid space.[23] The knowledge gained thereby encouraged him to insert a fine needle with a stylet into the lumbar interspace of an infant, a procedure which he thought might cause slight injury to a root fiber of the cauda but would not cause paralysis. With his presentation of the method at the Wiesbaden Congress of 1891,[24] spinal puncture became indispensable. It is to Quincke's credit that from the very beginning he utilized his puncture for diagnostic as well as for therapeutic purposes.[26] He insisted on accurate manometric pressure readings both at the beginning and at the end of the puncture, he studied the cells and measured the total protein, found tubercle bacilli in the fibrinous pedicle, noticed diminution of liquor sugar in purulent meningitis, identified bacteria, and gave consideration to the basis for the presence of blood. Of special neurological interest is the fact that in one of his very first patients, an infant, Quincke described the occurrence of a transient bilateral abducens paralysis following repeated removal of a considerable amount of fluid."[13]

". . . Fürbringer[10] in 1895 and Netter[21] in 1898 observed gross, chemical and microscopic changes in the fluid of patients suffering from meningitis, brain tumor and meningeal hemorrhage. Widal, Sicard and Ravaut[36] showed in 1901 that characteristic cytological changes occurred in the fluid as the result of disease of the nervous system. Froin[9] in 1903 described xanthochromia, increased cells and spontaneous clotting of the fluid in inflammatory disease of the meninges. With the introduction of the Wassermann test in 1906[34] and Lange's colloidal reactions,[14] examination of the spinal fluid became an important neurological diagnostic aid. The monograph of Mestrezat[19] in 1912 describing the constituents of the spinal fluid in health and disease marked the beginning of the scientific era of spinal fluid examination. . . .

"In 1913 Marie and his associates[17,18] introduced a two needle technique for examining the spinal fluid—one needle being placed above and one below the suspected lesion. Differences in color and protein of the fluid obtained from the two sources were considered significant. When cisternal puncture[1,35] was developed in 1919, Ayer compared the cisternal and lumbar fluids for differences in protein.[2] Much later the same principle was employed using only one puncture but examining the fluids collected in three tubes. The third tube was presumed to contain more fluid from rostral parts than the first tube and hence might have a much lower protein content[7] if the needle were caudal to the lesion."[33]

By these techniques much was learned about the static composition of human cerebrospinal fluid. Then in 1916, Hans H. G. Queckenstedt introduced a different line of investigation when he reported his studies of cerebrospinal fluid dynamics.[8,12,22,30]

Queckenstedt had been born in Leipzig-Reudnitz in 1876, the son of a teacher. He had attended the University of Leipzig, had trained under Ganser and others in Dresden and Zwickau, and had then moved to Rostock as assistant to Geheimrat Martius at the medizinischen Universitätsklinik. At that institution Queckenstedt carried out his important investigations until his untimely death in 1918 at the age of 42.[12,30]

"The number of Queckenstedt's publications was small. . . . Queckenstedt was highly gifted but never had the urge to write. But what he wrote had the touch of finality. Most of his attention centered on the spinal fluid. . . . From his youth, Queckenstedt had been keenly interested in physics and mathematics and thus by inclination turned to the problem of the dynamics of cerebrospinal fluid, which up to that time had been neglected. In his earlier experiences with lumbar puncture he was struck with the oscillation of the manometric fluid during respiration and he noted that the column of fluid fluctuated widely when the patient strained or coughed. What led him to study the effect of compression of the jugular veins on spinal fluid pressure is not known, but while carrying out this simple maneuver he observed that the pressure of the fluid sometimes failed to rise. . . . Such a failure, he concluded, indicated the presence of an obstruction of the subarachnoid space between the foramen magnum and the lumbar region in which the needle had been inserted. His test, announced in 1916 in an article . . . ,[22] in which three cases were cited (echinococcus infection of a lumbar vertebra, sarcomatous angioma of the conus medullaris, and cord tumor of undetermined

nature), was immediately recognized as a discovery of the first order. Interest in the liquor
was in the air and it was not long afterward that
Cushing, Weed and Dandy carried out their notable physiological studies in this field."[12]

Despite later modifications in technique
and equipment, Quincke's lumbar puncture[23-28] and Queckenstedt's test[22] are still
performed today much as they were when
they were originally described. Translations
of these original descriptions are reproduced
below.

References

1. AYER, J. B. Puncture of the cisterna magna. *Arch.
   Neurol. Psychiat., Chicago,* 1920, *4:* 529–541.
2. AYER, J. B. Spinal subarachnoid block as determined by combined cistern and lumbar puncture.
   With special reference to the early diagnosis of cord
   tumor. *Arch. Neurol. Psychiat., Chicago,* 1922, *7:*
   38–50.
3. BAILEY, P. Introduction. In: Lups, S. and Haan,
   A. M. F. H. *The cerebrospinal fluid.* Amsterdam:
   Elsevier Publishing Co., 1954, xv, 350 pp. (see pp.
   xi–xv).
4. BING, R. Medicohistorisches über den Liquor
   cerebrospinalis. *Schweiz. med. Wschr.,* 1954, *84:* 181–
   183; 204–207.
5. COBB, S. One hundred years of progress in neurology, psychiatry and neurosurgery. *Arch. Neurol.
   Psychiat., Chicago,* 1948, *59:* 63–98.
6. CORNING, J. L. Spinal anaesthesia and local medication of the cord. *N.Y. med. J.,* 1885, *42:* 483–485.
7. FABING, H. D. Progressive fall in protein content
   of cerebrospinal fluid withdrawn above a tumor of
   the cauda equina. A diagnostic aid. *Arch. Neurol.
   Psychiat., Chicago,* 1939, *41:* 373–374.
8. FAY, T. An apparatus to demonstrate the Queckenstedt phenomena for teaching purposes. *Res.
   Publ. Ass. nerv. ment. Dis.,* 1929, *8:* 161–163.
9. FROIN, G. Inflammations meningées avec réac-
   tions chromatique, fibrineuse et cytologique du
   liquide céphalo-rachidien. *Gaz. Hôp., Paris,* 1903,
   76: 1005–1006.
10. FÜRBRINGER, P. Zur klinischen Bedeutung der
    spinalen Punction. *Berl. klin. Wschr.,* 1895, *32:* 272–
    277.
11. GRAY, H. History of lumbar puncture (rachicente-
    sis). The operation and the idea. *Arch. Neurol.
    Psychiat., Chicago,* 1921, *6:* 61–69.
12. HAYMAKER, W. Hans Heinrich Georg Quecken-
    stedt (1876–1918). In: *The founders of neurology.*
    W. Haymaker, Ed. Springfield, Ill.: Charles C
    Thomas, 1953, xxvii, 479 pp. (see pp. 353–356).
13. HILLER, F. Heinrich Irenaeus Quincke (1842–
    1922). In: *The founders of neurology.* W. Haymaker,
    Ed. Springfield, Ill.: Charles C Thomas, 1953,
    xxvii, 479 pp. (see pp. 356–359).
14. LANGE, C. Die Ausflockung kolloidalen Goldes
    durch Zerebrospinalflüssigkeit bei leutischen Affek-
    tionen des Zentralnervensystems. *Z. Chemother.,*
    1913, *1:* 44–78.

15. LEVINSON, A. History of cerebrospinal fluid.
    Amer. J. Syph., 1918, *2:* 267–275.
16. MACINTOSH, R. Lumbar puncture and spinal
    analgesia. *Edinburgh: E. & S. Livingstone, Ltd.,*
    1957, 2nd ed., viii, 142 pp. (see pp. 1–9).
17. MARIE, P., FOIX, C., and BOUTTIER, H. Double
    ponction sus-et-sous-lésionnelle dans un cas de
    compression médullaire: xanthochromie, coagula-
    tion massive dans le liquide inférieur seulement.
    Rev. neurol., 1914, *27:* 315–316.
18. MARIE, P., FOIX, C., and ROBERT, F. Service que
    peut rendre la ponction rachidienne pratiquée à des
    étages différents pour le diagnostic de la hauteur
    d'une compression médullaire. *Rev. neurol.,* 1913,
    25: 712.
19. MESTREZAT, W. Le liquide céphalo-rachidien,
    normal et pathologique, valéur clinique de l'examen
    chimique, syndromes humoraux dans les diverses
    affections. *Paris: A. Maloine,* 1912, xvi, 681 pp.
20. MORTON, C. A. The pathology of tuberculous
    meningitis with reference to its treatment by
    tapping the subarachnoid space of the spinal cord.
    Brit. med. J., 1891, *2:* 840–841.
21. NETTER. Diagnostic de la méningite cérébro-
    spinale (signe de Kernig, ponction lombaire). *Sem.
    méd., Paris,* 1898, *18:* 281–284.
22. QUECKENSTEDT, H. H. G. Zur Diagnose der
    Rückenmarkskompression. *Dtsch. Z. Nervenheilk.,*
    1916, *55:* 325–333.
23. QUINCKE, H. Zur Physiologie der Cerebrospinal-
    flüssigkeit. *Arch. Anat. Physiol., Lpz.,* 1872, 153–
    177.
24. QUINCKE, H. Ueber Hydrocephalus. *Verh. Congr.
    inn. Med.,* 1891, *10:* 321–339.
25. QUINCKE, H. Die Lumbalpunction des Hydro-
    cephalus. *Berl. klin. Wschr.,* 1891, *28:* 929–933;
    965–968.
26. QUINCKE, H. Ueber Lumbalpunction. *Berl. klin.
    Wschr.,* 1895, *32:* 861; 889–891.
27. QUINCKE, H. Die Technik der Lumbalpunction.
    Berlin: Urban & Schwarzenberg, 1902, 15 pp.
28. QUINCKE, H. Die diagnostische und therapeu-
    tische Bedeutung der Lumbalpunktion. Klinischer
    Vortrag. *Dtsch. med. Wschr.,* 1905, *31:* 1825–1829;
    1869–1872.
29. SQUIRES, A. W. Emanuel Swedenborg and the
    cerebrospinal fluid. *Ann. med. Hist.,* 1940, *2:* 52–63.
30. STENDER, A. Concerning Queckenstedt and his
    test. *J. Neurosurg.,* 1949, *6:* 337–340.
31. TIMME, W. Presidential address. Historical résumé
    of the knowledge of the human cerebrospinal fluid.
    Res. Publ. Ass. nerv. ment. Dis., 1926, *4:* 3–6.
32. VIETS, H. R. Domenico Cotugno: his description
    of the cerebrospinal fluid, with a translation of part
    of his *De Ischiade Nervosa Commentarius* (1764) and
    a bibliography of his important works. *Bull. Hist.
    Med.,* 1935, *3:* 701–738.
33. WALKER, A. E. Diagnostic procedures. In: *A his-
    tory of neurological surgery.* A. E. Walker, Ed.
    Baltimore: Williams & Wilkins Co., 1951, xii, 583
    pp. (see pp. 23–39).
34. WASSERMANN, A., NEISSER, A., and BRUCK, C.
    Eine serodiagnostische Reaktion bei Syphilis.
    Dtsch. med. Wschr., 1906, *32:* 745–746.
35. WEGEFORTH, P., AYER, J. B., and ESSICK, C. R.
    The method of obtaining cerebrospinal fluid by

puncture of the cisterna magna (cistern puncture). *Amer. J. med. Sci.*, 1919, n.s. *157*: 789–797.

36. WIDAL, SICARD, and RAVAUT. Cytologie du liquide céphalo-rachidien au cours de quelques processus méningés chroniques (paralysie générale et tabès). *Bull. Soc. méd. Hôp. Paris*, 1901, s.3, *18*: 31–33.

37. WOOLLAM, D. H. M. The historical significance of the cerebrospinal fluid. *Med. Hist.*, 1957, *1*: 91–114.

38. WYNTER, W. E. Four cases of tubercular meningitis in which paracentesis of the theca vertebralis was performed for the relief of fluid pressure. *Lancet*, 1891, *1*: 981–982.

ABOUT HYDROCEPHALUS*

BY

GEH. MED.-RATH PROFESSOR DR. H. QUINCKE
(KIEL).

Hydrocephalus is a general term, and in each case in which fluid is increased in the ventricles we should define the cause, but at present it is not only necessary but also practical to talk about hydrocephalus because even if the causes of the increase in fluid in the ventricles may be different, at least very frequently the pressure itself creates the damaging effect. This is similar to other serous effusions, in which very often because of the mechanical disturbances a therapeutic procedure is indicated, regardless of the cause of the liquid in the peritoneal or pleural cavity. As in these cavities the resorption of an effusion is difficult because of the extension and compression of blood and lymph vessels and the resulting tension on their thin walls, so also it seems in an hydrocephalus having a certain degree of tension, the existence of the effusion is favored because with the pressure of the brain substance against the skull the passages from the subdural and subarachnoidal spaces into the pacchionian granulations are obliterated and in this way there is a vicious circle that can only be interrupted through the decompression of the serous cavity. Because of the occasional occurrence of spontaneous rupture (for instance through the nose), the chronic hydrocephalus of children often was treated by puncture, usually only with transient relief, but sometimes, like in the case that was presented a few years ago by Rehn, with prominent success.

I would like to report here two cases in which I did punctures, partly because of certain changes in the procedure, and partly because of other observations I made.

The first case was a twelve-year-old boy who came under my observation 3 years ago. He always had had a

* Translation of: Ueber Hydrocephalus, by H. Quincke, *Verhandlungen des Congresses für innere Medicin*, 1891, *10*: 321–339.

rather large head and suffered frequently with headaches. In his fifth year of life he fell from a staircase on his forehead. In his ninth year he was hit by a stone in the back of his head. However, his physical and mental development was normal, and the only thing unusual according to his mother was that frequently when he was walking he fell forwards. In January 1888 the headache increased, especially after school, then in the spring he started vomiting.

The father and 4 brothers of the child died with tuberculosis, one brother died with meningitis.

He was admitted in May 1888 and physical examination showed a well-developed, moderately well-nourished boy whose skull was large, sensitive to pressure, the horizontal measurement 59 cm., the distance from the root of the nose to the occipital protuberance 38 cm. The spontaneous headache was especially marked in the posterior part of his head. Sensation was normal, his gait insecure, neck rather stiff with active and passive movements. Pupils reacted to light, the left one somewhat more than the right, and optic neuritis on both sides.

Temperature normal; pulse ranging between 64 and 80. No abnormalities in the organs of the chest or abdomen.

With the treatments with potassium iodide, leeches on the mastoid processes, and tartaric acid ointment to the skull only a transient improvement was noted. There was frequent vomiting, paresis of the left abducens, and a flexion contracture of the legs. On the 23rd of June a puncture of the ventricles was done and this was repeated five times up to the point of death on the 13th of August.

In order to puncture the completely closed skull, I used two methods. One was that I made a defect in the bone with a crown trephine of approximately 12 mm. diameter without damaging the dura, and after healing of the skin incision I punctured twice through the hole in the bone just as through a fontanel. This method has the disadvantage of being very elaborate and requiring the repeated use of the same place in the brain for the punctures. The other four times an incision down to the bone of about 2 cm. length was made and then the bone was perforated with an angled awl and each time a puncture cannula was inserted into the burr hole 4–6 cm. deep.

The places of puncture were all within the area of the parietal cortex, 4–6 cm. on both sides of the midline. The puncture was done with needles from 1.1 to 1.3 mm. in thickness. In order to avoid the penetration of brain substance into the opening each had a matching stylet. This was removed immediately after the puncture, the cannula was connected with a rubber tubing to a glass manometer, and in this way the pressure of the fluid at the site of the puncture was measured. Through a connecting glass T-tube a certain amount of liquid could be drained, and in between the pressure could be measured again.

The table records the observed figures.

June 24—The head was shaved. The headache is more

Day	Hour	Total Amount	Specific Gravity	Partial Amount	cm. Water	mm. Hg	Pulse	
June 25 First Puncture								
	4.42	40 cc	1002	—	40 (45–36)	29	96	4 cm. from midline, 14 cm. behind frontal tuberosity. Opening with awl. Needle 4 cm. deep. In beginning, pulsatile oscillations in water pressure.
	4.47	—	—	—	22	16	78	
	4.49	—	—	—	15	11	—	
	4.50	—	—	—	10	7	108	
	4.55	—	—	—	—	—	104	
	4.59	—	—	—	—	—	90	
	5.4	—	—	—	—	—	106	
	5.6	—	—	—	−11	—	98	Glass manometer depressed 10 cm. below puncture opening.
	5.11	—	—	—	—	—	102	Removed. No pressure for the last 5–10 minutes.
July 11 Second Puncture					over	over		
	10.56	60 cc	1001	—	50	37	72	6 cm. from midline. Opening with awl.
	11.—	—	—	—	40	29	—	
	11.2	—	—	—	35	25	—	Flowing out.
	11.3	—	—	—	30	22	72	Systolic rises of 1–2 mm.
	11.13	—	—	—	27	20	—	
	11.15	—	—	—	36	26	—	Manipulation of manometer.
	11.19	—	—	—	10	7.5	—	
	11.22	—	—	—	9	7	66	
	11.26	—	—	—	7	5	—	
	11.28	—	—	—	1	—	—	
	11.29	—	—	—	−0.5	—	84	
	11.30	—	—	—	—	—	96	Cannula removed.
July 19 Third Puncture					over			
	4.17	75 cc	—	—	50	37	108	Through the hidden trephine opening, without anesthesia. Needle 5 cm. deep.
	4.20	—	—	—	20	14	100	
	4.27	—	—	—	12	9	—	Respiratory oscillations in pressure.
	4.38	—	—	—	6	4.5	—	The copious initial flow from the puncture opening diminished, so that suction was applied with a pressure of −10.
	4.40	—	—	—	8	6	92	
	4.44	—	—	—	passing −6	−4.5	—	
	to 57	—	—	—	−2	−1.5	100	
July 27 Fourth Puncture								
	1.11	70 cc	1006	—	50–60	37–44	—	Through the trephine opening.
	1.14	—	—	10 cc	35	25	82	
	1.15	—	—	10	18	13	—	
	1.16	—	—	10	11	8	92	
	1.18	—	—	10	6	4	—	
	1.20	—	—	10	1–2	1	—	
	1.22	—	—	—	4–5	3–4	—	
	1.24	—	—	10	−5	−4	—	Suction with −15.
	1.26	—	—	—	−2	−1.5	—	
	1.27	—	—	—	0	0	—	Suction.
	1.29	—	—	10	−10	−7	—	
	1.30	—	—	—	−5	−4	—	
	1.34	—	—	—	0	0	—	
August 1 Fifth Puncture								
	10.1	55 cc	—	—	50	37	—	Opening with awl.
	10.5	reddish	—	10	20–27	15–20	—	

Day	Hour	Total Amount	Specific Gravity	Partial Amount	Pressure cm. Water	Pressure mm. Hg	Pulse	
	10.7	—	—	10	12–15	9–11	—	
	10.10	—	—	10	9–13	7–10	—	
	10.13	—	—	—	4–8	3–6	—	
	10.16	—	—	—	—	—	—	Flow with −2.
	10.20	—	—	—	1	—	—	
August 8 Sixth Puncture								Anesthesia.
	12.30	70 cc reddish	1004	—	—	—	—	Somewhat behind both previous awl openings. Cannula 6 cm. deep.
	12.50	Trace, more albumin.			over 70	51	70–80	Respiration poor at first, becoming better with flow of fluid.
	—	—	—	30	36	23	—	
	12.55	—	—	30	−1	—	60	Suction.
	12.57	—	—	—	7	5	—	
	12.59	—	—	10	—	—	—	
	12.60	—	—	—	6.5	—	88	End. Cannula left in place. Dressing applied.
	4.—	—	—	—	35	25	—	

marked in sitting position than lying down. The occipital region is especially sensitive to pressure, but even hurts spontaneously. There is a remarkable optic neuritis. The vision is not disturbed.

June 26—Since the puncture yesterday the sleep is good. No headache lying down. Pain in the occiput as soon as the patient is sitting up.

June 29—No vomiting in several days. The paresis of the left abducens is much less. The patient is much more awake.

July 4—Under chloroform anesthesia a piece of bone about 12 mm. in diameter (3.5 mm. thick) was removed with a crown trephine, symmetrical to the first puncture opening. The tenseness of the intact dura allows the vessels to be only faintly visible.

July 12—The skin incision over the trephination opening is healed. The second puncture on the right, with awl perforation was performed.

July 20—After the third puncture yesterday, general condition is better. The patient can sit up without being dizzy. The flexion contracture of the hip and knee joint had caused lordosis of the lumbar spine which is now almost not noticeable. However, the patient is too weak in his legs to walk.

July 23—The contracture is not noticeable.

Because of increasing headaches and vomiting the punctures were repeated at shorter intervals.

August 4—The headache is sometimes so strong that the patient cries. It is especially pronounced in the back of his head. Pressure on the skull does not produce pain. However, pressure on the cervical spine and the lifting of the constantly drooping head produce pain. Also the flexion contracture in the hip and knee joints returns and with this the lordosis of the lumbar spine. The pupils react, are of medium width, the left one somewhat larger. Pulse is somewhat irregular between 72 and 92.

August 7—Contracture of neck and hip more marked. The lower extremities are slightly spastic. The tendon reflexes are increased. Leeches on the neck are without

influence. Apathy increasing.

August 8—Sixth puncture performed. Anesthesia achieved with little chloroform. A sudden cessation of breathing with a good pulse. Puncture completed with artificial respiration. After drainage of the fluid there was spontaneous respiration again, in the beginning Stokes type.

The contracture in the neck and in the hips disappeared immediately. After drainage of 70 cc. the cannula was left in place for another three hours. The pressure was 35 cm. = 25 mm. mercury. Then a permanent cannula with a flat head was inserted and covered by a dressing consisting of a moss pad which absorbed approximately 300 to 400 cc. during the first 24 hours, and after that approximately 150 cc. During these days patient is very thirsty.

August 9—The patient was feeling fine, less apathic, no vomiting, no headache. During the day the temperature went up to 40° C with chills. Pulse is 156 and all the symptoms of pressure return.

August 10—Temperature 39.8° C, pulse 132, sensorium clear, the cannula was removed.

August 11—Temperature 39.5° C, pulse 132, Stokes type of breathing. Patient rests on his left side. Eyes deviated to the left and upwards, with intermittent downward nystagmus. Patient is in coma.

August 12—Coma continued. Contracture in the neck and the legs had improved somewhat. The whole vertebral column was sensitive to pressure. In the evening the temperature was 40° C, the pulse was 158. The patient expired during the night.

Autopsy performed by Prof. Heller shows (after the examination of the hardened brain) severe chronic hydrocephalus, hypertrophy of the brain, a large blood clot between dura and skull, mild fresh meningitis, infiltrations of the lungs and residuals of pleuritis.

The skull is very large, 4 to 6 mm. thick. On the inside it is smooth. Only in the area of the burr holes there are osteophytes with multiple vessels. Between dura and skull in the right parietal area is a dark cherry-red layer of clotted blood 1.5 cm. thick, 7–9 cm. in diameter, which flattens the brain. The dura is very thin, tense, and the inside smooth. On the left side corresponding with the opening for the trephination, it is paler and surrounded by an area with reddened and partially hemorrhagic infiltration. The arachnoid is very thin and tense. The gyri of the brain are flattened, the sulci less prominent. In the area of the punctures on the right there are pieces of the brain substance approximately as large as rice throughout the arachnoid area. One puncture pierces through a larger vein whose surroundings are infiltrated with blood. In the very large ventricles are about 600 to 800 cc. of reddish cloudy liquid with a specific gravity of 1.008 containing protein (evidently the product of the maceration) which contains endothelium and pus particles. The brain weighs (without liquid) 1315 grams.

All four ventricles are enlarged, the lateral ones especially, the anterior horns only a very little, the posterior horns, and not at all the temporal horns which are very pinpointed. The brain substance over the lateral ventricles is up to 2.7 cm. thick, in parietal thickness 1.2 to 0.9 cm., and in the occiput 1.3. The ependyma is thickened and can be removed as a membrane. The septum is like a spider's web. The cavum septi pellucidi is wide. The corpus callosum and fornix are very thin with a fixed defect in the middle.

The third ventricle is very wide especially towards the floor. The middle commissure is white and granular.

The lamina quadrigemina is very flat and thin. The sylvian aqueduct is 5 mm. wide. The superior vermis of the cerebellum has completely disappeared except its anterior white matter so that the roof of the very enlarged fourth ventricle almost consists only of the arachnoid. The tonsils are displaced into the fourth ventricle on its lateral wall. The foramen of Morgagni is preserved.

The spinal dura is attached to the bones more firmly than normal, in some parts attached to the pia, but easily removed. In the pia are occasional yellow hard enclosures. Under the microscope, after fixation and staining with carmine, a large amount of cellular infiltration of the pia is demonstrable, especially posteriorly. The transverse section of the spinal cord is normal.

I would like to summarize the most important facts of this case and I start with the pressure.

The opening pressure during the first punctures was 40 then 50 to 60 and with the last ones over 70 cm. water pressure, corresponding to 29 to 51 mm. mercury. This is much less than the 100 mm. mercury at which the symptoms of direct compression of the brain began to appear in a test that Naunyn and Schreiber did with dogs.

With the drainage of the liquid, the pressure was lowered very quickly. With the first 10 cc., approximately 20 to 30, with the second, 10 to 15 cm. water, and then gradually slower—very different in the closed skull, than in a puncture of hydrocephalus in a brain that is partly covered with skin, whose elastic walls are able to contract around the diminished contents.

Usually I drained the liquid until the pressure was one or just a few cm., sometimes I added a little suction by lowering the glass tube, however,

the liquid always rose again in a few minutes up to or past the opening level; the liquid in the glass tubing showed the systolic and expiratory fluctuations which are known through experiments and which can be over 10 cm. during straining and crying.

The pulse was not influenced through the punctures in a definite or constant way; even before there was never an abnormal slowing of the pulse, only occasional irregularity. But the respiration which was irregular and sometimes even stopped under the influence of anesthesia was improved immediately when the high opening pressure was lowered with drainage of the fluid.

While the punctures with burr holes were done under anesthesia, the punctures with trephine holes were done without; the patient had no special sensation during drainage except the sensation of the stitch. But usually there was an improvement for one or several days after the puncture and a decrease of especially irritating symptoms, like a decrease in the headache and vomiting, the possibility of sitting up without being dizzy, and improvement in the mood and psychic functions. Particularly remarkable was that several times the flexion contractures of the lower extremities as well as the painful contracture of the neck disappeared immediately after the puncture, so that they were considered, at least in this case, not directly a symptom of the inflammation but a direct symptom of the pressure. Perhaps these positions had the same significance as flexion occurring with exudates in the knee joints, which means in this case the position associated with the maximum capacity of the dural sac.

True success through the punctures was not achieved in this case, the disproportion between secretion and drainage of the fluid had developed into a permanent state. The drained fluid was, as usual, clear as water, and had no traces of albumin except for a little increase with the last puncture. The punctures themselves were usually not dangerous procedures; only the last one was followed by fever and it may well have been the reason for the demonstrated mild meningitis. Attempts to culture the ventricular fluid showed no organisms and so the inflammation was regarded as aseptic; perhaps the invasion of leukocytes was favored by the strong transudation which was noticed while the permanent cannula was in place.

The perforation of the pial vein is regarded as an unfortunate incident, which, however, may occur again in the future; because of the pressure, the walls of the vein were pressed into the tract formed by the perforation of the dura to such a degree that the hematoma was extradural; and this also affected the pressure inside the skull.

Remarkable is the apparently normal mental development of the boy, because, even if the total weight of the brain was relatively high, there were several parts partially or totally missing, for instance, especially the corpus callosum and fornix, the lamina quadrigemina, and the posterior part of the vermis of the cerebellum;—possibly the latter was the reason for the tendency to fall forward?—

In the second case, we dealt with a $1\frac{3}{4}$-year-old boy who had been perfectly healthy, but who became sick and restless suddenly during his sleep on the 5th of December, 1890, was drowsy and had fever during the following days, and on the 8th of December, was completely comatose, had intermittent apnea, uncontrolled motions of the extremities, and vomiting.

He was admitted on the 9th of December. He was a well-nourished boy who was lying still, did not react to calls or stimuli of the skin, but who apparently was still swallowing normally. Intermittent strabismus, convergence, the pupils reacted equally. There was no stiff neck. No paralysis in the face or extremities. He had moderate changes consistent with rickets in his rib cage and joints. Temperature 39°. Pulse 112. Over the right upper lobe, he had a pneumonitic consolidation with changes in percussion and auscultation consisting of increased breath sounds and rales. No cough.

December 10—Temperature 39.5. Pulse 136. Stiff neck. In the evening, the respirations were intermittently irregular.

December 11—Temperature 37.2. Pulse 124. Otherwise, his condition remained the same.

The consolidation in the lung could have been recent or older, but the over-all picture of the illness was suspicious for severe impairment of cerebral activity, most probably caused by a fresh hydrocephalic exudate which could have resulted from either a simple inflammatory hyperemia or meningeal tuberculosis. Relief of the compression of the brain seemed indicated. To puncture a ventricle which was only slightly enlarged through the normal brain, however, seemed to me worthy of some consideration and a procedure not completely safe. According to an experimental paper[1] I knew that in the dog and the rabbit it is easy to inject fluids into the subarachnoid space with a Pravaz syringe without opening the bony part of the spinal canal. Therefore I punctured the subarachnoidal sac in the lumbar area, passing a very fine cannula 2 cm. deep between the third and fourth spinal arches, and drop by drop I drained a few cubic centimeters of water-clear cerebrospinal fluid. With the drops in the beginning dropping 8 and later 4 per minute, one could see clearly increases with expiration and decreases with inspiration. The puncture wound was closed with iodoform, collodion and cotton.

In the afternoon, the child was definitely less drowsy and could swallow much better. The respiration was regular. There was still a stiff neck.

During the following days, the condition was un-

[1] H. Quincke, Zur Physiologie der Cerebrospinalflüssigkeit. Du Bois u. Reichert's Archiv 1872.

changed. Temperature normal. Pulse 120–130. The urine contained some protein.

December 14—A second puncture between the third and fourth arches of the lumbar vertebrae was performed. In the beginning there was a flow of about 8 drops per minute, later less; therefore a careful suction with a Stroschein syringe was applied. Within 20–30 minutes a total of approximately 10 cc. of clear cerebrospinal fluid was drained. A short time later, the child became less drowsy, could fix objects and call his mother during the night.

December 15—Because the child was able to fix, it was possible to realize that there was a bilateral abducens paresis. The lungs were unchanged.

During the following days, the patient began to talk and to pay attention to what was said to him, he ate bread and took it in his hand. A mild left paresis of the facial nerve became apparent. The neck was still somewhat stiff.

December 17—A third puncture was done below the arch of the fourth lumbar vertebra. The cannula was connected immediately to a narrow rectangular glass pipe with rubber tubing. With the patient in the horizontal partially prone position, the pressure at the opening was 13–15 cm. water (equal to 10–11 mm. mercury). With crying it was 20, decreased rapidly again to 15 and soon after there was a drainage of 8 drops per minute through the cannula. Only a total of approximately 5 cc. were drained because the drainage soon became slower and the suction was somewhat difficult (possibly an unfavorable position of the cannula?).

The improvement increased. The consolidation of the right lobe decreased slowly, the child started to play, could sit alone in bed on the 23rd of December, and then learned to walk.

At discharge on the 10th of January, his gait and mental behavior seemed completely normal to his parents. His face was completely straight. Only the left abducens seemed somewhat paretic. Up to now the child has stayed healthy, the paresis of the abducens has disappeared.

I have to add that during the illness the child received 8 injections of Koch's fluid (from $\frac{1}{2}$ to 5 mg.). A single rise of temperature to 38.4, a slightly increased restlessness and an increased pulse were the only symptoms that could possibly be regarded as the effect of these injections. The tuberculous nature of the meningitis, which had to be suspected because of the symptoms, and because of which I first tried the injections, can almost certainly be rejected. This case has to be regarded as leptomeningitis infantum (Huguenin) or as a cerebral hyperemia with exudation (hydrocephalus acutus simplex). It is almost certain that in this case there was a true increase of fluid in the brain and spinal canal; in favor of this is the observed pressure of 10–11 mm. mercury during the third puncture which could have been considerably more during the first punctures,[2] but even

[2] I myself determined a normal pressure in the horizontal position in the lumbar spine of 4 mm. in a three-month-old child. Leyden determined the normal tension of the cerebrospinal fluid in the dog to be 8 mm. mercury.

more the improvement of the symptoms after each puncture, so that we got the impression that the favorable change in the apparently hopeless condition was indeed initiated and accelerated by the punctures.

This success, gentlemen, seems to me to create hopes for therapy even in other cases.

Anatomical research and animal experiments have shown that the subarachnoidal spaces of the brain and spinal cord are connected with each other and with the cerebral ventricles, and that the manifestations of pressure on the brain are best demonstrated experimentally by injecting liquid into the subarachnoidal sac of the cauda equina. Naunyn and Schreiber therefore prefer to talk about cerebrospinal compression instead of cerebral compression. In autopsies of acute and chronic hydrocephalus with cerebral compression, I have always found an increased tension in the lumbar part of the dural sac, and in chronic hydrocephalus frequently also have found an enlargement of the spinal canal.[3]

Usually as the result of a lumbar puncture, we can expect a decrease in cerebral compression; only in cases in which communication is disturbed by partial sclerosis of the subarachnoidal tissue or by occlusion of the sylvian aqueduct is the procedure useless.

The best result of the puncture is naturally to be expected in an acute increase of pressure, either if this appears in a normal individual or develops in addition to a chronic, asymptomatic increase of the cerebrospinal pressure. In an acute increase there is the most hope of full recovery if it is possible to help the patient over the momentary threat to life.

Of great importance for lumbar puncture is the fact which was discovered by Naunyn and Schreiber in experiments, that if there is an acute increase of pressure in addition to a previously asymptomatic increase, the now apparent symptoms of pressure continue even if the pressure is decreased to its former level, and only disappear if the pressure is decreased considerably (in this case more than 30 mm. mercury).

Lumbar puncture will be indicated most frequently in children, in tuberculous meningitis as well as in benign acute hydrocephalus, the leptomeningitis serosa simplex. The latter is regarded as a relatively rare disease, but perhaps some cases

of "cerebral hyperemia" and "convulsions" in children have a fatal outcome because of an acute effusion into the ventricles. The anatomical findings in these cases are not always clear and satisfying; in these cases lumbar puncture would probably bring more understanding, and in some cases, probably a cure.

I certainly believe that the puncture also will bring success in some cases of meningeal tuberculosis; I have in mind such cases which have only a small number of gray nodules and a delicate pia, but very marked ventricular effusion, and which evidently are taking a rapidly fatal course because of the cerebral compression. Just these cases gave me the initiative for the procedure, because it is not unlikely that after subduing the threat of the acute transudation the tubercles in many cases can become encapsulated.

According to my observations, adults not infrequently expire after an exacerbation of an existing chronic hydrocephalus. The hope of possibly bringing some help to these cases may also contribute to making this diagnosis, which is so vague at present, more secure in the future.

In one of these cases, I did a lumbar puncture several days ago.

A 25-year-old river shipman was suffering frequently with headaches starting in December of 1889, and dizziness starting in the spring of 1890. In June of 1890 a physician made the diagnosis of optic neuritis.

The patient stated that he never had been sick before, but he pointed out that he never could tolerate tobacco or alcoholic beverages even in very small amounts; he always became dizzy.

Admitted on the 7th of November 1890. The large and heavily built man is complaining about headache and dizziness, and walks with an uncertain gait as a drunkard. He has a moderate edematous swelling of the eyelids bilaterally, less of the conjunctiva; diplopia caused by bilateral paresis of many of the eye muscles and a very distinct optic neuritis. There are no other abnormal findings, especially no paralysis of the extremities.

Over a period of time the diagnosis vacillated between tumor, chronic meningitis and exacerbation of a preexisting chronic hydrocephalus.

Application of ice, and administration of laxatives, potassium iodide and mercury were without evidence of lasting success, despite the fact that the headache almost completely disappeared and the dizziness was intermittently less severe. The rigorous application of tartaric acid ointments to the head brought some relief; but the development of a left amaurosis and atrophy of the left optic nerve showed that the cerebral compression still existed.

I attempted a puncture on the 21st of March, but did not find the space between the arches, but I succeeded easily in a second attempt on the 3rd of April (each time under chloroform anesthesia). When the needle was inserted 6 cm. deep there was a drop of cerebrospinal fluid; the pressure over the puncture opening was 50 cm. water or 37 mm. mercury. Within one hour 80 cc. of

---

[3] With increased cerebrospinal pressure and existing cerebral symptoms usually no symptoms can be noticed in the spinal cord. The reason for this is probably that the spinal cord is more strongly built and is physiologically used to higher pressure (in the erect adult, the distance from the cerebral ventricles to the lumbar spine is approximately 50 cm. which is equivalent to 37 mm. mercury pressure).

completely clear liquid were drained which had a specific gravity of 1.015 and contained a large amount of protein.

The following day the patient noted that when he was walking he felt less dizziness than before.

I come to the technique of performing the puncture:

The patient lies on his left side with a markedly anteriorly flexed lumbar spine; with coma, especially in the child, anesthesia is not necessary. The puncture is done with a thin cannula below the third and fourth lumbar arches. The shape and size of the openings between the arches and their relation to the spinal processes in the different ages is demonstrated in the following illustrations.[4] In younger children, it is possible to puncture in the midline between two spinal processes, but because of the strong interspinal ligament it is better to puncture some millimeters lateral from the midline and to direct the needle in a way that it reaches the midline on the posterior wall of the dural sac. In the adult (and sometimes even in older children) the spinal processes are directed more inferiorly so that they cover a part of the inter-arch space, and this can be reached best by starting at the level of the lower third of the spinal process and a little lateral to it in the above-mentioned way and in pointing the needle somewhat upward. In addition, these things vary individually in adults. It is necessary to be led somewhat by sensation during this puncture. The emergence of the fluid shows that one has reached the subarachnoid space. In the nearly two-year-old child, the needle was inserted 2 cm.

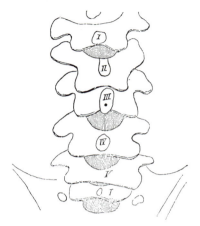

FIG. 28. No. II.

deep and in the adult it had to be inserted 4–6 cm.

In removing the needle—probably because of the structure of the fascia—it is sometimes necessary to overcome more resistance than with the insertion.

The spinal cord cannot be hit with this puncture because according to Ravenel, the conus medullaris in the newborn already reaches only to the third lumbar spine.[5] Also the cauda equina

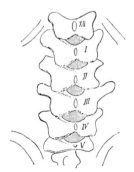

FIG. 27. No. I.

[4] Figures I to IV are drawn according to dry skeletons (Nos. I to III in perspective with the focus on the third lumbar spinal process. No. IV geometrically projected on a glass plate and later copied). No. V is copied after Luschka.

No. I. A one-year-old child (skeleton length 51 cm.)
No. II. A six-year-old child (skeleton length 75 cm.)
No. III. A ? twelve-year-old child (skeleton length 94 cm.)
No. IV and V. Adults

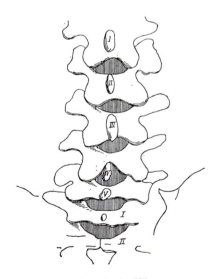

FIG. 29. No. III.

[5] Examining the bodies of eight children, I found the end of the conus at the level of the third lumbar spine up to the end of the first year, and at the level of the second lumbar spine after the end of the third year; only in one case in a four-year-old child at the level of the fourth lumbar spine.

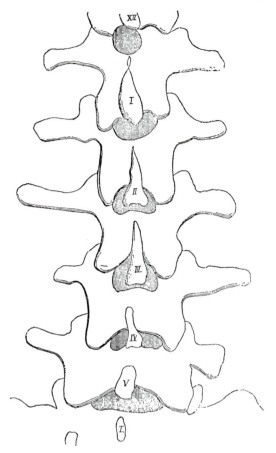

FIG. 30. No. IV.

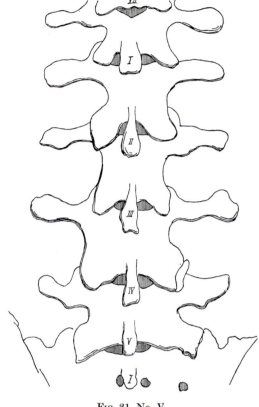

FIG. 31. No. V.

apparently is not easily entered, probably because the nerve roots which are floating in the fluid avoid the needle. In children, the circumstances are especially favorable because the diameter of the dural sac is much greater in proportion to the total of the nerve roots than it is in the adult, and frequently there is a medial free space of 5 mm. width or more between the roots of the two sides.[6]

In the adult where the cauda equina forms a much thicker bundle, injury of a root occurs more easily; this has to be accepted when compared with the greater danger of pressure on the brain.

There also arise the questions: How much fluid should be drained? How fast? How often could or should the puncture be repeated?—The answers can be given only after further experience.

Better than by simple punctures, the dangers of cerebrospinal pressure could be prevented if an

opening in the dural sac of some duration could be made. To achieve this goal, an opening to the outside would probably not be successful, because the permanent asepsis of the wound is in danger, from the constant drainage onto the dressing material. A successful procedure might be to insert a lancet-shaped needle into the space between the arches, to split the dura (and arachnoid) on their posterior aspect in the horizontal direction for some millimeters. From this subcutaneously located slit the fluid would drain into the loose epidural fat and soft tissue and would be resolved. I don't think one would have to fear an injury of the epidural veins, which is possible, because the pressure in the subarachnoid space would in the beginning remain greater and the tense dural sac would close the veins.

---

[6] Evidently there are considerable individual differences on this point which are independent of age.

AN AID TO THE DIAGNOSIS OF SPINAL CORD COMPRESSION*

By

Privatdozent Dr. **Queckenstedt**,
Oberarzt der Klinik.
Aus der medizinischen Universitätsklinik zu Rostock
(Direktor Prof. Martius).

In the many publications during the past few years regarding the composition of the spinal fluid in diseases producing compression of the spinal cord, the mechanical behavior of the spinal fluid has found very little consideration. In particular, as far as I can see, nowhere is there a simple experiment considered which allows direct proof of the reduction in space at the site of compression, thereby demonstrating without difficulty the character of the illness:

Each limitation of space in the vertebral canal usually reduces the space between the dura and the spinal cord. This diminution is almost always considerably greater than it would be from only the immediate local effect of the disease process, because in that region a swelling of the spinal cord also regularly occurs. Long before an actual compression is considered there is edema of that organ and its membranes which is generally considered to be a congested edema, even though it is not entirely explained as such. It corresponds to an "edema of the cerebrospinal fluid," i.e. an isolated increase in the albumin (without an increase in cells), which represents the essential characteristic change of the spinal fluid in diseases producing compression. The fusiform swelling of the spinal cord is often, as one can convince oneself especially during operations, so pronounced, with moderate reduction of the dural transparency, that it fills the subarachnoid space compactly, resembling a tampon cannula for the trachea. If such a blockage takes place very low, then the often described signs of intensive yellow coloring and total coagulation associate themselves with the increase of albumin in the cerebrospinal fluid, appearances which had first been generally recognized through their extraordinary characteristics in those special cases, but even so the occasional cell increase is of little significance to the character of the underlying changes.

Whenever the dural tube is so displaced, an exchange of the lumbar fluid cannot easily take place between the two spaces formed by the displacement. And also with each slight progression in the described condition, the narrowed passage opposes with greater resistance every movement of the cerebrospinal fluid. If there is an increase in fluid pressure above the point of compression, then according to the degree of the blockage, the fluid will either not shift at all or will escape inferiorly with reduced speed. Such an increase in pressure can be made possible simply by quickly squeezing the neck on both sides, or just on one side. Because of resulting increase of blood in the brain, the space for the cerebrospinal fluid is diminished inside the skull, and by equalization of the blood flow over the upper vertebral venous network, space may also be diminished from the outside, and therefore a pressure increase is created, which normally is transferred inferiorly with great speed and which can be demonstrated when a lumbar needle is inserted with a manometer. The beginning of the rise of the fluid in the manometer almost immediately follows compression of the neck, within less than a second, and the fluid rises very quickly, by interrupted movements, up to a preliminary maximum; one soon gets an idea of the normal time if the procedure is done a few times. In diseases with spinal cord compression, the rise itself is slowed down, and especially its beginning is delayed; frequently the neck must be strongly squeezed in order to demonstrate it; in addition, the pressure falls abnormally slowly or not at all when the neck compression is released.

In order to read all these signs accurately on the manometer, no obstruction to the pressure balance can be present in the lower part of the subdural space itself, including the lumbar needle. One has to convince oneself that this is not the case. It is important to notice that the (often very prominent) breathing fluctuations promptly follow respiration, and, of greater importance, that straining and coughing increases the pressure immediately and quickly. The distinction between the result of this pressure test and the outcome of the obstruction of the head is then very striking, whereas under normal circumstances this difference seems minimal by direct observation.

A complete, entirely impassable occlusion of the dural canal frequently is demonstrated by the obstruction experiment when the cord lesion is caused by vertebral disease. The reason for this may be that, especially in diseases of the vertebrae, the process of the illness itself is affected to a large degree by space limitation, and furthermore the hypothesis is given that, through displacement of the descending intervertebral veins, marked disturbances of the circulation occur, causing a severe edema of the spinal cord. The following case history serves as an example:

D., wife of a shipping agent, 35 years old.

In August, 1910 and January, 1911, the patient had temporary pains for some weeks in the right hip, in the

---

* Translation of: Zur Diagnose der Rückenmarkskompression, by Dr. Queckenstedt, *Deutsche Zeitschrift für Nervenheilkunde*, 1916, *55*: 325–333. Printed with the kind permission of Springer-Verlag, Berlin, Germany.

buttock, and in the lateral aspect of the upper part of the thigh when walking or working. After February, 1911, the same pains on the left side, occasionally and to a lesser extent on the right side, and in addition, constipation. Toward the end of August, 1911, within a few days, a rapidly advancing weakness over all of the left leg and in the right ankle, transitory urinary retention and inability to control thin stool. By the time of admission, also complained about pains over all the left leg and pains in the right hip.

Report on September 12, 1911.

Average height. Well nourished woman. Chest and abdominal organs, especially the lungs, clear. No fever. Wassermann reaction of the blood negative.

Spinal column from the mid thorax to the sacrum somewhat deviated to the right side and held rigid when bending forward. No tenderness to tap or jolt. At the dividing line between the thoracic and lumbar vertebrae, minimal edema of the skin, on the right side next to the last thoracic and first lumbar spines, a flat swelling; pressure on it gives a little local tenderness, and creates radiating pains in the buttocks, especially on the left side.

Slight incontinence of bowels and urine.

Bilateral pes equinus. Right ankle and joints of the toes completely motionless; in knee and hip joints all motions much diminished and ataxic.

Completely paralyzed on the left side, except for minimal extension in the hip, and very weak, ineffective contractions in flexion and extension of the thigh.

Hypotonia of the leg muscles; circumference smaller left than right, especially of the thigh. Reduction of direct and indirect excitability in the muscles of both upper and lower thigh is, in general, moderate, in the small foot muscles extremely marked (left side more than right), minimal degeneration in adductor groups and knee flexion on both sides is minimal, in the peroneus group is a prominent reaction of partial degeneration with a sluggish contraction, more prominent on the left than right side.

Knee reflexes equally poor. Achilles tendon reflexes increased with clonus, more on right. Plantar reflexes missing, no Babinski.

Effect of the lowest back extensor diminished. Abdominal wall muscles good. Abdominal wall reflexes present, equal on both sides.

Extreme damage of all sensory perception from the region supplied by the fourth lumbar root inferiorly, left side gradually reduced up to L2. Below L5, pressure and pain sensitivity almost completely gone on both sides.

The roentgenogram showed the first lumbar vertebral body on the right side destroyed and replaced by a diffuse cloudy shadow which extended over to the right vertebral border.

On September 18, the result of lumbar puncture was:

Pressure = 0 cm. (by sitting down, 6 cm.), breathing fluctuations up to 3 cm. By straining a rise up to 15 cm. By firm neck compression, no pressure increase, even after 30 seconds.

Fluid light, lemon color, contains some erythrocytes, 3 lymphocytes per cmm. Nonne-Apelt reaction: heavy cloudiness. Albumin content by the Nissl method, $6 \times 20 = 120$ units.

The operation on September 27 showed an echinococcal cyst of the first lumbar vertebra associated with many small daughter cysts, with an intact dura. The pa-

tient expired after two months from a streptococcal infection at the site of operation.

A very analogous result was shown by the lumbar puncture on a 62-year-old man with total paraplegia, etc. due to caries of the eighth thoracic vertebra: The pressure of 7.5 cm. (with breathing fluctuations of 2 cm.) showed no change even after one minute of obstruction of the head, while by straining it went up immediately to 14.5 cm.; the somewhat yellowish green liquid showed about 350 erythrocytes, 3 lymphocytes per cubic millimeter, an albumin content of $5 \times 10 = 50$ Nissl units, and therefore showed heavy cloudiness in the globulin reaction; Wassermann reaction negative.

In contrast to the total obstruction of the dural canal by the above-mentioned vertebral disease, when the cord lesion was caused by masses in the vertebral column, we found in all other observed instances only a delay in the shift of the cerebrospinal fluid which, by the way, was very marked, as for instance in the following patient with a tumor in the vicinity of the spinal cord:

S., laborer, 60 years old.

Since 1908, decreased continence of urine and stool, pain and lameness in the back and legs, "sleep" in the popliteal areas, especially on the right side, decrease in intelligence.

Findings at the end of January 1912:

Tolerable state of nutrition, extraordinarily round, large (60 cm.) skull. Dementia of a considerable degree.

Marked arteriosclerosis, heart enlarged toward the left. Decreased ability of the lungs to expand.

Vertebral column somewhat stiff in the vicinity of the hips.

Spastic gait. By passive movement, no distinct spasms.

Knee reflexes increased, on left side more than right. Achilles tendon reflexes absent, on left side paradoxic dorsal reflexes. No Babinski.

Musculature of the legs, especially the calves, thin, more on right than left.

Knee-heel test steady bilaterally.

Cremasteric and abdominal wall reflexes maintained.

Sensory tests very difficult because of dementia: Sensibility of the movement in the primary joints of the big toes uncertain. Romberg positive. Also, perhaps greater disturbances of the surface sensibility on the perineum and feet.

Urine dribbling and involuntary flatus.

Patient soon left the clinic and came back on February 13, 1913. According to the statement of his wife he had become more and more idiotic; because of increased weakness, he often fell down.

Patient could neither stand nor walk, fell backwards with legs stiff. However, movements in all joints of the legs possible. Distinct spasm, increasing distally.

Reflexes as before.

Calves thin and flaccid. Peroneus group flattened on right side.

Fibrillations in all lower leg muscles, not in the thigh muscles.

Incontinence of bowels and urine.

Extreme dementia (Arteriosclerotic in nature?)

Three lumbar punctures showed the following:

February 6, 1912.

Pressure 10 cm. By neck compression, very slow increase up to 30 cm., after release, extremely slow decrease.

Fluid lemon color, shows delicate coagulation, no cell increase, 120 Nissl units of albumin, heavy flaky cloudiness in the globulin reaction, negative Wassermann reaction.

March 4, 1912.

Pressure 14 cm., after draining off 4 cc., 12.5 cm. Marked breathing fluctuations up to 10 cm.! By neck compression, a slow increase up to 22 cm. pressure after a couple of seconds, even 8 minutes after the release of the obstruction, 19 cm. After drainage of fluid and after repeating the test, the same results. Liquid quickly congeals. Histological and chemical findings, aside from greater albumin content (200 Nissl units), as before.

March 25, 1913.

Pressure 8 cm., marked breathing fluctuations, fast increase with coughing. By jugular compression after a long latent period, slow intermittent increase up to 17 cm., no decrease, after a pressure fall to a pressure of −3 cm., by another neck compression, increase from −3 to 12 cm. in 5 seconds, to 17 cm. in 15 seconds, no decrease. In the third test the time between the neck compression and the beginning of the pressure rise is 4 seconds, otherwise analogous behavior. Fluid greenish yellow, noncoagulating, lower albumin content than before (36 Nissl units), otherwise essentially the same.

Patient finally expired after increasing cystitis and septic phenomena. The autopsy showed the suspected tumor (sarcomatous angioma) which compressed the conus medullaris from its anterior aspect, over which it extended inferiorly, and which had surrounded or destroyed some of the caudal roots. In addition, marked atrophy of the brain, especially in the frontal and temporal lobes. (Microscopic examination has not yet been completed.)

It is clear, that in the above-mentioned case the closure of the dural canal was demonstrable, and was a complete one. Even so, the fluid could be forced by an artificially raised pressure from the higher part of the subarachnoid space into the lower part, although differences in pressure of such magnitude and duration do not normally occur between these two parts. Frequently in instances of much less pronounced changes in fluid movement, hardly more than a capillary cleavage between spinal cord and dura could be presumed; one need only to visualize how little resistance such a relatively small and long tube as a lumbar needle exerts against the equalizing pressure. This demonstrates that a great disturbance in function may be present, which is perhaps equal to the above-mentioned echinococcosis, with absolute blockage of the dural tube, yet the sign is recognizable only in a mild form; a proportionality does not exist here. If one deals with cases involving the vertebrae of the neck, perhaps another phase comes into play. One must realize that

when the point of cord compression is so high, the blood which flows over collaterals because of the compression of the neck, also overfills the spinal venous plexus below the site of compression and, by its effect on the outside of the dura, increases the pressure of the cerebrospinal fluid below the site of compression; thus an overflow of spinal fluid to the lower part could be simulated, whereas in fact a complete blockage exists. However, the basic utilization of the experiment is not impaired. Experience teaches that this kind of pressure increase does not occur suddenly, but occurs gradually, if at all; it remains recognizable that the path for the fluid is not entirely free, which the following cases may verify:

L., tenant, 66 years old.

Since November, 1910, patient had continuous severe throbbing pain behind his left ear down to the shoulder, later a feeling of deafness. After the beginning of 1912, weakness in left leg, sensation of heat in right leg, numbness in left hand, and soon thereafter, increasing lameness of left leg and arm. In July 1912, the following condition was observed, which was unchanged from about March on:

Well nourished, healthy looking man. Sclerosis of the palpable arteries, enlargement of the heart to the left.

Gait spastic on the left. Spasm in all joints of the left leg with reduction of the basic strength. Patellar clonus, ankle clonus, left Babinski. On the right, knee and Achilles tendon reflexes somewhat increased.

Cremasteric and abdominal wall reflexes not clearly recognizable.

Left arm hangs with extended elbow (not in hemiplegic position), completely limp. Marked stiffness of left shoulder.

Triceps and biceps reflexes bilaterally increased, on left more than right. Radial periosteal reflex on left weaker (!) than on right.

Shoulder and arm muscles weak on left (!). Even wasting of the muscles of the forearm and hand without marked atrophy of single groups. More severe and prominent wasting of the biceps, triceps, latissimus dorsi, deltoid, and rhomboid muscles. In the muscles examined electrically (trapezius, deltoid, triceps, biceps) no marked difference of the faradic and galvanic excitability between the right and left, no sluggish contractions. No fibrillations. In the left shoulder joint no movement possible, in the elbow minimal flexion; with an attempt to make a fist, minimal finger flexion and dorsal flexion of the hand. Shoulder shrugging weaker on left than right.

Marked impairment of breathing on left. Movement of diaphragm on left only momentary, on right abundant and easily visible.

Sensibility:

Sensitivity to temperature markedly decreased on right side to the second rib, in back to the spine of scapula and on the arm, least on the outside of the latter, irregularity in sensitivity to pain, but less change than in sensitivity to temperature.

Inadequate distinction of pinhead and pinpoint on legs and trunk up to clavicle, and on the arms, without distinct bilateral differentiation.

Minimal reduction in sensitivity to touch on trunk

and inside of arms, also bilaterally about equal.

Position sense almost gone in left wrist, marked loss in elbow, distinctly decreased in shoulder.

Decreased in sensitivity to pressure and touch in the left anterior cervical triangle.

No disturbance in the bladder and rectum.

Rigidity of neck, head cannot be flexed to chest. Pain in neck on passive extension.

Roentgenograms of the cervical vertebrae showed no abnormalities.

Temperature normal. Blood Wassermann reaction negative.

The lumbar puncture gave:

Pressure 8 cm. On neck compression, very slow increase up to 30 cm. Fluid light yellow, clear.

Nonne-Apelt reaction: Cloudiness. Albumin content 10 Nissl units. Cell content: 3 per cubic millimeter.

Wassermann reaction with increased quantities (to 4 cc.) negative.

Diagnosis:

Compression from the left by a tumor at the level of the highest mark on the neck in the vicinity of the 3rd cervical segment.

The patient refused the proposed operation.

On another patient, who died because of the operation, whose diagnosis was left anterolateral cord compression at the 4th to the 5th cervical segments and in whom a neurofibroma of the left 5th cervical root was found which was the size of an almond, extradural and completely excisable, the following findings were derived by lumbar puncture: Pressure 13.5 cm., on straining, immediate increase to 24 cm. On neck compression, slow increase to 18 cm. In the fluid: Nonne-Apelt reaction strongly positive (flaky clouding), albumin content increased to $8 \times 10 = 80$ Nissl units, cell increase to 40 per cubic millimeter, negative Wassermann reaction.

Besides the mentioned cases, we have also found in a number of other patients with cord compression the sign of difficulty in displacing the cerebrospinal fluid. Without question this is a common finding and thus is of diagnostic value. It is most important in cases where few other symptoms or signs are present in the beginning to indicate cord compression—like in vertebral disease—thus it is especially useful as an aid in the diagnosis of tumors, and occasionally may even be decisive. Therefore it is an advisable principle to perform the obstruction test in each instance of cord compression—we perform it during all lumbar punctures—furthermore, the obstruction test is also advisable in those cases when definitively characteristic, yet isolated appearances, i.e. unilateral root pain and the like, are revealed, which make the experienced professional think of a tumor in its early stages. I am not aware of the degree to which the displacement of the fluid is restricted in such an early stage, since I myself have made no observations in this stage.

Be it noted that our sign does not allow the differentiation between extramedullary and intramedullary tumors, at least not always. Also, intramedullary tumors may be analogous to extramedullary ones in the development of collateral edema as we have learned from our own observed case of a glioma of the lumbar portion of the spinal cord. This is also quoted in the pertinent literature. On the other hand, there is generally no marked swelling of the spinal cord in other instances of cord compression like meningomyelitis, etc. Theoretically of course it is possible: We ourselves once saw a chronic case of tuberculous meningitis in which the spinal cord was affected mainly; in the cerebrospinal fluid a very unusual increase of the albumin content which was distinctly disproportionate to the cell increase, which was only minimal; the autopsy findings therefore showed an enormous edema of the pia which in such cases is probably secondary and which is related in its behavior to the edema of obstruction. Yet surely there are exceptions.

Finally it may be pointed out that the obstruction test occasionally may also be used advantageously for the orientation of operations. With all the certainty which the diagnosis of spinal cord tumors has reached, it still often happens that the expected tumor is not immediately found, which may be because the diagnosis of the level of involvement was incorrect or was only an approximation from the start. In such cases, compression of the neck veins may help one to recognize by the filling of the dural sac, this filling being either prompt or retarded or not occurring at all, whether one is above or below the tumor, and indicates to the surgeons how to continue the operation.

Neurosurgical Classic—24

I N 1895 Wilhelm Konrad von Röntgen revolutionized medical diagnosis by the introduction of roentgenography.[13,14] Two years later the hope was expressed that brain tumors might cast shadows in roentgenograms of the skull,[9] but it was soon found that no differentiation could be made between noncalcified tumors and the surrounding tissues.[2] Furthermore, calcification could be demonstrated in only a small proportion of intracranial tumors.[7] For these reasons, despite the occasional demonstration of bony erosion from intracranial neoplasms (such as Oppenheim's observation of changes in the sella turcica[10]), roentgenography had little use in the diagnosis of neurological diseases until the second decade of the twentieth century.

This lag was followed by the rapid introduction of ventriculography,[21] pneumoencephalography,[22] myelography,[23] angiography,[24] and a variety of special techniques for the demonstration of the cranial orifices.[2–4,11] Also during this period it was predicted by Arthur Schüller,[16] and verified by Howard Naffziger[8] that the pineal gland frequently is displaced laterally by an expanding mass in the opposite cerebral hemisphere.[1,3,4,11,12,15,17,20] Each of these two men was outstanding in his field, and working independently in different countries, they contributed an important sign for the diagnosis of intracranial disease.

"Without any shadow of doubt Arthur Schüller . . . was the father of neuroradiology. He was born in Brünn, the capital of Moravia in the old Austria, in 1874. . . . Schüller, qualifying in medicine in Vienna just after Röntgen's discovery, graduated with the highest honours—*sub summis auspiciis imperatoris Francesci Josephi*. This was a prize awarded by the Emperor Franz Joseph and was only given twice during his long reign of 68 years (1848–1916). Schüller immediately became interested in the radiology of the skull and in 1912 published a text-book on the subject: *Röntgendiagnostik der Erkrankungen des Kopfes*. This work was translated into English in 1918 by an American, F. F. Stocking. . . . One has only to glance at this text-book to see how far in advance of others was Schüller. . . . He differentiated many types of normal and pathological intracranial calcifications, but perhaps his greatest contribution was his work on the pituitary fossa. . . .

"More than 300 publications—books, monographs and papers—came from his pen, mostly while he was in Vienna. They covered not only the radiology of the skull but various aspects of neurology, surgery and psychiatry. He described three diseases and devised three operations, though he was not a surgeon. . . . "[3]

The ideas of Schüller about pineal displacement, which he thought should be evaluated routinely on anteroposterior roentgenograms of the skull, were expressed in the 1918 translation of his text-book as follows:

" . . . One can also, for example, in case of a displacement of the shadow of a pineal gland to the right or left of the median line, in symmetrically formed skulls, conclude the cause of its displacement to be pressure on the part of a tumor or traction on the part of a brain scar, as the following case shows:

"R.F., male, thirty-six years old. Trauma to the skull two years previously. At the time of examination he was suffering from hemiplegia of the right side following an apopleptic stroke. Internal organs normal. Wassermann negative. Suspicion of cerebral tumor.

"The roentgenogram showed that the pineal gland, the shadow of which was plainly recognizable, was displaced several millimeters to the left from the middle line, from which fact one was able to draw the conclusion that no large tumor of the left hemisphere could be the cause of the hemiplegia, but, rather, that there was probably a contraction present, perhaps in consequence of an area of softening."[16]

Howard C. Naffziger, an outstanding neurosurgeon, was born and educated in California. His surgical training was received under William S. Halsted and Harvey Cushing at the Johns Hopkins Hospital, and in 1929 he became Chairman of the Department of Surgery at the University of California. During the following quarter of a century he contributed many original concepts and useful techniques. Among other things, Naffziger emphasized the role of the anterior scalenus in compression of the brachial plexus, and devised a method of orbital decompression for exophthalmos.[18]

The recognition of pineal displacement by Schüller and by Naffziger was followed by the more detailed studies of others on the charting of the normal position of the pineal gland.[5,6,19] As an indication of the importance of this sign, pineal position has for many years been evaluated routinely in patients with suspected intracranial lesions.

References

1. BROWDER, J. Advances in neurological surgery during the past fifty years. *Amer. J. Surg.*, 1941, n.s. *51:* 164–187.
2. BROWN, P. Radiologic diagnosis. In: *The science of radiology.* O. Glasser, Ed. Springfield, Ill.: Charles C Thomas, 1933, xiii, 450 pp. (see pp. 139–186).
3. BULL, J. W. D. History of neuroradiology. *Brit. J. Radiol.*, 1961, *34:* 69–84.
4. DAVIDOFF, L. M., JACOBSON, H. G., and ZIMMERMAN, H. M. Neuroradiology workshop. *New York: Grune & Stratton*, 1961, *1:* 1–9.
5. DYKE, C. G. Indirect signs of brain tumor as noted in routine roentgen examinations: displacement of the pineal shadow. A survey of 3000 consecutive skull examinations. *Amer. J. Roentgenol.*, 1930, *23:* 598–606.
6. FRAY, W. W. A roentgenological study of pineal orientation. III. A comparison of methods used in pineal orientation. *Amer. J. Roentgenol.*, 1938, *39:* 899–907.
7. KALAN, C., and BURROWS, E. H. Calcification in intracranial gliomata. *Brit. J. Radiol.*, 1962, *35:* 589–602.
8. NAFFZIGER, H. C. A method for the localization of brain tumors—the pineal shift. *Surg. Gynec. Obstet.*, 1925, *40:* 481–484.
9. OBICI, G., and BOLLICI, P. Applicazione dei raggi X alla diagnosi di sede die corpi estranei della testa e dei tumori intracranici. *Riv. Pat. nerv. ment.*, 1897, *2:* 433–440.
10. OPPENHEIM. Discussion at Berliner Gesellschaft für Psychiatrie und Nervenkrankheiten, Nov. 13, 1899. *Arch. Psychiat. Nervenkr.*, 1901, *34:* 303–304.
11. PENDERGRASS, E. P., SCHAEFFER, J. P., and HODES, P. J. The head and neck in roentgen diagnosis. *Springfield, Ill.: Charles C Thomas*, 1956, 2nd ed., 2 vols. (see 2: pp. 1027–1033).
12. PILCHER, C. Fifty years of neurosurgery. *J. Tenn. med. Ass.*, 1945, *38:* 370–373.
13. RÖNTGEN, W. C. Ueber eine neue Art von Strahlen. *S.B. phys.-med. Ges. Würzburg*, 1895, 132–141.
14. RÖNTGEN, W. C. On a new kind of rays. A. Stanton, Transl. *Nature, Lond.*, 1896, *53:* 274–276. Also: *Science*, 1896, n.s. *3:* 227–231.
15. SACHS, E. The history and development of neurological surgery. *New York: P. B. Hoeber, Inc.*, 1952, 158 pp. (see p. 65).
16. SCHÜLLER, A. Roentgen diagnosis of diseases of the head. F. F. Stocking, Transl. *St. Louis: C. V. Mosby Co.*, 1918, 305 pp. (see pp. 156, 253).
17. SOSMAN, M. C. Radiology as an aid in the diagnosis of skull and intracranial lesions. *Radiology*, 1927, *9:* 396–404.
18. STERN, W. E. Obituary. Howard Christian Naffziger, 1884–1961. *J. Neurosurg.*, 1961, *18:* 711–713.
19. VASTINE, J. H., and KINNEY, K. K. The pineal shadow as an aid in the localization of brain tumors. *Amer. J. Roentgenol.*, 1927, *17:* 320–324.
20. WALKER, A. E. Diagnostic procedures. In: *A history of neurological surgery.* A. E. Walker, Ed. Baltimore: Williams & Wilkins Co., 1951, xii, 583 pp. (see pp. 23–39).
21. WILKINS, R. H. Neurosurgical classic—VII. *J. Neurosurg.*, 1963, *20:* 450–458.
22. WILKINS, R. H. Neurosurgical classic—VIII. *J. Neurosurg.*, 1963, *20:* 531–536.
23. WILKINS, R. H. Neurosurgical classic—X. *Neurosurg.*, 1963, *20:* 721–727.
24. WILKINS, R. H. Neurosurgical classic—XVI. *J. Neurosurg.*, 1964, *21:* 144–156.

A METHOD FOR THE LOCALIZATION OF BRAIN TUMORS— THE PINEAL SHIFT*†

By HOWARD C. NAFFZIGER,
SAN FRANCISCO, CALIFORNIA

From the Division of Neurological Surgery,
University of California Medical School

THE pineal shift as determined by X-ray examination will frequently localize a brain tumor. This method has been of great value in confirming opinions based on neurological examination, and it alone has frequently made the diagnosis possible.

It has also resulted in widening the range of diagnosis by X-ray examination. Formerly the minority of cases of intracranial pressure yielded X-ray evidence of the location of the lesion. Diagnostic information of a localizing character can now be obtained in the majority.

The percentage of brain tumors and of other gross intracranial lesions which cannot be localized by clinical methods of examination alone is considerable. It varies greatly if one considers the length of time the case is studied. It has been estimated at various figures. Dandy has made the statement that only 50 per cent of the tumors could be located with accuracy sufficient to guide the surgeon. This is probably a low figure for the clinical neurologist. Others have given much smaller percentages, but it seems reasonable to suppose that in a short period of observation there will remain something like 20 per cent which cannot be localized. In these, additional diagnos-

* Presented in part before the meeting of the Nevada State Medical Society, September 13, 1924.

† Reprinted from *Surgery, Gynecology and Obstetrics*, 1925, *40:* 481–484, with the kind permission of the Editor.

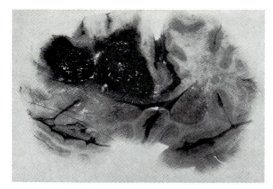

FIG. 1. Frontal section of brain showing a metastatic tumor with fresh haemorrhage into it. Note the great increase in volume of this hemisphere and the dislocation of the mid-line to the opposite side.

tic methods are required. We have found that, by simple and safe means, the number in this small and difficult group can be reduced.

It is a matter of common observation at autopsy that the portion of the brain in which a growth is situated increases greatly in volume. This is not only due to the presence of the lesion itself but to an increase in the fluid content of this hemisphere. To a less extent the brain as a whole becomes oedematous. In such conditions it is not uncommon to find the affected hemisphere even one-third larger than the opposite one (Fig. 1). The dislocation of the falx and of all mid-line structures to one side and the accompanying distortion are very striking.

Shueller [sic.][1] refers briefly to the displacement of the shadow of the pineal gland due to pressure from tumor or traction on the part of a brain scar. He quotes a case of right hemiplegia, presumably from circulatory causes, in which the pineal shadow was displaced to the left. He concludes that there was contraction of the left hemisphere perhaps from softening and that the pineal was drawn to that side from scar. No autopsy findings or confirmation of the diagnosis were mentioned.

Under the constantly improving methods of roentgenography and particularly with the use of the Bucky diaphragm, greater definition of structures is being obtained and more details are visible. Calcification in the pineal gland which occurs under normal conditions in a large percentage of individuals is often noted in lateral views of the skull. It occurred to us that the position of this structure might be of diagnostic value if variations in it occurred with gross lesions. The pineal shadow is seldom seen in the anteroposterior or postero-anterior view of the skull. This is chiefly owing to the position in which the film is taken. Ordinarily the pineal shadow is obscured by the accessory sinuses. When, however, the direction of the ray is parallel to a line drawn between the

external canthus of the eye and the external auditory meatus, the pineal shadow is seen to be projected well above the sinuses. We have found it more advantageous to have the patient in a face up position with the occiput against the film, as the pineal gland is somewhat closer to the back of the head than to the front. If with the head in this position (Fig. 2) the tube is carefully centered so that the central rays pass along the mid-sagittal plane, one can readily determine the relation of the pineal shadow to this plane. Developmentally the pineal is a true mid-line structure. There is little to indicate that its calcification has any pathological significance. A study of a large number of normals has shown that the shadow lies exactly in the mid-line (Fig. 3).

In all conditions associated with intracranial pressure and in the presence of a calcified pineal, our cases have been studied from films taken as described. It has been shown in the presence of intracranial pressure that where the lesion is located in the right cerebral hemisphere the pineal shadow has been shifted from its position in the mid-line toward the opposite side. The degree of pineal shift, as we have termed it, varies considerably. A common shift is a distance of about 1 centimeter (Fig. 4). We have, however, found it displaced away from the lesion for a distance of 2.5 to 3 centimeters (Fig. 5). When the gross lesion is on the left side, the pineal shift occurs to the right. The shift has been present whether the growth has been frontal, parietal, or occipital. With lesions of the posterior fossa or base which produce a high degree of intracranial pressure from an internal hydrocephalus, the lateral ventricles, both right and left, have been uniformly dilated. The pressure is so uniformly distributed, that the mid-line structures have not been dis-

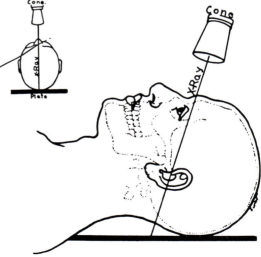

FIG. 2. Diagram showing the position of the head.

torted and the pineal retains its true mid-line position. No shift occurs. These experiences have been true in 15 cases proved by operation or autopsy.

ILLUSTRATIVE CASES

The following illustrate the pineal shift in cases with obvious signs of localization:

CASE 1. Pineal shift away from tumor (Fig. 4). E. W. University of California Hospital. No. 46667. Female, age 37. Diagnosis: glioma right frontal—cystic partly calcified. Cyst evacuation. This patient had a proved cystic glioma of the right frontal region. The roentgenogram is of interest in showing both the tumor partly calcified and the pineal shift toward the opposite side.

CASE 2. Marked shift of pineal to right with left temporoparietal tumor (Fig. 5). M. L. J. University of California Hospital. No. 46035. Female, age 55. Brain tumor left parietal, not proved. Patient entered hospital with a right hemiplegia and complete aphasia of gradual onset over several months. Choked discs and stupor were present. Neurological examination showed no involvement of cranial nerves, but the usual findings of a hemiplegia. Localization of lesion presented no problem but marked shift of pineal shadow to right was of interest.

CASE 3. No shift of pineal shadow with internal hydrocephalus. F. V. University of California Hospital. No. 45892. Female, age 27. Acoustic neuroma proved. Tumor removal. This patient gave the characteristic chronologic sequence of symptoms with typical findings. The fifth and seventh nerves were involved along with

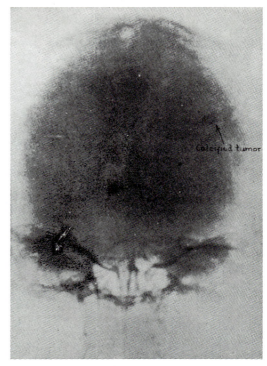

FIG. 4. Showing pineal shift away from the side of a calcified tumor.

the eighth. The cerebellar signs were pronounced and a high degree of intracranial pressure evidenced by highly choked discs. Marked internal hydrocephalus was proved by ventricular puncture.

The X-ray report noted—Pineal shadow in mid-line. No shift.

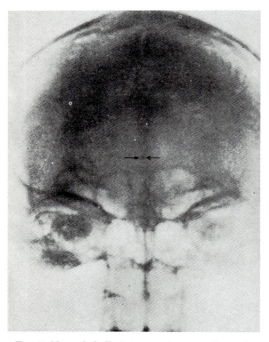

FIG. 3. Normal skull. A true postero-anterior projection showing the calcified pineal in the mid-line just above the frontal sinuses.

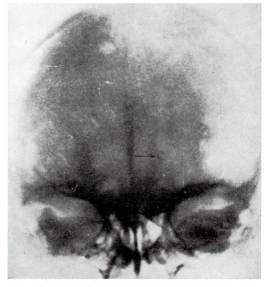

FIG. 5. Marked shift of the pineal shadow.

As an indication of the determining value of the method, the following is one instance.

CASE 4. E. F. Patient seen in consultation, May 22, 1924 with Drs. Fred Fairchild and Harbinson at the Woodland Sanitarium, Woodland, California. The patient was in stupor with slightly swollen optic discs and evidence of intracranial pressure. From the history his condition was presumably due to brain abscess. His state prevented perimetric fields, sensory tests, etc. There was a story of difficulty in the use of the left hand. It proved impossible for us to determine by examination of the patient whether we were dealing with an involvement of tracts in the right cerebral hemisphere or with a left cerebellar lesion. The roentgenograms previously taken in the usual manner gave no localizing information. It was noted, however, that these plates showed a calcified pineal. The patient was returned to the X-ray room. Films were taken in the manner here described, and it was found that the pineal shadow was in the exact mid-plane. Its position argued against a right cerebral lesion and for an internal hydrocephalus. With this aid a diagnosis of a left cerebellar abscess was made, found at operation and evacuated with recovery.

Reviews of a considerable number of X-ray plates have been undertaken with a view to determining in just what percentage of individuals the pineal gland is calcified. Various factors affect these figures, principally the age of the patient and the character of the roentgenogram itself. The percentage of calcified pineals is, of course, much decreased if any large number of children is included. In patients of greater age, a larger percentage of positives is obtained. The following figures are based on a study of 215 consecutive cases:

		Per cent
Total skulls	215	....
Pineal calcified in	97	45
In 45 cases under 20 years of age, 7 were calcified, or		15.5
In 96 cases over 20 years of age, 56 were calcified, or		58

In general it has been found that in something like 50 per cent of cases, the pineal gland is sufficiently calcified to be of diagnostic value. The two essentials for the use of this method of diagnosis are of course, first, that there is sufficient pineal calcification to cast a shadow; and, second, that intracranial pressure is present. It is doubtful whether any considerable dislocation of the gland will occur if there is not sufficient pressure to give intracranial signs. If, however, intracranial pressure is present as indicated by papillitis or choked discs, or possibly in more acute cases by an actual rise in the spinal manometer reading, it offers

great help. Subacute and acute conditions such as abscesses and haemorrhages, have given the characteristic shift. Stereoscopic plates are of decided help and permit one, without any great difficulty, to recognize even slight dislocation of the shadow from the mid-line. Studies are now being made from lateral views of the skull to determine the normal position of the gland in horizontal and vertical planes with reference to the skull as a whole. It is hoped that further observation and study may enable us so to standardize the lateral roentgenograms of the skull that we can detect an anterior or posterior or an up and down deviation of the gland from its normal position. It is also possible that if such conditions as transient oedema or swelling of one-half of the brain occurs, this method may be of value in detecting it.

Inasmuch as about 50 per cent of all cases showed calcified pineals and possibly 20 per cent or more of the intracranial gross lesions cannot be localized by clinical methods alone, this method will give us localizing information in one-half of these.

CONCLUSIONS

When the pineal gland is calcified (in about 50 per cent of all skulls), its position gives diagnostic information in cases *with intracranial pressure.* The shift has been found with brain tumors, brain abscess, and in certain cases of brain swelling consequent upon a vascular block.

A position of the pineal to the right of the mid-sagittal plane indicates a left sided lesion above the tentorium.

A position of the pineal to the left of the mid-sagittal plane indicates a right sided lesion above the tentorium.

A position of the pineal in the mid-sagittal plane in the presence of intracranial pressure indicates equal pressure on the two sides. In the chronic form of intracranial pressure as due to tumor or abscess this means internal hydrocephalus. This has been found occurring in lesions of the posterior fossa and distortion of the third and fourth ventricles.

In the roentgenological development of this method and the observations on most of the proved cases, I desire particularly to thank Howard Ruggles and Lloyd Bryan for their interest and aid. For additional observations and statistics on pineal calcification, I am indebted to James Thom, J. Rehfisch, and A. E. Elliott.

REFERENCE

[1. Schüller, A.] Roentgen Diagnosis of Diseases of the Head. Translation by Stocking. St. Louis: C. V. Mosby. 1918 Chap. II, p. 156.

Neurosurgical Classics—25, 26 and 27

ONE of the most important problems which had to be solved before neuro-surgery could become practical was the matter of hemostasis.[3,6] Even when the introduction of anesthesia and antisepsis had made intracranial operations feasible, the degree of hemorrhage which was usually encountered seriously limited the extent of these operations. Surgeons rapidly became aware that ligatures could not be used to control cranial and intracranial bleeding, and they depended mainly on patience and pressure. It was natural that this problem was among the first to be attacked by the early developers of neurosurgery. The success of their first innovations, as represented by Horsley's use of bone wax[1,4] and tissue stamps,[5] and Cushing's introduction of silver clips,[2] played a vital role in the subsequent evolution of modern neurosurgery.

References

1. BAILEY, H., and BISHOP, W. J. Notable names in medicine and surgery. *London: H. K. Lewis & Co.,* 1959, 3rd ed., xiii, 216 pp. (see pp. 155–156).
2. CUSHING, H. The control of bleeding in operations for brain tumors. With the description of silver "clips" for the occlusion of vessels inaccessible to the ligature. *Ann. Surg.,* 1911, *54:* 1–19. Also: *Trans. Amer. surg. Ass.,* 1911, *29:* 389–410.
3. GREEN, R. E., and STERN, W. E. Techniques of cranial surgery. In: *A history of neurological surgery.* A. E. Walker, Ed. Baltimore: Williams & Wilkins Co., 1951, xii, 583 pp. (see pp. 40–76).
4. HORSLEY, V. Antiseptic wax. *Brit. med. J.,* 1892, *1:* 1165.
5. HORSLEY, V. Note on haemostasis by application of living tissue. *Brit. med. J.,* 1914, *2:* 8.
6. LIGHT, R. U. Hemostasis in neurosurgery. *J. Neurosurg.,* 1945, *2:* 414–434.

ANTISEPTIC WAX.*

SIR,—The antiseptic wax which Mr. Rushton Parker refers to on page 1076 of the BRITISH

---

* Reprinted from Correspondence, The British Medical Journal, 1892, 1: 1165, with the kind permission of the Editor.

MEDICAL JOURNAL of May 21st has the following composition: beeswax, 7 parts; almond oil, 1 part; salicylic acid, 1 per cent. It is the outcome of experiments made in 1885, when, remembering the practice of Magendie and others at the commencement of the century in stopping the sinuses with wax, I tried the effect of "smudging" modelling wax worked soft in the fingers on the free bleeding cut surface of the cranial bones in dogs. As such a proceeding instantly arrested the bleeding, I tried to make an antiseptic compound for operations on man, and the formula was published. It was not, however, satisfactory in my opinion, and I asked Mr. P. W. Squire kindly to make experiments so as to arrive nearly at the tenacity of modelling wax. This, I think, he has perfectly succeeded in with the above formula. I have very often used it, and without the least inconvenience. I need hardly say that it is always sterilised by boiling before use, and kept in covered stoppered bottles.—I am, etc.,

VICTOR HORSLEY.

Cavendish Square, W.

NOTE ON HAEMOSTASIS BY APPLICATION OF LIVING TISSUE.*

BY

SIR VICTOR HORSLEY, F.R.S., F.R.C.S.

MANY years ago, acting on a hint obtained from Magendie's *Physiologie,* I showed that it is very easy to arrest bleeding from bone by the use of an aseptic plastic wax which can adhere to the cancellous spaces and to their walls. This method is now, I believe, in general use.

On the other hand, it is difficult to stop bleeding and haemorrhagic oozing from soft tissues except by the employment of a ligature, or pressure with a gauze tampon, or by irrigation with hot liquid (110° F. to 115° F.). For a long time I employed amadou for this purpose in experimental investigations where asepsis was not required, and with good results, as it adhered well to the bleeding point. To obtain, however, the same result in aseptic operations is not so simple. The factors which had to be obtained were:

1. Asepticity.

---

* Reprinted from The British Medical Journal, 1914, 2: 8, with the kind permission of the Editor.

2. Adhesiveness.
3. Thrombokinesis.

In view of my personal experience of the work of the late Dr. Wooldridge, it occurred to me that probably the best material would be living vascular tissue—that from the (injured) surface of a cut fragment of muscle, in all probability, thrombokinetic processes would most readily start; not merely on account of the plasma and plasmatic corpuscles of the tissue, but also the thrombokinetic by-products in the effused blood and the development of so-called blood platelets.

Such a fragment of the animal's own muscle offered all these advantages, and also asepticity. I was rather surprised to find that the necessary factor of adherence was also satisfied in a very remarkable degree.

If the bleeding point—for example, from the cut surface of the brain, liver, or any soft tissue—be gently pressed with gauze, and this instantly replaced by a piece of living muscle, and pressure again applied from fifteen to twenty seconds, it will be found that the muscle fragment closely adheres to the tissue it is applied to.

Such adhesion is necessarily limited by the pressure at which the blood is escaping from the bleeding point. By direct experiment on divided arteries (including the aorta) in the cat and dog, I found that a muscle haemostasis would resist as much as 60 to 80 mm. Hg blood pressure.

Further histological investigation of the exceedingly thin viscous layer occupying the plane of contact of the two masses of tissue shows that it contains blood platelets, fibrin fibrils, etc., in a considerable degree, and within a short space of time (five to ten minutes) of commencing the preparation.

To estimate the degree of active thrombokinesis I also tested the utility of the muscle after it had been boiled for five minutes at 100° C. Such boiled tissue had a very poor haemostatic effect. It seemed as if this was partly owing to the great loss of adhesiveness which is caused by the heat coagulation completely altering the physical surface of the muscle tissue.

Of other tissues I have only exhaustively tried fascia fully, and with the result that it has not proved satisfactory. It has not the factor of adhesiveness sufficiently well marked, though it can be employed where it is not convenient to take a piece of muscle. When experimental research had shown the remarkably rapid haemostatic effect of living tissue I used it freely in operations—above all, where it was necessary and convenient to leave a resting plug or tampon in a wound. Where an operation has been performed in two stages, I have occasionally had the opportunity of examining the isolated muscle tissue, and found it firmly attached and "organized." In no instance has any ill effect followed its employment.

THE CONTROL OF BLEEDING IN OPERATIONS FOR BRAIN TUMORS.*

WITH THE DESCRIPTION OF SILVER "CLIPS" FOR THE OCCLUSION OF VESSELS INACCESSIBLE TO THE LIGATURE.†

By HARVEY CUSHING, M.D.,

OF BALTIMORE,

Associate Professor of Surgery in The Johns Hopkins University.

ALL surgeons who make for themselves opportunities to observe the manipulative work of their fellows must appreciate the present general tendency toward the abandonment of the applauded methods of comparatively few years ago. The conditions under which Cooper, Pott, and Abernethy worked have long since changed, and though the by-the-clock methods which were essential to operative success in their day are still emulated in some of our present clinics, the stirring, slap-dash, and spectacular is rapidly giving way to the quiet, patient, and undramatic performance.

The elimination of pain has made hurry unnecessary; due respect for the principles which have grown from Listerism has made it inadvisable; the emphasis laid by Halsted on detailed blood-stilling during major operations has proved a further check, and lastly, an expectation of the reactionless healing which occurs only in tissues handled with the greatest delicacy and coapted with scrupulous care is prohibitive of haste and the old-time thrills for the bystander which accompanied it.

There are special reasons why the utmost precaution in anaesthetization, the gentlest methods of handling tissues, and the most accurate closure of wounds, accompanied by as painstaking haemostasis as possible, should be observed during the more difficult intracranial procedures. Neighborhood oozing obscures the clear view essential to the safety of such delicate manipulations as are required for the removal of, let us say, a lateral recess tumor or the trigeminal ganglion; whereas a more general loss of blood with the consequent lowering of arterial tension is a cordial invitation to its near relative shock, favors the onset of respiratory paralysis in cases associated with medullary pressure, makes anaesthesia more dangerous, and lowers resistance to infection through secondary anaemia.

These are premises, I am aware, which are not accepted by all surgeons, for many still feel that high-geared methods of operating can outdistance these largely imaginary risks, and there is a wide-

* Read by title before the American Surgical Association, June, 1911.

† Reprinted from *Annals of Surgery*, 1911, *54:* 1–19, with the kind permission of the Chairman of the Editorial and Advisory Board.

spread apprehension lest observation of these minutiae engender a reputation of being a slow and fussy surgeon. For, after all, what do these details amount to, with another patient awaiting his turn and an assistant who can close the wound, put on the dressing, and administer stimulants and infusions. But for those who grant the premises and agree that every effort should be made, even at the expense of time, to respect the tissues and to minimize the loss of blood by whatsoever methods one can summon to his aid, there are certain "tricks" which may be found useful, particularly in cerebral surgery.

It is necessary to bear in mind that two fairly distinct vascular systems will be encountered—internal and external. On the arterial or carotid side these systems are quite distinct, but on the venous side the communications between them are so free that, under conditions of intracranial stasis brought about by a growth producing an increase of tension, the venous return from the internal system is in large part shunted into the extracranial field. For this reason—though the "tricks" to be spoken of apply chiefly to the internal system of vessels with a cerebral and meningeal distribution—it may not be out of place to preface a few remarks concerning ways of combating loss of blood from the external coverings, through which the approach to the more important structures must be made.

Throughout this paper the more critical cases will be considered. If precautions are taken to meet the serious problems of haemostasis which the critical cases present, the simpler and less complicated ones can be more often carried through to a successful termination at one sitting. Furthermore, the discussion will be largely restricted to the osteoplastic type of operation on the cranial vault; for if its principles are mastered, operations in situations which forbid the use of a tourniquet or those in which a bone flap is prohibited may be conducted with comparative ease.

The Scalp.—That a trifling wound in a normally vascularized scalp may bleed abundantly is familiar enough. But when stasis of the extracranial vessels has been produced by a cerebral tumor, the loss of blood incidental to the long incision needed for an osteoplastic resection may be disproportionately excessive, unless precautionary measures are taken. Many devices have been suggested to control bleeding from the scalp, none of them in the long run being as efficient as a properly applied tourniquet. This, in any event, will control the arterial supply to the operative field, and if there is no cyanosis under the anaesthetic and no unusual widening of the emissary venous communications between the internal and external systems, not a single haemostatic adjunct may be required. When, on the other hand, venous stasis has long existed and wide communications have

formed between extra- and intracranial veins, the scalp will fill with blood and require the placement of clamps, no matter what device be employed. But even under these circumstances, the convex side of the incision towards the flap remains dry—a desirable result, as it avoids the risk of stripping scalp from bone through the weight of pendent instruments. When it is necessary to place clamps on the concave edge, even though the bleeding points may lie in the tough scalp proper, it is best to catch the galea and allow the mere weight of the clamps to close the bleeding points. This precaution will avoid superficial points of tissue necrosis which militate against the subsequent reactionless healing. The flat T-shaped clamps which have been devised for the scalp are, I think, undesirable, for the reason that they are difficult to place and are likely to damage the tissues.

As many of these more desperate cranial operations must require two or more stages before their end, it is essential that the utmost pains be taken in closing the wound to assure an epithelial approximation which will permit early removal of the external sutures. Needless to say, if there are points of staphylococcal stitch infection, or even granulating edges owing to inaccurate closure, the reopening of the wound after a few days, and possibly the later re-reopening after a subsequent interval, is accompanied by especial risks of infection.

Our local method of closing these wounds is to bring the edges of the galea together by a series of interrupted and buried fine black (iron-dyed) silk sutures. This row of buried sutures oftentimes so closely approximates the overlying tough scalp as to render the placement of cutaneous sutures hardly necessary, were it not for the fact that they are destined to control the arterial bleeding which would otherwise ensue on the final removal of the tourniquet. A satisfactory method of placing these sutures before they are tied, by a row of round, fine intestinal (cambric) needles, has heretofore been described.[1] They should be removed after thirty-six or forty-eight hours; and by the fourth or fifth day the incision is hardly visible, there are no points of reaction due to suture constriction, and epithelium covers the entire field.

The present paper is not an essay on wound closure, though such an essay might well be written, for many, I am aware, regard this step as so unimportant a detail of an operation that its performance is beneath the dignity of the operating surgeon himself. It is, however, a deserving detail of these measures, not only when a subsequent reopening is premeditated, but for the reason that in the case of a fresh first-stage wound, especially when clamps have been necessitated owing to

[1] Keen's System of Surgery, 1908, vol. iii, Fig. 152, p. 272.

venous stasis, some further loss of blood will occur during the closure. For it is inadvisable to attempt to ligate the bleeding points in the tough scalp, as the external approximating sutures may be relied upon to effectually control them; and to place and tie these sutures accurately and rapidly requires a full and not a crippled operative team.

Impatience to attain results is characteristic of the species surgeon and often leads to the taking of unjustifiable risks—one of the reasons for the high mortality ascribed to major intracranial procedures, those for tumor in particular. The writer is no exception and constantly finds it necessary to curb himself in the desire to do just a little more. But far more tumor operations have been carried to a successful outcome by the courage to temporarily withdraw after a bad start than by banging at hazards. Annoying though it is, it may improve one's score when in difficulties to play back with the loss of a stroke.

Postponement may thus be justifiable merely in view of a badly taken anaesthetic—and no tumor patient in whom pressure is considerable takes the anaesthetic any too well, even with the most skilful administration. At a subsequent trial circumstances may be more fortunate, or a preliminary dose of scopolamin with morphia or atropin, or a combination of chloroform and ether, may serve to offset the earlier difficulties. For cyanosis increases intracranial pressure by accelerating cerebrospinal fluid secretion,[2] which adds to the venous obstruction and so to the loss of blood—a bad cycle all around. But rare though it may be to have to abandon progress toward the final stage owing merely to a badly taken anaesthetic, postponement is not infrequently advisable because of excessive loss of blood from scalp and bone, and such a postponement would hardly seem an advance at all were it not for the fact that a blunt reopening of the uniting superficial wound after a few days is attended with relatively little bleeding.

The Skull.—All grades of vascularity may be encountered, and chief reliance must be placed upon the proper use of proper wax, for the intro-

duction of which Horsley deserves the lasting gratitude of us all. The cases which present the greatest difficulties are those in which a superficial tumor of long standing receives or discharges much of its blood supply through the diploetic spaces of the bone. This is particularly true of the large dural endotheliomata, which are often associated with extreme vascularity of the adjacent skull, even though the immediately overlying bone may be thinned by pressure atrophy. The enlarged diploetic channels, in these cases, sometimes the size of a radial artery, are often traceable on the radiographic plates, which in this way may be useful even though they rarely show actual shadows of the tumor. At times the very surface of the exposed skull may be so roughened and vascular that it must be rubbed with wax to check the extensive oozing from countless points.

But even with the generous use of wax, considerable loss of blood may be unavoidable in the process of outlining the bone flap under these conditions of abnormal vascularity with extreme venous stasis. For though extravasation from the bone edges may be controlled, it is less easy to combat the free bleeding due to the separation of meningeal emissaries, particularly if the incision be carried into an area of new-formed arachnoidal villi with a distribution beyond the usual confines of Pacchionian granulations. In any case it is well to give the longitudinal sinus and its lateral lacunae a wide berth, and not to outline the mesial edge of the proposed flap nearer than two or three centimetres from the midline. Should an exposure of the foot area be deemed necessary the safest method of approach is to turn down a low flap and subsequently cut out a bay from the upper edge, leaving a permanent defect over this dangerous vascular area.

Whether one prefers to outline the bone flap with electromotor or hand-driven instruments,— and I regard the latter as much the safer,— bleeding is likely to occur from the lacerated osteodural communications at the upper margin. For this reason it is our custom, after making the primary large trephine opening and the secondary opening with perforator and burr, to immediately pass a dural separator between the two, so as to break up the vascular attachments at this early stage. For when the instrument is withdrawn, the cerebral tension is sufficient to again plaster dura against bone and effectually check the bleeding, so that by the time the lateral margins of the flap have been cut, many of the emissary vessels will have become spontaneously occluded.

Postponement at this stage owing to loss of blood may sometimes be desirable, even before the flap, though thoroughly outlined, has been lifted away from the adherent dura. The advisability of this can often be gauged by the anaesthetist better than by the operator, and by a blood-pressure tracing better than by a finger on

---

[2] This is particularly true of ether, which, though the safest drug to employ, is unquestionably the most difficult to administer; and needless to say, its use should be in expert hands. There is less bleeding with chloroform, owing to the fact that it lowers arterial tension; but this in a way is comparable in its consequences to an actual loss of blood and so must be regarded as hazardous, as has been emphasized heretofore. And there are other hazards in the use of chloroform which formerly we did not recognize, namely, the hepatic necroses which in greater or less degree are a constant feature of chloroform administration and are particularly extensive after a readministration, when, as Dr. George A. Whipple has found, there is an especial tendency even to spontaneous bleeding, owing to the loss or diminution of one of the elements necessary to clot formation.

the pulse. The procedure up to this point has been a brief one, there will be a quick recovery from the anaesthetic, and a certain amount of pressure relief will be experienced through the slight elevation of the still adherent flap.

It is of course far more often possible to elevate the bone flap; for conditions such as may have rendered postponement advisable at a stage earlier than this are naturally rare. One must realize, however, that it takes nearly as long to get out of as it does to get into the intracranial chamber, and as there is likely to be about as much bleeding during the process of withdrawal as during entry, such blood as may be lost during further advance must be multiplied by two. And one should not wait for a profound upsetting of the pressor mechanism, for it does not go to pieces gradually, but suddenly. This is well exemplified in transfusions, for a large amount of blood may be given up by the donor with no appreciable change in his condition, until a little pallor, increased respiration, and restlessness indicate the need of uncoupling. Checking the flow at this stage is followed by complete readjustment within a few moments, and one is often thus misled into the thought that more blood might safely have been withdrawn; but this extra straw will often so upset the regulatory mechanism that hours or days are needed for a complete restoration.

The Dura.—We have come to a stage of the osteoplastic operation which calls for especial tricks of haemostasis, and the following adjuncts have been found useful: (1) *Small pledgets or "tips" of gauze* of various sizes secured by a black ligature, so that though blood-stained they can be easily located—minute Mikulicz pads as it were. (2) *Sterile absorbent cotton* to be used *dry* and plastered on an oozing surface, or *wet* in hot saline solution, a bowl of which at a temperature of 100° to 105° F. should be on the instrument tray immediately at hand. This dripping cotton is the best material for washing meningeal surfaces, and, when wrung out into flat pads, is the safest and most effectual substance for sponging or for temporary placement in deep cerebral wounds. (3) *Bits of living tissue*—supplied, for example, from the exposed temporal muscle—which serve admirably as a means of checking venous extravasation from points on the dura, and *fragments of partially organized blood-clots*, obtainable at a second-stage performance, are similarly useful. Finally (4) *silver wire "clips"* for placement on inaccessible vessels, which, though within reach of a clamp, are either too delicate or in a position too awkward for safe ligation.

On first elevating the flap there may be, particularly in cases with stasis, quite an abundant loss of blood from the raw surface of the dura. This bleeding comes from two sources, arterial and venous; that from the latter being by far the more troublesome; for only in case of a torn me-

ningeal at the lower anterior angle, due to its having deeply channelled the bone where this has been broken in turning back the flap, will arterial bleeding give trouble. When this occurs it is naturally the first thing to need attention, and if there is venous bleeding from the raw dural surface, it can meanwhile be temporarily controlled by promptly covering the whole surface with a large pad of the hot and dripping cotton, which is immediately dried out against the oozing dural surface by pressure with a gauze sponge. The arterial bleeding should then be checked without attempting to catch or ligate the vessel, which may be torn back "hang-nail" fashion. Some of the prepared gauze pledgets of proper size can be tucked under the bone, separating the dura from it until a point is reached where the vessel no longer channels the bone. Then the pressure of the pledgets against the tense dural surface will control the bleeding until later in the operation, when with an open dura the vessel can be caught by a "clip" if it proves to be inaccessible to a ligature.[3]

Permanent control of the venous bleeding is a more difficult matter. The artery, as its branches approach the upper part of the exposed area, is accompanied by many dural veins which have a more or less intimate connection with the bone, and many raw, bleeding points may be left after their separation. These points, especially if associated with Pacchionian granulations, may give a great deal of trouble during the further procedure, and indeed may continue to ooze after replacement of the flap and closure of the wound; and thus in the course of a few hours a thick extradural clot may form and give pressure symptoms. In our earlier experiences this was an occasional postoperative complication, and even now the possibility of its occurrence is always considered. The fact that dura and bone have been separated makes the formation of such an extradural clot possible, as the result of slow venous oozing, whereas in the ordinary extradural hemorrhage of traumatic origin, the extravasation comes necessarily from a ruptured artery. In other words, the tension of a purely venous extravasation under the latter circumstances would not suffice to peel the adherent membrane from the bone.

Even when the venous oozing seems at the

---

[3] Loose gauze pledgets of minute size, possibly a centimetre in circumference, are particularly valuable in ganglion operations. For one of them can be plastered against a bleeding point, say at the foramen ovale, and its anchoring ligature led out of the wound, leaving a sufficient exposure of the remaining field to allow for further progress in separating the dural envelopes. By using the proper tricks to control hemorrhage, in none of our last seventy-five cases has it been necessary to postpone a ganglion operation until a second session, and in none has it been necessary to place a drain.

close of the operation to have been effectually checked, postoperative vomiting or straining may start the bleeding anew by dislodgement of terminal thrombi, and for this reason in all cases in which the performance has been a bloody one the patient should not be lifted from the operating table until he has recovered in large measure from the anaesthetic. The table therefore should be made sufficiently comfortable by having a thick mattress covering, for it may be inadvisable to move the patient for two or three hours, and, indeed, it is not exceptional for critical cases to be kept in the adjoining recovery room over night before they are transferred to the ward. With such precautions, in addition to skilful administration of the anaesthesia, postoperative retching and vomiting are rare.

Oftentimes the gauze "tips" or pledgets of cotton, which, during the progress of the operation, have been used to cover and which have become adherent to bleeding points in the dura, cannot be removed without starting the bleeding afresh, so that one is occasionally tempted to leave the foreign material plastered against the dura in the hope of its becoming safely organized. This, of course, is undesirable (though we have found in animal experimentation that the cotton pledgets as a rule are well cared for) and also unnecessary, for an alternative has been discovered in *bits of living tissue* or *well-solidified blood-clots*. Small snips of tissue may be cut from an exposed raw surface, such as the temporal muscle—and muscle seems to be particularly valuable as a haemostatic—and when held for a moment on the bleeding point by a smooth instrument they will adhere more promptly and check further extravasation far better than gauze or cotton. Since this device for checking bleeding was first hit upon some two years ago, we have made frequent use of it, with most satisfactory results.[4]

It is possible that any living tissue will suffice. In a recent case of extirpation of a cerebellopontine tumor a troublesome point of venous bleeding was left at the side of the pons. It was controlled by a small piece of dura which, as the most available tissue, was cut off and plastered against the side of the brain-stem, adhering and effectually checking the bleeding after a few moments of gentle pressure. Organizing clots may also be utilized. They are particularly available in second-stage procedures; and at present, instead of scraping away the clots from primary trephine openings and discarding them, they are carefully preserved in saline gauze, and sections of them utilized in the same way as the bits of muscle tissue. Doubtless it will be found that tissue fragments can be prepared beforehand and kept sterile for this purpose.[5]

It is at this period—with a reflected bone flap and all bleeding from the dura checked—that postponement is most often advisable, not only on account of the loss of blood up to this stage, but more particularly should the membrane be so tense that cerebral protrusion of a dangerous degree is likely to occur through an immediate dural opening. Under these circumstances, even in the bone-flap operation, the principles of decompression come into play; for it cannot be emphasized too strongly that a rapidly forming hernia, comprising functionally important areas of a tense cortex which protrude through an immediately superimposed dural defect, often leaves irrecoverable paralyses. Hence, unless a tumor is obviously subjacent and there is every prospect of its removal at the first sitting, recourse should be had to a temporary palliative measure with a dural defect over a silent and preferably over the subtemporal area.[6]

In the making of a palliative subtemporal defect, whether a primary operation or one to be combined with a temporary osteoplastic resection, it is important that the fibres of the overlying muscle be preserved as intact as possible. This necessitates, particularly in the case of a primary decompression, the careful rongeuring away of the thin bone of the temporal region far under the edge of the split muscle, with an exposure of an area of dura carrying the main branches of the middle meningeal artery. Hence, when the dura is incised radially from a primary central opening to the margins of the bone defect, some of these branches, particularly the posterior radicle of the artery, are likely to be divided, and unless precautions are observed, bleeding may be troublesome. If the spoon-shaped spatula[7] is used

---

[4] Since this paper was put together I have learned from Dr. Lund's interesting report of the visit last summer of the Society of Clinical Surgery to Great Britain that Sir Victor Horsley demonstrated "the haemostatic action of a fragment of muscle" on the exposed brain during the progress of a laboratory experiment. It is not unlikely, therefore, and is indeed probable, that one or all of the "tricks" which I have here set down have been in use by others who have not regarded them of sufficient importance to record.

[5] If Bernheim's conclusions (*Jour. Am. Med. Assoc.*, 1910), that the walls of the blood-vessels possess more active clotting elements than do other tissues, prove to be correct the walls of preserved vessels may be applicable for this purpose; or the fibrin from whipped blood might be so prepared that it could be immediately plastered on bleeding surfaces, just as cotton is now used, and thus obviate the necessity for any subsequent replacement. Or, as Carrel has suggested (*Jour. Exper. Med.*, 1910, xii, 460) for the preservation of blood-vessels we may be able to preserve tissues *in vitro* for these purposes in a condition of "latent life."

[6] A useful method of combining at this stage a decompression with the exploration has been elsewhere described (Surg., Gynaec., and Obst., vol. iv, 1909, pp. 1–5). It has been put into practice in some thirty or forty cases with uniform satisfaction in the results.

[7] Surg. Gynaec. and Obst., 1909, vol. iv, p. 3, Fig. 2.

to hold the tense brain away from the dura while the radial cuts are being made, the arterial branches can usually be seen before they are divided, and a delicate clamp of the Halsted pattern can be applied on each side of the incised membrane even in the deeply overlain parts of the wound inaccessible for ligation. But what to do with these deep bleeding points after they were thus caught often gave us great concern in our earlier operations; and on one or two occasions it was necessary to divide the muscle transversely in order to obtain sufficient exposure for ligation. These difficulties have been overcome by means of silver "clips"—a device which possibly deserves the especial description given to it later in this paper.

The Brain.—The central nervous system can be seriously damaged in the attempt to employ the usual methods of haemostasis with gauze, clamp, and ligature commonly used for other tissues. From its first exposure, every effort should be made to avoid any injury to the pia-arachnoid until the actual moment of entry to the subcortex for the purpose of exploration or enucleation of an obvious growth, and such entry and proposed enucleation must be carefully planned out in accordance with the disposition of the cortical vessels. A safe enucleation may be completely frustrated by gauze sponging or otherwise roughly handling a brain under tension, by the protrusion and rupture of the tense cortex through the primary dural opening, by the accidental injury of a cortical vein carelessly wounded during the enlargement of the dural incision. The struggle to control the consequences of these seemingly trifling matters, which leave in the end a large patch of broken and infiltrated cortex through which ligatures have cut and against which gauze sponges have been held, is only too familiar, and operations for tumor are usually terminated by such an occurrence.

Familiarity with the tricks of lessening tension is all-important in the prevention of these accidents, and the different methods of dealing with a "dry" or "wet" brain by primary decompression, by pricking arachnoid spaces, by ventricular or lumbar punctures, by changes of posture and what not, is a subject too large to be dealt with in the present paper, though indirectly bearing a close relation to loss of blood incidental to manipulations of the nervous tissues themselves. The whole matter hinges more on the disturbances of cerebrospinal circulation than upon the size and position of the tumor. For with a smoothly taken anaesthetic there may be little or no difficulty in manipulating a brain holding the largest of growths, whereas cyanosis with increase of stasis may make the exposure of a brain, under previously normal conditions of tension, hazardous in the extreme. A small growth of the brain stem, on the other hand, may lead to a great stasis of fluid, the embarrassments from which can be promptly set aside by a ventricular puncture. In any event, a satisfactory subdural exploration can only be made after a considerable diminution in tension has been brought about in one way or another.

The question of tension, furthermore, is quite apart from the actual primary vascularity of the growth, for some of the most vascular lesions, which consequently are difficult to handle, fortunately may be uncomplicated by tension, just as tense brains may hold relatively non-vascular growths which are readily enucleable. However this may be, great care should be exercised in attacking a growth when once it has been brought into view and has been given the wide exposure essential to a safe attempt at extirpation.

Notwithstanding the statement of physiologists to the contrary, one rarely if ever sees "shock" in cerebral operations as a thing apart from hemorrhage or injury to some vital centre. This is abundantly supported by certain of our experiences with extensive cerebral manipulations at second-stage operations in unanaesthetized patients. Hence, with careful choice of the stage at which an extirpation may be attempted—meaning largely an unbled subject—an abundance of time and patience should be expended in the careful and slow manipulations necessary for the dislodgement of the tumor. The tearing out of a growth by the insertion of the fingers means a fragmental removal, extravasation and oedema from unnecessary damage, and blind points of hemorrhage most difficult to identify. On the other hand, it is astonishing how dry the subcortex may actually be if care has been taken in respect to the superficial vessels. One can usually find a safe point of entry through the cortex; and much of the remainder of the operation consists in the slow separation of brain from tumor, working now here, now there, leaving small, flattened pads of hot, wrung-out cotton to control oozing for the time being from a given area, until it can be again attacked. I know of no better training in such procedures than can be gained by the experience of making clean-cut extirpations on the lower animals—let us say of the motor territory of the canine brain.

A few fine silk (bead) ligatures may be passed on delicate curved needles to secure some of the vessels crossing the line of proposed cortical (circumferential) incision if one is necessary, but care should be taken not to include the large *Venae anastomoticae* or important branches of the middle cerebral artery, lest outlying areas of softening result and leave unexpected and unexplainable palsies to be answered for. Indeed, it is often surprising how widely one can push aside many of these vessels in the pia-arachnoid which at first would seem unquestionably to need ligation.

The actual tilting out of a tumor is largely a

one-man performance, and the operator's left hand is necessarily occupied in holding and guarding the tissue in process of separation. The manipulations meanwhile are carried on by slow, blunt dissection with the right hand, while an assistant keeps the field clean by the careful use of wet cotton pledgets. During the progress of the measure, particularly in the case of a deeply seated tumor, vessels may be encountered passing from brain to tumor and lying in tissues in which it is obviously futile to place an ordinary haemostatic forceps. Under these circumstances the silver "clips" to be described may be found to be useful, just as they are in the presence of dural bleeding from points awkward of access; for the jaws of the instrument holding the clip will pick up the visible vessel or bleeding point just as would the ordinary clamp, the "clip" being left to take the place of an actual pendent instrument.

Despite the rapidity with which the surrounding brain tends to fill up the gaping hole left by the final dislodgement of the growth, the raw surface of the cavity may continue to ooze. This condition can best be controlled by filling the hole with a wad of dry absorbent cotton which is replaced as it becomes saturated. Ultimately the contracting cavity will be left sufficiently dry to justify closure without drainage, for a drain leading from the nervous tissues to the external world should never be used if it can possibly be avoided. The cavity, even if large, should be filled with normal salt solution, and the dura closed as accurately as possible over it. Even if it has been necessary to leave a defect in the dura overlying the cavity, the same principles are to be adhered to.

It was formerly our custom, in order to draw off the excess of bloody fluid as the brain tended to swell and fill the cavity, to leave one or two folded protective wicks, which were led from the cranial chamber through the primary trephine opening to a puncture in the scalp, outlying the

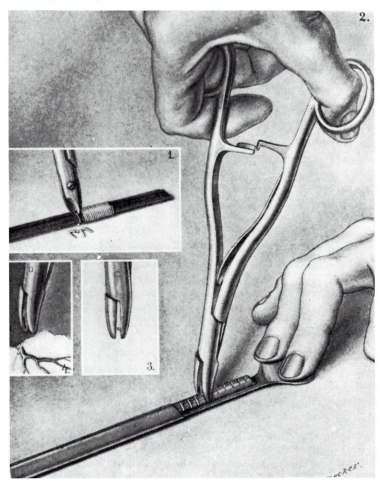

Fig. A. Drawing to show (1) silver wire loops being cut after wrapping on grooved steel pencil; (2) one of the clips being picked up from the loaded magazine; (3) clip in position in jaws of holder; (4) clip placed on meningeal vessel at the edge of a dural incision, the empty instrument showing the mould for the clip. (Reduced one-third.)

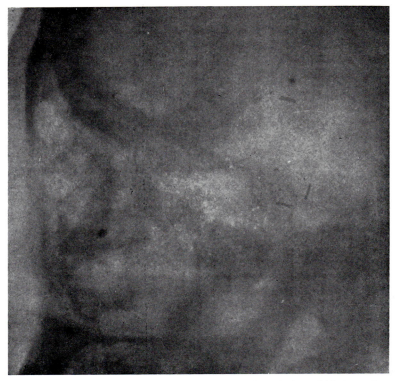

Fig. B. X-ray of a patient's head after subtemporal decompression, during which four clips were placed on bleeding points in the dural margin. Showing unobstructed view of normal sella turcica, two of the clips being in line with its posterior border.

original line of incision. For in this way an oblique passage is insured, and one which is easily occluded by pressure after the withdrawal of the wicks. But particularly in second-stage performances we have found this to be less and less necessary as we have learned how to leave a dryer wound. In the case, for example, of the tumor pictured in Fig. C., the huge cavity left by the removal of the growth was merely filled with salt solution, the flap replaced, and the wound closed with no drainage whatsoever.

SILVER-WIRE CLIPS AS LIGATURES

The thought has doubtless occurred to many that much time and trouble would be saved in major operations could there be devised some form of haemostatic clamp, the mere placement of which would leave a fine, knotted ligature on the bleeding point so as to obviate the alternatives which we now possess, either of leaving a pendent instrument or taking the time necessary for ligation. Some one will probably have the ingenuity to construct an instrument of this kind, which will be useful not only for such extensive performances as complete breast amputations, where many delicate vessels must be secured along the axillary vein and where the temptation is great to leave dangling a heavy mass of clamps, but

also in operations during which vessels are necessarily divided at depths easily reached by a clamp but in positions awkward for ligation. It was doubtless this thought, coupled with a knowledge of the ingenious instrument used by some surgeons for closing skin wounds by the superficial placement of removable, toothed metal bands, that led to the device which we have come to employ.

Some three years ago a small U-shaped bit of wire held in the jaws of an ordinary clamp was first successfully used to check bleeding from a troublesome meningeal vessel divided in a subtemporal operation. As further trials were made on subsequent occasions, the difficulties of holding the small bit of wire in position were overcome by an indentation (Fig. A, 4) in the blades of the clamp in which the wire could securely lie. The wire U's have finally come to be made in large numbers and of equal size by cutting them from a flat metal pencil, around which the wire has been previously wrapped (Fig. A, 1). In order to furnish clips which will not slip easily from the tissues on which they are placed, the metal pencil is longitudinally grooved, so that by lightly tapping the wire, after winding, the inner surface of the loops becomes transversely ridged. A deep median groove allows the pointed wire-cutters to snip the

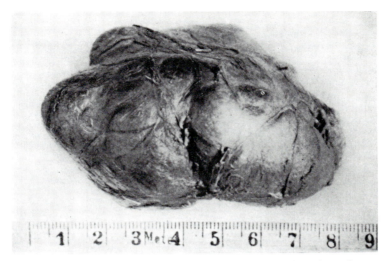

Fig. C. Dural endothelioma (actual size) with adherent clips. Tumor successfully extirpated at second stage, weighing 200 grammes. Bone-flap operation; closure without drainage; uncomplicated recovery.

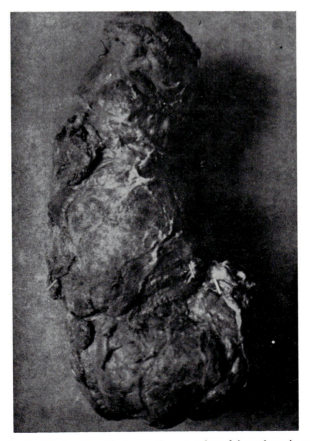

Fig. D. Clips adhering to the inferior thyroid stump of an enucleated intrathoracic goitre (slightly reduced).

several loops (Fig. A, 1) of the same size. They are then loaded on a magazine and picked up individually, as needed, by the holder (Fig. A, 2). The first "catch" of the holder locks its sprung handles at a point which closes the jaws sufficiently to enable them to take up the loop from the magazine without deforming the easily compressed wire, and the instrument unlocks itself when the U has been flattened against the bleeding point (Fig. A, 4). These matters are made sufficiently clear by Mr. Becker's excellent drawing without further description.

The instrument in its present form has been put to use at some stage or another in almost all of our operations on the brain for the past year or two. Like any tool, however, a certain amount of experience is necessary before it can be used with facility. In the hands of some ingenious mechanic it would doubtless be capable of much greater perfection; it would be well to have a self-loading tool if one could be constructed without its being too cumbersome.

The "clips" have been found useful for the occlusion of inaccessible vessels divided in the dural incisions of decompressive operations (Fig. B), for the occlusion of the meningeal at the foramen spinosum if its division is advisable during the operation for trigeminal root avulsion, and, as has been stated, during the enucleation of cerebral tumors for the occlusion of the vessels passing from cortex to tumor—vessels the position and delicacy of which often make ligation well-nigh impossible (Fig. C).

Though from the present character of my operative work I have had little opportunity to test the value of these silver "clips" in operations other than those on the brain, I can recall occasions in intra-abdominal work when the instrument would have been most useful—occasions when a bleeding vessel, such as the artery of the cystic duct, in the depth of the wound could be caught by a clamp but in a position difficult for ligation, particularly if the operator's left hand was occupied in holding the viscera aside to secure the necessary exposure. The "clips," however, have been utilized in a recent enucleation of a large intrathoracic thyroid tumor (goitre plongeant) in a case of acromegaly. The tumor, the descent of which had doubtless been encouraged by the skeletal enlargement of the upper thorax, had exerted pressure against the superior vena cava, and venous stasis of the entire upper body was so extreme as to give an appearance of a malignant mediastinal growth. During the process of dislocating and delivering the growth from its subclavicular position, many of the inferior thyroid vessels below the clavicular level were clipped before their division in positions which would have made ligatures very difficult to apply and the placement of a number of clamps out of the question (Fig. D). "Clips" similarly have been successfully used by Emil Goetsch in such delicate procedures as the experimental occlusion of the canine hypophyseal stalk, and by L. J. Crowe for securing the bleeding points after a tonsillectomy. It is not improbable that similar instruments fashioned to carry loops of stouter wire and of larger calibre might prove useful in occluding vessels larger than those for which we have heretofore used the device.

Summary.—One of the chief objects of concern in intracranial surgery should be the avoidance of any unnecessary loss of blood, for at best, in many cases of brain tumor associated with venous stasis, bleeding is likely to be so excessive as to necessitate postponement of the final steps of the procedure until a second or even a third session.

The common methods of blood stilling by sponge, clamp, and ligature are largely inapplicable to intracranial surgery, particularly in the presence of bleeding from the nervous tissues themselves, and any device which serves as an aid to haemostasis in these difficult operations will bring a larger number of them to a safe termination at a single sitting, with less loss of blood and less damage to the brain itself.

In addition to the more familiar tourniquet for the scalp, and wax for diploetic and emissary bleeding, suggestions are offered as to the use of gauze pledgets, dry sterile cotton, fragments of raw muscle and other tissues, as well as sections of organizing blood-clots for superficial meningeal bleeding, and silver "clips" for inaccessible individual points either in dura or brain.

The successful consummation of any critical operation often depends upon seeming trifles. It is, however, the scrupulous observance of surgical minutiae that makes possible the safe conduct of major intracranial performances—performances which a few years ago were attended in most cases by a veritable dance Macaber.

Neurosurgical Classic—28

Oﾠne of the most significant contributions to the development of modern neurosurgery was the introduction of electrosurgery by Cushing and Bovie.[1,3,5,8–10,14–16,18,19,21–24]

"Cautery with the hot iron was used to some extent in Hippocratic times and it became the paramount tool of the surgeon, to the point that it replaced the knife, in the degraded medicine of the middle ages—'any one could apply the cautery, practically no one the ligature,' remarks Harvey. Selective use of the cautery to sear an artery and promote tight coagulation of its edges was recommended by Albucasis (11th century). It was the achievement of Paré (1552) to make clear the great advantage of the ligature over the cautery, yet surgeons were loath to relinquish a practice that derived authoritative support from Hippocrates and Galen, and about which had grown up a huge ritual, so that two hundred years later the cautery was still in spotty use. Ultimately it died out to await rejuvenation in the guise of electrosurgery.

"The discovery by d'Arsonval (1891)[2] that electrical currents of high frequency alternation are devoid of the physiological stimulation (muscle twitching and pain) long known to be associated with the low frequencies used in power transmission, set the stage for the twin fields of medical diathermy and electrosurgery. . . .

"In view of the critical dependence of neurosurgery upon methods of hemostasis that do not involve implacing and tying a ligature, it is difficult now to explain the long delay of that specialty to investigate and adopt what has become the number one device in the list. The d'Arsonval apparatus was used for destruction of skin lesions by Rivière[20] as early as 1900, and Doyen[12] in 1907 supplied the important improvement of a large indifferent 'ground' plate. By altering the design of the circuit, W. L. Clark[6] in 1910 obtained what proved microscopically to be tissue dehydration, and for this mild type of electrosurgery he proposed the term desiccation. Clark also added considerably to the power and quality of the instrument by installing multiple spark gaps in the place of the single gap then in vogue. Meanwhile Lee de Forest, in 1908, using his newly invented 3-electrode thermionic valve, had supplied the first radio tube high frequency apparatus capable of furnishing a cutting current, with which Neil and Steinberger, experimenting on dogs, 'made

fine, clean incisions with little bleeding.'[17] That this was not an isolated example of the use of electrosurgery in the role of the scalpel, is revealed by two reports issued in Europe in 1910[11,13] describing electrical methods of cutting tissue. Finally, the tuned frequency of the circuit was increased from the 500,000 cycles common to the diathermy apparatus, to the more effective 2,000,000 to 3,000,000 cycles of electrosurgery not, as Cushing[9] remarks, by Bovie in 1926, but by Doyen in 1907–1908.[12] Thus the essential features of electrosurgery as we know it today were all at hand by the end of the year 1910, including the choice between the multiple spark gap machine and the vacuum tube oscillator, the determination of the most suitable frequency, and a knowledge of the effect of electrical heating upon tissues, including the terms *fulguration, coagulation, desiccation* or *dehydration* and *cutting current*. It is true of course that one could scarcely thumb through a catalogue and order a 'Burdick' or a 'Bovie' but the experimentive surgeon of the day could and did find equipment builders who produced passable models for his use. It is a matter of record that electrosurgery was early extended from the lesions of the skin to internal surgical fields, being adapted to hemorrhoids in 1907,[7] the tumors of the bladder in 1910[4] and by its outstanding advocate, W. L. Clark,[6] to a large variety of applications, including the breast, cervix, tongue and throat, being found especially useful in the highly vascular structure of the angiomata.

"Thus it is scarcely creditable to neurosurgical acumen that it was not until 1926 that the accidental proximity of an electrophysicist working in a cancer hospital on one side of Van Dyke Street in Boston, and a pioneer neurosurgeon on the other, brought about the long awaited trial of electrosurgery in what was to be its most perfect application, hemostasis in the field of brain surgery. . . . "[18]

According to Dr. S. C. Harvey, in a letter to Dr. R. U. Light:

" 'John Morton and I were attending a session of the American Medical Association in Atlantic City in June, 1925 and were watching a demonstration of the use of a desiccating and cutting diathermy machine on a big block of beef. . . . Dr. Cushing came along, stopped to speak to us, and in a purely jocular fashion, one of us, I am not sure which, said, 'Here's something you ought to use on the brain!' Not that we had any idea it was applicable there, but I think with the mischievous purpose of stirring Cushing up at the thought of employing such a gross and disgusting procedure as was evidenced in the demonstration. We did not get the reaction we expected from him. He seemed rather thoughtful, and we separated after a time, with no further thought about the incident. He apparently returned to Boston, and being aware that they were trying out Clark's method of removing malignancies at the Huntington, established contact there. Bovie of course was the physicist, and was working at the time on improving the high frequency apparatus and was in the process of developing a better machine than had been manufactured before. It may have been that Cushing had this in the works before he went to Atlantic City, but he gave no evidence of it at the time, and I cite it as evidence—scarcely necessary—of his alertness and aggressiveness in picking up a new idea.' ''[18]

Fortunately, the efforts of Cushing and Bovie were successful and established the use of electrosurgery in neurosurgical operations. As a result, innumerable patients have been benefited since that time.

References

1. ADSON, A. W.   The evolution of neurosurgery. *Surgery*, 1949, *25*: 91–100.
2. D'ARSONVAL, A.   Action physiologique des courants alternatifs. *C. R. Soc. Biol. Paris*, 1891, *43*: 283–286.
3. BALLANCE, C.   The dawn and epic of neurology and surgery. *Glasgow: Jackson, Wylie & Co.*, 1930, 40 pp.
4. BEER, E.   Removal of neoplasms of the urinary bladder. A new method, employing high-frequency (Oudin) currents through a catheterizing cystoscope. *J. Amer. med. Ass.*, 1910, *54*: 1768–1769.
5. CALVERT, C. A.   The development of neurosurgery. *Ulster med. J.*, 1946, *15*: 123–140.
6. CLARK, W. L.   Oscillatory dessication in the treatment of accessible malignant growths and minor surgical conditions. A new electrical effect. *J. adv. Ther.*, 1911, *29*: 169–180.
7. COOK, F. R.   The high-frequency metallic discharge. A new treatment; its possibilities. *Med. Rec., N. Y.*, 1907, *72*: 1017–1020.
8. CUSHING, H.   Macewen Memorial Lecture on the meningiomas arising from the olfactory groove and their removal by the aid of electro-surgery. *Lancet*, 1927, *1*: 1329–1339.
9. CUSHING, H.   The meningiomas arising from the olfactory groove and their removal by the aid of electro-surgery. *Glasgow: Jackson, Wylie & Co.*, 1927, 53 pp.
10. CUSHING, H., AND BOVIE, W. T.   Electro-surgery as an aid to the removal of intracranial tumors. With a preliminary note on a new surgical-current generator. *Surg. Gynec. Obstet.*, 1928, *47*: 751–784.
11. CZERNY, V.   Ueber Operationen mit dem elek-
trischen Lichtbogen und Diathermie. *Dtsch. med. Wschr.*, 1910, *36*: 489–493.
12. DOYEN, E.   Surgical therapeutics and operative technique. H. Spencer-Browne, Transl. *New York: William Wood & Co.*, 1917, *1*: 439–452.
13. EITNER, E.   Ueber eine neue Art von Kaustik. *Wien. klin. Wschr.*, 1910, *23*: 168–169.
14. GREEN, R. E., AND STERN, W. E.   Techniques of cranial surgery. In: *A history of neurological surgery*. A. E. Walker, Ed. Baltimore: Williams & Wilkins Co., 1951, xii, 583 pp. (see pp. 40–76).
15. GURKOW, H. J.   The history of neurosurgery. *Marquette med. Rev.*, 1961, *27*: 49–54.
16. HORRAX, G.   Neurosurgery. An historical sketch. *Springfield, Ill.: Charles C Thomas*, 1952, xi, 135 pp. (see pp. 98–99).
17. KELLY, H. A., AND WARD, G. E.   Electrosurgery, *Philadelphia: W. B. Saunders Co.*, 1932, xxii, 305 pp. (see pp. 4–5).
18. LIGHT, R. U.   Hemostasis in neurosurgery. *J. Neurosurg.*, 1945, *2*: 414–434.
19. OLIVECRONA, H.   Neurosurgery, past and present. *Acta neurochir.*, 1951, *2*: 4–7.
20. RIVIÈRE, J. A.   Action des courants de haute fréquence et des effluves du résonnateur Oudin sur certaines tumeurs malignes et sur la tuberculose. *Gaz. Gynéc.*, 1900, *15*: 241–247.
21. SACHS, E.   The most important steps in the development of neurological surgery. *Yale J. Biol. Med.*, 1955–1956, *28*: 444–450.
22. SCARFF, J. E.   Fifty years of neurosurgery, 1905–1955. *Int. Abstr. Surg.*, 1955, *101*: 417–513 (see pp. 443–444).
23. SEHGAL, A. D.   History of neurological surgery. A brief review of the men and achievements which have contributed to the development of this expanding surgical specialty. *Med. Times, N. Y.*, 1962, *90*: 868–870.
24. VINCENT, C.   Chaire de neuro-chirurgie. Leçon inaugurale. *Pr. méd.*, 1939, *47*: 761–766.

ELECTRO-SURGERY AS AN AID TO THE REMOVAL OF INTRACRANIAL TUMORS*[1]

BY HARVEY CUSHING, M.D., F.A.C.S., BOSTON
WITH A PRELIMINARY NOTE ON A NEW
SURGICAL-CURRENT GENERATOR[2]
BY W. T. BOVIE, PH.D., CHICAGO

A NEW ELECTRO-SURGICAL UNIT (W. T. BOVIE)

THE apparatus here described has been developed with the idea of making instantly available to the surgeon the various kinds of currents which have proven most useful for his purposes, delivering them through a single lead

* Reprinted from *Surgery, Gynecology and Obstetrics*, 1928, *47*: 751–784, with the kind permission of the Editor.
[1] From the surgical clinic of the Peter Bent Brigham Hospital, Boston.
[2] From the Biophysical Laboratory of the Huntington Memorial Hospital for Cancer Research, Boston.

into operating instruments of practical design. No use is made of electrically heated cauteries, wires, or scalpels. The effects obtained depend entirely either upon the heat developed by the current in passing from the active electrode *into* the tissues, or upon the ohmic heat developed by the current in passing *through* the tissues.

As is well known, comparatively large amounts of an alternating current, if the frequency of the alternations is sufficiently high, can be passed through the tissues without producing any physiological effect other than that of heating. The amount of heat developed by a high-frequency current is proportional to the square of the current density.

In electro-surgery, a high current density is obtained by making the active ("operating") electrode small, whereas the inactive ("indifferent") electrode, through which the electrical circuit between the patient and machine is completed, is made large so that the current density in its immediate vicinity will be sufficiently low to permit the small amount of heat developed to be readily dissipated by the blood stream.

For certain purposes (biopsy) it is possible, as in the original procedure termed "fulguration," to dispense with the indifferent electrode entirely, no complete electrical circuit being made between the two terminals of the machine. Under such circumstances, the patient's body becomes charged and discharged with each alternation of the current; and with the high frequencies used, the amount of the current passing from the active electrode into and out of the tissues is sufficient to produce the desired effects.

This preliminary report is not a suitable place for a discussion of the characteristics of the various currents employed. The physical principles involved are complicated, since the currents used change their direction of flow from one to three million times per second and distribute themselves in the electrical circuits in a manner very different from that of steady currents or alternating currents of far lower frequency, such as those employed in a lighting circuit. Thus the simple relations between voltage and amperage which hold for steady currents and for alternating currents of lower frequency are upset by what the physicist terms phase shifts. Our purpose will be better served if, instead of giving a description of the physical characteristics of the currents, we catalogue such characteristics in terms of the effects which they produce in the tissues.

There are three distinct ways in which the various high-frequency currents delivered by the Unit are used in electro-surgery: (1) *superficial dehydration;* (2) *cutting;* (3) *tissue coagulation.*

1. For *superficial dehydration* the active electrode is held, not in actual contact with, but sufficiently close to, the tissues to be dehydrated, so that sparks are sprayed across the intervening space. The very high temperature of the sparks is sufficient completely to dehydrate a thin outer layer of tissue.

2. For *cutting purposes,* the active electrode is energized by a different type of current. The cutting is not done by the electrode, which has no sharpened edge, but actually by the current which forms ahead of the electrode an electrical arc which by volatilizing the tissues separates them as though they were cut. Further, by a suitable modification (variable amount of damping) of the same current a greater or a lesser degree of coagulation or dehydration may be produced at will at the edges of the severed tissues. When the tissues are not particularly vascular the current is so modified as to produce the minimum amount of dehydration, but when the blood supply is greater the amount of dehydration is correspondingly increased.

The apparatus is provided with control switches so that the active electrode can be instantly energized with the particular kind of cutting current which the surgeon requires; for sometimes he wishes a strong current to make deep incisions rapidly, at others weaker currents, by which delicate bloodless dissections may be carried out.

3. For *heating the tissues en masse* (the so-called electro-coagulation), the kind of current used differs widely from that employed for cutting. An electrode energized with coagulating currents instead of having cutting properties cannot be moved through the tissues. The tissues surrounding the electrode become heated to a depth depending on two factors, the density of the current and the length of time it is permitted to flow. If a large tissue mass is to be coagulated, a comparatively weak current must be used for a prolonged period, until it becomes heated throughout. For should a stronger current be used the tissues in the immediate vicinity of the active electrode would become so quickly dehydrated or even carbonized that the current would cease to flow and the deeper tissues would not be affected. If, on the other hand, a small tissue mass is to be coagulated, one uses a strong current for a brief length of time, so that surrounding tissues are not affected.

It has been sufficiently emphasized in the foregoing paragraphs that the usefulness of this electro-surgical unit lies in the possibility it offers of varying at will the character of the cutting current so as to secure different degrees of dehydration.

The apparatus. The usual electro-surgical apparatus is provided with a foot-control for turning on and off the current. But since it has been found in practice that a foot-control limits the surgeon too much to one position, a convenient hand-control has been added. This not only gives the surgeon increased freedom of movement but greatly facilitates his co-ordination.

Because of its shape, the hand-control has become known about the laboratory and hospital as the "pistol grip." It consists of a special handle designed to hold the operating electrode, the current being under the control of the surgeon's index finger which presses a small trigger. A number of operating electrodes have been constructed for special purposes, all of them interchangeable in the pistol grip. For obvious reasons, such accessories as retractors, and so on, which the surgeon needs to employ in the operating field, should be constructed out of insulating materials.

NEUROSURGICAL EXPERIENCES WITH THE BOVIE UNIT (HARVEY CUSHING)

The surgery of intracranial tumors has grown from its small and unsatisfactory beginnings to a specialty of unquestioned importance. Tumors of the brain of one sort or another are extremely common, and as experience accumulates they are coming to be treated with increasingly favorable results. Such notable progress indeed has been made in recent years that the dismal attitude regarding these operations, widely held at the turn of the century, has gradually been replaced by one of comparative confidence and optimism.

This transformation has come about through the contributions of many. An improvement in the operative procedures which would serve to prevent herniations and the dreaded fungus cerebri of the early days was the first necessary step to be taken. A better understanding of the cerebrospinal fluid circulation in its relation to intracranial tension and to choked disc soon led to the establishment of the principles of decompression. Without serious secondary complications, the surgeon could at least make openings in the cranium usually with alleviation of suffering and oftentimes with preservation of vision. There soon followed a vast improvement in methods of tumor localization; and on the heels of this has come a rapid increase in our knowledge of the histopathology of the lesions themselves.

In consequence of this notable progress in three directions—*a more refined technique, more precise methods of localization, a better understanding of tumor histogenesis*—we begin to have some clear ideas of the natural history of tumors of particular types as they arise in their favored situations. Those who have a live interest in the subject accordingly are beginning to think and to write in terms of particular tumors and their behavior, rather than of tumors in general and their pressure effects as measured by the old-time cardinal symptoms of headache, vomiting, and choked disc.

As the outcome of all this, what now chiefly concerns us is the ability more often to foretell not only the locus but the probable nature of the growth before its exposure; for this foreknowledge will not only be an aid to prognosis but will modify our preparations to meet the particular hazards of the task that lies ahead. Since the methods of getting in and of getting out of the cranial chamber have become more or less standardized, it is oftentimes easier to expose a tumor than to know just what to do with it when brought to view. The appropriate treatment will depend, of course, upon many factors which will often put the skill and judgment of the surgeon to a severe test; but the ideal is extirpation of the lesion in one session if possible, and in accomplishing this no technical element is more important than the control of bleeding.

So far as I am aware, the principles of electrosurgery have heretofore not been utilized in cranio-cerebral operations. Three or four years ago, with a form of diathermy apparatus then on the market, I essayed to make incisions in the brain with an electrified needle, but either from lack of experience or lack of imagination I did not see how for cutting or hæmostasis the novelty could possibly supersede the more familiar methods in general use. Not until the autumn of 1926, when, in the Huntington Hospital nearby, I happened to see Dr. Bovie's electrified wire loop being used for the purpose of bloodlessly scooping out bits of malignant tissue for examination, did I realize that here was a new tool which might possibly be utilized for the piecemeal removal of some of the more inaccessible intracranial tumors.

The results have exceeded all expectation and the methods of brain tumor extirpation have been so largely revolutionized by these new principles that a report of some of our experiences seems to be called for even though improvements and alterations in the apparatus and in our understanding of its possibilities are being so rapidly made that the developments of tomorrow can hardly be foreseen.

The surgeon, however, need not be expected to know the full details of the electro-thermic principles which are involved, though it behooves him to have some familiarity with them if he is to do more than merely run the machine. One may learn to pilot a motor-driven vehicle without necessarily knowing the principles of the internal combustion engine, but it will add to his efficiency in emergencies if he does so.

Our initial experience with the current-generator and its wire-loop electrode may appropriately serve as a starting point for this paper. The question involved was merely one of its possible aid as a hæmostatic agent in a case in which we had gotten into trouble just two years ago this October.

The patient (Surgical No. 27271), a paper maker, aged 64, entered the hospital *September 23, 1926*, with a history of having first noticed a swelling on the right side of his head five months previously when he was recovering from a severe attack of pneumonia. The lesion slowly enlarged until it reached a large size (Fig. 1). It was painless, had a increased surface temperature and was soft, almost fluctuant, in consistency. The X-ray showed that the bone underlying the tumor was highly vascularized and defective. Various diagnoses were made, such as a cyst, a chronic osteomyelitic abscess, a cholesteatoma, a meningioma, a syphiloma, and a melanoma, but a rapidly growing sarcoma was favored. The physical and neurological examination apart from the visible tumor was negative. No primary lesion was detected in lungs, prostate, or kidneys.

On *September 28*, the tense scalp with some difficulty was reflected from over the surface of the tumor. An attempt to remove the extracranial portion of the growth by scraping it away from the roughened and highly vascularized bone led to excessive bleeding which was finally got under control by the implantation of muscle and of cotton pledgets wet in Zenker's fluid. Though the patient's condition became precarious from loss of blood, enough of the growth was finally removed to permit the reflected scalp to be replaced and closed. The pulsations of the brain were transmitted to the raw base of the tumor in the pathological bone defect, and it was the operator's impression that he was dealing with a malignant type of meningioma.

On *October 1*, Dr. Bovie came to our rescue and, with a damped dehydrating current, the remaining extracranial portion of the growth was removed with surprising ease by the loop-electrode and the bleeding points checked by coagulation. The large area of the skull invaded by the tumor was then encircled by a series of performations which were connected up by Montenovesi forceps. Bleeding was profuse and a transfusion was necessary. The flap was again closed without drainage.

On *October 11*, at a third-stage operation, the scalp

was again reflected and the entire block of involved bone together with the adherent dura measuring about 10 by 8 centimeters in circumference was removed (Fig. 2), bleeding from the dural margins being easily controlled by the application of clips and by coagulation.

The *pathological diagnosis* was a myeloma of plasma-cell type. Subsequent X-ray study of the entire skeleton failed to reveal other foci of disease.

The patient made an excellent recovery from the operation (Figs. 3 and 4) and showed no evidence of local recurrence four months later when, according to report, he died of an acute nephritis. There was no postmortem examination.

It may have been an error in judgment to have undertaken this operation, but the diagnosis was uncertain and with the procedure once started there was no backing out. The operation could in all probability have been completed in a single sitting had we known as much then as we do today of electro-surgical methods of attacking a lesion of this type; but as things stood two years ago we were fortunate enough to get safely through the critical second session without a fatality. During the course of this second operation the raw central surface of the tumor had been thoroughly coagulated, and it was a matter of great satisfaction to find at the final session ten days later that there had been no unusual reactions from the large area of superficially charred tissue that had been so long buried.

Shortly after this another patient, a twelve year old child with a midline extracranial tumor of similar sort (Fig. 5) entered the clinic. The preoperative diagnosis in this case also was uncertain. The extracranial lesion in spite of its vascularity was without difficulty cleanly removed in a single session, and what might otherwise have been a serious operation proved to be a simple matter. Healing was reactionless (Fig. 6). The growth, unfortunately, was a metastatic sympathicoblastoma, and the child had begun to show evidence of a spinal metastasis by the time of her hospital discharge.

Encouraged by the technical success of these operations, we began step by step with Dr. Bovie's moral support to engage in the more serious business of attacking tumors that lay wholly within the cranial chamber. We were, of course, dealing with a novel procedure and were utterly ignorant of the immediate physiological or remote pathological effects that might be produced by electrical dehydration or charring of the nervous tissues.[3]

[3] It may not be out of place for the writer to express here the great obligation he is under not only to Dr. Bovie for his sacrifice of time in personally attending a great number of the many prolonged operative sessions during the first six months of our use of the apparatus which he had assembled but also to the officials of the Huntington Hospital who, until Mr. G. H. Liebel of the Liebel-Flarsheim Company of Cincinnati kindly pro-

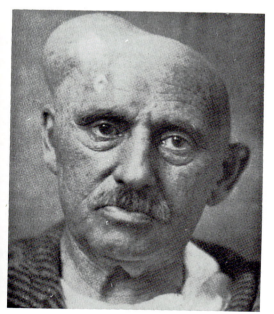

Fig. 1. Case 1. Rapidly growing tumor of skull (myeloma) before operation.

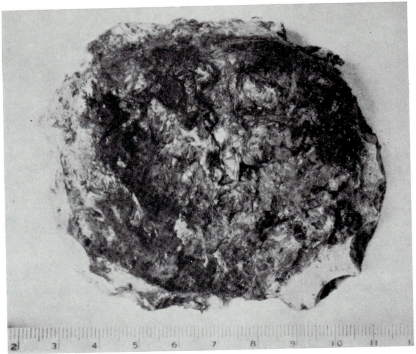

Fig. 2. Case 1. External surface of remaining block of tumor with encircling bone removed with subjacent dura at the third session.

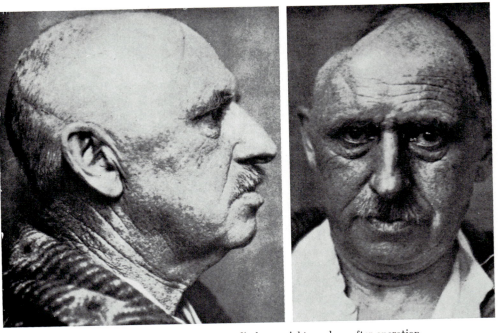

Figs. 3–4. Case 1. The patient on discharge eighteen days after operation.

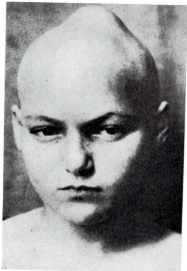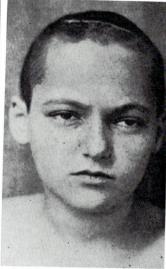

Figs. 5–6. Sympathico-blastoma before and after its electro-surgical removal. Pre-operative
diagnosis meningioma, sarcoma, or myeloma.

Many shifts and adjustments from our customary methods of procedure were found to be necessary, but we fortunately avoided any serious accidents other than an occasional infection which crept in to mar our generally irreproachable wound healing. These few infections were due, as we have since learned, to faulty technique rather than to any lowering of the resistance of the tissues to which we at first were inclined to ascribe them.

The whole question of the anæsthetic had to be carefully reviewed, for though most intracranial operations today are carried through under local anæsthesia, a supplementary inhalation narcosis may sometimes be necessary if the patient is mentally unco-operative or made physically uncomfortable. On certain occasions in the course of prolonged operations, the body became so heavily

charged that the anæsthetist on accidentally touching the patient's face could get a spark, which might well enough have caused an ether explosion under the hood. Only once, however, did anything of this sort occur. It was a case in which a small opening had been made into the frontal sinus in the course of a transfrontal osteoplastic operation. This led to a direct communication between the respiratory passages and the field of operation; and suddenly the ether vapor was sparked and went off in a blue flame, fortunately without any injurious effects. The experience, however, was sufficiently disconcerting to lead us for a time to substitute for inhalation narcosis the rectal administration of ether to tide patients, when necessary, over the more uncomfortable period of a prolonged session.

Other difficulties experienced at the outset were due to the fact that epileptiform attacks were occasionally produced (cf. Case 6) when the electrode was used to check bleeding from the surface of the dura. For though these high alternating currents are not supposed to have any stimulating effects on irritable tissues, apparently under certain circumstances they could become so diffused from the point of discharge that their "overtones" were capable of producing physiological responses; and a Jacksonian fit or a convulsion in the course of an operation when the dura is open may lead to serious consequences.

We were also troubled at the beginning by the tendency of the current to become grounded through the table, through the metal retractors, and so on. Once the operator received a shock which passed through a metal retractor to his arm

---

vided us with our own machine a year later, uncomplainingly permitted their apparatus to be daily transported on loan to the Brigham Hospital at what inconvenience to their own operating schedule can well be imagined.

In his all-too-brief introductory note, Dr. Bovie fails to say that he was led to take an interest in the subject purely on account of the biophysical principles involved in getting an answer to the question of why an alternating current of one type can separate the tissues as though they were actually cut, while another will merely coagulate them and cannot be used for cutting. The original apparatus was assembled with Mr. Liebel's collaboration solely out of interest in the electrical problems raised in its construction and with no expectation that it would ever be marketable. If the mention of the manufacturer's name should prove in the nature of an advertisement, it is no less deserved than it is unsolicited.

and out by the wire from his headlight, which was unpleasant to say the least. On another occasion (Case 4), owing to the improper application of the indifferent electrode during a prolonged operation, a second-degree electrical burn was produced which was slow to heal. Some of these complications were due to inexperience; some of them lay at the door of the apparatus itself, and we were temporarily forced to employ a wooden table, wooden spatulae and so on; but one by one the difficulties have been wholly eliminated by progressive modifications in the design of the current generator. Further improvements will unquestionably follow, but as things now stand those who come to use the apparatus will be spared from much that we have gone through and will find it possible without risk to utilize their ordinary operating table equipment and customary methods of procedure.

During this two years' period, we have with growing confidence come to utilize electro-surgical methods for increasingly difficult surgical problems and have even sent for old patients who have either been refused operation in the past or whose tumors on exposure have been regarded as inoperable. In all of this we have undoubtedly increased our operative mortality, for the sense of security due to the vast improvement in the technique of hæmostasis, which electro-surgery makes possible, has led us into undertakings that would have been foolhardy to say the least in other days.

By no means does the introduction of this adjunct to cranio-cerebral surgery mean the entire abandonment of the established principles of osteoplastic intracranial procedures. It is chiefly revolutionary in that it enables the surgeon to excavate the central portion of many tumors, particularly those that are encapsulated, with greatly lessened bleeding so that the growth may be collapsed and its shell more safely and with less contusion than formerly be brushed away from the enveloping brain. This is no new principle, to be sure, for it has been long applied in the intracapsular attack on the tumors of the cerebellopontile angle that arise from the *Nervus acusticus*. But it has been far less commonly utilized for the removal of other tumors, it having been the surgeon's ideal to remove the growth, when possible, intact rather than in separate fragments owing to the risk of inoculation of the field by tumor cells which the piecemeal method favors. But when the electrical loop is used for the purpose, the risk of sowing viable cells is negligible.

These principles of primary intracapsular enucleation by electrical methods apply more obviously to the treatment of the meningeal tumors which were among the first to be successfully, though in the beginning somewhat crudely, attacked. They consequently deserve primary consideration, and the case reports may well be restricted to our experiences in the spring of 1927 as they are more likely to illustrate technical errors and accidents that have since come to be largely avoided.[4]

The Meningiomas. From the standpoint of their relative benignity, these of all intracranial tumors are regarded as the most favorable for operation. However, they often attain a huge size before they are recognized; their environment is apt to be excessively vascular; their attachment to one or another of the large dural sinuses supplies an element of especial danger, and if the area of attachment is not removed a recurrence is inevitable; they often arise in inaccessible regions of the base of the brain, and even when more favorably situated their removal intact is likely to be followed by cerebral œdema and by circulatory disturbances on the part of the cerebrospinal fluid that delay convalescence. Hence, they are possibly in the long run the most difficult of all tumors safely to attack and completely to remove without secondary complications.

Fortunately, however, the most serious of all postoperative complications, namely a wound infection with secondary meningitis, has long been wholly eliminated; and consequently when a fatality from an infection followed the prolonged use of the current in our first serious case, we were greatly disheartened even though there were extenuating circumstances. The tumor which had been unsuspected was an extremely large and fibrous one which arose from the angle of falx and tentorium; the operation was long drawn out; there were strangers unfamiliar with the fastidious ritual of the operating room who were running the apparatus that had been borrowed in the emergency; and there may possibly have been some slip in the proper sterilization of the pistol and electrodes that came to be handled by the operating team. At the same time there was an equal possibility that the electro-thermic effects of the current might have so lowered the resistance of the tissues, ordinarily capable of combating a mild infection, as to have been responsible for the patient's death from meningitis nine days later.

As chance would have it, soon after this disheartening experience with the primary excavation of a meningioma in the manner mentioned, two patients entered the hospital at almost the same time, each of them with a large subfrontal tumor originating from the meninges of the olfac-

---

[4] The mere description on paper of the elaborate ceremony incidental to the safe extirpation of a brain tumor under any circumstances falls far short of the actual performance; and when a description of the novel electro-surgical methods of dehydrating and coagulating the tissues of the central nervous system is called for in addition, one despairs of doing justice to the subject.

tory groove. The account of the operation on the first of these patients (Surgical No. 28026) was made the basis of the Macewen Lecture[5] some five months later and the report of the other may serve our purpose here to illustrate the method of procedure.

CASE 2. The patient (Surgical No. 28046) was a married Jewess 36 years of age who had a fairly typical olfactory groove syndrome. Following an injury five years before her admission she began to appreciate a diminution in the sense of smell which soon became wholly lost. Of late she had been having curious attacks of numbness and stiffness in the left side of the face suggestively Jacksonian in character. There was evidence of loss of memory, and her relatives were aware of dispositional changes.

Objectively there was nothing to show except a complete anosmia and bilateral papillœdema of low grade. A slight enlargement with erosion of the sella turcica and a minute area of calcification to the left of the midline just above the olfactory groove slightly back of the crista galli were apparent on the stereoscopic roentgenograms.

On *February 15, 1927* under novocain anæsthesia the usual right frontal osteoplastic flap was reflected to the side laying bare an extremely tense dura. An unsuccessful attempt was made to empty the ventricle, the puncture needle encountering a large resistant tumor in the depths. The tension was so great that it was impossible to elevate the frontal dura from the orbital plate in

[5] Cushing, H. The meningiomas arising from the olfactory groove and their removal by the aid of electrosurgery. University of Glasgow Publications IX, 53 pp. Extract in Lancet, June 25, 1927, 1329–1339.

order to get to the base of the tumor before we opened the membrane. The patient was therefore given an intravenous injection of hypertonic saline which promptly reduced tension sufficiently to permit the dura to be incised along the sphenoidal ridge, which was found to be in an advanced stage of pressure absorption.

The under surface of the frontal lobe was then elevated and brushed away from the growth until its lower edge was well enough exposed so that "scallops"[6] of the tissue could be scooped out with the electrified loop. A sufficiently deep furrow was thus made to let the spatula-elevator be inserted under its upper edge so as to overcome the tendency of the tense brain to extrude into the wound (Fig. 7, I). The growth was then excavated still further until the shell of that portion which lay to the right of the falx could be collapsed and withdrawn in the manner shown (Fig. 7, III, IV).

The only period of real anxiety in this tedious performance was caused by a sharp arterial hæmorrhage which followed the dislodgment of the posterior nodule of the growth which overlay the pituitary fossa. Because of the great depth of the cavity and the anatomical distortion of the structures, it was difficult to tell what vessel may have been injured, but it presumably was the anterior cerebral. The vessel was allowed to bleed into the sucker and, after two or three unavailing attempts to pick it up by silver clips, it was caught between the blades of dissecting forceps and by good fortune successfully coagulated by passing the current along the instrument. In the flurry of this procedure it was greatly feared that the chiasm might have been contused or 'cooked' by the current, but on clearing away the clot

[6] For want of better terms, the peculiar worm-like strips of tissue that are scooped out by the loop may be called "scallops" and the procedure "scalloping."

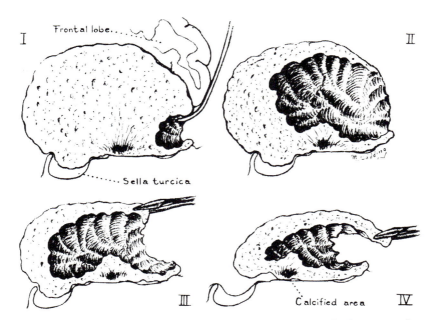

Fig. 7. Case 2. From surgeon's postoperative sketches indicating the steps in the process of excavating a large olfactory groove meningioma and of withdrawing its shell. (Reduced ⅓.)

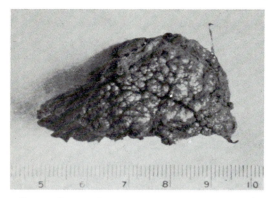

Fig. 8. Case 2. Last fragment of tumor to be dislodged from left frontal lobe and withdrawn from under divided falx. Note characteristic nodular surface of a basilar meningioma in this situation.

the compressed chiasm and nerves could be seen cleanly exposed and apparently uninjured.

The process of removing this right-sided half of the tumor had permitted fluid in large amounts to escape from the meninges in the exposed right Sylvian region so that tension had become wholly reduced. It was, therefore, possible more easily to expose and to attack the equally large mass of tumor to the left of the falx which was freely excavated with the loop after first removing the crista galli and making a cross section of the falx. Finally the remaining shell of this half of the tumor which contained the calcified area was freed from the left olfactory groove, dislocated out of its pocket, and drawn out from under the falx in one piece (Fig. 8). As a last step, the site of the dural attachment of the growth

along each olfactory groove was dehydrated by brushing it with the electrode with the purpose of destroying so far as possible any remaining nests of cells. The flap was replaced without drainage.

From this five-hour operation, during the last stages of which ether had been necessitated, the patient made a perfect recovery. There was no evidence of injury to any of the exposed nervous structures apart from a temporary diplopia due to a third nerve palsy on the right side (Fig. 9), which had probably been produced in the process of checking the bleeding vessel. Vision remained unimpaired. She has recently been examined (*February 15, 1928*) and except for her residual anosmia she remains symptom-free (Fig. 10).

The charred fragments of the tumor which were collected and saved, possibly representing not more than half of the growth, weighed 35.5 grams (Fig. 11).

The outcome of this operation was more satisfactory than in the similar case described in the Macewen Lecture, for normal vision has been preserved. But the brilliant results in these two cases were soon offset by two other unsuccessful operations in one of which we were wholly baffled, from inexperience, by uncontrollable bleeding, and in the other by an indolent wound infection which ultimately proved fatal. In both instances, though the tumors had reached a large size with marked mental changes and near blindness, the diagnosis of an olfactory groove meningioma was unmistakable. The first of the cases, in which bleeding got beyond our control, follows:

CASE 3. A young man (Surgical No. 28338), 32 years of age, sustained contusions in an automobile accident in *1918*, six years before his hospital admission. To this

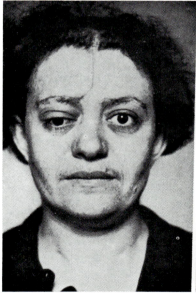
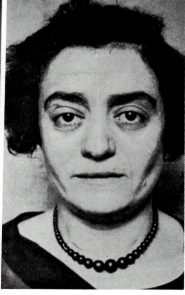

Figs. 9–10. Case 2. (Left) Photograph of the patient on her discharge showing the inconspicuous scar and the slight residual palsy of the right third nerve which had been contused during dislodgment of the posterior fragments of the growth. (Right) Photograph a year later, to show recovery of the third nerve palsy and invisible scar.

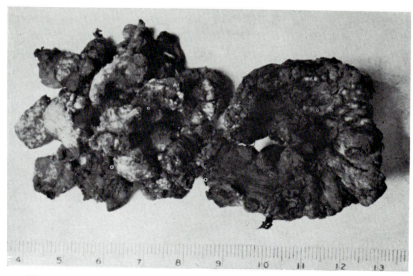

Fig. 11. Case 2. Photograph of such fragments of the tumor as were preserved. The large, partly excavated block of the growth shown on the right lay wholly to the left of the falx and was the last fragment to be dislodged. (cf. Fig. 8.)

were attributed the symptoms of an unmistakable left olfactory groove tumor, which in the course of time had begun seriously to affect vision.

He was first operated upon *October 10, 1924*, when the lower anterior margin of the tumor was exposed but its unusual vascularity prevented more than a fragmentary removal of tissue for verification. As a result of the decompression he did extremely well for nearly two years when pressure symptoms began to reappear. Consequently on *July 2, 1926*, a second operation was undertaken and a larger portion of the growth was removed than at the first session, but the operation again had to be abandoned owing to excessive bleeding from the surface of the excavation.

The case was given up as surgically hopeless and recourse was had to radiation which accomplished nothing. Mental symptoms became progressively more pronounced during the succeeding 8 months, and on the bare chance that the lesion might be amenable to electrosurgical methods it was again attacked on *March 8, 1927*. At this time in the course of a nine-hour operation wholly under local anæsthesia the chief mass of the growth to the left of the falx was thoroughly scalloped, but interstitial bleeding in the depths became increasingly difficult to control and withdrawal with a transfusion was necessary. On the following day we were forced by undue bulging of the flap to re-elevate it and to remove by suction a sufficient amount of the infiltrated and dislodged growth to restore normal tension; but bleeding was started afresh and in spite of another transfusion he succumbed some 12 hours later.

At autopsy it was found that only the left half of the large growth had been in large part removed. The median section of the brain shows (Fig. 12) the dimensions which one of these tumor growths may attain.

Our experience with electro-surgical methods was wholly insufficient at the time to enable us to deal with such a highly vascular and formidable

lesion. Bleeding was, if anything, accelerated rather than checked when the attempt was made to coagulate the raw surface after removal of each scallop of tissue, for the growth was soft and the charred surface tended to cling to and come away with the electrode.

The growth nevertheless might possibly have been removed without undue difficulty in 1924 when it was first exposed had it been approached from the right rather than the left side, had we uncovered the tumor more fully by removing the overhanging shelf of the frontal lobe, and had we known at the time that the vascularity of such a lesion could be reduced by the slow process of surface coagulation before its piecemeal extirpation was begun.

The story of the other olfactory groove tumor, in which a postoperative fatality from infection occurred is briefly as follows:

CASE 4. The patient (Surgical No. 28344) was an obese Jewess, 56 years of age, who had been practically blind from primary optic atrophy for two years, and who had complete anosmia and advanced mental changes. The X-ray showed the telltale spot of calcification in the stalk of the tumor over the olfactory groove.

At the operation on *March 26, 1927*, a huge growth much larger than expected was disclosed by the usual transfrontal procedure. The lesion was excavated with the electrified loop in much the same piecemeal fashion (Fig. 13) described in the operative note on Case 2. In this process the frontal horn of the ventricle was opened, and though this was unintentional the escape of fluid gave an abundance of room in which to work. The growth finally, so far as could be told, was removed in its entirety, the depressed chiasm and flattened optic tracts being left fully exposed. The patient, though in

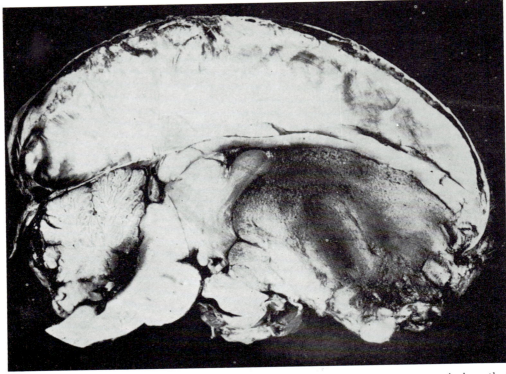

Fig. 12. Case 3. To show, on median section, a large symmetrically placed olfactory groove meningioma the left half of which had been attacked by electro-surgical methods which proved ineffective from the excessive vascularity of the lesion.

good condition at the conclusion of the prolonged eight-hour procedure, the last part of which had required a general anæsthetic, was transfused with 250 cubic centimeters of blood.

She made an excellent immediate recovery, but unhappily the convalescence was complicated not only by a temporary diabetes insipidus but by *an extensive electrical burn over the abdomen* where the negative electrode had been insecurely applied. There was also a superficial wound infection in which a cerebrospinal fluid leak ere long developed. This leak persisted for some seven weeks during which time the patient remained in fairly good condition but on its spontaneous closure she rapidly went down hill and finally died two months after the operation. The autopsy showed a suppurative staphylococcus ependymitis. No residual of the tumor was to be found (Fig. 14).

The lesion in this case was a large, symmetrically placed meningioma estimated at *circa* 70 grams (the collected fragments weighed 51 grams), but it fortunately was not particularly vascular. The prolonged session was due largely to apprehension lest damage be done to the vessels and chiasm enveloping the tumor in the depths of the wound. The infection was unquestionably attributable to some slip in technique during the unduly long exposure of the open wound rather than to the secondary effects of tissue coagulation to which we at the time were inclined to ascribe it.

These four cases represent, then, our first essays to attack the large olfactory groove lesions which have been ordinarily regarded as inoperable, though many surgeons have, of course, exposed them at operation and have removed them in part. We have since had six other wholly successful operations of the same kind, some of them with total removal of tumors as large as the last described. They, however, add nothing more from an electro-surgical standpoint to the records given above, apart from the fact that the operations, owing to accumulated confidence, were much less time-consuming, some of the more recent cases having been conducted throughout under local anæsthesia.

The discouragement produced by these two fatal operations for olfactory groove tumors recorded above had meanwhile been offset by the more favorable outcome of operations for large meningiomas in other situations less difficult of approach. One of them was a subtentorial lesion that had once been given up as inoperable as will be told:

CASE 5. The patient (Surgical No. 28262), was a woman 46 years of age whose symptoms suggesting a cerebellar tumor had begun in 1920. In 1922 a subtem-

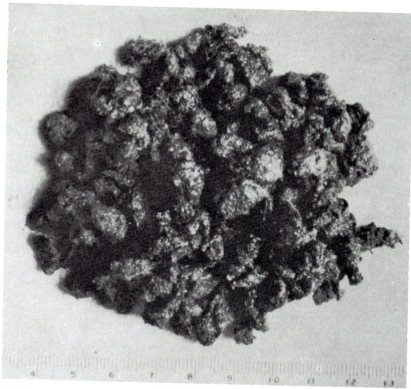

Fig. 13. Case 4. The collected fragments (scallops) of a symmetrically placed olfactory groove meningioma removed at a single session with ultimate fatality from infection.

poral decompression had been made by a surgeon in Montreal. This relieved her headaches for a time but on their return a year later she was referred to the Brigham Hospital where one of my assistants explored the cerebellum and exposed what was thought to be a large, inoperable glioma.

She made an excellent recovery and was free from further symptoms of any serious import for the next four years when headaches began to return and cerebellar ataxia gradually became so pronounced she could not freely get about. A fragment of the tumor removed at the operation for histological examination had meanwhile been shown to be an actively growing meningioma. In the belief that the growth might be favorable for removal by electro-surgical methods she was encouraged to return and on *February 23, 1927*, the cerebellum was again exposed and under local anæsthesia a *circa* 60-gram meningioma, which almost filled the posterior fossa and had its main attachment to the lateral sinus and lower surface of the tentorium as far forward as the incisura, was successfully extirpated piecemeal in its entirety by the process of scalloping with the electrified loop (Figs. 15 and 16). The wound as usual was closed securely in layers without drainage of the huge cavity. Recovery was uneventful and healing perfect (Figs. 17 and 18) in spite of the temporary tendency of the cavity to fill with xanthochromic fluid which made an occasional postoperative puncture necessary.

Another case of precisely this same sort, in which an exceedingly dense fibroblastic meningioma had been once exposed and abandoned as inoperable, has since been similarly and successfully operated upon, the patient who was doing well enough as the result of the decompression having been induced nevertheless to return for another trial.

We may now pass to another far more accessible type of meningioma but one nevertheless whose very exposure may prove to be attended with exceptional risks. Possibly none of these tumors are more difficult safely to uncover than those which take their origin from the meninges at the outer end of the sphenoidal ridge near the pterion where the middle meningeal vessels groove or perforate the lower corner of the parietal bone. The region may be excessively vascular and even the preliminary ligation of the external carotid has little influence on the bleeding that may be set going. Moreover, there are apt to be cranial endostoses that project into the core of the tumor and should these be torn out when the flap is elevated, the bleeding may at times be most difficult to get under control.

A good example of such a tumor that had progressed to a fatal issue without surgical intervention is the famous case so often referred to in the

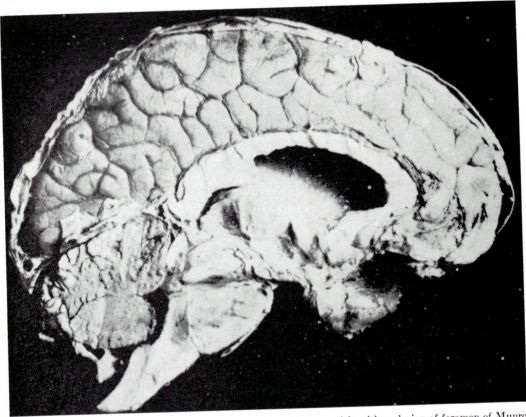

Fig. 14. Case 4. Median section of the brain showing dilated left ventricle with occlusion of foramen of Munro from suppurative ependymitis. No trace of tumor found. For comparison with Figure 12.

writings of Byrom Bramwell (Fig. 19). We have had a number of typical examples of these tumors in our series, some of them successfully enucleated in successive sessions, but I had particular reason for being gun-shy of them, having had the shocking experience a little more than two years ago of losing a colleague, a young Boston physician who had died on the operating table from the loss of blood caused by the mere reflection of the ragged and tumor-involved bone flap which adhered to the vascular surface of the tumor. While this harrowing episode was still vividly in mind, the patient whose history follows entered the clinic.

CASE 6. A married woman (Surgical No. 28364), 44 years of age, had the classical symptoms and signs of a low left Sylvian fissure meningioma associated with contralateral Jacksonian seizures beginning in the face. There was aphasia with slight right facial palsy and a right homonymous hemianopsia. The X-ray showed the typical endostosis projecting into the stalk of the tumor at the outer end of the sphenoidal ridge with enormous environmental diploetic sinuses and deepened meningeal channels.

Preparations were made for a critical operation with a donor prepared for transfusion and masses of pectoral

muscle secured from a breast amputation scheduled for the same hour.

On *March 18, 1927,* under local anæsthesia, a left osteoplastic flap was outlined with some difficulty, and when elevated it broke off only partly exposing the highly vascular dura over the tumor. Bleeding was excessive in spite of pressure and the abundant implantation of muscle which was at hand. Since these measures were insufficiently effective, they were abandoned and with the field kept reasonably dry with the sucker, the effort was made to coagulate the dural vessels. This had the desired effect on the bleeding but *the current caused a severe convulsion* beginning in the right face and necessitating the inhalation of ether for its control. After some delay and after consciousness had been regained, *a second convulsion was produced by the further coagulation of the meningeal vessels,* and from this time the patient was kept under ether. The remainder of the tumor-involved bone overlying the core of the lesion and extending down into the sphenoidal ridge was then removed piecemeal, each bite of the rongeurs being followed by sharp bleeding fortunately controllable by coagulation. Finally the subtemporal area of involved dura was fully uncovered.

The patient's blood presssure by this time had fallen off markedly, and preparations were made for refusion of the collected blood. Meanwhile with the purpose of

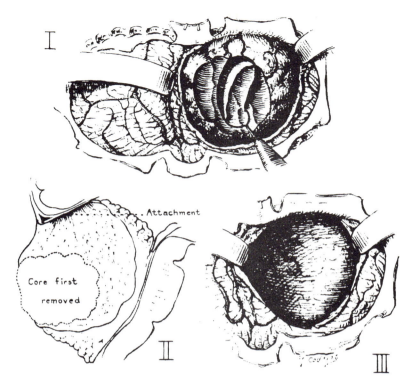

Fig. 15. Case 5. From the immediate postoperative sketches, to give an idea of situation and extent of the lesion. *I* Shows tumor in process of scalloping; *II*, partial excavation before forced collapse of shell; *III*, cavity after final extirpation.

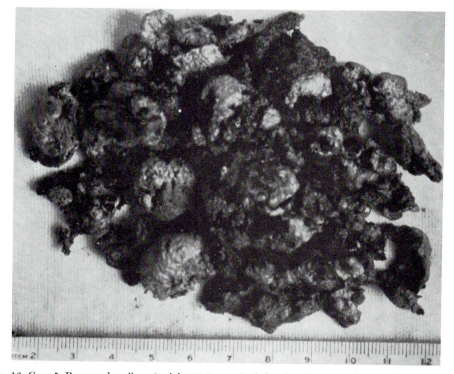

Fig. 16. Case 5. Preserved scallops (weight 50.5 grams) of the *circa* 60-gram subtentorial meningioma.

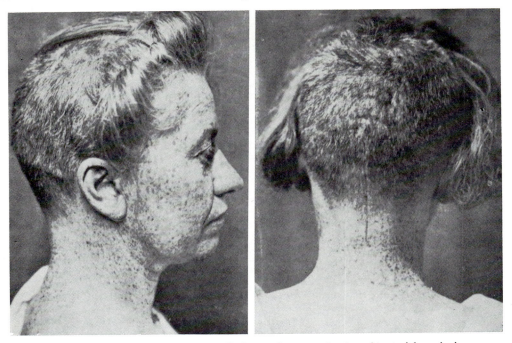

Figs. 17–18. Case 5. The patient on her discharge after operation for subtentorial meningioma,
to show inconspicuous scar of the usual cross bow incision.

getting some idea of the surface extent of the lesion, in anticipation of the probable necessity of a second-stage performance, one or two small incisions were made through the dura supposedly beyond the periphery of the lesion. On each occasion, soft tumor rather than brain was exposed, for the growth proved to be unexpectedly large, fully ten centimeters in its surface diameter. The idea of encircling the area of adherent dura with the intent of allowing the lesion to extrude between two operative periods was therefore abandoned.

The attempted transfusion had been a failure, from inability to get into a sufficiently large vein, but as the pressures by this time had begun spontaneously to return, the chance was taken of at least starting with an intracapsular enucleation. Accordingly, with the desiccating current the dura was incised directly into the heart of the tumor from which generous scallops of tissue were successively scooped out with the electrified loop. The center of the lesion fortunately proved to be of low vascularity, and the excavation was carried sufficiently

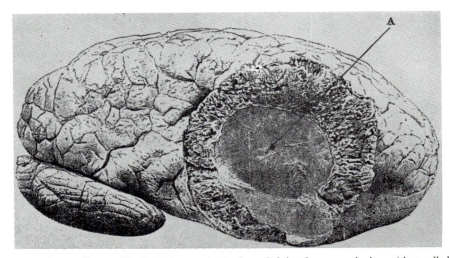

Fig. 19. Byrom Bramwell's classical example of a large Sylvian fissure meningioma (then called sarcoma) found at autopsy. A points to the center of the adherent disc of dura mater.

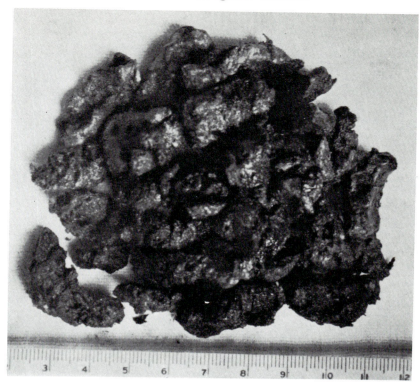

Fig. 20. Case 6. The clustered scallops so far as they were preserved that were excavated from the heart of the tumor (cf. Fig. 21) before its collapse permitted removal (weight 58.5 grams).

far to permit of the partial collapse of its shell.

The growth was then encircled by an incision through the intact outlying dura. The chief difficulty lay in getting a free dural margin in the deeper, more vascular and more inaccessible sphenoidal region without further loss of blood which the patient could hardly have stood. But this difficulty was overcome by making the division of the membrane between a succession of curved clamps and by sealing the severed margins with the current passed along the clamps before their removal.

The shell of the growth, thus freed, began promptly to extrude and it was a simple matter to collapse it as it was brushed away from the nervous tissue forming its nest, such small vessels as were found to enter the surface of the growth being picked up and coagulated as the enucleation proceeded. The shell of the growth was finally dislodged from its huge pocket with scarcely any injury to the pia arachnoid, the greatly enlarged and dislocated Sylvian vessels lying exposed in the depth of the cavity. While the osteoplastic flap was being replaced and the wound closed a transfusion of 500 cubic centimeters of whole blood was given. All told, it was a seven-hour session.

The photographs of the preserved tissues (Figs. 20, 21, and 22), which weighed 128 grams and probably represented a *circa* 150-gram tumor, together with photographs of the patient (Figs. 23 and 24) who made a prompt and uninterrupted recovery will tell all that is additionally needed to complete the story.

Few operations in surgery are likely to be more

hazardous, to offer more technical difficulties, or to put a greater strain on the judgment and resourcefulness of a surgical staff. To be sure, procedures of this sort have in the past been successfully carried through by other than electro-surgical methods, but hardly in one sitting. The steps of the operation have possibly been given in unnecessary detail for those who have had personal experience with similar tumors and who are already aware of the difficulties. The principal reason, however, for including the case here is to call attention to the fact that epileptiform seizures were produced by the passage of the coagulating current through the dura, and to give warning of this possibility. Fortunately, the convulsions occurred before the dura was opened else they might have caused serious trouble from the accentuation of bleeding and cerebral protrusion.

To show that the successful outcome of this case was not exceptional, a few weeks later the outer margin of another still more deeply situated meningioma (Surgical No. 28598) arising from the sphenoidal ridge was stumbled upon in the course of an exploration for a presumed tumor of the right frontal lobe that had been wrongly localized by misinterpretation of the ventriculograms. The *circa* 100-gram growth shown in the

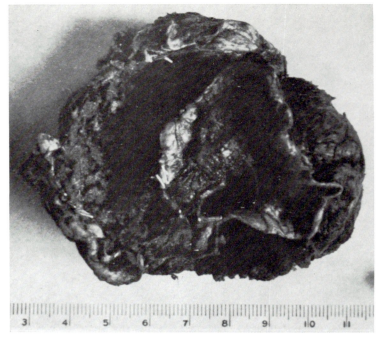

Fig. 21. Case 6. The outer surface of the thoroughly gutted tumor to which at one
margin the flap of adherent dura is still attached (weight 70 grams).

accompanying photograph (Fig. 25) in the course
of an eight-hour session including the ventriculography was thoroughly excavated, collapsed, and

cleanly removed, after which the residual dura
which could not be removed on account of its
dense attachment to the wing of the sphenoid was

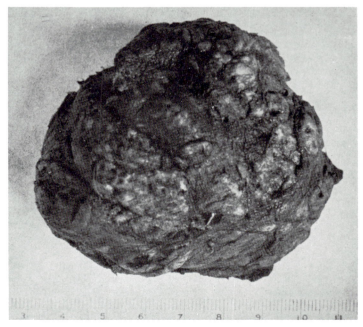

Fig. 22. Case 6. The intact inner surface of the tumor shell that lay in the widely expanded Sylvian pocket.

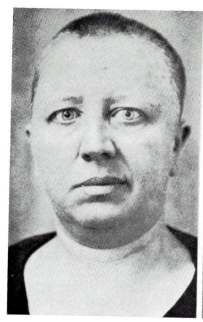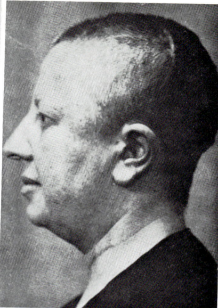

Figs. 23–24. Case 6. The patient on her discharge showing slight residual right facial palsy which soon disappeared.

thoroughly dehydrated by spraying with the ball electrode. Recovery was perfect.

In another place and in another connection[7] has been described how electro-surgery may be of aid not only in the primary attack on smaller meningiomas in inaccessible situations but as a means of destroying the sometimes irremovable cell nests in the adherent dura and bone. But what has already been said will perhaps be enough to show what may be done with these particular lesions.

During the two years we have had an unusual number of meningiomas, thirty-nine patients having been admitted for their primary operation and twelve for a secondary operation or for recurrent symptoms. In all but four of the cases the tumor was removed in a single session with six (11.7 per cent) fatalities, four of which have already been mentioned. This is a high mortality percentage but many of the operations would not have been even ventured upon at all or would have been given up in course as unduly hazardous or impossible of accomplishment by other than electro-surgical methods. As four of the fatalities were due to infection, it must be confessed that on this score the electro-surgical methods served temporarily to increase operative risks, but this

of late appears to have been wholly overcome.

The Blood Vessel Tumors. What has been said above regarding the risks from loss of blood in dealing with the larger meningiomas applies still more to the tumors that are actually of angioblastic origin, for many of them are truly formidable lesions even when attacked with the aid of electro-coagulation, as we soon found to our cost. On March 19, 1927, the day after the successful extirpation of the large Sylvian meningioma that has been described, we ventured to attack a rapidly enlarging capillary hæmangioblastoma of the fourth ventricle. An account of the case has been included in a monograph[8] which deals with the subject of the blood-vessel tumors as a whole and a brief résumé will suffice for our present needs. It was the first occasion in which we had used the highly damped desiccating current for the purpose of superficially dehydrating and shrinking a vascular growth before its removal.

CASE 7. After many vicissitudes from mistaken diagnoses the patient (Surgical No. 28406), a young woman of 23 years, had finally been operated upon in *September of 1925* at which time a large cerebellar cyst was evacuated and a highly vascular nodule disclosed in its base. An attempt to remove even a small fragment of the lesion for histological identification led to bleeding that was checked with great difficulty. She did well for a year when owing to a return of symptoms the cerebellum was

[7] Cushing, Harvey, and Eisenhardt, Louise. The meningiomas arising from the tuberculum sellae, with the syndrome of primary optic atrophy and bitemporal field defects combined with a normal sella turcica in a middle-aged person. Arch. Ophthal. (Chicago), vol. 1, 1929 (in press).

[8] Cushing and Bailey. Tumors arising from the blood vessels of the brain. Angiomatous malformations and hemangioblastomas. C. C Thomas, Springfield, Ill., 1928. (Case XXIV)

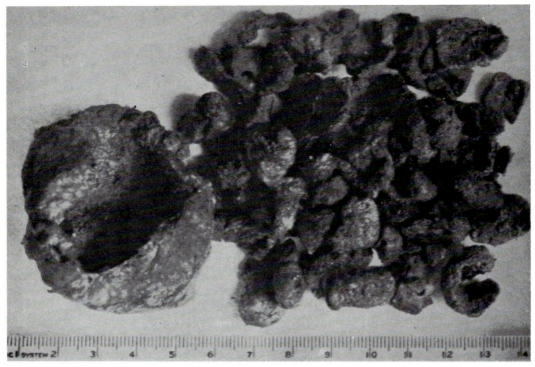

Fig. 25. Showing the characteristic scallops of tissue and the residual shell of a meningioma
(Surgical No. 28598) arising from the sphenoidal ridge in the deep Sylvian region.

again exposed in *August, 1926*, and the cyst evacuated, but the tumor nodule had doubled in size and efforts to deal with it again led to alarming hæmorrhage. The relief afforded by this second operation lasted for only six months and though under ordinary circumstances the case would have been regarded as surgically hopeless, Dr. Bovie felt that we might conceivably slowly carbonize a lesion of this type, and the chance was taken. The growth as shown by the operative sketches in the article referred to had by this time (*March 19, 1927*) come completely to fill the central portion of the posterior fossa.

It was found by spraying the highly vascular surface of the tumor with the coagulating current, the ball electrode being used for the purpose, that the surface could be shrunken and charred as the cerebellum was gradually brushed away from it, no physiological effects being produced. By this method, what represented possibly the outer half of the lesion was gradually brought into view and coagulated. The central portion of the exposed growth was then partly scalloped, but such a degree of bleeding soon began to occur from the raw cavity that it was necessary to take muscle from the patient's leg for purposes of implantation before it could be controlled. The headward portion of the lesion was finally tilted out sufficiently to permit cerebrospinal fluid to escape from the dilated iter; and as the patient had by this time begun to complain of the discomforts of her position on the table, the flaps were replaced and closed in the usual detail after what had been over a five-hour session.

We were at this time unaware of what effect the heat engendered by this long process of coagulation might have upon the medulla. Nor did we know how well the large eschar which was left behind would be tolerated by the enveloping tissue. Our apprehensions on these scores happily were ungrounded; she made an immediate excellent recovery and showed no signs of reaction. At the end of a week's time, fearing to wait longer lest we should be unable to unfold the tissues easily, the tumor was again exposed, this time under ether anæsthesia; and after the remainder of its surface had been treated in the same fashion as before, it was possible to tilt outward the charred mass, thereby exposing the full length of the dilated and naked floor of the fourth ventricle. The base of the tumor was then clamped off, dehydrated, and removed from its attachment just above the calamus scriptorius (Fig. 26). The patient made an excellent recovery from her anæsthetic and passed a good night; but early the next morning she began to have some respiratory difficulties from which she succumbed on the morning of *March 28.*

In this case we had made a desperate throw and failed, whether from poor judgment or inexperience need not be discussed. Had the same methods been employed when the tumor was smaller, the operation might well enough have been carried through to a successful issue. This we have had the good fortune to demonstrate in a more recent case. As was explained in our monograph on the subject of these blood-vessel tumors, the true

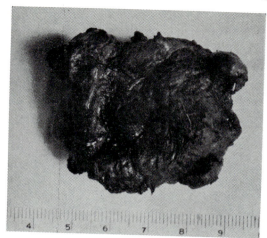

Fig. 26. Case 7. The remains of a large capillary haemangioblastoma of the fourth ventricle charred and shrunken by electro-desiccation before its removal at a second session with fatality from pneumonia.

hæmangioblastomas are invariably found in the cerebellum, some of them being cystic and some of them largely solid lesions. And a month after the fatal operation described we had made sufficient progress to encourage us to send for an old patient known to harbor one of these formidable lesions of the latter type.

CASE 8. The patient's history (Surgical No. 28582) occurs as Case 21 in our monograph on the blood-vessel tumors, and it will suffice to say here that she had first been operated upon for an emergency cerebellar syndrome in 1923, the tumor not being brought to view. She had pulmonary tuberculosis, and a cerebellar tuberculoma was suspected.

As a result of the decompression she did well for nearly three years. In July of 1926 at a secondary exploration, a huge, unmistakable hæmangioma occupying the larger part of the right cerebellar fossa was exposed. Because of its vascularity, it was not even possible to remove a fragment of the lesion for histological verification. From this operation she had received but little if any benefit and aware that she was rapidly losing ground she was encouraged to return.

At the third operation on April 19, 1927, under local anæsthesia and in spite of her highly advanced cerebellar symptoms, the desperate procedure of slowly attacking the huge angiomatous growth by the process of desiccation and coagulation was successfully carried through in a seven-hour session with three transfusions in course.

She made all-told a satisfactory surgical recovery, and had it not been for her by this time advancing pulmonary tuberculosis the prognosis would have been favorable. She died at her home from some obscure cause without autopsy seven months later.

Two other patients with a growth of precisely this same formidable sort have since been seen through with better success: one of them a young boy whose tumor had been previously exposed

and considered inoperable; the other an adult in whom the vascular growth was successfully and radically attacked by dehydration methods on its first exposure.

We had hoped that the angiomatous malformations, a discussion of which comprised the first part of our aforementioned monograph, might be similarly attacked by electro-surgical methods, but in the single case in which the attempt was made we had the misfortune to "spark" through one of the superficial vessels of the aneurysmal lesion thereby causing troublesome bleeding. Without further experience it is impossible to tell whether vascular malformations of this nature can be effectively attacked. We have found experimentally, however, that vessels of considerable size may be sealed by compression with the ball electrode and the employment of a slowly coagulating current. All of this needs very careful further study.

Cerebral Gliomas. Our early electro-surgical experiences as already stated were largely restricted to the development of the methods of treating the meningiomas in the manner described, and our first essays to deal with the tumors composed of elements of the nervous system were unsatisfactory. However, what we might some day learn to do was foreshadowed by an occasional experience like the following in which the exposed surface of the lesion lay uncovered in the wall of a large cyst.

CASE 9. The patient (Surgical No. 28547), a young man seventeen years of age, had been previously operated upon in June, 1924. At that time he presented unmistakable symptoms of a left temporal lobe lesion and at the operation a massive subcortical glioma of a comparatively benign type (astrocytoma) was, for the day, radically attacked and in large part removed though because of bleeding a visible portion of the tumor in the depth of the lobe was left behind. The flap was replaced leaving a subtemporal defect.

The patient made an excellent recovery and had been steadily at work as a farm-hand until a month before his re-admission at which time the subtemporal decompression began slightly to protrude and some of his former symptoms to return. He reported this fact and was requested to re-enter the hospital for examination.

He proved to be in such excellent physical condition that under ordinary circumstances one would have felt inclined to advise delay, for in spite of an occasional headache he was well able to continue earning his livelihood.

At the operation on April 14, 1927, on once more reflecting the old bone flap under local anæsthesia, a huge temporal lobe cyst containing at least three hundred cubic centimeters of xanthochromic fluid was encountered and evacuated. With the cutting current a long incision was then made quite bloodlessly through the overlying fibrotic tissues at the site of the old decompression. In the floor of the widely opened cyst was seen a solid mass of recurrent tumor the size of a hen's egg. This large mural tumor was removed in two large fragments (Fig. 27) with extraordinary ease by the aid of the dehydrating current. The growth appeared to lie in the

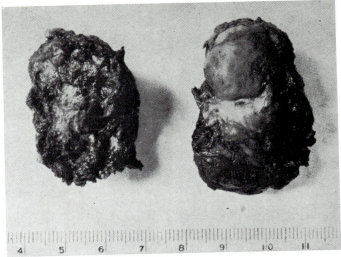

Fig. 27. Case 9. Two large fragments of a fibrillary astrocytoma which was electrically dissected from the crotch of the lateral ventricle and which constituted the mural nodule of a large temporal lobe cyst.

fork of the dislocated ventricle which was widely opened in the process of its removal. The tissues actually melted away miraculously before the sparking point in a manner that would not have been possible by ordinary methods of tissue division. The boy made a prompt and excellent recovery (Figs. 28–29), a few taps of the subtemporal region having been required because of the accumulation of cerebrospinal fluid due to the opened ventricle.[9]

This happens to have been the first case in which a wooden table and wooden spatulæ were employed, and the avoidance of any discom-

[9] In other cases of this sort when the wall of the lateral ventricle has been widely opened by such a procedure, the exposed choroid plexus has been removed, a procedure which is greatly facilitated by electrical dissection.

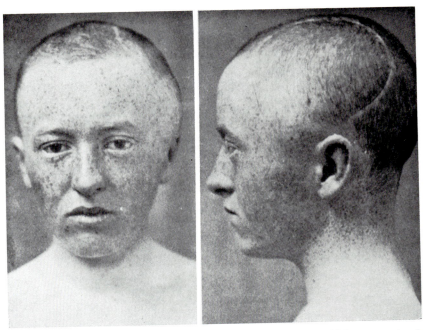

Figs. 28–29. Case 9. The patient 14 days after operation for a recurrent temporal lobe tumor, showing fullness of subtemporal region due to temporary tendency of cerebrospinal fluid to accumulate because of the widely opened ventricle.

forts or physiological reactions was ascribed to these accessories. Their importance was unduly emphasized, as we now know, but under the encouragement of this experience we began gradually to gain confidence in attacking cerebral gliomas of varied sorts and in time learned with properly modified currents how to make transcortical incisions with comparative bloodlessness and without getting the electrode "gummed" with tissue in the process. As a result of this we have become even more radical than heretofore in the removal of these tumors for the former methods of block dissection were apt not only to be somewhat messy and bloody, but there was always the likelihood of inoculating the raw tissue with viable tumor cells—a risk greatly lessened when electrical methods of dissection are used. The details of procedures of this type need hardly be gone into for they differ greatly from case to case and they are unquestionably capable of vast improvement in technique, which will doubtless come to be perfected given time and experience.

It may suffice to say that the removal of glioma-containing lobes of the brain (frontal, temporal, or occipital) may be enormously facilitated by electro-surgical manipulation, and should one apprehend that the nervous tissues lining the raw cavity still contain tumor or have been infected by implantation of tumor cells, as a last step in the lobectomy the raw surface may be gone over by the loop and as many additional thin layers of tissue be scalloped out as may seem necessary.

Cerebellar Gliomas. Gliomas which arise from or involve the roof of the fourth ventricle are very common lesions particularly in childhood, as the writer has elsewhere taken pains to point out.[10]

Even before we began to employ electro-surgical methods of operating, we had begun radically to attack these tumors and many of them had been successfully removed, the ultimate prognosis varying in accordance with the pathological nature of the lesion, whether a highly malignant medulloblastoma, a less malignant ependymoma, or a relatively benign astrocytoma. It is perhaps incorrect to speak of them as fourth ventricle tumors rather than as tumors of the vermis, though in their removal as was described above in connection with Case 7, the widened ventricle is usually laid bare from the distended iter to the calamus.

The operations are time-consuming, technically difficult, and demand full bilateral exposure of the cerebellum oftentimes with removal of the laminæ of the atlas. It is impossible to carry out the necessary manipulations through the single vertical or transverse incisions that have recently come to be advocated for cerebellar operations. The crux of the enucleation lies in the control of bleeding from the choroidal branches of the posterior cerebellar arteries in the tonsillar region adjacent to the calamus, for it is from this source that these median tumors appear to receive their main blood supply. Should one of these vessels fail to be clipped or coagulated before its division, it is often most difficult to secure the bleeding point, and interstitial bleeding in this region is attended with great danger.

The posterior end of many of these tumors lies exposed between the tonsils so soon as the cisternal arachnoid is opened. Others are only exposed by drawing the tonsils up out of the foramen and separating them so as to bring the calamus and triangle of Magendie into view. Still others are not visible on the surface, but their presence is betrayed by an unnatural prominence or widening of the uvula. Under these circumstances the electro-surgical methods can be effectively utilized in place of the scalpel or blunt dissector in making the long median incision through the vermis down to the tumor which, even when large, often lies at a surprising depth.

When the surface of the growth has been well exposed by brushing each of the divided cerebellar hemispheres to the side, it may be primarily excavated in various ways depending largely upon its consistency. When it is too soft to be handled, as is true of most of the medulloblastomas, the sucker must be largely resorted to; but even under these unfavorable circumstances electrical methods are constantly called for to control bleeding points, more particularly as one approaches the vascular stalk of the tumor in the region of the calamus.

These operations for fourth ventricle tumors are relatively common ones, there having been thirty-five examples verified during the past two years,[11] few, however, of such seriousness as that for the fourth ventricle hæmangioma (Case 7) described above. One or two of the cases in which the electro-surgical adjunct was first employed may serve in illustration.

CASE 10. The patient (Surgical No. 28604), a child eight years of age, was admitted on *September 27, 1926*, with a choked disc of 5 diopters, secondary hydrocephalus, and a full-blown cerebellar syndrome so advanced that an operation was performed without the customary delay for detailed study. During the course of the usual exploration under local anæsthesia with a

---

[10] The intracranial tumors of preadolescence. Am. J. Dis. Child. April 1927, xxxiii, 551–584.

[11] The figures are approximately as follows: out of five hundred forty-seven operations for tumor during the twenty-four months, exactly four hundred tumors were surgically verified or reverified. Of these, approximately three hundred were cerebral tumors and about one hundred cerebellar tumors (including acoustic neurinomas), thirty-five of them having been fourth ventricle tumors, the great majority occurring in children.

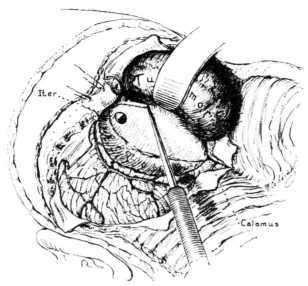

Fig. 30. Case 10. From postoperative sketch showing on an oblique view the final step of electrically separating the line of attachment of the dislodged tumor along the right side of the ventricle. (Reduced ⅓.)

ventricular puncture to diminish venous stasis, a highly vascular median tumor was exposed. It was thought to be a hæmangioma and was considered to be inoperable. A small fragment of tissue removed for verification, proved subsequently to be too greatly infiltrated to determine the histological type of lesion. She was nevertheless given a series of X-ray treatments and did extremely well for the next six months during which she remained free from symptoms.

Her mother reported in *April, 1927* that she had begun again to have occasional attacks of morning vomiting, and in the hope that the tumor might possibly be removed by electrical methods and believing that it would be better not to delay until the beneficial effect of the decompression had been wholly lost, the child was readmitted for a secondary operation.

The clinical history contains the following note which was dictated immediately after the operation on *April 21, 1927*, when the sketches (Fig. 30) were made and the steps of the procedure fully described. It tells more vividly than would now be possible or permissible the impressions of the case at the time.

"Of the extraordinary and revolutionizing experiences we have been having in the past month this case I think exceeds them all.

"The child since her re-entry to the hospital after a former decompression with subsequent radiation has been so absolutely free from any evidences of tumor I had almost begun to feel that we had better postpone further intervention as unnecessary on the assumption that the tumor must have been absorbed by the X-ray. I had not the slightest suspicion that we were going to find a far larger tumor than was originally exposed.

"I am not at all sure whether the tumor that was found is a hæmangioma after all; it may possibly be a medulloblastoma or indeed an astrocytoma. There was no evidence of the great vascularity which caused us to cut short the primary operation and which may possibly have been due solely to stasis.

"Even so, without the electrical devices I probably would not have done more than to give this growth a partial removal by suction and probably would never have gotten it very fully in view, particularly in the neighborhood of its lower pole, for here the attachments were dense and vascular and bled at a touch, but they simply melted away before the dehydrating current.

"So far as I could see, for the first time one of these fourth ventricle tumors was removed intact without leaving behind even a suspicious tag of tissue. In the process a new manœuvre was employed in that the growth, after being freed as effectively as possible on the near side well up under the tentorium, was then pressed to the opposite side by the wooden spatula. The lateral wall of the dilated ventricle, thus put on the stretch, was then electrically opened by a bloodless incision the full 6 centimeter length of the ventricle. This made it possible for the tumor to be tilted out until the opposite wall, as shown in the sketch (Fig. 30), was in its turn similarly divided, thereby permitting the growth to be lifted out in its entirety (Fig. 31).

"There is one important point which should be mentioned in that the dehydrating current proved distinctly a better method of separating the growth from the adjacent cerebellum than the ordinary method of brushing it away, for, owing I presume to their relatively greater content of water, the nervous tissues melted away before the sparking current, leaving the surface of the growth cleanly exposed. In the customary procedure of dissecting the brain from a lesion of this sort, one is likely sometimes to get more deeply into brain than is desirable or, on the contrary, and what is still worse, occasionally to break through the surface of the tumor."

This brief preliminary statement, as it occurs

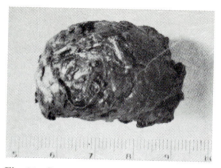

Fig. 31. Case 10. The shrunken nodule of fourth ventricle tumor after fixation.

in the record, tells about as much as does the detailed account of the operation that follows it, apart from the fact that it dismisses with slight reference the difficulties of re-exposing the growth because of the dense adhesions due to the old operation, in the separation of which the cutting current proved infinitely superior to the scalpel. Nor does it mention the fact that the vascular surface of the growth was sprayed and shrunken with the damped dehydrating current as it was gradually brought to view. The tumor proved to be an astrocytoma composed mainly of protoplasmic elements which gives the case (Figs. 32–34) a most favorable prognosis.

When these fourth ventricle astrocytomas are accompanied by a cyst, the problem is greatly simplified, particularly if the cyst lies superficial to the mural nodule so that it lies fully exposed. Examples of the manner in which these lesions may be dealt with under these favorable circumstances are shown in the accompanying sketches:

one (Fig. 35) shows a comparatively small mesially placed nodule attached to the roof of the ventricle; the other (Fig. 36) shows a larger mural tumor which was laterally placed in the right hemisphere.

In past years surgeons were apt to congratulate themselves on the mere evacuation of a gliomatous cyst, which of course leads to an immediate brilliant operative result. But painful experience has shown that the cyst is not an evidence of degeneration of a lesion and that somewhere in its wall lies a tumor nodule from the surface of which the xanthochromic fluid exudes and in time the tumor, unless it is removed, may come wholly to replace the former cyst. Under these circumstances its total removal at subsequent operations becomes increasingly difficult with each attempt because of the tissue adhesions which form. I have under continued observation a patient who as a lad of nine years was first operated upon in 1907 when I jubilantly enucleated a cerebellar cyst. Since then he has grown to young manhood, but in the intervening twenty years, owing to recurring symptoms due to the progress of his slowly infiltrative astrocytoma, he has been subjected to six operations until there is little of his cerebellum remaining. Had the nature of the process been appreciated in 1907 it might even at that early day have been removed at a primary session, and both patient and surgeon been spared much tribulation.

When these fourth ventricle astrocytomas are found at their first exposure to be unaccompanied by cysts, the problem is quite another one. It is rare that they can be removed in their entirety as in the operation on Case 10 that has been re-

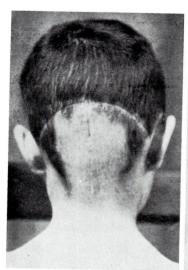
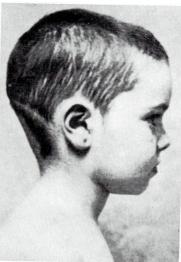
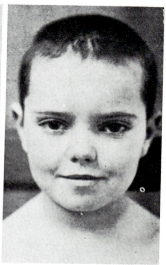

Figs. 32–34. Case 10. Patient May 20, 1927 at time of discharge. The bald patch was due to the former radiation which so far as known is ineffective for astrocytomas.

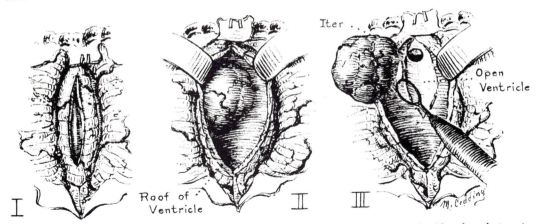

Fig. 35. Operative sketch (Surgical No. 30509) showing: *I*, the primary incision through widened uvula to outer surface of cyst; *II*, the opened cyst showing thin roof of ventricle on which lies a flat mural nodule; *III*, loop being used for cutting last attachment of nodule to ventricular roof after its dislocation outward.

corded in detail. It is usually necessary partly to excavate the tumor before it can be brushed away from the cerebellar hemispheres without producing undue contusion; and so far as possible during the manipulation of the tumor, pressure upon it must be avoided because of its position over the medulla, the respiratory mechanism, in many cases already compromised, being easily upset.

An example of one of these solid tumors which happened to be an unusually firm medulloblastoma but which on May 17, 1927, had been thus treated by primary electrical excavation before removal is shown in the accompanying photograph (Fig. 37), and the operative sketches (Fig. 38) give some of the stages of its removal. In the case shown in Figure 39, the tissue was electrically split and its two halves removed in successive stages. On other occasions it may be found difficult or impossible to remove the posterior portion of the lesion owing to its dense attachment to the region of the calamus. An example of this is shown in Figure 40; the removal of the residual nodule was given up as too hazardous.

The general run of soft medulloblastomas that occupy this same region are less suitable for electrical scalloping and are most effectively attacked by suction. The technical problems necessarily differ considerably from case to case and each tumor has to be surgically manipulated according to its peculiarities. Fourth ventricle tumors are alike merely in the fact that the chief point of particular danger lies, as may be re-emphasized, in the method of controlling the chief vascular attachments which lie alongside the calamus, for which purpose electrical coagulation is more likely to be effective than the employment of clips.

The Acoustic Tumors. Because of their characteristic symptomatology the acoustic neurinomas are possibly the most easily recognized of any intracranial tumors. Moreover they are inherently benign lesions. And yet from a technical standpoint, particularly when they have attained a large size, they offer greater difficulties than almost any other tumor with which the neurosurgeon is obliged to deal. Though the usual run of these patients came to operation during the first few months when we were grounding ourselves in the first principles of electro-surgery, difficulties were experienced owing to the spread of the current to the nerves enveloping the tumor, physiological responses being produced which were most disturbing to the patient. Consequently about all that the electrical adjunct could be used for was as a purely supplementary measure for coagulating dural margins and possibly for making the primary incision into the tumor and sealing some of its surface vessels.

However, during the past six months we have come to modify our traditional method of exposing these awkwardly accessible growths, and as a matter of fact we were forced into the manœuvre owing to the urgent postoperative complication in the case to be described.

CASE 11. The patient (Surgical No. 30497), a foreigner, was admitted with an advanced cerebellopontile syndrome. On account of marked mental changes he was wholly uncooperative. He was bedridden because of his ataxia, nearly blind from secondary atrophy, and there was extreme dysphagia. The operation had to be begun under ether narcosis which he took badly. His respiratory embarrassment was such that in spite of a ventricular puncture there was sufficient stasis to cause undue loss of blood.

The tumor, a large one, was finally well enough exposed to permit of a partial intracapsular enucleation, a slow process as the growth was firm and vascular. Owing to the patient's condition it was necessary to withdraw without having accomplished much more than a decom-

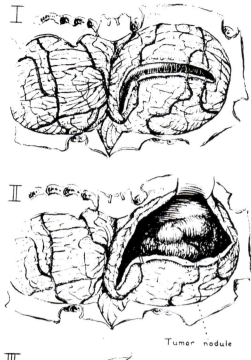

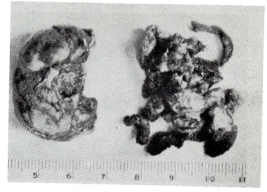

Fig. 37. An unusually firm medulloblastoma of fourth ventricle (Surgical No. 28754) removed after primary excavation by scalloping to reduce the size of the lesion.

This was accomplished with amazing ease and quite bloodlessly with the dehydrating current. The tumor, which previously had been awkwardly exposed under the margin of the retracted hemisphere, then lay fully bared to view. It was radically excavated with the loop-electrode until its capsule could be so fully collapsed that the anterior portion of the growth, which was wedged alongside the pons in the tentorial opening, could be released.

Though the loss of blood had been considerable and though the two operations had consumed over five

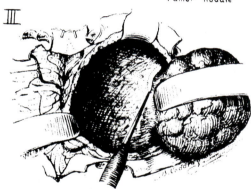

Fig. 36. Operative sketch (reduced ⅓) illustrating the steps of the electro-surgical removal of a large laterally placed mural astrocytoma (Surgical No. 31096).

pression. The wound was closed none too easily and, as is customary, the patient was left face-down on the table to await the full recovery from the anæsthetic. This he failed satisfactorily to do. Gradually respiration became still more embarrassed with increasing cyanosis, a falling blood pressure and rising pulse rate. It was evident, if life were to be saved, that the desperate chance would have to be taken of re-opening the wound —always a most disheartening procedure.

Preparations for resuming the operation were made, and the carefully closed wound was reopened. The evident cause of the compression was a swollen, oedematous, and infiltrated cerebellar hemisphere overlying the growth, for on its release the patient's respiration and color almost immediately improved. There was nothing for it but to remove a large crescent of the hemisphere.

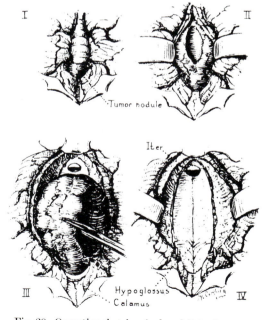

Fig. 38. Operative sketches (reduced ⅓) to show steps in the electro-surgical removal of a solid fourth ventricle tumor (Surgical No. 28754): I, shows appearance at primary exposure; II, after splitting the vermis and removal of primary scallop; III, the partly scalloped tumor being dislodged; IV, the bed of tumor with widely opened ventricle after removal of its roof together with tumor.

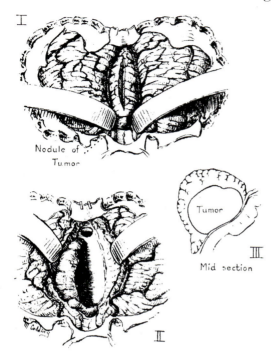

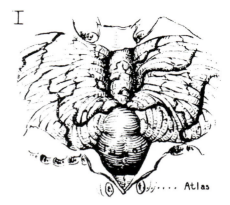

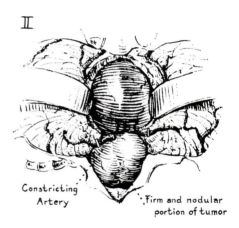

Fig. 39. Operative sketch (reduced ⅓) of a solid fourth
ventricle tumor, the two halves of which were removed
at separate sessions (Surgical No. 30945). In this case
the situation of the tumor would have been betrayed by
the bulging uvula even had its lower pole not been
brought to view by separating the tonsils.

hours, the patient began immediately to improve, and a
month later he was able to walk out of the hospital in
unusually good condition for the victim of an acoustic
tumor that had attained such a large size.

What was particularly unexpected in this man's
case was the fact that the postoperative cerebellar
symptoms were, if anything, less marked than one
usually sees in comparable cases when the cerebellar hemisphere has merely been retracted and
left in place. We had fully anticipated that the
removal of what must have amounted to practically the lower third of the hemisphere would
leave the corresponding leg and arm so ataxic
that they would be practically useless.

Since this illuminating experience we have
adopted this method as a preliminary step in exposing other acoustic tumors (Fig. 41) and have
not only been able thereby to get a far better
primary view of the lesion but have come to feel
that in advanced cases a partial cerebellar extirpation is, in the long run, less likely to accentuate
pre-existing ataxia than did the inevitable contusion of the lobe that was formerly produced by
the method of retraction.

How far one may go with the adoption of this
principle of removing the uninvolved shelf of

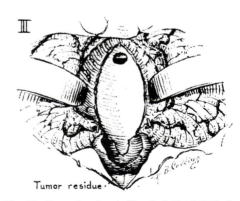

Fig. 40. Operative sketch (Surgical No. 32102) showing: I, a fibrillary astrocytoma projecting through the
foramen magnum necessitating removal of the arch of
the atlas; upper extension of tumor shown in II, unsuspected until electrical incision through vermis; in III
is shown the remaining adherent and irremovable posterior end of tumor after removal of lesion by scalloping.
(Reduced ²⁄₉.)

brain that overlies a tumor rather than merely
retracting it or incising through it down to the

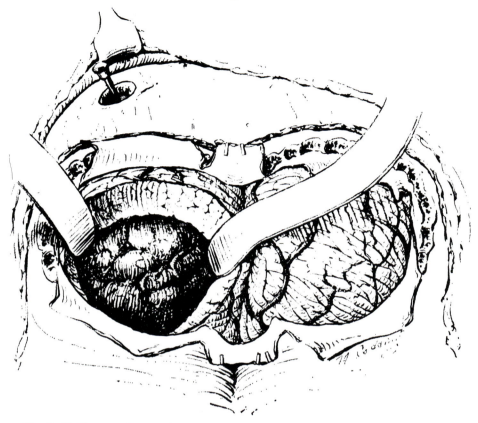

Fig. 41. To illustrate the procedure described in the text of uncapping an acoustic tumor by electrically excising a generous portion of the overlying cerebellar hemisphere.

surface of the tumor with subsequent separation of the incised edges, remains to be seen. The temptation will be great to extend the principle in regions where cortex registers no important function now that the excision of tissue is so greatly facilitated by electro-desiccation. And the same thing applies as well to lobectomies for the mass extirpation of gliomas—a principle which should of course not be carried too far. The mere prolongation of life unless it can be made better worth living is not an accomplishment for the surgeon to pride himself upon, as has often been emphasized.

As Dr. Bovie's preliminary note was written in May, 1927, it has seemed appropriate to restrict the case reports in this paper, so far as possible, to an account of our early experiences which had begun to accumulate during the spring of that year. In all of these operations the active electrode was used while attached to the hand-made pistol-grip which he had devised and carved out of bakelite (Fig. 42), the current being "shot" by the surgeon. Meanwhile a second person, Dr. Bovie himself in those instructive days, controlled the switchboard and modified the character of the current in ways he thought appropriate to

the surgeon's particular needs of the moment.

We had originally discussed the possibility of having keys on the handle of the pistol-grip which would enable the surgeon himself to change and modify the currents employed so that an operator at the switchboard of the apparatus would no longer be required. But as a matter of fact, we have tended in quite the other direction. For we have come more and more to dispense with the pistol altogether and to use the electrode as a pencil, and this for reasons to be explained has made it necessary to take on an additional assistant instead of eliminating one as we originally planned to do.

For gross work the pistol does well enough and it is of course a great convenience for the surgeon to have the current under the immediate control of his trigger finger. But for delicate dissection in dangerous places, around the optic nerves and chiasm, for example, the movement of the electrode with the pistol in hand, compared to the movement of an instrument held in the fingers like a pencil, is exceedingly awkward. One need only attempt to write his signature with a pencil inserted in the muzzle of a revolver to appreciate the difference. We consequently have been obliged to take recourse to a foot switch, which has been supplied with the newer models of the apparatus, or, better still, to have an extra assistant cleaned up who not only holds the pencil when not in use but who often plays a far less passive rôle than this as may be explained.

On one occasion (on April 26, 1927, to be exact), a large right frontal glioma of a somewhat unusual type was exposed and attacked by electrical methods. In this process which necessitated the removal of the larger part of the lobe and the laying bare of the anterior falx, an unusual number of vessels were encountered; and since the operator's left hand was engaged in careful retraction of the brain while the right was holding the pistol, the coagulation of these vessels, though they were plainly brought to view, was difficult to compass. The need was felt for some sort of a split pointed electrode that could be used for making incisions when closed and yet could be opened, in the fashion of the usual duck-billed forceps, so as to pick up a bleeding point for purposes of coagulation. Dr. Bovie promptly acted on this suggestion and constructed an ingenious instrument for the purpose that could be controlled with the thumb while the pistol grip was being held.

Meanwhile, however, we had hit upon a more practical method of accomplishing the same end though it necessitated having an additional assistant who intermediated between the surgeon and the operator of the machine, and to whom the pistol could be handed when not in use instead of its being hung on the rack which had originally been devised for the purpose. In this way the surgeon's operating hand or hands might be quickly freed so that an exposed vessel could be picked up by the long, smooth-bladed, and slender dissecting forceps along which the intermediary assistant could then "shoot" the current after bringing the active electrode, which he was holding, into gentle contact with the end of the forceps.

For an operation which at best requires many assistants, to have two more thus crowded in, not to mention a cumbersome piece of apparatus, seems a needless expenditure of personnel as well as of space; but it is difficult to see how this can be well avoided if advantage is to be taken of the very important rôle these extra hands may be called upon to play in an emergency.

One hesitates to make suggestions to others who will come to, or have already begun to, employ electro-surgical methods for tumor removal. Novel manœuvres will doubtless be hit upon by them that have not yet occurred to us. There are a few things, however, from our own experience to which attention may be called. A suction apparatus with a long bent glass nozzle (not a metal one as seems to be commonly used) has long since come to be an almost indispensable part of our neurosurgical equipment. For though it is not a fool-proof instrument and may do damage in awkward hands, it is useful in many ways: it serves as a means of keeping the wound free of blood and irrigating fluids so that sponging is no

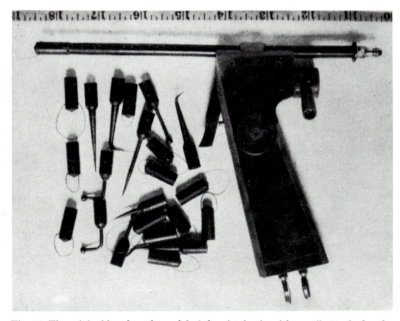

Fig. 42. The original hand-made model of the pistol-grip with pencil attached and a cluster of terminal electrodes of various types.

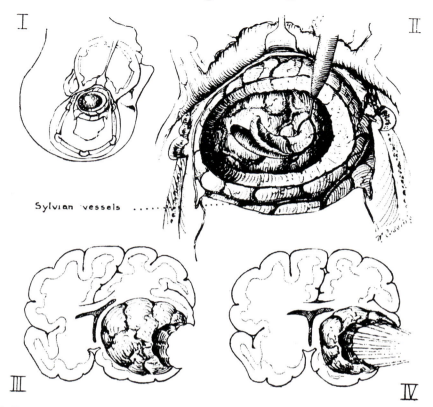

Fig. 43. To illustrate the successive stages of the electro-surgical removal of a large vascular meningioma occupying the temporal fossa and arising from the tentorium. After the primary uncapping of the lesion by electrical removal of the oval disc of overlying cortex, and after brushing the vascular surface of the exposed tumor with a ball electrode and coagulating spray, the sketch *II* shows the primary scallop in process of removal; *III* shows the condition at the end of the first session; *IV*, at the end of the second session. The shell of the tumor was finally removed at a third session (Surgical No. 32127).

longer employed; it serves as a means of sucking out the bulk of the softer tumors; and nowadays in connection with electro-surgery, since the active electrode cannot be used in a bloody field, it serves to keep dry the point at which the current is to be applied. Even should a vessel of considerable size, too large to be sealed by the dehydrating current, happen to be divided in the process of incising the brain or of scalloping a tumor, it can, without flooding the wound, be allowed to play directly into the sucker while the point is picked up by the forceps down which the current is allowed to pass in the manner described.

A beginner, if his experience coincides with ours, will often have difficulty in regulating the current so as to seal the bleeding point properly without so damaging it as to start bleeding afresh. At times when too strong a current is used to coagulate a naked vein of considerable size, the steam caused by the dehydration may actually lead to an explosive rupture of the vessel wall. Until we learned largely to overcome these diffi-

culties, we continued to place reliance, as of old, on silver clips and though for the control of the larger vessels clips cannot be wholly superseded, they are used less and less frequently and the current more and more for hæmostasis. Even a fairly large artery may be effectively occluded without risk of opening into its lumen, provided some tissue is picked up by the forceps on each side of the vessel and included in the dehydration process.

There are times when solid tumors of the meningioma type (cf. Case 3) may be in themselves so highly vascular that when they are scalloped with the loop, even with a highly damped cutting current, bleeding from the base of the furrow may be serious. And if this process has to be repeated over and over again without waiting to control the bleeding after each scallop is removed, the patient will shortly have become too exsanguinated to permit further progress.

We have recently been dealing with a huge deep-seated meningioma of angioblastic type, with an audible bruit, that required three separate stages before the shell of the tumor could finally be collapsed and dislodged (Fig. 43). The growth, which was approximately a 150-gram lesion, lay deep in the left temporal fossa and was exposed by electrically excising the oval disc of temporal lobe that overlay it. In spite of a superficial preliminary treatment of the surface with a coagulating spray, when the growth came to be scalloped with a damped dehydrating current (Fig. 43, II), it was necessary owing to excessive bleeding to keep the raw groove, from which each piece of tissue had been looped out, clean by suction and to shift from the loop to a ball electrode and from the cutting to the coagulating current before the surface could be sufficiently dried safely to permit the removal of the next fragment. Finally it was found that if the scallop of tissue was allowed to remain in its bed for a time or was held in place by the slight pressure of a cotton pledget, it could be removed shortly with practically no bleeding.

There is no gainsaying that the employment of the Bovie unit or any other form of current generator as an aid to the removal of a brain tumor adds a complication to an already highly complicated procedure. Yet in making a review of the early histories for purposes of this present communication, I find it expressly stated over and over again that the particular procedure in question, though an extremely prolonged and arduous performance, was one which without the electrosurgical adjunct would have been impossible to carry through to a safe conclusion.

During the two years that have elapsed since we hesitatingly began to employ the currents in cranio-cerebral surgery, five hundred and forty-seven operations for tumor have been performed. Though for some of these operations the electrical methods were not essential, there were few of them, even when no tumor was found, in which they could not advantageously be employed. The currents are useful even for such trifles as brushing the surface of the dura with the ball electrode in order to seal the torn meningeal veins from which persistent oozing may sometimes try one's patience, or similarly for checking the persistently oozing points on the under surface of the reflected bone before its replacement, or for coagulating some refractory vessel on the incised dural margin. To be sure, muscle implantation, bone wax, and silver clips have long been used for these several purposes and they cannot be wholly dispensed with even now, but on the whole electrical methods usually serve to accomplish the same ends more expeditiously.

Nearly twenty years have passed since Pozzi announced to the Academy of Medicine in Paris a method for the cure of malignancy by the action of sparks from the terminal of an Oudin resinator, a procedure termed "fulguration" as Dr. Bovie mentions in his introductory note. Slowly and gradually this original procedure has been modified and extended until for the treatment chiefly of cutaneous lesions and of orificial malignancy, it has gained enthusiastic advocates. The possibilities of electro-desiccation and coagulation, nevertheless, have not as yet come to be sufficiently appreciated by the general surgeon who has been prone to regard what are called surgical endothermy or diathermy as merely refined methods of tissue cauterization.

Surgery is a conservative art. It takes to novel methods reluctantly as an old dog to new tricks. It was slow to adopt the ligature; slow to adopt the principles of antisepsis; slow to adopt the fastidious technique and painstaking hæmostasis that have largely put a stop to operating by the clock. It has been equally slow to adopt the principles of electro-surgery which, from a technical standpoint, are likely to be no less revolutionizing.

Neurosurgical Classic—29

ROBERT H. WILKINS, M.D.*

National Cancer Institute, Bethesda, Maryland

THE present republication of the "Case of Cerebral Tumour" by A. H. Bennett and R. J. Godlee initiates a new series referred to in the Editorial Comment in this issue of the *Journal of Neurosurgery.* The classical works, selected for republication from time to time, usually will be accompanied by pertinent comments based on various authoritative works in the field of neurosurgical history.

CASE OF CEREBRAL TUMOUR†

BY

A. HUGHES BENNETT, M.D., F.R.C.P.,

PHYSICIAN TO THE HOSPITAL FOR EPILEPSY AND PARALYSIS, AND ASSISTANT PHYSICIAN TO THE WESTMINSTER HOSPITAL.

THE SURGICAL TREATMENT

BY

RICKMAN J. GODLEE, M.S., F.R.C.S.,

SURGEON TO UNIVERSITY COLLEGE HOSPITAL.

Received January 13th—Read May 12th, 1885.

THE chief features of interest in the case, to which the attention of the Society is directed, are, that during life the existence of a tumour was diagnosed in the brain, and its situation localised, entirely by the signs and symptoms exhibited, without any external manifestations on the surface of the skull. This growth was removed without any immediate injurious effects on the intelligence and general condition of the patient. Although he died four weeks after the operation, the fatal termination was due, not to any special effects on the nervous centres, but to a secondary surgical complication. The case, moreover, teaches some important physiological, pathological, and clinical lessons, and suggests practical reflections which may prove useful to future medicine and surgery.

* With the assistance of the Division of Neurosurgery, Duke Medical Center, Durham, North Carolina.

The technical assistance of the Library Branch of the Division of Research Services, National Institutes of Health, and especially the Circulation Section under the direction of Thelma P. Robinson, is gratefully acknowledged.

† Reprinted from *Medico-Chirurgical Transactions,* London, 1885, *68:* 243–275.

History.—The patient was a farmer, æt. 25, who applied for advice to the Hospital for Epilepsy and Paralysis, Regent's Park on November 3rd, 1884. His chief complaint was paralysis of the left hand and arm, which incapacitated him from work. He stated that his family history was unimportant, that he had always been temperate and in robust health, and that he never had suffered from syphilis or a day's illness of any kind in his life. About four years ago, while in Canada, a piece of timber fell from a house, struck him on the left side of the head and knocked him down. He thinks he lost consciousness for a few moments, after which he so far recovered as to be able to resume his work. On the following day he was quite well. With the exception of occasional slight headaches he afterwards remained in good health for a year, at the end of which time he first began to experience a feeling of twitching in the left side of his mouth and tongue. This soon developed into attacks of a paroxysmal character, which gradually became more pronounced and frequent, and continued to occur at irregular intervals. Some months afterwards he had a "fit" which began with a peculiar feeling in the left side of the face and tongue, and turning of the head to the left side. The sensation ran down the left side of the neck to the arm and leg, and culminated in loss of consciousness and general convulsions. For a few days subsequent to this the patient suffered from headache, and felt generally unwell, but ultimately regained his former condition. For two and a half years, although maintaining his robust health, he was subject to daily recurrences of the paroxysmal twitchings of the left side of the face without loss of consciousness, and also to the more severe general convulsive seizures with loss of consciousness, which occurred on an average about once a month. Six months before admission spasmodic twitchings of the left hand and arm, without loss of consciousness, were observed and these have continued daily, alternating with the already mentioned twitchings of the face, the two, however, rarely occurring at the same time. Shortly afterwards weakness of the left fingers, hand and forearm was experienced, which gradually increased to complete paralysis. Since the upper extremity began to be affected, there had been no recurrence of the general convulsive attacks with loss of consciousness. The patient was able to continue at work till August, 1884, when the weakness of the arm prevented him using his tools. Since then twitching of a like nature has taken place in the left leg, which usually supervenes upon, and is accompanied by, similar attacks in the arm on the same side. Quite recently the left lower extremity has been weak and the patient has walked a little lame.

Present condition.—On examination the patient was found in robust general health. His intelligence was unimpaired. All his organs and functions were normal except those about to be described. He suffered from frequent violent paroxysmal attacks of lancinating pain in the head, not localised but diffused over the vertex. There was nothing abnormal to be detected on the scalp or skull, and there was no special tenderness. On deep and hard pressure there was an area, not strictly defined, which seemed to be more sensitive than the neighbourhood. This was situated in the parietal region, close to the right of the sagittal suture, on a level with a line drawn vertically from the anterior portion of the external meatus of the ear. The movements of the eyeballs and pupils were normal; vision was normal, the patient being able to read No. 3 of Jaeger's types at twelve inches with the left, and No. 5 with the right eye. Examination of the fundi showed all the usual appearances of optic neuritis on both sides, most marked on the right, in the retina of which a number of small haemorrhages were discernible. There was slight comparative immobility of the left side of the face, chiefly elicited by attempts at forced movements. The tongue when protruded pointed slightly to the left. Articulation was normal. The hearing was asserted by the patient to be normal, but was less acute in the right ear. A watch which on the left side was heard at threee feet, was only detected on the right at eight inches. The common sensibility of the head, and the other special senses were normal. There was complete paralysis of the left fingers, thumb and hand. The movements of the elbow-joint were very limited, and those of the shoulder impaired. There was no attempt at supination or pronation of the forearm. There was no trace of rigidity or wasting of the muscles. The irritability to mechanical stimulus of those of the forearm was markedly increased, and the temperature of the skin was lower on the left as compared with the right side. The left lower extremity was stated to be weaker than the right, but, when the patient lay in bed, its movements seemed much the same as those of the other, but were performed with more hesitation and less alacrity. When walking there was slight lameness, the toes were not completely cleared from the ground, so as to necessitate slight swinging of the leg in progression. The limbs were of equal size and the muscles of normal appearance. Their mechanical irritability and the knee-jerk phenomenon were greater on the left side, though somewhat excessive in both. The temperature of both legs was equal. The sensibility of the skin was everywhere normal, and the appearance of both sides of the body was the same.

Progress of the case.—While under observation in the hospital the condition described continued. The patient suffered frequently from paroxysmal attacks of lancinating pains in the head. These lasted sometimes for twelve or more hours at a time, and they were so violent that the patient was occasionally delirious and kept the whole ward disturbed with his cries. There were intervals during which he was entirely free from pain. He also suffered from seizures of very severe sickness not specially associated with the headaches. During these he vomited all food, and when the stomach was empty continued to retch with great violence. This would sometimes last for several days, causing great distress, and much reducing the strength of the patient. During residence in the hospital the attacks of paroxysmal twitchings of the muscles were frequently observed. These occurred many times every day. The most common form was a rhythmical tremor which began in the first, second, and third fingers of the left hand, which afterwards spread to the thumb and wrist as far as the elbow. This continued for perhaps a minute, and then ceased, generally by the limb being held or rubbed.

Another form began in the left angle of the mouth and side of the face, and a feeling as if the tongue was being contracted. These parts also continued to twitch for a minute or two. These two kinds of attacks rarely occurred at the same time, but took place independently of one another. Sometimes, but not commonly, the movements began in the face or arm, extended from the one to the other, and from thence down the side of the neck and body to the leg, so that the whole left side was convulsed without any loss of consciousness. The leg was never observed to be affected by itself.

Diagnosis.—The sequence of events described, with all the circumstances of the case, led to the diagnosis that there was an encephalic growth, probably of limited size, involving the cortex of the brain, and situated at the middle part of the fissure of Rolando.

Treatment.—The patient was ordered the bromide and iodide of potassium, twenty grains of each, thrice daily, which he took for a month. Ice to the head gave no relief, and the vomiting was unrelieved by any treatment. The severe pain was ameliorated by hypodermic injections of morphia.

The terrible sufferings of the patient rendered life intolerable to him. All remedial measures having failed, and as it was obvious that his symptoms were extending, and that a fatal termination was not far distant, it was determined that an attempt be made to remove the morbid lesion. It was hoped that even if such a proceeding was not permanently successful it might alleviate some of the more pressing symptoms. The novelty and risks of the proposed treatment having been fully placed before the patient and his friends, they readily consented to the adoption of any measures which offered any prospects of mitigating the urgent distress or of averting a certain death.

Operation.—In order to expose the cortex of the brain at the middle third of the fissure of Rolando the following procedures were adopted. A longitudinal line was drawn between the frontal and occipital protuberances, down the middle line of the scalp (Fig. 1, *1*). A second line was drawn at right angles to this at the level of the anterior border of the external meatus of the ear (Fig. 1, *2*). Parallel to this a third line was drawn at the level of the posterior border of the mastoid process, which reached the longitudinal line about two inches behind the second (Fig. 1, *3*). From the junction of the first and third lines, a fourth was drawn diagonally downwards, reaching the second at a point two inches above the external meatus (Fig. 1, *4*). This diagonal line was believed to represent the direction of the fissure of Rolando. The spot where theoretically the centre of the trephine should have been placed was about half an inch behind the diagonal, and about one and a half inches from the longitudinal line (Fig. 1, +). As there was a tender point on the scalp about two inches anterior and to the inside of this (Fig. 1, *), it was determined to make the first opening in the skull between the two. (The order and position of the trephine openings are seen in Fig. 1, *a b c*.)

On November 25th, a trephine one inch in diameter was applied to this region (Fig. 1, *a*) and a circle of bone removed. The centre of the aperture was one and a quarter inches from the middle line and half an inch behind a line drawn vertically from the meatus of the ear. The dura mater was found normal in appearance. In this a crucial incison was made, through which the brain substance bulged, as was thought, abnormally. The sur-

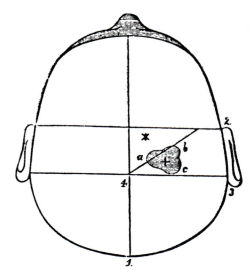

FIG. 1. External surface of scalp. 1, 2, 3, 4. Lines to determine position of fissure of Rolando. + Theoretical and actual position of tumour. * Tender spot on scalp. a, b, c. Position and order of trephine openings.

face appeared somewhat more yellow in colour than natural, but was otherwise apparently as in health. A second trephine opening was made, slightly overlapping the first (Fig. 1, b), external and slightly in front of it, and the angles thus left were rounded off with a chisel and hammer, the brain being protected by a copper spatula. The incision in the dura mater was prolonged, exposing an increased surface of brain but without further revelations. The trephine was applied a third time so as to join the two former openings posteriorly (Fig. 1, c), and when the edges were chipped off a triangular aperture with rounded angles was left, measuring two, by one and three quarter inches. The incision in the dura was then prolonged, exposing a surface of brain nearly the size of the opening in the skull, which presented the same appearance as that already described. Occupying most of this space and crossing it obliquely from above and behind, forwards and downwards, was a convolution, down the posterior aspect of which ran a large blood-vessel. Into the centre of, and parallel with this convolution, an incision about three quarters of an inch in length was made with a scalpel. From an eighth to a quarter of an inch below the surface, a transparent lobulated solid tumour was seen, thinly incapsulated, but perfectly isolated from the surrounding brain substance. After prolonging the incision in the cortex, the surface and sides of the growth were easily separated by means of a narrow spatula of steel so tempered that it could be bent into any shape required. The mass was conical in shape the base being upwards. After its superficial portion was isolated, the finger was, as far as possible, inserted behind the tumour, and attempts made to enucleate it. In doing so the upper half broke across. A large Volkmann's sharp spoon was then employed to scrape out the deeper parts of the growth; and this was continued till all the morbid material was removed and apparently healthy brain matter only remained. This part of the operation was

rendered difficult by the rapid welling of blood into the wound. No artery of any size spouted but there was a general oozing, which accumulated rapidly as soon as the sponge was removed. The cavity thus left was about one and a half inches in depth and of a size into which a pigeon's egg would fit. The hæmorrhage was arrested by applying over the cut surface a suitable electrode from an electro-cautery. The dura mater was then drawn together at its anterior part by a few carbolised silk sutures, and a drainage-tube of moderate calibre, made of india rubber, was inserted into the wound beneath the dura at its posterior border. The skin was brought accurately together, except where the tube lay, by silver wire and silk sutures. During the entire operation the carbolic spray was used, and both before and after, all the ordinary antiseptic precautions were taken.[1] The wound was dressed with carbolic acid gauze, completely covering the scalp, and firmly fixed in position with bandages. During the entire operation, which lasted two hours, the patient took chloroform without a bad symptom, and no nervous phenomena were developed. Subsequent examination proved the tumour to be a glioma about the size of a walnut, presenting the usual microscopical appearances of that disease (Fig. 2).

Progress of the case after operation.—Half an hour after the operation the patient was in the usual drowsy condition which follows the administration of chloroform. He answered questions rationally and comprehended what was said to him. There was no increase of paralysis of the face or tongue, and articulation was as before. There was no trace of movement in any part of

[1] The antiseptic precautions were as follows:—The patient's head having been previously shaved, except the very lowest part of the scalp quite below the occiput, the whole was thoroughly soaked with carbolic acid lotion (1–20), but particular attention was not directed to the sores left from some blisters at the upper part of the neck, which were not noticed till afterwards. After the patient was placed on the table the parts were again washed with 1–20 lotion, and the upper portion of the body was surrounded by carbolised towels, one being also placed beneath the head. Instruments and hands were soaked in the same lotion and the spray was used throughout the operation.

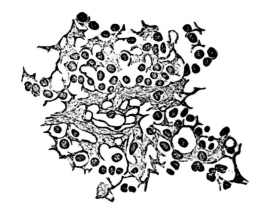

FIG. 2. Structure of glioma, from section by Dr. Hebb, about 400 diam.

the left upper extremity, but the left leg could be moved at will, but to what extent it was not judged advisable to determine. Six hours afterwards the patient was quiet and comfortable. He had taken small quantities of milk and soda water, and had not been sick. Pulse 80, full and regular; temp. 98°. There was no pain in the head and only slight soreness of the wound was complained of. There was slight paresis of the left side of the face and occasional twitchings of both angles of the mouth, the cheeks, and the alæ of the nose. There had been no movements elsewhere.

November 26th (the day after the operation).—Pulse 56, of good strength and regular, morning temp. 98.4°. The patient had recovered from the effects of the anæsthetic, and was now quite sensible and intelligent. There had been occasional vomiting, shooting pains in the head, and twitchings on the left side of the face. During the night a fair amount of nourishment had been taken. The wound was dressed. A small amount of serum had soaked down to the edge of the dressing behind. The edges of the incision were in perfect apposition, and the scalp was quite flat.

27th.—The patient had passed a good night, and slept well. Had no return of vomiting; had occasional twitching of the left arm and side of the face, as well as occasional shooting pains in the head. The morning pulse 54, temp. 97.6°. Passed water, and the bowels acted freely after an enema. Took plenty of fluid nourishment. The patient was quiet, and at time of visit without pain. He was somewhat drowsy and apathetic, but perfectly intelligent, and answered questions with promptitude and accuracy. Articulation was normal. The movements of the eyeballs were natural. The pupils were somewhat dilated, equal, and contracted to light. There was distinct but slight paresis of the left side of the face. The tongue, when protruded, inclined somewhat to the left. The left upper extremity was throughout immovable. The left leg could be raised and pulled up when desired, but for fear of disturbing the patient, the amount of this was not fully tested. The left knee-jerk was markedly increased. The sensibility of the skin was everywhere normal. There had been nowhere any twitchings for the last twenty-four hours. During the day there were occasional shooting pains in the head. The wound was left untouched as there was no appearance of discharge.

28th.—During last night the patient slept fairly well, but was occasionally disturbed by sharp pains in the head. Morning pulse 60, temp. 98.6°. The patient was bright and cheerful. He has had no twitchings of the face or limbs, but had suffered from occasional pains in the head. The paresis of the face was very slight, the articulation natural, and the condition of the limbs as before. He had taken plenty of nourishment. When the wound was dressed the discharge was found to consist of a small amount of thickish pink serum, with an obvious though faint smell. There was a distinct bulging of the scalp at the seat of operation, where it was slightly tender.

29th.—The patient had passed a good night. Morning temp. 98.6°, pulse 76. During the day there was no return of the pains in the head, or twitchings of the limbs. The general condition was as before. The patient was in good spirits, intelligent, and took food well. The left leg could be moved at will. During the evening there was some swelling of the eyelids and face, accompanied with smarting pain. On changing the dressings

the lips of the wound was found swollen, and the discharge had a decidedly putrefactive smell. The lower lateral incision was opened up, and the drainage-tube removed and washed. From the openings some thick brown pus was squeezed. The scalp in the neighbourhood of the wound was somewhat œdematous. Dressings were re-applied as before.

30th.—The general condition was as before, except that to-day there were no movements of the left lower extremity. Morning temp. 99.4°, pulse 88. The swelling of the face and scalp was very considerable. In the morning the drainage-tube and several stitches were removed, and a dressing of wet boracic lint substituted for the gauze. The wound was freely syringed with carbolic lotion (1–20) in which iodoform was suspended. The dressings were changed twice during the day, and on the last occasion all the stiches were removed. By this time there was hardly any trace of putrefactive smell. A hernia cerebri as large as half an orange, consisting of granular looking matter mixed with blood-clot, had protruded through the lips of the wound. Towards evening the swelling of the face and scalp had considerably diminished. At midnight the patient felt quite comfortable.

December 1st.—To-day an extended examination was made. Morning temp. 98.4°, pulse 88. The patient felt well in every respect. He was cheerful, perfectly intelligent, conversed freely, and took an interest in the details of his case. For some time there had been no trace of twitchings of the limbs or pains in the head. The swelling of the face and scalp had almost disappeared. The pupils were equal and normal. Vision was normal. The movement of the eyeballs was natural. The skin was cool and moist. The mouth and face were drawn slightly to the right on forced movement, and the tongue was protruded slightly to the left; articulation and hearing were as before. There was no movement whatever of any part of the left upper or lower extremities. The sensibility of the skin of the left limbs was considerably diminished to touch, but not lost. The left knee-jerk was still considerably exaggerated as compared to the right. The plantar reflex was the same on both sides. The general condition of the patient was excellent, and his appetite good. The urine was loaded with urates, but otherwise normal. The wound was dressed morning and evening. The hernia, which somewhat increased in size, was freely treated with carbolic acid, iodoform, and a solution of chloride of zinc (gr. xl–℥j). The discharge had almost lost its offensive smell.

2nd.—The general condition as before. Now there was no trace of œdema of the face or scalp. Morning temp. 98.6°, pulse 88. The hernia cerebri appeared to be somewhat larger.

3rd.—The general condition as before. Morning temp. 97.6°, pulse 54. The greater portion of the hernia, which had now reached the size of half a cricket ball, was clipped away with scissors. The parts removed consisted chiefly of granular matter and blood-clot, and apparently contained little true cerebral matter. They had a faint offensive smell. This removal was continued till a surface was reached where the tissues bled freely, which was only very slightly above the level of the scalp. This was freely treated with a strong solution of chloride of zinc and iodoform. The stump was dressed with boracic lint soaked in carbolic lotion, which was tucked under the edges of the flaps. The whole as at former dressings was enveloped in a mass of salicylic wool and firmly bandaged. Immediately after the dressing the temperature was 100°. In the evening when the wound was dressed again the discharge was found copious and watery.

4th.—The general condition as before. Morning temp. 98.4°, pulse 88. A cap of block tin was fitted over the hernia which bled slightly from small points all over its surface. The discharge was diminished and now quite odourless.

13th.—During the last ten days the general condition of the patient had continued to improve. On examination to-day he felt well in every respect. There had been no pain in the head or twitchings in the face or limbs. The appetite was excellent and all the organic functions were normally performed. The disposition was cheerful and the intelligence perfect. The patient conversed all day with the nurse, who could detect no signs of mental failure. There was still slight paresis of the left side of the face and tongue. The movements of the eyeballs were normal. The pupils were equal, and contracted normally to light and accommodation. Vision was apparently normal, and No. 7 of Jaeger's types could be read with the right and No. 4 with the left eye at twelve inches in rather a bad light. The optic neuritis still existed in both eyes, but was distinctly improved, the hæmorrhages in the right having almost completely disappeared, and the swelling of the left disc being almost gone. The sensibility of the face was normal and all the special senses were as before the operation. The entire left upper extremity still remained completely paralysed, the muscles being limp and flaccid and without trace of rigidity. The left lower limb was also without voluntary movement. The sensibility of the skin of the entire left side, below the neck, was diminished to touch, but not altogether lost. The temperature of both sides was nearly the same. The mechanical irritability of the muscles and the tendon-reflexes on the left side were increased as compared to those on the right, and on the left there was well-marked ankle clonus. There was nowhere any rigidity or wasting of the muscles.

During the last ten days there was no essential change in the wound, except from day to day a gradual increase in size of the hernia. This now projected about an inch above the scalp. Its surface was smooth and clean, and the discharge was copious, colourless, and odourless. The margins of the mass were clipped away so that no mechanical obstruction might be offered to the contraction of the flaps, which process seemed to be in progress. In doing so a vascular part was soon reached, and a clear fluid in considerable quantity exuded. The deep surface of the flaps was covered with healthy granulations.

16th.—The patient continued well till last night, when he was restless, and felt his left arm and leg very cold. About six this morning he was seized with a rigor which lasted five minutes. Soon afterwards he suffered from shooting pains in the head and was very sick. Five hours after, the temperature was 100.2°, the pulse 100. The patient complained of severe pain in the frontal region. He was dull, apathetic, and nauseated. There were twitchings in the right arm and leg, and occasionally slight ones on both sides of the face. Until to-day there had been little change in the wound, except that the flaps were gradually drawing together and tending to cut off the superficial part of the hernia. This

morning it was found that the hernial mass had greatly increased in size. It was now rugged and of a dark colour. Attempts to remove portions of it were prevented by the profuse hæmorrhage. There was no putrefactive smell. In the evening it was found that the patient during the day had suffered much from pain in the head and vomiting. A hypodermic injection of morphia had been given in the afternoon, which had produced sleep for several hours. The temp. was 102.2°, the pulse 100. Later the temp. was 104.6°, the pulse 140.

17th.—Morning temp. 102.6°, pulse 140. Passed a very restless night, suffering much pain in the head, and in the right arm and leg. Was found pale and dull and very feverish. The patient understood what was said to him, but was slow to answer, and his replies were not easily understood. Another injection of morphia was given without inducing sleep or relieving pain. The hernia was found to have greatly increased in size, and was again about the size of half a cricket ball.

18th.—The patient passed a fairly quiet night. Morning temp. 101.2°, pulse 140. Has had little or no pain in the head, was quite intelligent and answered questions sensibly. There were no twitchings or increase of paralysis. He was feverish and very thirsty, but continued to take a good amount of fluid nourishment. The hernia was breaking down by a sloughing process, and a considerable quantity of semi-fluid detritus flowed from the cavities forming in the mass. This had again a slight putrefactive smell.

19th.—The general condition was the same as yesterday. The hernia was clipped off almost to a level with the bone, and a flat plate was placed and secured over the stump. In the evening the patient was very feverish and very talkative. He volubly related incidents in his past life, and carried on conversations quite sensibly with imaginary persons. He was very restless and had no sleep. He was intelligent and answered questions correctly. Articulation was somewhat thick and indistinct. There was no apparent increase of paralysis, and the right limbs moved freely as before. He still continued to take plenty of nourishment. Evening temp. 103.6°, pulse 150.

20th.—Has had no sleep for twenty-four hours. Was still very restless and feverish, but had no pain. Was evidently weaker, but there were no new symptoms. Temp. 104°, pulse 150. When the eyelids were opened both eyes were seen deviating to the left, but could be voluntarily fixed in a straight line. No change in the wound.

21st.—The patient was evidently sinking. He was emaciated and a bedsore had developed on the right gluteal region. Still feverish, restless, and sleepless. He continued to talk volubly with a thick indistinct utterance. Temp. 104.4°, pulse 144, very weak. Was perfectly sensible. Bowels relaxed and motions passed involuntarily in bed. There was a general tremor of all the limbs, and the right side occasionally twitched.

22nd.—Had gradually become weaker. The breath had a sweatish smell and the skin a yellowish waxy appearance. The articulation was so indistinct as to be unintelligible. Had no pain, no sleep, was very feverish, and now refused food. Was still perfectly sensible.

23rd.—Since last report gradually sank, and died at 8 a.m. this morning. No new symptoms occurred and the patient was sensible to the end. The condition of the wound continued as last described.

The post-mortem examination (December 24th, thirty

hours after death).—The body throughout was thin but not greatly emaciated. There was no special muscular wasting, the rigor mortis was well marked, and the skin was everywhere of a pale yellow colour and of waxy appearance. On the most prominent part of the left gluteal region was a circular patch three inches in diameter, of black discolouration. On cutting across and into this, it was found to extend an inch in depth into the tissues, including a portion of muscle. On the right parietal region was an open wound of the scalp. This was of an irregular quadrilateral shape and measured three by two and a half inches. It reached to within half an inch of the middle line of the skull and its direction in its longest axis lay between this and the posterior margin of the ear. The edges were somewhat raised, everted, covered with healthy granulations, and for a quarter of an inch free, beyond which the skin was adherent to the bone. Elsewhere the scalp was healthy, and there were no signs of pus or putrefactive smell. The space between the edges of the wound was filled up by the base of the hernia which had been shaved off. This spread over the surface of the bone to which it was adherent, and had to be cut away with the knife. The removal of this exposed the aperture in the skull made by the trephine. This was of triangular shape with blunt rounded angles and measured two, by one and three quarter inches. Its longer axis lay almost exactly between the parietal protuberance and the central line of the skull, reaching to within about half an inch of both. The edge of the bone was perfectly healthy and presented the appearance of a clean cut. The skull cap was removed in the usual manner and the brain and cord were taken out, when it was seen that the inner aspect of the arachnoid at the base of the cranium was lined by a layer of pale yellow, coagulated, recent lymph. This was most abundant in the right middle fossa and over the base of the sphenoid bone. It also extended for a short way down the spinal canal. The dura mater of the base was somewhat thickened but otherwise normal.

The brain.—On inspecting the base of the brain a thin layer of lymph was found spread over the surface of the arachnoid. This was most abundant over the base of the right temporo-sphenoidal lobe, over the pons and medulla, and down the upper part of the spinal cord for about an inch. It reached forwards, but less in amount, to the bases of the frontal lobes, sideways to the inner edge of the left temporo-sphenoidal lobe, and backwards as far as the anterior border of the cerebellum. The outer edges of the cerebellum, most of the left temporo-sphenoidal lobe, and the under surface of the frontal lobes were entirely free from the effusion. This deposit of lymph extended from the base of the brain over the right temporo-sphenoidal lobe, and could then be followed by a tract about an inch wide to the under surface of the wound, from which it evidently emanated. The membranes covering the under surface of the right temporo-sphenoidal lobe were markedly congested and their vessels dilated. There was also slight injection of those at the under surface of the cerebellum. Elsewhere the membranes of the base were healthy. The convolutions of the base of the brain were everywhere normal in appearance, except that those of the right temporo-sphenoidal lobe were somewhat more flat and the sulci less deep than those of the opposite side. The consistency of the cortex was here everywhere intact, except a patch of slight softening about the size

of a sixpenny piece at the most anterior extremity of the temporo-sphenoidal lobe. The external surface of the dura mater covering the hemispheres was on both sides normal in appearance, except over the right parietal region, where the wound had been made, through which protruded the base of the hernia cerebri. This corresponded almost exactly in size, shape, and position with the aperture in the skull and measured two and a half by two inches. The free edge of the dura was adherent all round to the cut surface of the bone. On reflecting this from the brain it was found normal in every respect on the left side. On the right it was somewhat thickened throughout, and very considerably so immediately round the wound, especially behind and below. Here also in several places there were recent adhesions of the two layers of the arachnoid which were readily torn across without force. Traces of lymph were found scattered over the whole hemisphere, but chiefly over the occipital and temporo-sphenoidal lobes. It was most abundant in a narrow tract stretching from the lower border of the wound, proceeding downwards to the base of the brain as already described. Above and in front of the wound there was no appearance of inflammatory exudation. Throughout the left side there was slight subarachnoid effusion. The anterior lobes were pale and normal in colour. Behind a vertical line drawn through the bases of the frontal convolutions the membranes at the upper part of the cerebrum were of a pinker colour, and their vessels more injected with blood, than in front and below; otherwise their appearance was normal. The convolutions on this side appeared to be slightly flattened and the sulci somewhat shallow, otherwise they were normal. On the right side the membranes above and in front of the wound were precisely the same as on the left. Behind and below, and especially over the superior part of the temporo-sphenoidal convolutions, they were intensely congested. The convolutions of the frontal and parietal regions on this side, both in appearance and consistency, were in all respects the same as those on the other, and they were equally voluminous on both sides, but the parietal area had a shrunken appearance as if it had fallen inwards. In the centre of this, and occupying the position of the fissure of Rolando, was the wound in the brain. It corresponded in position to the hole in the skull, but was a trifle larger, measuring two and a half by two inches, the longest axis being directed somewhat obliquely from above downwards.

The destruction of the cerebral cortex is illustrated in the accompanying diagrams (Figs. 3 and 4), and will be seen to involve, first, the entire length and thickness of the ascending parietal convolution with the exception of a small portion of its superior and inferior extremities, both of which remained intact; secondly, almost the entire upper third of the ascending frontal convolution, and the posterior portion of its upper half; and thirdly, the anterior third of the gyrus supramarginalis. This deficiency in the grey matter was occupied by the rough material constituting the stump of the hernia cerebri which projected about half an inch beyond the surface of the brain. Surrounding and closely adjacent to this on its anterior, superior, and posterior aspects, the cerebral cortex was normal in appearance and firm in consistency. The margin of the aperture in the grey matter was sharply cut, slightly folded inwards, and its inner edges were adherent to the hernia. At the

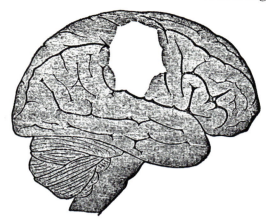

FIG. 3. Diagram showing position and extent of cerebral cortex destroyed as seen from without. The white space occupied by stump of hernia cerebri.

inferior border of the wound the convolutions, although normal in appearance, were slightly softened to the touch, and this softening extended as so to include the superior temporo-sphenoidal convolution, below which the cortex was of firm and normal consistence. On the inner aspect of the right hemisphere there was a circular depression, about the size of a sixpenny piece, without softening, and which appeared as if the part had fallen inwards. This involved the terminal portion of the fissure of Rolando, and a part of the sulcus caloso-marginalis, a small portion of the gyrus fornicatus, the posterior part of the marginal convolution, and the anterior border of the quadrilateral lobule. A transverse section was made across the brain through the ascending parietal convolution in the direction of the fissure of Rolando. The deficiency in the cortex is seen in Fig. 4 to consist of complete absence of that part which corresponds to the middle parietal fasciculus with the inferior portion of the superior, and the superior portion of the inferior parietal fasciculi. The spaces thus left had partially collapsed, and were filled with new formation from which the hernia cerebri sprang. This morbid condition had in an irregular and unequal manner spread inwards, reaching as far as the upper margins of the corpus callosum and internal capsule. The brain having undergone the process of hardening it was not easy to exactly limit the softening, which seemed to be confined entirely to the centrum ovale. The lower portion of the inferior, and the inner portion of the superior parietal fasciculi were uninjured. So also were the insular lobe, the internal and external capsules, the corpus callosum, the optic thalamus, and the lenticular and caudate nuclei. Whether the lateral ventricle had been opened into it is difficult to say. There was no collection of foreign matter in its interior; at the same time the morbid process had extended in close proximity to it.

A histological examination of the different tissues was made by Dr. Hebb, who reported their condition to be as follows:

"The appearance of a section of the glioma has already been referred to (Fig. 2). The hernia cerebri and subjacent tissues consisted of blood-clot, granular matter, and disorganised nervous tissue. The cortex in the neighbourhood of the wound presented the appearance of inflammatory change in its pia mater and superficial layer, but was otherwise normal. Elsewhere the structure of the brain was healthy, and nowhere was there any evidence of gliomatous disease. The retinæ and optic nerves presented all the usual appearances of neuroretinitis in a well marked but not advanced stage. The membranes of the cord had undergone marked change. The inter-meningeal space at the upper cervical region was filled with pus. In the cervical and dorsal regions the membrane was considerably thickened, which condition gradually diminished from above downwards. In the grey matter of the cord there was evidence of nuclear activity, apparently of quite recent origin, otherwise it was healthy. There was no trace of descending sclerosis."

Commentary.—In commenting on the preceding series of facts it will be convenient to discuss the points of interest under the following heads: (1) Diagnosis, (2) the surgical treatment, (3) the clinical phenomena after the operation, (4) revelations of the autopsy, physiologically and pathologically considered.

1. *Diagnosis.*—All the circumstances of this case pointed to an encephalic growth on the right side. This was more especially evidenced by the slow and insidious invasion of the symptoms, the gradual progress and special distribution of the paralysis, the violent intracranial pain, the uncontrollable attacks of vomiting, and the double optic neuritis. Whether a tumour on the right side of the brain was caused by the blow on the left side of the head a year previous to the development of the first signs of ill-heath, must remain uncertain.

It was also concluded that the morbid lesion involved the cortical substance, because certain motor phenomena were developed, and certain motor districts implicated after a definite method and in definite order; the paralysis was unaccompanied by any alterations in sensibility; and above all, because of the existence of certain paroxysmal seizures of local convulsion, without loss of consciousness, which were eminently suggestive of irritation of cerebral grey matter.

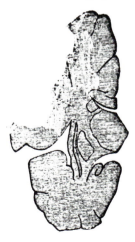

FIG. 4. Diagram of transverse section through ascending parietal convolution showing destruction of cerebral cortex and corona radiata. The white space occupied by granular matter of hernia cerebri.

The special seat of the lesion was further believed to be the middle part of the right fissure of Rolando. This conclusion was arrived at by the consideration of the combined revelations of physiological experiment and clinical observation. After centuries of doubt and confusion on the subject of cerebral localisation, quite recent investigations have at last rendered it certain that around this sulcus are grouped those nervous areas which preside over the movements of the other side of the body. Adopting the topography of the brain constructed by Professor Ferrier as the result of his well-known researches, it may be said in general terms, that the motor centres which govern the voluntary movements of the lips and tongue are situated in the lower portions of the ascending parietal and frontal convolutions. Higher up in the same gyri are the areas for the muscles of the face. Occupying the middle portion and nearly the whole extent of the ascending parietal convolution are the centres of the fingers and hand. In the middle of the ascending frontal convolution are those elements which originate movements of the arm and upper arm, including flexion, pronation, and supination of the forearm. At the superior and posterior aspect of the ascending parietal convolution is the centre for the lower extremity, and at the upper and anterior portion of the ascending frontal convolution are centres for complex movements of both the upper and lower limbs. Now, in the case before us there was complete paralysis of the fingers and hand, with inability to pronate and supinate the forearm, there was partial paresis of the movements of the elbow, and weakness of those of the shoulder-joint. There was also slight paresis of the leg and one side of the face. Accompanying all these there were paroxysmal convulsions in all these regions, occurring either singly or in definite order one after the other. These phenomena were to be accounted for by an extensive but not absolutely complete destruction of the motor centres of the fingers, hand, and forearm, with slight encroachment on, and irritation of, those of the face, upper arm, and leg. A very definite localisation of the disease was thus permitted, and the tumour was pronounced to have occupied the whole thickness of the middle two fourths of the ascending parietal convolution, and a portion of the adjoining upper half of the ascending frontal convolution. The morbid lesion, whilst almost completely destroying these areas, in addition modified the functions and caused irritation of those in their neighbourhood, without seriously involving their structure, namely, the superior and inferior extremities of the ascending parietal and frontal convolutions, and the postero-parietal lobule.

Having thus accurately localised the position of the tumour its size could as a consequence be approximated. Assuming the disease to be limited to the cortex at the point already indicated, the fact that the centres of the leg above, of the face and tongue below, of the sense of sight behind, and of the movements of the eyeballs in front, were not seriously involved, proved that the growth was of limited size. A glance at the relative position and size of the convolutions of the human cerebrum indicate that a foreign body occupying such a position could not, roughly speaking, exceed some two inches in diameter. It was probable that the growth took its origin in the lower third of the ascending parietal convolution, and as it increased in size spread upwards and backwards, further involving its substance

and part of the ascending frontal convolution, finally reaching the lower edge of the postero-parietal lobule. Such disease might therefore be represented by an ovoid mass the size and shape of a pigeon's egg, lying obliquely in the fissure of Rolando. This theoretical reasoning arrived at before the operation, subsequently proved to have been substantially correct.

The question finally arose whether the tumor was confined to the cortex or whether it was situated in the centrum ovale below, and from thence invaded the grey matter. It was not forgotten that a slowly-growing mass, reaching considerable dimensions, might develop in the conducting elements of the brain, without causing symptoms capable of exact definition. It was also fully recognised that a small tumour immediately under the cortex and involving its under surface might cause precisely the same symptoms as one limited to the grey matter. From an operative point of view the existence of even a large growth, which in this case was improbable, would not necessarily interfere with the procedure, because in that case little harm could be done to the life of the patient, and his urgent symptoms, on the other hand, might be relieved by the simple process of trephining. If the tumour was small the grey matter could be incised and the mass removed. As a matter of fact this last is what actually was done in the case under consideration, the growth being found in the centrum ovale, under the cortex, involving the convolutions before determined.

As to the probable nature of the tumour, the age of the patient, the absence of syphilis, and the slow growth of the disease suggested glioma, but on this point no definite conclusions were hazarded.

2. *The surgical treatment.*—For the purpose of removing the tumour from the brain, three trephine holes were made in the skull, because after the first piece of bone was taken away and no superficial disease discovered, it was thought advisable to enlarge the opening, to further expose the brain and to make room for completing the operation. The aperture made by the three removals, even when the angles were chipped off, only measured $2 \times 1\frac{3}{4}$ inches. The tumour was found exactly in the centre of the opening, and in the position corresponding with theoretical calculation and measurement. It had no relation whatever to the tender spot on the skull, and, had attention been confined exclusively to that, the result would have been entirely misleading. The process of trephining involved no difficulties, but it exemplified the advantages of the chisel and hammer over Hay's saw for rounding off corners of bone. In similar operations it might be advisable in the future to employ a larger trephine. One convolution only being exposed during the operation, there was at the time some question as to whether it was the ascending frontal or parietal. This doubt arose from the circumstance that in the attempt to approach the tender spot, the theoretical position had been slightly departed from, and the trephine advanced and raised, so as to come between the two. Accordingly for the moment this convolution was thought to be the ascending frontal, the aperture in the bone being so small that its relations could not be seen. After death, however, it was apparent that the convolution which had been incised was that in which from the first the disease had been diagnosed to exist, namely, the ascending parietal. There was no external appearance of disease about this part of the cortex except that it seemed swollen, less

glossy, and less vascular than natural. An incision into this showed the morbid growth to be immediately under the surface, and almost completely involving the entire thickness of the cortex. On clearing the superficial parts of the growth, a small spatula, neither sharp nor blunt, and so tempered that it would keep any shape given it, was found a most serviceable instrument. Such is preferable to the use of the cautery, as the latter so chars the parts as to modify their natural appearance, and thus prevent a differentiation between healthy and diseased tissues. It may be questioned whether it was advisable to arrest the hæmorrhage from the interior of the wound by means of the galvanocautery. Such a proceeding leads of necessity to the formation of a considerable amount of detritus which may afterwards prove detrimental. The bleeding moreover was not severe and would no doubt have become arrested by natural means. The advisability of introducing a drainage-tube may also be questioned. It was not judged safe to completely close so large a wound, distended as it must have been with accumulated serum and blood. Moreover, had putrefaction not occurred it is not likely that the soft india-rubber tube would have caused any serious irritation. The argument in favour of complete closure of the wound, so strongly advocated by those whose experience is confined to operations on the brains of monkeys, is, it is maintained, not convincing when applied to a large injury in the human subject, the more rapid healing of the tissues of the lower animals being a matter of common knowledge. Another point of doubt is the propriety of introducing sutures into the dura mater. The most important matter for discussion, however, is the occurrence of putrefaction, which undoubtedly appeared in the wound some days after the operation. This, it may be maintained, was the cause of the inflammation and consequent hernia cerebri. All the usual antiseptic precautions were taken during the operation, and the only flaws in its strict application which suggest themselves are, first, that the scalp was not sufficiently purified prior to the operation, and second, that no special measures were taken to carbolise the galvanocautery apparatus. In future operations of this nature it is strongly urged that surgeons should not only employ carbolic acid, but also a solution of corrosive sublimate as antiseptics, and that the scalp should not only be rubbed with these, but soaked with them for some hours previously. There may have been other sources of septic contagion in the washing of the sponges, or from the blisters on the neck which escaped observation. It may be doubted whether the putrefaction was ever completely subdued; the fact of the meningitis occurring at last, and that of a smell having again become apparent after the attempt at removal of the second protrusion, point probably to a continued septic infection. As to the hernia two observations only have to be made. First, it was remarkable that the discharge continued for such a long time to be so copious and so watery, which suggested the idea of its being cerebrospinal fluid. Secondly, there was a difficulty in shaving if off owing to the enormous size of its base, and to the danger of serious hæmorrhage.

3. *Clinical phenomena following the operation.*—The patient, on recovery from the effects of chloroform after the operation, was found perfectly intelligent, the former pain in the head, and violent twitchings in the limbs, had disappeared and never returned, there was no increase of the paralysis of the face or leg, and all the organic functions remained normal. The only change which had taken place was completion of the paresis of the upper extremity, which was now paralysed throughout. This was evidently due to the unavoidable destruction of the remaining arm centres in the removal of the tumour. Otherwise the neighbouring brain matter had not been injured, as was evidenced by all other functions remaining intact. The surgical operation itself in no way injured the nervous centres with the exceptions mentioned, while it immediately relieved all the distressing symptoms. This satisfactory condition remained unchanged for four days, when the discharge from the wound was found to have a putrid smell. Coincident with this began the hernia cerebri, and following its development, arose fresh symptoms in the shape of paresis of the left leg and partial anæsthesia of one half of the body. These were probably due to the effects of simple pressure, and possibly to the subsequent secondary softening of the conducting fibres caused by it. That the inflammatory condition which led to this was purely local was shown by the fact that, with the above exception, the condition of the patient remained in all respects as before the operation. The temperature never reached 100° or the pulse 100 beats per minute. The intelligence was absolutely intact and the appetite and general condition in every respect satisfactory. The patient had lost all pains in his head, all traces of twitchings of the limbs, and all his severe attacks of vomiting. Even the double optic neuritis had markedly diminished. This state continued daily to improve till the twenty-first day, when suddenly the patient was seized with a rigor followed by fever and all the symptoms of meningitis from which he died a week afterwards. This inflammation was afterwards seen to be local and due to septic matter from the wound causing irritation of certain areas of the cerebral membranes. If putrefaction was the sole cause of this condition, hope may be entertained that by its prevention in other cases a more satisfactory termination may be looked for. Although meningitis continued to a fatal end, no new nervous symptoms supervened, the absence of which was probably due to the presence of a hole in the skull, through which excess of pressure was relieved.

4. *Revelations of the autopsy.*—After death, inspection of the parts showed that the brain was practically everywhere healthy except the area injured by the operation and the membranes in its immediate neighbourhood. From its lower border a narrow tract of recently effused lymph extended downwards by the temporo-sphenoidal lobe towards the base of the skull, over a large portion of which it spread, leaving the adjacent parts heathy. It was therefore obvious that this condition was produced by irritating matter from the interior of the wound, flowing downwards between the layers of the arachnoid, accumulating at the base, and by its presence causing meningitis in its track. The local inflammation of the wound had so opened out the parts and separated the adhesions as to permit the discharge to percolate into the cranial cavity, but not till three weeks after the operation. Had this not occurred there is no reason why the healing process should not have been maintained, and the entire wound become ultimately cicatrised. The patient would then have continued permanently in a satisfactory condition, and escaped the secondary and fatal complication. The recovery from serious surgical injuries to the brain-sub-

stance of man, as well as experimental researches on that of animals, show that such a termination is perfectly possible.

The cortical substance at the edges of the wound in the brain was firm and healthy, except at the inferior border, which was slightly softened, probably from infiltration of the meningeal effusion. The deficiency in the grey matter was clearly defined and the portions of absent convolutions could be accurately limited. On the subject of central localisation only general conclusions can be drawn, as the destruction was not limited to the cortex, but in great part was situated in the centrum ovale below. The fibres, however, thus injured were those corresponding to the grey matter above, and may therefore be said to represent the conducting media of the higher centres. The symptoms immediately before the death of the patient, as far as they go, entirely harmonise with those which have already been determined by experimental inquiry to arise from corresponding lesions of cortical matter, with others superadded, which can be easily explained by the processes of pressure and softening in the neighbourhood. The inferior extremities of the ascending frontal and parietal convolutions being found only very slightly involved, accounts for the almost total absence of orolingual symptoms during life. The almost total destruction of the remainder of the ascending parietal convolution explains the complete paralysis of the fingers and hand, and the partial paresis of the face. The lesion of the middle third of the ascending frontal convolution produced the immobility of the elbow- and shoulder-joints, and the loss of pronation and supination in the forearm. The almost complete immunity from disease of the lower part of this gyrus permitted the nearly natural movements of the face, lips, and tongue during life. The bases of the three frontal convolutions were perfectly healthy, but a day or two before death temporary conjugate deviation of the eyeballs was observed, both being turned towards the left, which was probably due to irritation of these regions by the neighbouring disease. At no time was there any paralysis of the muscles of the eyeballs. The postero-parietal lobule was found almost intact, its anterior margin only being involved in the wound. For some days after the operation the patient moved his left leg freely, and it was only after the appearance of the hernia that the limb became paralysed. This was therefore due not to destruction of the cortical centre of the lower extremity, but to pressure and softening within the wound. This was evidenced by the sinking in of the healthy convolutions on the inner aspect of the hemisphere at a point exactly corresponding with the situation of the conducting fibres of this region. The anterior portion of the supra-marginal gyrus was absent. This convolution Professor Ferrier associates with the sense of sight. In this case there was no evidence of any serious impairment of vision or hemiopia, although the patient saw better with the left than with the right eye. There was, however, double optic neuritis, most marked on the right side. The deficiency in sight was evidently due to this and not to a central lesion, in which case the weakness of vision would have been chiefly in the opposite or left eye. It is therefore probable that no appreciable loss of function could be attributed to the disorganisation of a portion of the right supra-marginal gyrus. It is, however, to be observed that the convolution was only partially destroyed, and Professor Ferrier has shown

that even when it is completely obliterated on one side the consequent blindness on the other is only temporary, the opposite centre apparently rapidly compensating for the loss. Shortly before death the patient, though sensible, talked very volubly, carried on conversation with imaginary persons, and recited the most elaborate and yet perfectly coherent adventures. May these not have been the result of visual hallucinations, and due to irritation of this centre?[1]

Although the right superior temporo-sphenoidal convolution was somewhat softened it was not so to any great extent, and it was probably recent and due to mechanical infiltration. During life the hearing of the left ear was perfect. The comparative deafness on the right side was due to deficiency in the auditory apparatus and not to a central lesion.

The destruction of the centrum ovale for the main part corresponded with that of the cortical substance above. Its exact limits were difficult to define owing to the gradual softening in the neighbourhood. The internal capsule, corpus callosum and basal ganglia were, however, intact. So also was the remainder of the brain. The intellect, other senses, with all the organs and functions of the body except those already detailed, remained normal till the last.

Such are the main points of interest and reflections concerning a case which throughout has been a source of great anxiety and responsibility. This has chiefly been due to the fact that we have not had the advantage of any precedent of a like nature to guide us in our methods of procedure. Operations on the brain-substance have not been uncommon in the history of medicine, but these have hitherto been performed either for the relief of surgical injuries, or for disease indicated by local manifestations. We have nowhere been able to discover the recorded example of a case where a cerebral tumour was diagnosed by the symptoms observed, without visible or tangible external signs, and was in consequence operated on and successfully removed. Since this has been accomplished in the present instance, the public papers have asserted that the same has already been carried out on several occasions in the Royal Infirmary of Glasgow. To this it can only be said that up to the present date no report of such proceedings is to be found in medical or scientific literature.

In conclusion, we would observe that, although unfortunately in this instance life was not permanently preserved, the experience we have gained by this case leads us to the belief that there is an encouraging prospect for the future of cerebral medicine and surgery, and that as a tumour of the brain can be diagnosed with precision and successfully removed without immediate danger to life, we confidently anticipate that under more favourable circumstances the operation will be performed with lasting benefit to the patient.

Although brain tumors had been removed prior to this one reported by Bennett and Godlee,[10–13,17,18] it is important because it was better publicized[2–7,19,22,23] and attracted more attention to the feasibility of the operative

---

[1] In connection with the sense of sight, the fact may be noted that the optic neuritis was most severe on the side of the cerebral lesion.

removal of intracranial growths, even when localized solely by neurological examination.[1,8,9,14–16,20,21] The abstracted discussion of this case by Hughlings Jackson, David Ferrier, William Macewen, and Victor Horsley,[5] as well as the reports by Macewen[18] and Francesco Durante[12] of their first tumor excisions, will be reprinted in a forthcoming issue of the *Journal of Neurosurgery*.

REFERENCES

1. ADSON, A. W. The evolution of neurosurgery. *Surgery*, 1949, *25:* 91–100.
2. BENNETT, A. H., and GODLEE, R. J. Excision of a tumour from the brain. *Lancet*, 1884, *2:* 1090–1091.
3. BENNETT, A. H., and GODLEE, R. J. Sequel to the case of excision of a tumour from the brain. *Lancet*, 1885, *1:* 13.
4. BENNETT, A. H., and GODLEE, R. J. Case of cerebral tumour. *Med.-chir. Trans.*, 1885, *68:* 243–275.
5. BENNETT, A. H., and GODLEE, R. J. Case of cerebral tumour. [Abst.] With discussion by Jackson, H., Ferrier, D., Macewen, W., and Horsley, V. *Brit. med. J.*, 1885, *1:* 988–989.
6. BENNETT, A. H., and GODLEE, R. J. Case of cerebral tumour. [Abst.] With discussion by Jackson, H., Ferrier, D., Macewen, W., and Horsley, V. *Proc. roy. med. chir. Soc. Lond.*, 1882–1885, n.s. *1:* 438–444.
7. BRAMWELL, E. Alexander Hughes Bennett and the first recorded case in which an intracranial tumour was removed by operation. *Edinb. med. J.*, 1935, n.s. *42:* 312–315.
8. BROWDER, J. Advances in neurological surgery during the past fifty years. *Amer. J. Surg.*, 1941, *51:* 164–187.
9. CALVERT, C. A. The development of neurosurgery. *Ulster med. J.*, 1946, *15:* 123–140.
10. DURANTE, F. Estirpazione di un tumore endocranico: (forma morbosa prima e dopo l'operazione). *Boll. Accad. med., Roma*, 1885, *11:* 247–252.
11. DURANTE, F. Estirpazione di un tumore endocranico. *Arch. Soc. ital. Chir.*, 1885, *2:* 252–255.
12. DURANTE, F. Contribution to endocranial surgery. *Lancet*, 1887, *2:* 654–655.
13. DURANTE, F. Contribution to endocranial surgery. *Trans. int. Congr. Med. [Wash.]*, 1887, *1:* 570–571.
14. GODLEE, R. J. On the antiseptic system, as seen in Professor Lister's wards at Edinburgh. *Lancet*, 1873, *1:* 694–695; 729–731.
15. GREEN, R. E., and STERN, W. E. Techniques of intracranial surgery. In: *A history of neurological surgery*. A. E. Walker, Ed. Baltimore: Williams & Wilkins Co., 1951, xii, 583 pp. (see pp. 80–110).
16. HORRAX, G. Neurosurgery. An historical sketch. *Springfield, Ill.: Charles C Thomas*, 1952, xi, 135 pp.
17. MACEWEN, W. Tumour of the dura mater—convulsions—removal of tumour by trephining—recovery. *Glasgow med. J.*, 1879, n.s. *12:* 210–213.
18. MACEWEN, W. Intra-cranial lesions, illustrating some points in connexion with the localisation of cerebral affections and the advantages of antiseptic trephining. III. Tumour of dura mater. *Lancet*, 1881, *2:* 581–582.
19. POWER, D. Some bygone operations in surgery. VIII. The first localized cerebral tumour. *Brit. J. Surg.*, 1932, *19:* 523–526.
20. SACHS, E. The history and development of neurological surgery. *New York: P. B. Hoeber, Inc.*, 1952, 158 pp.
21. SCARFF, J. E. Fifty years of neurosurgery, 1905–1955. *Int. Abstr. Surg.*, 1955, *101:* 417–513.
22. THORWALD, J. The triumph of surgery. R. Winston and C. Winston, Transl. *New York: Pantheon Books, Inc.*, 1960, xi, 454 pp.
23. TROTTER, W. A landmark in modern neurology. *Lancet*, 1934, *2:* 1207–1210.

Neurosurgical Classics—30, 31 and 32

In the August 1962 issue of the *Journal of Neurosurgery* the "Case of Cerebral Tumour" reported in 1885 by A. H. Bennett and R. J. Godlee was reprinted and relevant references were given. In the present issue the abstracted discussion of this case by Hughlings Jackson, David Ferrier, William Macewen and Victor Horsley is reprinted, together with the reports by Macewen and Francesco Durante of their first excisions of intracranial tumor, which preceded Godlee's operation.

ROYAL MEDICAL AND CHIRURGICAL SOCIETY*

Tuesday, May 12th, 1885

GEORGE JOHNSON, M.D., F.R.S., President, in the Chair

Case of Cerebral Tumour. By A. HUGHES BENNETT, M.D. *The Surgical Treatment.* By RICKMAN J. GODLEE, F.R.C.S.—The chief features of interest in this case were that, during life, the existence of a tumour in the brain was diagnosed, its situation localised, and its size and shape approximated, entirely by the signs and symptoms exhibited, without any manifestations of the growth on the external surface. The growth was removed by a surgical operation, without any immediate injurious results on the intelligence or general condition of the patient, who lived, relieved of his former symptoms, for four weeks, and at the expiration of that time died, not from any special failure of the nervous centres, but from the effects of a secondary surgical complication. . . . The general conclusion arrived at was that, although in this instance life was not permanently preserved, the fact remained that the operation at once removed all the painful and distressing symptoms, without causing any injurious effects on the general health or nervous system of the patient. From the experience gained by this case, as well as from observations in other directions, the authors expressed the opinion that there was a hopeful future for cerebral surgery; and that there was every prospect, in other cases of a similar nature, of permanent relief being afforded, and life prolonged, in a class of disease at the present very distressing, and uniformly fatal.

Dr. HUGHLINGS JACKSON congratulated Dr. Hughes Bennett on the accuracy of his diagnosis. The operation Mr. Godlee performed showed that Dr. Bennett was right in saying that a cerebral tumour might, so far as the operation itself went, be safely removed. The patient,

most unfortunately, died, but he died of a secondary surgical complication. Dr. Hughlings Jackson also warmly congratulated Dr. Ferrier, from whose researches the tumour was localised. Speaking more generally of localisation of cerebral tumour, with regard to trephining, Dr. Hughlings Jackson said that there was a kind of monoplegia, often passing into hemiplegia, which was almost decisive evidence of tumour; a paralysis beginning very locally, for example, in the thumb and index-finger, and spreading very slowly, week by week. In such a case he should not advise trephining, since there would be a great probability of a large tumour in the centrum ovale; not certainly, for he had seen hemiplegia in a case of tumour growing from the dura mater, pressing down on the cortex. The convulsive seizures of localising value were not cases of epilepsy proper, but epileptiform seizures—convulsions beginning one-sidedly and very locally, in the hand, or cheek, or foot. Whilst the seizures pointed with certainty to disease of the opposite cerebral hemisphere, they did not always occur from such gross disease as tumour. In some, there was local softening. When, however, there was also double optic neuritis, such gross disease as tumour might be confidently predicted. Even yet there was not evidence of exact position. Dr. Hughlings Jackson had not yet seen a case of epileptiform seizure caused by disease outside Ferrier's region; but such cases had been recorded by great authorities. Hence, repeating in effect what Charcot and Pitres had urged, we required also some local persisting paralysis of the part convulsed—persisting, since temporary paralysis after a seizure was no further help towards localisation. So far, then, three things were required; local persisting paralysis, epileptiform convulsions, and double optic neuritis. Dr. Hughlings Jackson mentioned the case of a man who had had convulsions and paralysis of one arm; a tumour, a cubic inch in bulk, was found involving the hindermost part of the uppermost frontal convolution. This was before Hitzig and Ferrier's researches; the exact position of the tumour was not diagnosed. That tumour might probably have been removed with safety; yet there was considerable softening. Moreover, there was a tumour in each lateral lobe of the cerebellum, although there had been no cerebellar symptoms. Another case, in which a woman had very many convulsive attacks of one arm (and later wider seizure), was mentioned. In this case Dr. Hughlings Jackson correctly predicted tumour of the hindermost part of the uppermost frontal and adjacent ascending frontal convolutions, but not with the confidence he should have done had Ferrier's researches then been made. The tumour was about an inch in diameter, and had it been removed, very likely the woman's life would have been saved. She had not double optic neuritis, but, making an exception to a former statement, were he to observe a case of repeated convulsions nearly always limited to one arm, exactly alike at each recurrence, he should, even

* Reprinted from *The British Medical Journal*, 1885, 1: 988–989, with the kind permission of the Editor.

without double optic neuritis, consider them to be, in all probability, tumours in the region mentioned. In another case he had correctly diagnosed tumour of the same region, but there were also other tumours in that half of the brain. Admitting difficulties—that the tumour might be very large; that there might be softening about it, that besides the tumour localised there might be others—yet, in a case where the tumour was evidently going to kill the patient, when there was intense pain in the head, and when, as sometimes happened, the patient had twenty or thirty fits a day, the patient would consent to risk something, and a surgeon might justifiably operate. Dr. Hughlings Jackson remarked that, after operation in such cases as he had mentioned, there would, he thought, be some permanent paralysis, but this was little in comparison with the misery of pain, the torment of repeated fits, and great danger of death. In conclusion, Dr. Hughlings Jackson said that in a case of convulsion limited to one arm, or beginning in one leg, with some persisting paralysis of the part first convulsed in the seizure, and double optic neuritis, he should diagnose tumour or other such gross disease of the upper part of the Rolandic region, and should seek surgical advice as to the propriety of trephining, not forgetting to state prominently the three difficulties mentioned.

Professor FERRIER had seen the case in question before, during, and after, the operation, and congratulated Dr. Bennett and Mr. Godlee on the large measure of their success. The operation, as an operation, was wonderfully successful, and was borne without any serious depression. He had always maintained that as possible; for he thought the operations on man not more or less serious than on animals, and his own experiments on animals had included many in which, with careful precautions, inflammation had not resulted. As bearing on treatment by trephining, he cited a case from his patients in King's College Hospital this year. The man had grave symptoms, gradually increasing to complete paralysis of the left side, pain in the right frontal region, double optic neuritis, and almost complete coma; the right eyeball was rather fuller than the left. The symptoms were attributed to some growth pressing on the sphenoidal fissure, whether from above or below could not be determined. Sir Joseph Lister agreed to make an exploratory operation. As soon as the dura mater was incised, the brain bulged out, and, as soon as he put in his finger, there was a rush of fluid out of what seemed to be a cyst, but was really a very greatly dilated anterior horn of the ventricle. There were great reduction of pressure and relief of paralysis, but no further operation could be attempted. The left arm gained some power, and for a time the coma lessened; but in a week death ensued, not from surgical complications, but from the tumour, which was found to press upwards on the sphenoidal fissure. It would have been reached if the finger had penetrated half an inch deeper, but was too large to be removed. The case, however, showed the safety from surgical complications.

Dr. WILLIAM MACEWEN called attention to some cases which had been referred to by the papers in connection with the case of Dr. Bennett and Mr. Godlee. In 1876, he had seen a case of wound of the frontal region, resulting in symptoms of abscess in the third frontal convolution. He failed to get leave to operate, but after death found that the operation he had planned would have reached the abscess. Since then, he had had a series

of cases, in which the researches of Dr. Hughlings Jackson and Professor Ferrier, and of MM. Charcot and Pitres had greatly assisted him. He read a detailed description of two cases. The first was of a woman aged 25, who had left hemiplegia from syphilis contracted about four years previously. There was first tingling of the left arm and then of the left leg, and afterwards a peculiar sensation of the parts, which the patient called numbness. Lastly, there was gradual loss of power of left arm and left leg; langour and dulness of intelligence. From these he inferred cortical lesions, probably gummata, in the parts controlling arm and leg, namely, the upper half of the ascending frontal convolution and paracentral lobule. After three weeks, he trephined over this region, and found the internal table of the bone removed to be rough, and the dura mater thickened in consequence. Over the surface of the ascending frontal convolution was a yellowish opaque effusion, very friable, this also bridged the fissure of Rolando. Towards the paracentral lobule was a resistant portion, into which incision was made, and followed by a gush of grumous fluid. On the internal table of the bone, osteophytic growths were found, and a second crown of the trephine taken out to remove them. The excised bone was broken up into small pieces, and reimplanted in the brain-tissue; the wound was supplied with a chicken-bone drainage-tube, and the whole carefully dried and dressed with iodoform. In forty-eight hours there was much relief; in a week she could move her toes and fingers, and, in a fortnight, could flex her leg a little. The temperature remained normal, and the dressings were not touched for three weeks; when they were changed, the wound was found to be almost healed, but fresh dressings were kept on for three weeks longer. After two months, she could walk easily, though with a slight dragging of the leg, and since then had grown strong enough for her ordinary household duties. The second case he had not time to describe in detail, but its essential points were the same as in the other. It was after an injury, round which arose an encephalitis and lepto-meningitis. The left arm was paralysed. The skull was trephined, and many minute clots were found in the left ascending frontal convolutions. The recovery was complete. Professor Ferrier had asked how many times he had had hernia cerebri in his cases; he had never had it as the result of an operation, but once it occurred immediately on opening the dura mater, under which there was encephalitis in the motor area. He had operated on seventeen cases for the relief of intracranial pressure; in fourteen by trephining, in three by elevation of the bone; fourteen had recovered. In eleven, he had divided and reimplanted the portions of the excised bone. He should hesitate to use a galvano-cautery to the brain-tissue.

Dr. HUGHES BENNETT thanked the Society for the kind reception they had given to his paper. He had been much interested with Dr. Macewen's cases, but felt obliged to say, with all due deference, that they did not appear to him completely analogous. The chief lesson to be learnt from his own case was that a small lesion could be diagnosed and cut down upon; in Dr. Macewen's cases, the injuries were much more extensive; they were, however, very encouraging to cerebral surgery. He wished to call the attention of the Society to a brain exhibited on the table, taken from a case treated by his colleague Mr. Richard Davy. The skull had been trephined, and eight pieces of bone were extracted from the cortical tissues that had been jammed into them by a severe accident. A cavity resulted, that was big enough to hold a pigeon's egg. The recovery was absolute, but no antiseptics at all had been used; the patient's head lay on a water-pillow, without any dressings; yet there was no encephalitis or meningitis, or softening, only a dense cicatrix. The subsequent death of the patient was in no way due to this injury or operation, but was brought about by an attack of pleuropneumonia.

Mr. VICTOR HORSLEY remarked that the last case Dr. Hughes Bennett had mentioned was not strictly analogous to those cases where the head had not been injured before; for, after injury, adhesion might take place, which would guard the brain against further inflammation. His experience in experiments on animals led him to agree with Professor Ferrier in thinking that animals were as liable to complications of cerebral operations as man. The subcutaneous use of morphia, however, in animals diminished the haemorrhage by about one-half, by inducing contraction of the arterioles, which generally bled freely; and that, he thought, was a hint for the management of cerebral operations in man.

Mr. GODLEE congratulated Dr. Macewen on his interesting and successful cases. His operations led to less haemorrhage, as involving incisions into abscesses, rather than into healthy tissue. He felt a doubt himself whether the use of the galvano-cautery did not lead to inflammation and hernia cerebri, though Dr. Ferrier's case showed that there might be hernia without inflammation. As to the deeper parts of the tumour, they had been lucky in finding a glioma so accurately limited. A salt-spoon would have been a more convenient instrument for removing it than a small and sharp-edged Volkmann's spoon. Professor Ferrier's and Mr. Horsley's experience furnished an *argumentum ad simiam*, but he could not feel justified in admitting that it applied exactly to man. He thought Dr. Macewen's system of drainage deserved consideration, and also his careful attention to the condition of the scalp before the operation. In his own case, he considered putrefaction to have occurred owing to a certain want of care in cleansing the head before the operation; and, if he had to do the same operation again, he should soak the scalp for twenty-four hours in a solution of corrosive sublimate, and afterwards of carbolic acid; and, under such conditions, should not hesitate to undertake a second similar operation.

INTRA-CRANIAL LESIONS,

ILLUSTRATING SOME POINTS IN CONNEXION WITH THE LOCALISATION OF CEREBRAL AFFECTIONS AND THE ADVANTAGES OF ANTISEPTIC TREPHINING.*

BY WILLIAM MACEWEN, M.D. GLASG.,

SURGEON AND LECTURER IN SURGERY TO
THE ROYAL INFIRMARY, GLASGOW.

III. TUMOUR OF DURA MATER.

Epileptiform convulsions; trephining; removal of tumour from dura mater and orbital cavity; recovery.—This patient was a girl about fourteen years of age, who was admitted into Ward 22, Glasgow Royal Infirmary, on July 22nd, 1879, suffering from a swelling at the upper and inner portion of the left orbital cavity. Her object in seeking hospital treatment was the removal of this small

* Reprinted from *The Lancet*, 1881, 2: 581–582, with the kind permission of the Editor.

tumour. It was about the size and shape of a kidney-bean, its flat surface lying against the roof of the orbit, and extending inwards under the orbital plate of the frontal. It seemed firmly fixed to the periosteum, and it had a fibrous feeling. The pupil of this eye was contracted, and exhibited little response to light. When the finger ran over the surface of the brow, a prominence about the size of a large barley-grain was felt about two inches and a half above the supra-orbital ridge. This little body was firmly fixed to the periosteum. She complained of a dull fixed pain confined to the left side of the brow. Her history showed that she had been treated for months previously by large doses of iodide of potassium, but, notwithstanding, the pain in the left side of the forehead became worse, and the tumour in the orbital cavity increased. The contracted state of the left pupil and the pains which she experienced over the front of the left side of the brow presented a probability of the presence of intra-cranial pressure, as the small tumour in the front of the orbital cavity could scarcely produce these. She was therefore advised to remain in the ward for observation. A few days after, while sitting at the bedside, she uttered a cry, and immediately the muscles of the right side of the face began to twitch, the right arm was firmly flexed, and violently twitched. The twitchings lasted for two or three minutes, and were entirely confined to the right side. An interval of ten minutes elapsed, when the spasms reappeared in the right side of the face and on the right arm, lasting for about fifteen minutes. Two minutes after a third attack ensued, this time involving the whole of the right side of the body. These attacks began to be more prolonged, and the interval between each shorter, until they became continuous, the whole body becoming implicated in a general convulsion. Simultaneously with the commencement of the convulsions she lost consciousness, which continued throughout the attack. Towards the end of the third hour from the commencement of the attack the face became livid; the respiration extremely slow; the pulse slow, irregular, and feeble. These symptoms were evidently increasing, and a fatal issue seemed imminent. Her temperature during the last two hours increased at the rate of a degree each hour. At 8.30 it was 103.4°.

Under these circumstances trephining was determined on. The barley-sized node over the left side of the frontal was selected as the seat of operation. In cutting through this node it was found to be gummatous in appearance, and to extend over the frontal in a flattened form continuous with the pericranium. The bone underneath this little tumour was found to be rough and imparted a softer feeling to the finger than usual. A trephine having a disc an inch in diameter was chosen and a portion of bone was elevated. The skull was thicker than normal, and attached to the under surface of the disc was a tumour of a gummatous aspect. A portion of the tumour adhered to the disc which was removed. The remainder was attached to the dura mater and spread over that membrane in a downward direction towards the base of the frontal lobes. At the trephine opening the tumour was fully a quarter of an inch in thickness and three-quarters of an inch in breadth. From this point it tapered down to about one-sixteenth of an inch in thickness, while its breadth increased, so that it appeared like a leaf spread over the surface of the dura mater. The tumour was removed from the dura mater as far down as the orbital portion of the frontal, the dura mater being gently pressed aside to permit of this. The supraorbital tumour was then removed. In doing so it was found to have a firm attachment to the orbital plate of the frontal, and it was seen to be continuous with the barley grain-sized nodule on the left side of the brow, the connexion between these two points being about a millimetre in thickness, but having a superficial square area of about two inches. It was difficult to separate this without removing the pericranium, which consequently was removed in several places. The skull was roughened and softer than usual over this portion. After the whole of the tumour was removed, drains were introduced and the parts were brought together by sutures.

After recovering from the influence of the anaesthetic the convulsions did not return. Next morning, twelve hours after the operation, the patient's temperature was 99.6°. She was perfectly conscious, answered several questions intelligently, lifted her head to get dressed, and stated that she felt well. Her right side, however, remained completely paralysed.

On the fifth day after the operation her temperature began to increase shortly after she had been dressed. In an hour after she became aphasic, and the convulsions returned. When this condition was made known to me I visited the hospital and removed the dressings, which had been applied with a little pressure over the wound, in order to reduce a slight bulging which appeared at the trephine aperture. An hour afterwards her condition was greatly improved, the convulsions had ceased, and consciousness was restored. From this time she gradually improved, the paralysis of the right arm and leg passed slowly away, and her intelligence became perfect. The wounds were firmly healed in a month from the date of the operation; but she was kept "assisting" in the ward for another month, after which she was dismissed. From that time till now she has visited the ward to report her condition at least once monthly, and she has continued in good health down to the present. She is engaged in regular employment.

The indications which led here to a probable locus of brain pressure were: (1) The contraction and fixity of the left pupil. (2) The presence of a supraorbital tumour of a gummatous character and of a small nodule of probably similar consistence on the left side of the frontal. (3) A fixed dull pain on the left side of the brow, between these two tumours. (4) Convulsions commencing on the right side of the face, and afterwards involving the right side of the body (though ultimately becoming general).

CONTRIBUTION TO ENDOCRANIAL SURGERY*[1]

By F. DURANTE

PROFESSOR OF SURGERY

In May, 1884, C. B——, a woman, thirty-five years of age and a native of Narni, came under my care. Her general appearance was good; she seemed well nourished,

* Reprinted from *The Lancet*, 1887, 2: 654–655, with the kind permission of the Editor.
[1] Paper read in the Surgical Section of the International Medical Congress held at Washington, U.S.A., September, 1887.

although not of a very robust constitution. Externally, she showed no abnormality, except as to her left eye, which appeared somewhat low and drawn outwardly, otherwise the movement as well as the functions of the globe were normal. This deformity had manifested itself only within the three months previous to her visit to me. For a year or more however, she had entirely lost her sense of smell, her memory had become impaired, particularly as to remembering names, and she experienced a peculiar sensation of vacuity which caused her to feel uncertain in her movements. Motion, sense of touch, and sensibility to heat and pain remained natural. From her husband I learnt that she had somewhat changed in disposition; that from being generally happy and bright, she had become sad, melancholic and taciturn, although she did not seem to brood over the state of her health. The senses of hearing and taste, and the functions of the chylopoietic viscera were perfect; also nothing abnormal was found on a close examination of the nasal and pharyngeal regions. The course of the disease, the loss of memory and of the sense of smell, and the objective and subjective state of the patient led me to believe in the presence of a tumour within the cranium, the pressure of which affected the anterior lobe of the brain and paralysed or destroyed the olfactory nerve. Moreover, the displacement of the globe of the eye led me to believe also that the tumour had penetrated the superior arch of the orbital cavity. Such being my diagnosis, I now proposed to the patient an operation that would remove the offending object, explaining to her the gravity of the operation without reserve. She was brave, and she consented.

To reach the tumour it was necessary to make a large opening in the left frontal bone; so with an incision commencing from the inner angle of the left orbit upwards nearly to the hair line as far as the temporal region, I raised all the soft tissue from the bone in a flap. The bone being exposed, with a sharp scalpel and hammer I removed a large portion of it, commencing at the superior orbital margin, inferiorly, and found that the internal parietes of the frontal sinus had been forced outwardly. The dura mater being now exposed, I examined it, and found that it had been perforated by the tumour just opposite the frontal eminence. With great care I now began to scoop out the tumour. As soon as a considerable portion of the tumour was removed, I detected that it did not adhere beyond the internal surface of the dura mater, and that therefore its enucleation was comparatively easy; and then removed it and carried with it all the adherent portions of the dura mater. The haemorrhage was slight and easily controlled by the haemostatic, a tampon treated with sublimate. The tumour was lobular, of the size of an apple, and weighed seventy grammes. It occupied the anterior fossa at the base of the left cranium, extending to the right and upon the cribriform lamina, which it destroyed. Posteriorly it extended to the glenoid tubercles before the sella turcica. The left anterior cerebral lobe was greatly atrophied; the orbital arch was much depressed, but not perforated by the tumour as I had anticipated. Having stopped the bleeding completely, I now united the wound by first intention, leaving in the cavity occupied by the tumour a drainage tube, which descended to the left nasal fossa through the opening made on the ethmoid by a prolongation of the neoplasm; then I closed the nasal cavity with an iodoform tampon. The operation lasted about an hour.

The patient bore the chloroform very well, showing only the weakness following the use of an anaesthetic and attendant upon loss of blood. On the third day she had fairly recovered, and the wound was healing without suppuration. The drainage worked well, a large quantity of serum tinged with blood flowing through it. On the fourth day, however, the patient was overtaken by sudden prostration, was inclined to sleep, exceedingly disinclined to talk, and complained of mental confusion. I then discovered that the drain had stopped during the night, so I at once removed the tampon, replacing it, however, further down the nasal cavity. The effect was good; the serous fluid began to drip again. Not satisfied with this, I applied a gum-elastic "pump" to the external opening, and drew off about thirty grammes of liquid. The flow was thus re-established, and continued all the following day and night. On the renewal of the flow the alarming symptoms disappeared as if by magic. On the seventh day I removed the stitches and the drainage tube, and on the fifteenth day the patient returned to her home, doing very well. She had lost that sensation of vacuity around her person which made her uncertain in her movements, but had not regained her memory or the sense of smell.

Three months after I presented my patient to the Chirurgical Society at its meeting in Perugia in 1884. She was in a happy frame of mind, and willingly related her experience. She stated that now all her faculties and moral conditions were normal, and that she had even regained her sense of smell. This greatly surprised me, for I felt sure that I had destroyed the left olfactory in removing the tumour, which had destroyed the cribriform lamina of the ethmoid. Upon experimenting, however, with aromatic substances, we found that she could only smell with the right, and that the left was totally insensible, its olfactory having been destroyed either by the pressure of the tumour or by the operation itself. The part of the bone which had been removed was now partially reproduced, the cavity in the region of the operation had disappeared, and the eye had regained almost entirely its normal position. The tumour, under the microscope, presented a multiform fibrocellular structure of sarcoma.

It is now four years since that operation was performed, and my patient is in perfect health. My diagnosis and the operation, apparently so hazardous at the time, are therefore justified by the result. And, though such operations have generally failed, the success of mine should secure proper consideration at the hand of modern surgery.

The progress of experimental pathology and of studies of cerebral localisation every day now smooths our way to the diagnosis of cerebral diseases, so that the cranial cavity may in future justly enter into the dominion of surgery. The frontal and parietal regions can now be successfully attacked by the scalpel of the surgeon, and many affections of the meninges become trophies of rational surgery.

Neurosurgical Classics—33 and 34

"One of the greatest advances in the method of opening the skull for surgical exploration of the brain and its investing membranes was that made in 1889 by Wilhelm Wagner of Königshütte."[10]

"Previous to this the skull had been opened by means of a trephine, and the area enlarged as necessary by mallet and chisel or by the use of bone forceps. The new method at once made large areas of the brain more easily accessible without leaving a large and troublesome cranial defect. At the same time it sounded the knell of the various elaborate and time-consuming methods of craniocerebral topography which were then in vogue. . . . In other words, it was now possible for neurosurgeons to visualize the underlying cerebral cortex sufficiently well so that with the wider exposure obtained by the osteoplastic flap the lesion was almost certain to be brought into view if the neurological localization had been at all accurate."[8]

"The experimental work of Wolff[13] in 1863 had shown that osteoplastic techniques were possible."[7] "In 1864 Ollier had suggested an osteoplastic resection of the skull, his idea being to lift up a piece of the skull adherent to a flap of soft parts,[1] but it was not until 1889 that Wagner first adopted this principle when operating upon the living subject."[10]

"On November 23 of that year, Wagner reported the case of a patient upon whom he had performed osteoplastic craniotomy, and entitled his paper 'On temporary resection of the vault of the cranium in place of trepanation.'[12] The operation had been performed on October 3, 1889 upon a laboring man aged twenty-seven, who was unconscious following a blow on the side of the head, and who two days after the accident developed signs and symptoms pointing to intracranial hemorrhage from the left middle meningeal artery. Wagner, who had previously experi-mented upon cadavers with the object of producing a bone flap attached at its base to the soft parts so that the flap could be turned down, a reasonably large area of the brain exposed and the flap subsequently replaced, now performed his operation for the first time on a living subject. A large bone flap was chiselled out and turned down with its base attached to the scalp, the bleeding meningeal artery secured and the flap re-placed. Wagner's patient died twenty-four hours later, but the operation had introduced a new technic in the surgical exposure of the brain, and it was not long before other and more successful attempts were carried out."[10]

"At the time of his original description Wagner stated, 'I only use small strong chisels and elevators. Perhaps some form of circular saw could be constructed which could be set in motion after the manner of a dentist's drill with which it would be possible to work more quickly and accurately.' He added a word of warning against the ham-mering necessary for chiselling, and the liability to cerebral concussion from hammer-ing the skull is of course obvious."[10]

"Because of the shock to the patient, Horsley objected to this method and con-tinued to use wide bony resections by remov-ing as much bone as necessary with forceps. The resulting defect undoubtedly served a useful purpose as a postoperative decom-pression until the later method of combined bone flap and decompression was advocated by Cushing[2] in 1909."[8]

"In 1891 . . . Toison[11] suggested that the bone be divided from within outward by a chain saw passed between burr holes. His saw, being fairly clumsy, was little used."[10] Prior to 1897 Leonardo Gigli[3,4] developed a wire saw which he used for cutting the sym-physis pubis in obstetrical procedures. "Obaliński[9] used the Gigli saw for the performance of a craniotomy following Toison's method. Gigli[5,6] himself then designed guides for his saw."[7] "Many craniotomies have been invented to facilitate the Wagnerian operation, but none so far has been sufficiently successful to supplant Gigli's saw completely. . . ."[10]

REFERENCES

1. COTTERILL, J. M. Note on a method of trephining. *Edinb. med. J.*, 1894–5, *40:* 633–636.
2. CUSHING, H. A method of combining exploration and decompression for cerebral tumors which prove to be inoperable. *Trans. Amer. surg. Ass.*, 1909, *27:* 565–572.
3. GIGLI, L. Über ein neues Instrument zum Durchtrennen der Knochen, die Drahtsäge. *Zbl. Chir.*, 1894, *21:* 409–411.
4. GIGLI, L. Zur praktischen Verwerthung der Drahtsäge. *Zbl. Chir.*, 1897, *24:* 785–788.
5. GIGLI, L. Zur Technik der temporären Schädelresektion mit meiner Drahtsäge. *Zbl. Chir.*, 1898, *25:* 425–428.
6. GIGLI, L. Über einige Modifikationen an dem Instrumentarium und der Technik der Kraniektomie mit meiner Drahtsäge. *Zbl. Chir.*, 1900, *27:* 1193–1199.
7. GREEN, R. E., and STERN, W. E. Techniques of cranial surgery. In: *A history of neurological surgery.* A. E. Walker, Ed. Baltimore: Williams & Wilkins Co., 1951, xii, 583 pp. (see pp. 40–76).
8. HORRAX, G. Neurosurgery. An historical sketch. *Springfield, Ill.: Charles C Thomas,* 1952, xi, 135 pp.
9. OBALIŃSKI, A. Zur Technik der Schädeltrepanation. *Zbl. Chir.*, 1897, *24:* 857–859.
10. ROGERS, L. The history of craniotomy: an account of the methods which have been practiced and the instruments used for opening the human skull during life. *Ann. med. Hist.*, 1930, n.s. *2:* 495–514.
11. TOISON, J. De la trépanation du crâne par résection temporaire d'un lambeau ostéoplastique (procédé de Wagner et procédé personnel). *P.V. Ass. franç. Chir.*, 1891, *5:* 325–338.
12. WAGNER, W. Die temporäre Resektion des Schädeldaches an Stelle der Trepanation. *Zbl. Chir.*, 1889, *16:* 833–838.
13. WOLFF, J. Die Osteoplastik in ihren Beziehungen zur Chirurgie und Physiologie. *Arch. klin. Chir.*, 1863, *4:* 183–294.

THE TEMPORARY RESECTION OF THE CALVARIUM INSTEAD OF TREPANATION*

W. WAGNER

The actual trepanation, if I mean by it only the removal of a piece of the intact bony calvarium or debridement in complicated fractures, and do not count as trepanation the removal of carious foci and the like, is always to be considered as mutilat-

ing surgery. The brain is deprived of a larger or smaller area of its natural protection and although in many cases a firm scar of connective tissue forms in the established openings which provides some protection, this is not always so, and the majority of the trepaned patients require that the defects be covered by artificial protective covers.

Therefore, with more or less success, recently attempts were made to reinsert the resected bony piece in its former place, to transplant bony pieces in the opening, etc.

My own effort was directed for some time to devising by anatomical experiments a method that would allow us to resect optionally and temporarily a large piece of the calvarium so that it could be removed completely from its opening, but at the same time remain in connection with the soft parts so that its healing would be assured.

After many attempts I have arrived at the following method:

By a cut in the form of the Greek Ω (omega), the soft parts of the pertinent sections of the skull are cut to the periosteum. When the flap retracts it is pressed firmly to the skull and along its edge a cut is made through the periosteum, running parallel to and inside of the first cut at the average distance of 0.5–1 cm. Then the bone is chiselled completely through along the arched portion of this inner omega cut, whereas in the two legs of the omega only a groove is chiselled, from the external side inward. Two narrow chisels are inserted into this groove and, without injuring the soft parts lying above, the bony bridges are chiselled through subcutaneously.

The bony piece enclosed by the arched portion of the omega can now be lifted easily with narrow elevators and folded back parallel to the legs of the omega, together with the overlying soft parts. Between these legs it and its overlying soft parts are connected with the remaining covering of the skull by means of a pedicle at least 3 cm. wide.

This folded piece then is simply reinserted in its place. The flap of soft parts which, in view of the difference in the cut made in the soft parts and in the bone, projects over the latter by about 1 cm., then is sutured carefully, as are the legs of the omega after the drainage of the angles. The bony piece always fits well in its gap, especially if the small edges of the inner lamina which remain in the bony opening are allowed to remain as a shelf in order to prevent the sinking in of the resected part.

After I had convinced myself sufficiently by anatomical experiments about the feasibility of the operation I had an opportunity recently to perform it on a living person. The case is as follows:

P. Chwolka, aged 27, had the misfortune on October 1, 1889, of being injured in an accident in which a

* Translation of: Die temporäre Resektion des Schädeldaches an Stelle der Trepanation, by W. Wagner, *Centralblatt für Chirurgie,* 1889, *16:* 833–838, printed with the kind permission of the Editor.

heavily loaded coal carriage crushed the side of his head. He lost consciousness immediately. Nothing else could be learned from his coworkers who brought him to the hospital. At the time of admission C. was completely unconscious and bleeding from both ears, particularly the right one, and also from his mouth and nose. The pulse was weak, accelerated but regular. With the exception of a relatively extensive and markedly fluctuating blood effusion in the left temporal region, no external injury was noticeable. When being bathed, C. opened his eyes, groped around, and was grasping convulsively the edge of the tub with both hands. However, he did not react at all to calls, etc. After the bath his pulse was somewhat weaker and several injections of camphor were administered. Ice packs were applied to the head. At first he lay quietly in the bed, but then turned over several times, always wrapping himself in the covers. Toward evening the pulse was completely normal, and so was the respiration. The patient voided into a pan placed under him, groped for it with his hands, but always without opening his eyes. Both pupils were wide, reacted poorly.

2 October. During the night the patient either tossed from side to side or for a short time remained in a completely curved-up side position. A large amount of blood flowed from his mouth and ears until midnight. The patient vomited greenish thin material several times.

In the morning he opened his eyes when called, turned his head, and stared blankly around. At the same time a pronounced left-side ptosis was revealed, the left pupil did not react to light stimuli, and the sclera was entirely covered with effusion of blood. After several attempts, the patient reached out with his right hand. The pulse was good, on the average 70. This condition persisted throughout the day. The patient continued to react to calling by movement of his eyelids. In the evening he voided in bed. Throughout the day he continually repeated the action of wrapping himself in the covers. With the exception of the mentioned manifestations of the left eye, no motor or sensory disturbances were noticed.

3 October. The night was passed as before. In the morning the pulse was only 60, the somnolence was deeper, the right arm was completely without any feeling and paralyzed; on the other hand, the right leg was moved and drawn when pricked with a needle. Toward noon the pulse dropped to 52 and in the afternoon was irregular and weaker. The patient himself lay more quietly.

In the afternoon at 3:30 the symptoms of cerebral pressure increased and were related to a hematoma of the left meningeal artery. It was decided to perform ligation.

At the typical area of ligation an omega cut was made to the periosteum so that the base of the flap was situated inferiorly and horizontally, and after the circumcised flap of the soft parts retracted, a cut was made through the periosteum within the first cut by about 1 cm. First of all the bone was chiselled through along the curved section of the cut and then a groove was chiselled in the posterior leg. The bony bridge then could be punched through easily subcutaneously and it was not necessary to chisel a groove also in the anterior leg. The entire flap with the bony piece was then folded back. The bony piece had a maximum length of 6.5 cm. and a

maximum width of 5.0 cm.; the base, a good 3 cm. The flap of soft parts projected over the bone 1 cm. in all directions. During the chiselling the blood flowed out in large amounts, especially when the bony piece was being lifted, and after its removal clots appeared. When these were wiped off completely, the main trunk of the middle meningeal artery presented itself and the dura mater was completely bloodless, while at the lower edge of the wound the torn vessel was shown spurting clear red blood. The bleeding stopped after a purse-string ligation of the vessel. In the temporal region, somewhat posterior to the edge of the wound, a deeply extensive fissure was found, which was clamping rigidly shreds of the temporal muscle inside the cranium. Small shreds of brain substance were rinsed out. After reinsertion of the bony plate the wound was sutured and drained at its lower angles.

During operation, both the strength and the count of the pulse increased (100–110) but it was not yet completely regular. During the entire afternoon and evening the patient was lying on his left, completely still, deeply somnolent, but breathing silently; his pulse was now regular and strong (80–100), he held his right arm bent at a right angle, and he was also moving and kicking. As on the two previous days liquid nutrition was allowed to drip in.

4 October. Throughout the night the patient lay still, breathing quietly. In the morning his condition was unchanged, his pulse was good, his right arm was moved, his somnolence increased. Toward noon his breathing became more superficial; his pulse became weaker and slower. In the afternoon, about 24 hours after operation, death occurred.

Autopsy (not performed until October 9 because of delayed authorization. Consequently the findings on the brain are inaccurate.)

The cutaneous flaps revealed nothing indicating disturbed nutrition; the bony piece fit firmly in its gap. After opening the cranial cavity an effusion of blood appeared outside in the entire length of the temporal muscle. The meningeal vessels were dilated; there was no trace of inflammation. The main trunk of the left meningeal artery was bound under and bloodless. After removal of the brain there was noted a fissure starting deep behind the operative bony gap, extending through the squamous portion of the temporal bone and across the petrous portion (from which a piece was chipped off), passing in the left wing of the sphenoid, penetrating the sphenoidal body so that the piutitary fossa was broken and shifted posteriorly, and disappearing across the large right wing of the sphenoid into the right petrous portion of the temporal bone. Small effusions of blood were seen at several places along the fissure. The fissure of the cranial base was so complete that with a slight pulling apart two fingers could be inserted into the gap.

In the brain, which was already very pulpy, there was seen next to this finding a corresponding crushing of the pons and of the cerebral peduncle. Furthermore there was found in the left temporal lobe in the region of the squeezed-in muscle a defect the size of a cherry pit. The right temporal lobe showed one slightly larger and several small extravasations of blood, penetrating more or less deeply.

Consequently this case concerned a severe fracture of the base of the skull with a rupture of the left middle meningeal artery. The indication for the temporary cranial resection was furnished by the gradually increasing hematoma of the dura mater. The effect of its removal was the elimination of the manifestations of severe cerebral pressure, but other severe cerebral injuries developed, so that death occurred after 24 hours.

It would serve no purpose to discuss the case further, since it concerns us only inasmuch as it is the first case in which I performed the temporary cranial resection on a living person. Of course, it furnished only a preliminary proof that the operation can be performed easily on a patient.

The fact that the flap of the soft parts was still intact after 24 hours does not prove yet reliably that nutritional disturbances do not occur later.

It can be assumed *a priori* that a flap having such a wide base certainly will heal, especially if—as I take it for granted—the necessary configuration has been given to the course of the vessels. It also can be expected that the bony piece which remains in connection on its entire external side with the soft parts will not suffer any nutritional damage, but will grow back smoothly into its gap. If this should not happen the surgical patient is no worse off than if the bony piece were removed as done in the past.

In addition, I would like to make the following remarks concerning the technique:

In the case described I chiselled a groove only in one of the legs of the omega, from which the bridge could be cut through easily subcutaneously.

I believe that it is better to make first only the cut through the skin, periosteum and the bone in the line corresponding to the arched portion of the omega, and only then to establish one or possibly the other leg. If the bony bridge which is to be punched through is very wide, which depends necessarily on the size of the piece to be resected, then one leg is not sufficient and it must be chiselled through from both sides. During the operation I used only narrow strong chisels and elevators. They are sufficient. For my first anatomical experiments I had made several small round saws (of the type used to cut plaster) and bayonet-shaped chisels to be able to chisel through the base of the bony piece easily.

I abandoned both of them. The work with the circular saw is very uncomfortable when smaller pieces are to be removed; they are suitable for the resection of very large pieces only. In such cases I also was considering a hammering procedure, delivering blows with a chisel. Perhaps circular saws could be constructed which could be set in motion similar to dentists' drills. This would allow us to work quickly and accurately. I am not aware of the existence of such a saw. (Professor Richter advised me while this report was in press that several such models were constructed in France by Collia and Péan and also by Ollier.) Aside from the generally unfavorable effect on the brain by the frequent blows with the chisel, I believe that the work with the chisel is the safest, since physiologically or pathologically thickened or thinned areas of the skull, or rapidly changing differences in the thickness can be noticed immediately during chiselling while in such cases the brain can be easily injured with the saw.

I abandoned the bayonet-shaped chisels since they bent too easily at the strength in which they were needed and since the ordinary chisel serves just as well.

As concerns the applicability of the method, in case it proves successful, it should be suitable for all cases of opening of the uninjured skull (excluding trepanation of the mastoid process)—that is, for the removal of hematomas of the dura mater, openings of brain abscesses, removal of tumors and foci in epilepsy, etc.

Foreign bodies such as knife blades, bullets, bone splinters, etc. lodged in the brain after having penetrated the skull could also be removed in such a way that an oval piece of the bone, in whose center the pertinent point of entry is situated, is cut around and temporarily resected.

A much larger view of the cerebral surface and the site of the foreign body is obtained than in simple trepanation of the area of entry.

ON THE METHOD OF TEMPORARY CRANIAL RESECTION BY MEANS OF MY WIRE SAW*

LEONARDO GIGLI

Having had the effectiveness of my saw for cranial trepanation pointed out to me by Professor Obaliński's paper in No. 32 (1897) of this journal, I turned my attention to the development of the method with the conviction that with no other instrument was it possible to cut out an osteoplastic flap of the desired size with such a degree of safety or to intervene at any point of the brain over a wide area.

The greatest difficulty of the method of craniectomy with my saw consists of introducing it under the bone of the cranium without exerting pressure and without damaging the membranes of the brain.

For this purpose I have developed a kind of grooved probe which is bent at almost right angles at the end (Fig. 1a, b).

In the groove of this probe a whalebone some 8 to 9

* Translation of: Zur Technik der temporären Schädelresektion mit meiner Drahtsäge, by Leonardo Gigli, *Centralblatt für Chirurgie*, 1898, *25:* 425–428, printed with the kind permission of the Editor.

Die Sonde, ²/₃ natürlicher Größe.

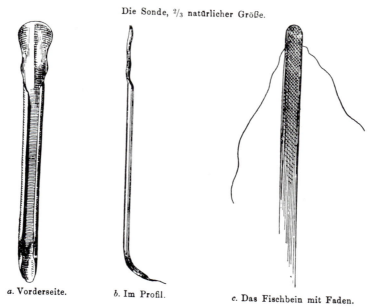

a. Vorderseite.   *b.* Im Profil.   *c.* Das Fischbein mit Faden.

FIG. 1. (*a*) Anterior side. (*b*) Profile. (*c*) The whalebone with thread.

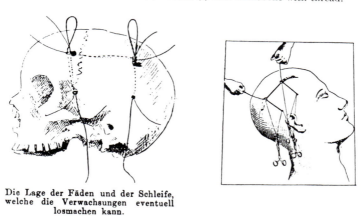

Die Lage der Fäden und der Schleife,
welche die Verwachsungen eventuell
losmachen kann.

FIGS. 2 and 3. Position of thread and loops, which can eliminate any possible adhesions.

mm. wide can be slid and pushed forward in a direction given by the end of the probe parallel to the surface of the brain.

I have preferred to use the whalebone, although it does not entirely meet modern requirements, because it is the safest. Wire springs, if too thick, are not sufficiently pliable and supple; if they are too thin they cut very easily. Watch springs such as those recommended recently by Lauenstein and Trnka, which are sharp, if they do not touch the dura mater parallel with their end or if they come up against the posterior surface of the bone, will be hindered in their forward progress. On the other hand, with the whalebone we are certain of not causing any injury, even if we force the instrument to overcome any resistance that might be encountered or to test for any possible adhesions. In such cases it can be pushed forward.

To bore through the cranium, like Obaliński, I used Collin's perforator with a trepanation crown measuring 1 cm. in diameter and a 5 mm. fraise recommended by Doyen and Braatz.

The operation takes place as follows: After establishing the site and the size of the flap to be formed, a cut is made at its upper and posterior corner down to the bone and this is exposed until the crown can be inserted.

After removal of the slice of bone the dura mater is loosened and the beak of the probe is inserted between it and the cranium in the direction of the triangular lobe to be formed. The probe itself is held firm by means of the left hand suported on the cranium and in its groove the whalebone is inserted and a thin, long, strong thread is threaded into the whalebone.

In very rare cases one encounters difficulties when pushing the whalebone forward; sometimes I was able to push the whalebone on the surface of the cerebral hemispheres from the occipital bone as far as the upper edge of the cavity of the eyes.

If any pathological conditions are encountered that might give rise to difficulties, these certainly can be overcome by suitable forced movement of the probe, since it is quite impossible to cause any injury by this means. At the inside end of the enclosed whalebone, the position of which easily can be determined by measurement, a second trepanation is made and by means of tweezers and a hook, the thread attached to the whalebone is caught and pulled forward and together with it also the whalebone. Of the double thread pulled forward in the manner of a loop, a section is cut which is twice as long as the stretch of bone situated between the two trepan crowns and the two ends of this thread are caught up in a pair of tweezers and the outer part of the much longer thread is left free in situ. Next the probe is led once more through the first bore hole with its bend pointing downward in the direction of the edge of the flap and the corresponding end of the longer part of the thread mentioned earlier is threaded in the whalebone and the whalebone is once again pushed farther down in the groove of the probe and farther forward. Where the end is found a small hole is bored in the exposed bone with a small fraise and through this hole the thread is pulled through and here again a section of thread is cut off in proportion to the length of the border in question, the threads are freed and the probe and whalebone are pulled back.

The same maneuver is repeated on the other trepan opening for the formation of the third border of the bone. Thus by means of four simple bores, of which two are very small, a silk thread is led under the three edges of the flap which are to be cut and another continuous thread is allowed to come out under all of these borders with the two ends through the last small bores. Now while care is taken that the two threads have not crossed one another, the ends of the thread are pulled under the segment of bone between the last two bores where the base of the flap is situated. By this means any possible adhesion of the dura mater with the internal surface of the osteoplastic flap is separated, so as to avoid the possibility that upon later development of the flap extensive tears might arise in the membranes of the brain.

Next the soft parts are cut from bore hole to bore hole, of course without severing the base of the flap, the silk threads are replaced by the wire saw and the protective whalebone and the corresponding stretch of bone is sawed completely through at the edges and partly at the base, until finally broken through.

By this means one obtains an osteoplastic flap of the desired size which very easily can grow back again completely.

It is also possible to operate with a simple fraise with a 5 mm. diameter in which case instead of the crown, two or three bores with the fraise, one beside the other, must be made in order to be able to introduce the probe through the greater opening made in this manner.

These are the principal outlines of the rapid and simple and satisfactory method proposed by me. I would have preferred to wait for this publication until after performing operations on live subjects, but the rapidly succeeding works on similar subjects and the great importance of the matter have prompted me to this publication at this early date in which I received the encouragement and urging of my students, to whom I express my warmest thanks.

Neurosurgical Classic—35A

O F Harvey Cushing's many contributions to neurological surgery, perhaps the most important was his development and standardization of neurosurgical operating technique. Dr. Cushing himself summarized this succinctly when he was questioned about his contributions. His reply was, "Tell them that I closed the galea."[6]

Aside from the development of many important surgical instruments, Dr. Cushing advanced neurosurgical operating technique by the introduction and adaptation of several basic principles.[1–5] Foremost among these were the principles of careful hemostasis, gentle manipulation of tissues, and meticulous attention to details, which had been taught to Cushing by the man who was chiefly responsible for his surgical training, Dr. William S. Halsted.

In an address to the St. Louis Surgical Society on December 16, 1907, parts of which are reproduced below, Cushing outlined his procedure for performing osteoplastic resection of the skull. It is an unwritten tribute that most of the steps in this procedure are still followed today.

1. Cushing, H. On routine determinations of arterial tension in operating room and clinic. *Boston med. surg. J.*, 1903, *148:* 250–256.
2. Cushing, H. Technical methods of performing certain cranial operations. *Surg. Gynec. Obstet.*, 1908, *6:* 227–246.
3. Cushing, H. Technical methods of performing certain cranial operations. *Interst. med. J.*, 1908, *15:* 171–187.
4. Cushing, H. Surgery of the head. In: *Surgery, its principles and practice.* W. W. Keen, Ed. Philadelphia: W. B. Saunders Co., 1908, *3:* 17–276.
5. Cushing, H. Some principles of cerebral surgery. *J. Amer. med. Ass.*, 1909, *52:* 184–192.
6. Horrax, G. Some of Harvey Cushing's contributions to neurological surgery. *J. Neurosurg.*, 1944, *1:* 3–22.

TECHNICAL METHODS OF PERFORMING CERTAIN CRANIAL OPERATIONS*,[1]

By Harvey Cushing, M.D.
Associate Professor of Surgery, the Johns Hopkins University, Baltimore

. . . On this particular occasion . . . I purpose to limit my remarks largely to a description of such technical methods as have come to be more or less habitual, in Dr. Halsted's clinic with which I am associated, in the routine performance of the simpler operations of craniotomy and craniectomy. . . .

From a purely technical point of view we are more indebted to the method of temporary osteoplastic resection, first attempted by Wagner in 1889, than to any other factor for the satisfactoriness of most of our present-day operations on the cerebral hemispheres. These trap-doors may be cut from the cranium with a variety of tools; the simplest armamentarium is a mallet and chisel, the most elaborate, a motor, with its trephines, burrs and saws, driven by electricity. . . .

Simplicity is a desirable quality in operative technique, but the blows of a mallet, even though transmitted in a glancing direction, are undesirable; and speed, the chief advantage of the motor-driven rotary tools, is invariably a source of danger, even in accustomed hands. It really matters little, except in saving time for the surgeon, whether an osteoplastic flap can be elevated by one method in seven minutes, or whether another requires twenty; and an operator who persists in taking dangerous corners at high speed will be the cause of a serious or fatal accident some day, whether he is driving an automobile or opening a skull. . . .

STEPS OF AN OSTEOPLASTIC RESECTION

Since this procedure may be taken as representative of any major operation on the skull, I shall, at the risk of being tedious, describe the general plan of preparation and performance to which I adhere . . .

General preparation. It is, I believe, a fairly universal custom to have the patient's head shaved and treated antiseptically in the ward on the day before the operation—some even advocate a double preparation of this kind. This I consider an unnecessary precaution, if not positively unwise; for the patient is apt to pass an un-

* Reprinted in part from *Surgery, Gynecology and Obstetrics*, 1908, *6:* 227–246, with the kind permission of the Editor.
[1] Read before the St. Louis Surgical Society, December 16, 1907.

comfortable night and, even with the most expert shaving, the scalp is likely to be a little "sore" the morning of operation. In something over 350 craniotomies I have never seen an infection, even a superficial stitch abscess, and have ceased to regard the chance of sepsis as a possible complication of these operations.

It is our custom, without previous ward preparation, to have the hair clipped and shaved just before the operation. . . . After a double shaving, once with and then against the direction of emergence of the hairs, there may be a preliminary cleansing of the scalp with green soap and a soft brush, the head then being wrapped in a towel wrung out of warm bichloride solution. The final preparation is deferred until after the anæsthetic.

Position on the table. It is a great advantage, though it does not appear to be a common practice, to place the patient on the table in the position most favorable for the operation before administering the anæsthetic. . . .

Many operators have a particular form of head-rest for all cranial operations, table extensions for this purpose having been described by Horsley, Frazier, Morestin and others. For the usual operations on the vault, however, small, flat, solid pillows or sand-bags seem to be all that are necessary to turn and hold the head in the desired position: on the other hand, I regard a head-extension with shoulder supports as essential for occipital work, chiefly to insure free respiration. Thus do surgeons' views differ. Whatever form of table be used, however, it is desirable to have the head-end capable of being raised or lowered at will.

The anæsthetic. Regardless of the drug to be employed, it is essential that it be administered by an expert— preferably by one who makes this his specialty. . . . Cerebral surgery is no place for a "Guck in die Luft" anæsthetist.[1]

In all serious or questionable cases the patient's pulse and blood-pressure, their usual rate and level having been previously taken under normal ward conditions, should be followed throughout the entire procedure, and the observations recorded on a plotted chart. Only in this way can we gain any idea of physiological disturbances—whether given manipulations are leading to shock, whether there is a fall of blood-pressure from loss of blood, whether the slowed pulse is due to compression, and so on. A further safeguard is an artificial respiration apparatus, to be immediately put into use in case there is failure of an already burdened respiratory centre, either from the anæsthetic, from loss of blood, or from additional medullary pressure due to cerebral manipulation. . . .

In this country, where chloroform is doubtless ad-

[1] We have, of late, in all of our cerebral operations followed the custom of having the etherizer constantly auscultate the heart. This is accomplished by strapping the transmitter of a phonendoscope to the precordium. From this a long tube passes to the aural receiver which is held against the auricle as is the receiver of a telephone operator. This is much more satisfactory than the usual supervision of cardiac action by the occasional palpation of the pulse for which a hand must be disengaged. It is surprising that the method has not come into general practice before this.

ministered less well than ether, the latter is the anæsthetic of choice at most hands, the primary stage usually being induced with ethyl chloride. . . .

The question of the anæsthetic in a two-stage operation is an especially serious one, and under these circumstances, the dangers from chloroform would possibly be less than those of a repeated etherization. Some years ago, however, having had a fatality from chloroform, I employ it far less frequently in cranial operations than ether, restricting its use largely to children.

Local anæsthesia may at times suffice, especially for such simple measures as ventricular puncture, though infiltration of the scalp is difficult. I have learned, furthermore, that in favorable cases no anæsthetic need be required in a second-stage operation limited to manipulations of dura and brain after re-reflecting an original bone-flap.

Preparation of the operative field. With the patient anæsthetized and in proper position on the table the final cleansing is done; for this, alcohol and 1 to 1000 bichloride solution are sufficient.

It is my practice at this stage, before the landmarks are obscured by the covering of operative sheets and towels, to outline the proposed incision on the scalp by a superficial scratch with the scalpel.

An operating neurologist should acquire the power of visualizing the brain, its main fissures, the insula, the ventricles, etc., through the intact skull; and those who have, by long practice, familiarized themselves with the rules of cranio-cerebral topography, learn to judge the position of the main fissures with no greater margin of error than when measurements are employed. . . .

With the proposed flap thus outlined and the head raised by an attendant's hand placed under the back of the neck, a broad square of wet bichloride gauze is thrown over the entire head; over this, in turn, is placed a *tourniquet*.

For the *control of hæmorrhage from the scalp* numerous forms of tourniquet have been advocated. Many use a simple rubber tube, or Esmark bandage, both of which are difficult to apply and to fasten without slips in the aseptic technique. Crile has employed a rubber dam which, being stretched over the entire scalp, renders it bloodless. I formerly used a pneumatic tourniquet, but have finally come to a form of rubber ring in which is inserted a buckle . . so that the tube can be made into a ring of any size and can be easily removed at the end of the operation. Practice enables one, with a given quality of tubing, to estimate the size of the ring, necessary in a given case, to shut off arterial supply from the scalp without causing undue pressure. The ring, furthermore, is provided with a median tape . . whose length—measured after the head is shaved—should equal the distance from glabella to inion, and the object of which is to prevent the ring from rolling over the orbits, as it is likely to do, especially if there is a prominent forehead. Having been boiled, the ring is applied by the operator and an assistant . . being snapped over the head from occipital to frontal regions (Fig. 4).

In the majority of cases all bleeding from the scalp is thus controlled, though in certain patients with tumor, in whom there is marked intracranial stasis, some of the veins on the concave side of the incision which receive blood through emissary vessels from within the skull may have to be clamped. . . .

Around and just above the tourniquet a small towel,

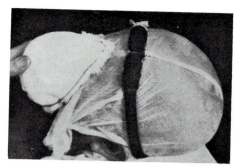

FIG. 4. Cranial tourniquet in position over gauze cap.

folded lengthwise and wet in bichloride, is tightly pinned, and to this is securely fastened the large sheet which covers the etherizer like a tent and leaves exposed little more than the area outlined by the preliminary incision . . If there is any likelihood of the slipping of these surrounding sheets, they may even be pinned directly into the scalp. . . .

The osteoplastic flap. With the operative field thus prepared, the incision is carried down to the skull, through gauze and soft parts, in the line previously scratched on the scalp. When the bone has been exposed it can be opened in a number of different ways. . . .

The "combined method," to be described, makes use of the following general principles: 1. Division of the bone between two or more primary openings (Toison). 2. Incision by an advancing instrument from a simple opening. 3. The making of all cuts from within outward. 4. The leaving of a beveled flap.

A primary opening through the thickest part of the exposed cranium, usually near the parietal eminence, is made with a hand-trephine . . which should be of generous size, with a crown fully 2 cm. in diameter. . . . Bleeding from diploëtic vessels, in certain cases of tumor, may be severe. . . . It may be controlled by the proper use of Horsley's wax, with which the beveled teeth of the trephine may be filled.

One or more secondary openings . . . at the upper edge of the incision are made with a Doyen perforator and burr . . Then, with a long-handled blunt dissector or dural separator, introduced through the large trephine opening, the dura between these openings is freed from its bony attachments. On withdrawing the dissector the cerebral pressure, in most cases, suffices to hold dura against bone again, and thus serves to control such bleeding as may have been occasioned.

From these two primary trephine openings the lateral edges of the flap are then cut downward toward the base in a line concentric with the skin incision. The first half-inch of these lateral cuts is made with Montenovesi forceps . . which leave a 2.5 mm. incision, followed by the weaker Dahlgren forceps . . as the thinner bone near the temporal region is approached.

A Gigli wire saw is then passed on a guide, of which there are numerous forms, between the two openings and the mesial edge of the flap is cut on a broad bevel . . (this is an important detail, for it enables the subsequent solid replacement of the flap without danger of its being driven inward by a snug pressure-bandage). The flap is then forced back by the insertion of blunt instruments around the edges, and is broken across at its base. . . .

Provided the flap includes the region of the pterion, the meningeal artery may be torn owing to its having channeled the broken bone. The vessel should be ligated at its lowest point of exposure by making at a distance a small opening in the dura, through which a grooved director can be inserted; on this the curved needle may be passed without danger of injuring even a tense cortex. Bleeding from the expansions of the lateral sinus, in case they have been exposed by a high flap, is best controlled by the pressure of sterile absorbant cotton, pledgets of which I find to be as valuable, as a hæmostatic agent for the intracranial part of the work, as is wax for the bone itself. . . .

The intracranial procedures. At this stage, if there has been a fall of arterial tension from loss of blood, the further progress of the operation, especially in tumor cases, may well be postponed for a second session. If there is no contra-indication on this score, the dura is opened in a line concentric with the bone incision . . leaving plenty of margin for subsequent suture. The membrane should be incised on a grooved director, especially if there is increased tension, for it is very important to avoid any possible injury to the pia-arachnoid. In case the tension is so great as to threaten this, a lumbar puncture should be performed at this stage of the operation.

The dural incision should not be made too near the median line, lest the edge of the parasinoidal expansions, or the veins entering them, be injured. If the mesial edge of the hemisphere is to be exposed it is best to open the dura in this direction by a separate radial cut, and if necessary to rongeur away some of the bone toward the median line. . . .

If the expected lesion is not disclosed and if the topography is not perfectly clear, the fissura centralis may have to be determined by faradization of the cortex. . . .

If an incision of the cortex is necessary, whether for exploration, for extirpation of a given area in cases of focal epilepsy, or for the removal of a neoplasm, such cortical vessels as will evidently have to be divided must first be ligated on each side of the proposed incision, which should, if possible, be confined to the exposed surface of a convolution, and should not cross a sulcus. The finest strands of split silk, preferably black, should be used for these ligatures, and they should be passed around the vessels with delicate curved French needles, which are introduced and emerge in non-vascular areas. . . . Subsequent dissections are carried out with blunt instruments, and the momentary pressure of cotton pledgets will usually check the oozing.

A brain which tends to protrude may sometimes be "dropped back" by elevation of the head and trunk, or by evacuating cerebrospinal fluid. This can at times be accomplished by pricking the exposed arachnoid spaces and by milking out the fluid; at other times a lumbar puncture may be necessary, and the removal of fluid in this way during the course of an operation is of the greatest possible help under many circumstances, being in large measure free from the dangers which attend a similar proceeding in the presence of great cerebral pressure when the skull is closed.

Closure. Unless there is reason for permanent decompression, in which case the dura somewhere should remain open, an accurate approximation of the membrane in its two layers should painstakingly be carried out, to prevent the formation of adhesions, or their reforma-

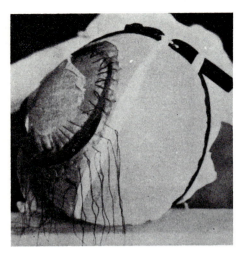

Fig. 18. Showing method of closure of
wound before removal of tourniquet.

tion if they have been found and divided as the presumed source of irritative symptoms. If a large cerebral
defect remains after the removal of a growth, or if the
brain has receded from its normal level owing to evacuation of cerebrospinal fluid, the space should be filled
with warm isotonic salt solution before closing the dura.

The bone flap is solidly replaced and the scalp is, in
turn, accurately approximated in a broad surface. It is
well to draw together the galea aponeurotica by a few
buried sutures before closing the outer layer. For the
latter many use a continuous suture which has the advantage of speed. Inasmuch as the closure, in many
cases, is completed before the tourniquet is removed, I
feel the need of a more accurate and solid approximation; this is accomplished by rapidly placing about the
incision a series of straight, round-pointed cambric
needles which serve to keep the edges everted as each
suture is tied, and thus to assure a ridge of tissue with a
flat apposition, which prevents subsequent bleeding
from the vessels of the scalp (Fig. 18). An approximation

of the divided epithelial edges which is beyond reproach
may be secured in this way.

Drainage is occasionally advisable—perhaps in 20 per
cent of the cases—but it should be avoided if possible. . . . I prefer to take advantage of the trephine
openings made in this method of resection at the upper
angles of the flap. The drains, of cigarette form, covered
with protective so that they may be easily withdrawn,
are led out, not through the original incision, but
through puncture wounds made in the scalp about 2 cm.
to its outer side; this insures for the drain an oblique
passage which can be occluded by pressure, in case there
should be a tendency for cerebrospinal fluid to escape
after their withdrawal. . . .

The wound, covered with silver foil, is partly dressed
and some pressure exerted before the tourniquet is removed, after which an abundant dressing with an outer
starched bandage is applied. The ears should be carefully protected with cotton to prevent discomfort from
pressure.

The first dressing is made in forty-eight hours, when
the drains, if used, and all the sutures are removed. The
silver foil and its thin inter-leaved paper, wet with alcohol, dries into a crisp protection which is particularly
ideal for a head dressing. . . .

. . . It may be said, in passing, that I have never seen
a bone flap lose its vitality, and indeed in one case reported with Dr. Thomas the flap was for one reason or
another elevated on six occasions and a tumor finally
removed at the last sitting.

My own experience does not accord with Frazier's, in
that removal of bone alone, without opening the dura,
will suffice for decompressive purposes in cases of tumor,
and believing that a dural opening is always necessary
I have come to make this opening in a situation where
the protrusion will be protected—under the temporal
muscle in cerebral, and under the occipital muscle in
suspected cerebellar lesions. . . .

It is not always necessary to leave a beveled flap;
indeed, it is not always possible. For example, in the
thin skulls of infants, more especially in the new-born,
it is not practicable, owing to the thinness of the bone;
hence in these patients the flap is usually made throughout by a biting tool. . . .

(To be concluded)

Neurosurgical Classics—35B and 36

THE March 1963 issue of the *Journal of Neurosurgery* contained Harvey Cushing's classical description of his procedure for performing osteoplastic resection of the skull. A continuation of that paper, which describes Cushing's techniques of subtemporal and suboccipital craniectomy, is reproduced below, together with his method of combined exploration and decompression for irresectable cerebral tumors. The illustration in Fig. 1 of the latter paper was drawn by Dr. Cushing.

TECHNICAL METHODS OF PERFORMING CERTAIN CRANIAL OPERATIONS

By Harvey Cushing, M.D.

Associate Professor of Surgery, the Johns Hopkins University, Baltimore

(Concluded)

I have thus far in the main considered only those forms of craniotomy in which a flap has been made and then replaced. There remains a large number of operations—craniectomies—in which it is either impossible or inadvisable to attempt an osteoplastic resection.

SUBTEMPORAL OPERATIONS. Many of these operations are characterized by the removal of more or less of the thin cranial wall underlying the temporal muscle, whether they are conducted for purposes of exploration, usually in traumatic cases; for purposes of decompression, in states of increased intracranial tension associated with tumor, hydrocephalus or œdema of one source or another; for the removal of growths or natural structures like the Gasserian ganglion, lying in the mid-cerebral fossa; or even for the still deeper exposure of the 3rd ventricle or the pituitary body. Not only is it difficult in this situation to make a satisfactory osteoplastic flap, but the precaution is unnecessary if proper use is made of the temporal muscle, fascia and galea in the closure.

In all of these operations, with a perfect technique and abundant experience in the proper disposition of gauze, towels and sheets, a small portion only of the head need be shaved. . . .

A tourniquet cannot be used in this low situation, but pressure of a finger on the temporal artery as it crosses the zygoma allows the vessels to be picked up in the scalp, after their division, without undue loss of blood. Otherwise, the preliminary preparation, the subsequent precautions in regard to securing a small, isolated and well protected field in which to work, the administration of the anæsthetic on the operating table, and other details, are the same as those which have been described under osteoplastic operations.

The steps of a subtemporal craniectomy, however, differ somewhat, particularly in the manner of approach through the temporal muscle, according to the nature of the case, whether (1) a ganglion operation, (2) a decompression for tumor, or (3) an exploration in cases of cranial trauma.

1. In the *Ganglion Operation*—Here the muscle fibres must be divided and scraped away from the bone well down to the base of the temporal fossa, in order, after making the small cranial opening, to give direct access to the base of the mid-cranial fossa without undue elevation of the temporal lobe. The operation is, of course, conducted outside of the dura, the subdural space being opened with escape of cerebrospinal fluid only when the sensory root is liberated and withdrawn from its pontine attachment.

At the present writing I have performed sixty-eight of these operations and have ceased to regard them as particularly difficult—no more difficult, indeed, than many of the extracranial procedures which are advocated and which give no certainty of permanent relief in cases of major neuralgia. Two of my early patients I lost through inexperience; in the last forty operations there have been no complications of any sort.

The small curvilinear skin incision, . . entirely within the hair margin, should be placed so as to avoid division of the upper branch of the facial nerve which innervates the occipito-frontalis muscle (pars frontalis). The muscle itself should be divided as in the older operation in horseshoe-shaped fashion, and scraped away from the bone so as to bare the lower part of the fossa. I still think it is essential for more reasons than one to remove the zygomatic arch, and this can be done by crowding forward the periosteum and fascia from the point at the temporal attachment of the zygoma where it is crossed by the incision, without risk of injuring the aforementioned twig of the N. facialis.

If the soft parts are painstakingly closed in layers—muscle, fascia, galea and skin—there will be no apparent sinking in of the temporal region in consequence of atrophy of the muscle. A drain is rarely needed. Without tests for sensation it should be impossible to tell subsequently, by inspection alone, upon which side the neurectomy has been performed. Experience first, patience second, and a proper kit of spatulæ and blunt dissectors third, are in descending sequence the essential requisites for success in carrying out this delicate operation.

2. *The Subtemporal Decompression for Symptoms of Increased Intracranial Tension*. Here I think it is wise to make a curvilinear skin incision, more or less concentric with the temporal ridge or line of attachment of the temporal muscle. . . . A flap of scalp alone should be reflected with careful preservation of the stout galea-aponeurotica, which in turn should be incised and reflected laying bare the temporal fascia. This fascia is then incised in line with its fibres in about the middle of the muscle. While the edges of the split muscle are carefully held apart, its attachments, together with the pericranium, are separated by an elevator from the bone under the entire muscle belly.

The bone is then entered in any way desired—I prefer a Doyen perforator and burr, followed by Montenovesi

forceps, and then by Horsley rongeurs as the opening is
enlarged. The chief difficulties lie in the fact that the
muscle cannot be elevated far from the skull without
tearing it—an undesirable accident in view of the subsequent closure. . . . Care must be taken not to injure the
meningeal artery, not to tear the tense dura by a sharp
spicule of bone, and above all to avoid cerebral contusion by rough manipulations with the rongeur forceps.

A generous area of bone having been removed, it
remains to slit the dura in stellate fashion to the edge of
the opening. In cases of great tension this is often a difficult thing to accomplish without injuring the pia-arachnoid—an accident which may lead to very undesirable
consequences. One can usually estimate the degree of
tension by palpation, but if this is not conclusive a very
small entering incision is made. If the brain tends to
forcibly protrude, especially if it is dry and there is no
escape of fluid with resultant lowering of tension, a lumbar puncture should be performed in order to accomplish
this end.

A dangerous, at times fatal, procedure, as I have often
reiterated, when the cranium remains closed and cerebral tension is great, lumbar puncture and withdrawal of
the cerebrospinal fluid from below loses its hazardous
features after the cranium has been opened: . . . In more
than half of my subtemporal decompression cases for
tumor—now nearly sixty in number—lumbar puncture
has been resorted to at this stage of the operation.

In this operation, again, the wound is painstakingly
closed in four layers—muscle, fascia, galea and skin.
There results more or less protrusion under the closed
muscle, though never a large hernia such as one sees in
cases of decompression protected by scalp alone. . . . In
the long run, for all cases of inoperable or inaccessible
cerebral tumors, this, in my experience, has proved to be
the most satisfactory method of decompression. . . .

There is one group of cases which are an exception and
which do not receive much benefit from temporal decompression alone—namely, those in which the condition is complicated by a hydrops ventriculorum due
most often to closure of the iter by the pressure of a
subtentorial growth. . . . Thus, although a subtemporal
decompression is not always effectual in relieving the
symptoms of pressure, it may be said that there have
been no fatalities in our rather large series of cases.

Not only for tumor, but for other conditions of tension, will a subtemporal decompression prove to be often
a helpful, sometimes a life-saving, measure. Among these
conditions may be mentioned thrombosis or embolism;
for when there is a large area of cerebral softening, the
lesion, in consequence of œdema, may lead to great
swelling. . . .

Other states for which the operation is suitable are
intracranial syphilis . . . and many forms of œdema,
more particularly in acute serous meningitis and in the
œdema of nephritis. . . .

3. *The Temporal Exploration in Traumatic Cases.*
Particularly in bursting fractures of the skull with general pressure symptoms and no external indication of the
character and situation of the cerebral lesion, no site for
an exploration is so likely to disclose the seat of trouble
as one in the temporal region, and no form of operation is
so likely to meet the needs of the conditions usually found
as the "split-muscle" operation with removal of bone.

As drainage is often indicated in these cases, I prefer
to make the skin incision parallel to the line of muscle
fibres, . . . there being less need here for a protecting flap
of scalp since the pressure of the traumatic œdema is an

acute process which subsides in the course of a few days.
Otherwise the operative approach to the lesion is similar
to that in the tumor cases.

The advantages of such an operation in these patients
may be briefly summarized as follows: An opening in
this situation will disclose the extradural clot of a ruptured meningeal, if this vessel or one of its branches as is
so often the case has been injured by a meridional fissure; similarly, this is the most common situation for an
isolated subdural clot to be found; again, in bursting
injuries associated with cortical laceration, it is the tips
of the temporal lobes which are most often affected;
further, in the larger number of basilar fractures the
fissures run into the middle cranial fossa, and hence free
bleeding from the base may be most effectively drained
by placing a protective wick under the temporal lobe
and leading it out at the lower angle of the split-muscle
incision; lastly, since a post-traumatic period of œdema,
which endures for some days after the injury (the wet
brain of our predecessors) and which through pressure
may prove serious in an unopened skull, is usual in these
cases, the subtemporal opening serves to ward off almost
completely the disturbances which otherwise appear.
The operation itself is simple and it is often desirable to
carry it out bilaterally.

SUBOCCIPITAL OPERATIONS. For the exposure of subtentorial lesions—tumors of the cerebellum or lateral
recess, a basilar meningitis to be drained, the freeing of
adhesions about the 4th ventricle resultant to an old
inflammation, etc.—the principles of tourniquet and
bone-flap are inapplicable, just as in operations conducted through the temporal region. In this situation,
also, owing to the possibility of subsequent firm closure
under muscle there is little reason for preservation of
bone.

Though many surgeons place the patient on the side
for these operations, I much prefer a symmetrical face-
down position particularly since I regard a bilateral exposure as desirable in all cases. A face-down posture, however, interferes greatly with respiration unless the
shoulders are held away from the table to allow of free
costal movements; consequently a table outrigger has
been devised for these cases, possessing shoulder supports and a separate crutch with a horseshoe-shaped top
in which the head comfortably and securely rests (Fig.
32). . . . The anæsthetic is sprayed against a mask
attached under the "horseshoe." . . .

In order to fully benefit from the "principle of dislocation" mentioned under osteoplastic operations, a bilateral
exposure of both cerebellar lobes is desirable to allow of
the outward dislocation of the lobe on the opposite side
during the manipulations of the other. . . . For this
symmetrical approach I find it advantageous to make,
in addition to the usual curvilinear cut over the occipital
ridge, a median incision with division of the soft parts
not only down to the occiput but to the spinous processes of the upper cervical vertebræ. This "cross-bow
incision" gives an exceptional view, owing to the possibility of lateral reflection of the flaps. [*] A fringe of
muscle and aponeurosis, together with the galea, is carefully preserved at the upper edge for subsequent union
by suture with the reflected muscle flaps.

[*] An illustration of the "cross-bow incision" is Fig.
154 in Dr. Cushing's article: Surgery of the head. In:
Surgery, its principles and practice. W. W. Keen, Ed.
Philadelphia: W. B. Saunders Co., 1908, *3:* 17–276.—
R.H.W.

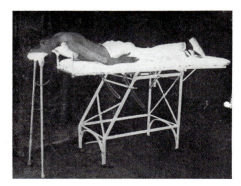

FIG. 32. Showing patient in position on table for cerebellar or high spinal operations.

Primary openings having been made in the bone thus laid bare, they are enlarged with rongeurs, upward so as to expose the lateral sinuses on each side, across the median line avoiding the bone over the torcular, and then downward so as to include the posterior half of the foramen magnum. The dura is then widely opened and the mid-occipital sinus, if present, is ligated.

. . . There are certain points in the bone where hæmorrhage may be met with in these operations, and especial care must be taken at the torcular and at the posterior margin of the mastoid processes. During the deeper manipulations, a large vein which bridges the subdural space at the side of the cerebellum is often encountered, and injury to it should be avoided if possible.

As foretold in my opening paragraphs, it has been my endeavor merely to picture some of the technical steps in these, the commoner cranial operations, in the hope that some operators, who may have had less opportunity for neurological work and whose interests nevertheless lie in this direction, may profit by some of my experiences. There are many of the more difficult procedures, as the operations on the pituitary body, drainage of the 3rd ventricle, extirpation of the Gasserian ganglion, removal of deep-seated tumors, operations for apoplexy and the like—the more dangerous and critical of the modern cranial operations—which for the time being and until their veriest detail is established on an unquestioned basis should rest in the hands alone of those specially trained, not only in neurology, but in the particular conduct of cerebral operations. The advance of operative neurology is greatly impeded by the prevailing impression in regard to its dangers and general futility— an impression due in large measure to the often reckless attempts made in this difficult branch of surgery by the untrained and inexpert.

A METHOD OF COMBINING EXPLORATION AND DECOMPRESSION FOR CEREBRAL TUMORS WHICH PROVE TO BE INOPERABLE[1]*

By HARVEY CUSHING, M.D.

Associate Professor of Surgery, Johns Hopkins University, Baltimore, Maryland

It is often impossible to judge from the neurological symptoms alone whether a growth, known to occupy one of the cerebral hemispheres, will prove to be accessible or suitable for surgical removal. Usually this cannot be determined until a thorough exposure and investigation of the cortex has been made. Hence, when reasonable uncertainty exists as to the operability of such a tumor one oftentimes hesitates to abandon a patient merely to the results of a subtemporal decompression, even though this simple palliative operation affords a large measure of relief in the great majority of cases.

Under circumstances, therefore, in which an exploration with an extensive exposure of the hemisphere seems justifiable, a temporary osteoplastic resection is doubtless the method of choice; but when such a resection has been made and an inoperable tumor or a tense brain without surface lesion is disclosed, there seems to be practically only one way to withdraw from the operative difficulties; namely, to leave the dura open and remove the bone-flap, closing scalp alone over the protruding hemisphere. . . .

The abandonment of an operation in this fashion, however, often leads to ill consequences, for the cerebral protrusion under the protection of scalp alone may, through œdema, . . . become so large as to jeopardize the solid union of the recent scalp wound, the parting of which is likely to be the forerunner of a fungus cerebri. . . .

Another equally undesirable sequel of a cerebral hernia which happens to include the important central gyri . . . is the contralateral palsy which may result from injury of the pyramidal tract fibres as the direct outcome of an extensive protrusion with œdema in cases of great tension. . . .

A further objection to the removal of the bone from an osteoplastic flap made directly over the seat of the lesion concerns the not infrequent rapid increase in size of a vascular growth owing to hæmorrhages in its substance; for some of the poorly supported, thin walled vessels may be ruptured during the change of position which occurs when the cortex protrudes through the open dura. Furthermore, even in the absence of any of these complications such a protrusion is unsightly and an uncomfortable thing for the patient to carry about.

To surmount some of these difficulties and at the same time not only permit of a thorough exploration of the hemisphere with preservation of the bone-flap, but also obtain the advantages of a subtemporal decompression —in other words, to restrict the subsequent hernia largely to the relatively "mute" temporal lobe under the protection of the temporal muscle—we have resorted to the simple device, which may doubtless have occurred to others, of making the subtemporal defect after the bone-flap has been reflected.

The particular steps of the procedure may be briefly summarized. An osteoplastic resection, whatever tools may be employed, has doubtless come to be made, in the hands of all, under some form of tourniquet, with the omega-shaped flap broken off across the thin squamous wing of the temporal bone. If the disclosed dura shows no evidence, through the transparent membrane, of a subjacent growth and proves to be so tense that caution speaks against opening it lest the pia-arachnoid become damaged and the cortex ruptured by a violent protrusion, a subtemporal area of bone is immediately removed as follows (cf. Fig. 1). From under the portion of temporal muscle which has been turned back with the flap, a

* Reprinted in part from *Surgery, Gynecology and Obstetrics*, 1909, 9: 1–5, with the kind permission of the Editor.

[1] Read before the American Surgical Association, June 3, 1909.

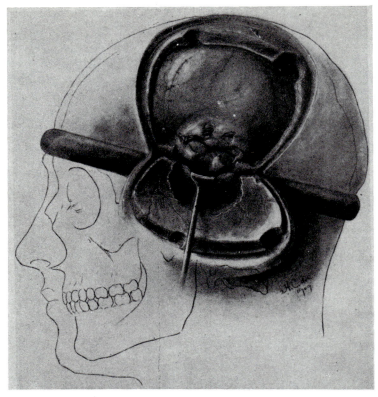

Fig. 1. To illustrate the method of combining a subtemporal decompression with an exploration of the hemisphere. Note: (1) Protrusion of temporal lobe through permanent dural opening destined to underlie bone defect after replacement of flap (dotted line indicates hidden area of bone rongeured away from side of skull while reflected edge of temporal muscle and tourniquet are held out by retractor). (2) Lines of partial closure of dura on its replacement following exposure of the hemisphere.

roughly semicircular area of bone is cut away with heavy rongeurs, which remove bone without jar and so without risk of stripping the remainder of the resected bone from the soft parts. This accomplished, a similar area is rongeured away from the side of the skull well down into the temporal fossa under the tourniquet, the temporal muscle being held away by a retractor. . . . If the base of the bone-flap has been made sufficiently broad a margin possibly a centimeter in width can be left on each side as a support for the flap after its replacement. A subtemporal bone defect is thus secured with even less difficulty than is experienced in making the usual subtemporal opening from without through a split-muscle incision.

The dura is then carefully opened and incised in stellate fashion to the margins of what promises to be a sufficient circle of denuded cortex for a generous decompression. (Cf. Fig. 1.) . . .

Further procedure may be abandoned at this stage and the flap replaced, but if it seems wise to temporarily reflect the dura in order to study the cortex of the hemisphere better than can be done through the transparent membrane, a lumbar puncture may be helpful at this period of the operation. . . . Usually, after the puncture, even when there is a large tumor present, the hemisphere will settle back so that on reflection of the membrane (preferably with its base toward the middle line in the

reverse position to the customary flap) a thorough exploration is permissible in all directions under the dural margin.

As an aid to this exploration I have found a spoon-shaped, round-edged spatula . . . a very helpful instrument, for by its use the cortex can be pressed away without the danger of injury to the pial vessels which exists when the usual flat, square-edged spatula is employed. . . .

In case no surface evidence of a lesion is found, and if there are no justifications for subcortical investigation, the lateral margins of the dural flap are resutured in position, and the osteoplastic window is replaced. . . .

This combined method of exploration and decompression was first employed in the fall of 1907 and I have since had about twenty operations of this type with fairly uniform satisfaction in the procedure. . . .

In a number of patients tumors have been unexpectedly disclosed in consequence of the wide exploration which is permitted by this method. . . .

The method is available also for cases in which a tumor may actually have been extirpated should there seem to be any reason for leaving a defect either to allow for the postoperative œdema which may occur, or to allow for a future protrusion should the growth not have been totally removed or, in case of a glioma, should there be apprehension of a possible recurrence. . . .

Neurosurgical Classic—37

ON JULY 21, 1876, an 11-year-old boy was admitted to the Royal Infirmary in Glasgow with the history of a head injury suffered in a fall 2 weeks previously. A small suppurating wound was present over the left eyebrow, and the boy was lethargic and febrile. Twelve days later he had a right-sided convulsion with a transient aphasia. William Macewen diagnosed a cerebral abscess, which he thought was located in the third left frontal convolution. He proposed to evacuate the abscess through a trephine opening, but the patient's friends refused to give permission. After the patient's death a short time later, Macewen received permission to perform the proposed operation just as he would have if the boy had been alive. Through a temporal trephine opening, the dura mater was incised and a narrow bistoury was inserted into the brain for an inch and a half in the direction of the third frontal convolution. Pus welled out along the bistoury, confirming the diagnosis, and a later postmortem examination revealed an abscess the size of a pigeon's egg in the white matter of the second and third frontal convolutions.[1,5,6]

Macewen was convinced that this boy died unnecessarily, as did most patients with brain abscess. Over the ensuing years he attempted to reverse this hopeless situation by energetically applying to the problem his considerable skill and judgement, basing his actions on the evolving principles of the new science of bacteriology. The extent of Macewen's success became apparent in 1893, when he published *Pyogenic Infective Diseases of the Brain and Spinal Cord.*[6] In this work, which has remained a classic for over 70 years, Macewen presented his results in 94 patients with intracranial infections. Of these there were 5 with extradural abscesses who were operated upon, with 5 recoveries, and 19 with brain abscesses who were oper-

ated upon, with 18 recoveries. Since then these results have remained a challenge for surgeons treating intracranial abscesses.[2-4,7,8]

In an evaluation of Macewen's work, Geoffrey Jefferson[3] stated:

"The magnitude of this achievement is enhanced if we remind ourselves that although surgeons had sometimes operated upon the mastoid, the first clear description of mastoiditis as a definite entity had been given only as recently as 1877 by Frederick Bezold. Its surgery had only just been released by Lister's work. Credit must be given to Macewen therefore as a pioneer in correct mastoid surgery, quite apart from his contributions to the complications that arise from middle ear disease. . . .

"My own views on the reasons for Macewen's success with abscesses are that he was his own operator both on the mastoid and the abscess. . . . At the same time a considerable experience of intra-cranial abscess convinces me that Macewen could not possibly have kept his record unless he had continued to remain firm enough to reject, as he did, twenty per cent of the cases."

Excerpts from *Pyogenic Infective Diseases of the Brain and Spinal Cord* are reprinted below.

References

1. BOWMAN, A. K. The life and teaching of Sir William Macewen. A chapter in the history of surgery. *London: W. Hodge & Co. Ltd.*, 1942, x, 425 pp.
2. GRANT, F. C. Brain abscess. Collective review. *Int. Abstr. Surg.*, 1941, *72*: 118–138.
3. JEFFERSON, G. Sir William Macewen's contribution to neuro-surgery and its sequels. *Glasgow: Jackson, Son & Co.*, 1950, 36 pp. (see pp. 27–29).
4. KING, J. E. J., and TURNEY, F. Brain abscess: evolution of the methods of treatment. *Ann. Surg.*, 1954, *139*: 587–610.
5. MACEWEN, W. Intra-cranial lesions, illustrating some points in connexion with the localisation of cerebral affections and the advantages of antiseptic trephining. IV. Abscess of brain. *Lancet*, 1881, *2*: 541–543; 581–583 (see pp. 582–583).
6. MACEWEN, W. Pyogenic infective diseases of the brain and spinal cord. Meningitis, abscess of brain, infective sinus thrombosis. *Glasgow: J. Maclehose & Sons*, 1893, xxiv, 354 pp.
7. WEBSTER, J. E., and GURDJIAN, E. S. The surgical management of intracranial suppuration. Methods in

diagnosis and management, and a report of 23 cases of civilian and 33 cases of military abscess. *Int. Abstr. Surg.*, 1950, *90*: 209–235.

8. Young, A. Sir William Macewen. An oration. *Glasgow: Jackson, Wylie & Co.*, 1926, 52 pp.

CHAPTER II. PATHOLOGY OF CEREBRAL ABSCESS AND MENINGITIS.*

The pathology of abscess of the brain is so closely interwoven with that of infective meningitis, and the one so frequently accompanies the other, that the pathological aspects of both are dealt with in the same chapter.

In a given case, where a cause of infective inflammation exists on the outside of the skull, from which the interior becomes affected, the alternative, whether meningitis or brain abscess results, depends partly on the anatomical arrangement of the structures, and partly on the intensity and rapidity of the inflammatory action: which again, may be dependent upon the nature of the micro-organism and the virulence of its action. One, or more, of several intracranial conditions—pachymeningitis, lepto-meningitis, ulceration of the brain, abscess of the brain, and necrosis of the cerebral tissue, besides the involvement of the intracranial sinuses with disintegrating thrombosis—may result therefrom. . . .

Lepto-meningitis and cerebral abscess may form independently of a visible tract of inflammation spreading inwards from the initial focus of irritation outside the cranial cavity. In such cases, the pathogenic cause has been conveyed through the vascular system by direct extension from the source of infection to the meninges or brain. This may be done by a thrombosis extending through the veins into the pia or the brain; or the veins may become blocked by a localized disintegrating thrombus, portions of which, containing pathogenic micro-organisms, may be carried inwards by the reversed blood stream. . . . If it should involve the arterial contents, a localized thrombus may result, of which, if it disintegrates, a portion may be carried from the larger vessel into the terminal capillaries in the white cerebral substance, where it would set up minute infective haemorrhagic extravasations, round which an abscess might form. . . . Inflammation may also spread through the lymphatic vessels to the brain. The perineural sheaths may likewise be the path along which the micro-organisms travel, though one very seldom finds cerebral abscess forming by perineural extension, lepto-meningitis being there the rule. . . .

In the great majority, if not in all cases, the peccant matter, which occasions both acute lepto-

* Excerpts reprinted from Pyogenic Infective Diseases of the Brain and Spinal Cord. Meningitis, Abscess of Brain, Infective Sinus Thrombosis. By William Macewen. Glasgow: J. Maclehose & Sons, 1893, xxiv, 354 pp.

meningitis and brain abscess, is organismal. Whether the various forms of intracranial disease have each a distinct specific organism which produces it, and it alone, is for the future to decide. It is, however, probable that the same organism may induce several of these intracranial lesions, the modifying circumstances being, the degree of intensity of its action, its opportunities of access to the intracranial contents afforded by the pathologico-anatomical condition of the parts, and the degree of the restraining force of the living tissues presented by the individual.

The free communication between the nasopharynx, the tympanum, and the mastoid antrum, is such that diseases due to micro-organisms arising in the first-named part, not infrequently affect the others, while, when the membrana is softened by disease and perforation ensues, organisms have free access to the tympanum directly from without. When the middle ear has become inflamed, and its mucous membrane is converted into granulation tissue and purulent exudation issues from it; then it forms a model incubating chamber for micro-organisms, which find there abundant pabulum, ever freshly poured out, and an even, temperature uniformly favourable for their development. Once they have penetrated into the mastoid antrum and the adjoining mastoid cells, they are so far removed from the influence of antiseptics applied to the middle through the external ear, that they rest secure and fructify uninterruptedly as long as pabulum is forthcoming. . . .

The pathogenic organisms found in suppurative lepto-meningitis and brain abscess, as tested both by the microscope and by careful plate cultivations in the author's cases, have most frequently been the streptococcus pyogenes and the staphylococcus pyogenes aureus. . . . When pus in the intracranial suppurative lesion has been compared with that emanating in the same case from the exterior wound or otorrhoea the same organisms have frequently been found in both. . . .

The mere chronicity of an otorrhoea, without extension of serious disease, is no guarantee to the individual of future immunity. Patients so affected are at any time liable to the rapid onset of dangerous sequelae. This may arise from fresh inoculation of the discharges in the middle ear, or from the exposure of fresh areas of the membranes, brought about by progressive disintegration and the implication of these fresh areas in the pathogenic process.

Though acute attacks of infective inflammation of the skull, such as from compound fractures, frequently lead to intracranial extension of the pathogenic process, yet primary acute attacks of otitis media are rarely followed by extension of the pathogenic process to the brain or its membranes. This immunity of the cerebral structures from implication in presence of primary though severe attacks of otitis media, is accounted for by the fact, that the bone and the mucous membrane of the middle ear are still intact, and present a barrier to infection travelling inwards. The virulence of the inflammation might, however, even under such circumstances produce thrombosis of a sinus or give rise to other intracranial complication. . . .

. . . Caries in the tympanic cavity does not usually affect the bone equally all round, but extends in certain directions. When it extends through the antrum and involves the mastoid cells the inner walls of some of which are very thin and contiguous to the sigmoid groove, the latter is apt to be involved and exposed. When it attacks the roof of the middle ear, the tegmen, though a dense plate of bone, yet is thin, and when once ulceration does secure a hold upon it, perforation of the middle fossa of the skull frequently results. When the tegmen is in this thinned brittle condition it is very apt to break on slight concussion, produced by blows on the head, or by vibration of the hammer and chisel when used in opening sclerosed mastoids. When the molecular disintegration of the middle ear proceeds inwards and forwards, the whole of the interior of the petrous bone may become, in extreme cases, hollowed out, leaving a shell externally. The labyrinth—the cochlea, and the semicircular canals—being encased in harder bone, often resist the distintegrating process, though they also are occasionally invaded. . . .

. . . The most frequent seats of perforation from middle ear disease are the tegmen over the tympanum or antrum and the sigmoid groove. When an abscess follows the former it is situated in the temporo-sphenoidal lobe, and when it follows the latter the abscess is generally located in the cerebellum. . . .

. . . When the dura mater has been exposed by osseous erosion it throws out in advance of this lesion a mass of granulation tissue from its external surface, which not only offers obstruction to the further inroads of the pathogenic process, but also assists in the absorption of the disintegrating bone. Such masses of granulation tissue, projecting into the middle ear from the dura through the erosion in the tegmen, have been mistaken for so-called "aural polypi" and have been abrupted or snared, and not infrequently serious intracranial inflammatory action has followed, apparently as the consequence. Similar granulation masses are to be found issuing from the layer of dura forming the wall of the sigmoid sinus through the sigmoid groove into the mastoid cells. These masses of granulation tissue are usually surrounded with pus, a portion of which is pent up intracranially, forming an extradural abscess, the contents of which ooze out if the neck of the granu-

lation mass, as it issues through the erosion, be pressed gently aside. Occasionally, however, the granulation tissue may be accompanied by very little pus, the erosion taking place with all the greater insidiousness. In not a few cases there exists a small necrosis of the bone in the tegmen tympani or sigmoid groove. The extradural abscess forming on the inner side of it. . . .

. . . the softened brain tissue, in contact with the infective nidus, is prone to purulent disintegration forming a cerebral ulcer, and the pus ensuing from the ulceration being confined between the soldered membranes and the brain will probably be described as an abscess, especially when met with during an operation. The formation of a true cerebral abscess, however, occurs by a further extension from this pial accumulation and softened cerebral tissue along the paths of the cerebral vessels, which penetrate the white substance of the brain. The infective virus acting upon the vessels, and causing oedema of the brain with leucocytal exudation, often mingled with extravasation of red blood corpuscles, soon forms an area of purulent encephalitis. In the majority of fully-formed abscesses in the temporo-sphenoidal lobe, an opening into the abscess cavity exists at the base of the brain, which indicates the point of brain indentation caused by the infected conical projection in the membranes. . . . These openings may be regarded as the area of initial invasion, and not merely as due to a secondary process of absorption of the abscess wall. Such openings in the base of the brain connected with abscess in the temporo-sphenoidal lobe are almost always located in the same place . . . so that, as a rule, in cases of cerebral abscess the path by which the infective processes spread from the tegmen to the brain can be traced, and the majority of abscesses develop by direct extension from the infective seat. It is therefore of great importance, in the treatment of such cases, besides dealing with the abscess, that the point of origin of the infective processes in the tissues should be sought for and their paths of extension traced, in order that they may be eradicated.

The statement that disease of the tympanum causes cerebral abscess chiefly, while disease of the mastoid cells causes cerebellar abscess, is misleading, inasmuch as the tympanum is diseased in both forms; and in the majority of cases in which the mastoid antrum and cells are affected, grave intracranial disease of the middle fossa results. The tegmen tympani is often eroded at the same time as the involvement of the sigmoid sinus occurs, and cerebral abscess in the temporal lobe is not infrequently met with, along with infective sigmoid sinus thrombosis. . . .

It must be admitted that there are cases in which abscess of the brain may find an exit through the erosions set up by the ulceration. . . .

As a rule these abscesses cannot empty themselves owing to the tortuous passages through the erosions filled with granulation masses, and on account of the resistance in their walls when encysted. Most of them end fatally when not relieved surgically. . . .

When a pathogenic embolism occurs in a cerebral artery or vein situated in the white substance of the brain, haemorrhagic extravasation ensues, accompanied or shortly followed by an exudation of leucocytes, which infiltrate the extravasation and the brain tissue in the vicinity. These leucocytes rapidly degenerate into pus, while the neighbouring nerve tissue disintegrates and liquefies. These emboli may be accompanied by anaemic or haemorrhagic necrosis, according as an artery or a vein has been blocked. This may be indicated by the appearance of the parts during operation: when they are oedematous and glistening they are anaemic, and therefore due to arterial thrombosis, and when they appear as reddish-brown sloughs they are haemorrhagic and due to venous thrombosis. When large arteries are blocked, necroses of extensive areas may occur which may be afterwards separated. Such large necrotic portions may also arise from very acute and infective inflammation of the brain. . . .

The tissue surrounding and forming the boundary of the acute abscess is actively inflamed. The vessels may be seen in all stages of inflammation, from hyperaemia in the outer zone to thrombosis in the inner. Surrounding the vessels are masses of exudation cells mingled with extravasated red blood corpuscles, and the glimpses of brain tissue which may be had in the less inflamed parts show it to be softened and disintegrating. When the inflammation has been great the vessels are scarcely recognisable on account of the exudation cells not only filling the surrounding parts, but also the vessel wall, and in great measure occupying its interior, the red blood corpuscles being faintly seen in some, while in others they have entirely disappeared. Irregularly distributed over the surface of the abscess are portions of minute sloughs of an oedematous greyish appearance, with pus in their periphery and in the pockets or the sinuosities in the abscess wall. The surface toward the abscess is flocculent, shaggy, and irregular in outline. Occasionally little naked thrombosed vessels project from its surface into the abscess cavity at parts where the molecular disintegration has proceeded more actively in the soft brain tissue surrounding the vessel. As in processes of ulceration in other parts of the body, the small vessels become thrombosed in advance of the molecular necrosis, and so haemorrhage into the abscess is prevented. Occasionally, however, the process of disintegration is more rapid than that of thrombosis, and bleeding occurs into the abscess cavity, giving rise to symptoms of apoplexy. The zone of brain tissue surrounding

the abscess is oedematous, and its vessels are hyperaemic. There is thus in the periphery of an acute abscess no other wall than a softened and disintegrated cerebral tissue filled with exudation cells and extravasated blood.

The pia mater and arachnoid tissue over an area of cerebral degeneration have often a milky and turbid appearance.

The encephalitis surrounding the abscess extends to a distance beyond the abscess itself. Were this zone of encephalitis to embrace a part of the brain whose function was known and capable of external manifestation, symptoms might arise which might lead one to localize the abscess at a distance from its actual seat.

. . . When the process of molecular disintegration which has produced the abscess ceases, and the brain tissue possesses sufficient vitality to assume a formative action, the debris of disintegrated tissue, granular cells, leucocytes, blood, and inspissated pus become entangled in the meshes of fibrin, the elements for the formation of which are poured out from the living tissue. Into this mass large numbers of leucocytes penetrate. Some of these form into elongated spindle cells, bundles of which may be seen interspersed throughout the membrane. At an early period it contains no bloodvessels, and, therefore, secretion from its surface must be limited to the few leucocytes which have travelled through it from the living tissue. Later a few bloodvessels may project from the living tissue into the membrane at a point where it is abundantly penetrated by leucocytes. These vessels are, however, of the most primitive description, such as may be seen in imperfectly developed granulation tissue. They are at first so small and imperfectly developed that they can only supply nutriment to the leucocytes in their immediate neighbourhood. As they are generally to be seen on the side of the encapsulating membrane next the living tissue, they cannot provide many exudation cells for fresh pus formation.

The pus in the abscess thus becomes encapsulated by a layer of membrane of very low vitality which shuts off the living brain tissue from the dead pus within. When this capsule is complete on all sides the abscess becomes to a great extent stationary. First, because the process of molecular disintegration has ceased. Secondly, as the leucocytes which penetrate for some way into the living wall of the abscess, and which might be converted into pus were they shed on the inside of the capsule, are principally caught by the meshwork of fibrin, so that few pass into the abscess cavity; and as the lining membrane increases in thickness the difficulties of transmigration of the leucocytes increase, both on account of the greater distance they have to travel, and the increasing formation of fibrous tissue bundles, which are interspersed throughout it. Thirdly, this same membrane, although it does permit the passage of serum from the pus cavity to the vessels in the living tissue, yet prevents the absorption of the particulate portions of the disintegrated pus. The thickness of the abscess capsule varies considerably, from one to five or more millimetres. It is generally smooth internally, and rather ragged and flocculent externally—next to living brain tissue. It is for the most part rounded or ovoid, while the boundary of the acute abscess is generally irregular in outline. The time required for the formation of the abscess capsule is indefinite, and depends on the condition of the part and the character of the inflammation. Some abscesses of at least three weeks' duration were found to be without capsules. . . .

. . . This wall may not, however, remain permanently in the condition described. Changes take place in it from the side of the living tissue. The circumferential pressure of the brain upon the abscess may facilitate the absorption of the fluid portion of the pus. Well-formed vessels may be thrown out from the living brain tissue, and penetrating the capsule, may thus aid in the absorption of pus debris through phagocytic action. In this way it is possible for a considerable portion of a small cerebral abscess to become absorbed.

. . . On the other hand, if the capsule be replaced in part by a layer of vigorous granulation tissue, a fresh supply of pus may be formed which may augment the size of the abscess and exercise pressure from within upon the capsule which is thus apt to become thinned at parts. The abscess may then burst either into the ventricles or into the subdural space. In either case very serious symptoms ensure. . . .

. . . The tissues in the vicinity of the encapsulated abscess are not always tolerant of the foreign body in their midst. They suffer from an amount of compression, which is apt to induce degeneration and atrophy. Slight causes may then occasion in them fresh oedema and inflammation, just as encephalitis occurs round a tumour. If this encephalitis becomes purulent, a new abscess may form in the periphery of the old one, leaving the latter intact within its capsule. It is probable, however, that a leakage of the contents of the abscess into the compressed tissues in the vicinity may set free from imprisonment inflammatory elements (micro-organisms) which, meeting with fresh pabulum, regain their former vitality, and start afresh the inflammation in the tissues on the outside of the capsule. In such a case, an extramural abscess develops in the circumference of the old one, which it may set so completely free from its attachments that the encapsulated abscess may be found floating in the pus of the peripheral or secondary abscess. This was observed in one of the author's cases, in which the primary abscess contained in its cyst-like sac was seen floating in a pool of pus.

. . . The size of a cerebral abscess cannot always be estimated by the degree of pressure produced. It is not like a solid tumour, which, to the extent of its bulk, pushes aside the living tissue in its vicinity. The molecular disintegration by which the abscess is formed hollows out an aperture in the brain which is filled by the molecular debris and pus. The abscess will, therefore, not produce the same amount of pressure on the adjacent structures as a solid tumour of the same size, so that pressure symptoms occasioned by an abscess would be less than would be produced by a tumour of corresponding bulk. On the other hand, the symptoms due to oedema and inflammatory action would probably be greater in the acute stage of abscess formation than in most tumours. . . .

There can be no doubt that the pulse is slowed in cerebral abscess owing to the pressure exerted, as after the abscess has attained a certain size its rate decreases as the abscess increases, and the moment the pressure is relieved by evacuation of the pus there is a sudden bound in the pulse rate, from for instance 40 to 120 per minute. . . . The point referred to above must here be remembered; the pus in the cerebral abscess *may* only occupy the area destroyed by the molecular disintegration, and, if so, little pressure can be exerted on the brain, and therefore little alteration occurs in the pulse rate. . . .

Pyaemic abscess of the brain may arise from infective matter originating in some source of infection in any part of the body. This peccant matter entering the blood is carried by the bloodstream until it is deposited in a small vessel producing infective embolism. The diseases which have been known to give rise to this condition in the brain are, among others, disintegrating pneumonia, foetid bronchitis and empyema, foetid pericarditis, infective compound fractures, seldom acute infective periostitis, and occasionally infective ulcers of the intestines and abdominal cavity. Infective peritonitis generally ends fatally so soon after its onset that cerebral abscess has no time to form. . . .

It is well to remember that pyaemia, though generally the cause of multiple abscesses, may itself arise from intracranial suppuration, especially when the sinuses are also involved.

. . . Abscesses are rarely multiple saving when they originate in pyaemia, in which case they are in two-thirds of the cases multiple, and generally very numerous, and invade both brain and cerebellum. . . . 93 per cent of abscesses from traumatism are single: 87 per cent are single when due to otitis media. . . .

. . . After an abscess has been evacuated the brain tissue tends to fill the gap left by the removal of the pus. If it be an acute abscess, the resiliency of the brain is retained and its expansion is rapid, a few minutes to a few hours sufficing to close the gap. After evacuation of chronic encysted abscess, the expansion is much slower, taking days before the cavity is obliterated. When the wound has been at once closed after evacuation and the dura replaced, there is a probability of the brain remaining free from adhesions, but as a rule it becomes more or less fixed to the dura. When the wound has to heal by granulation tissue, the opening into the brain meanwhile being kept patent for pus evacuation, the pia mater adheres to the cicatrix, soldering the brain to what becomes a rigid wall. Such anchoring of the brain is subsequently apt to produce a shock on sudden movement of the patient, as on sudden rising from a recumbent or sitting posture. This physical effect directly applied to the brain itself, though acting like a drag or pull, is akin in its physiological result to a blow applied to the cerebrum. It is apt to cause unconsciousness, generally of very brief duration. The man may fall, but is able to pick himself up in a few seconds. In some few instances the unconsciousness lasts longer. When very frequently repeated, even when the effect is so slight as to be only slightly perceptible to the patient, this frequent dragging is apt, months or years afterwards, to produce encephalitis over an extended area of the brain. This cerebral irritation might lead to epileptic fits, though the author is not aware of any undoubted instances following operation for cerebral abscess. There are, however, many such cases resulting from traumatisms, in which the brain has been soldered to the unyielding parietes. . . .

CHAPTER III. SYMPTOMS OF ABSCESS OF BRAIN AND MENINGITIS.

The elicitation of a differential cranial percussion note* as an aid to cerebral diagnosis in certain gross changes of the intracranial contents, especially in children, has been practised by the author as opportunity offered during the last ten years, and as it has been found to be useful in diagnosis the following may assist those desirous of practising it.

The percussion note is obtained by the cranial walls vibrating when struck, the note being modified by the consistency and volume of the contents and their relative position to the bone. The sound elicited depends first on the susceptibility of the skull to vibrate, and secondly on the effect which the intracranial contents exert on these vibrations. When struck, a thin cranium vibrates more easily than a thick one. A skull may be so thick that it vibrates little, if at all, to ordinary digital percussion. In the cranium of an infant, whose bones are only united by a membrane, and where they lie somewhat loosely on the brain, the percussion note elicited is so slight, dull, and flat, as scarcely to be perceptible. Should, however, the contents of such a cranium increase sufficiently to

* This was later named "Macewen's sign"—R.H.W.

produce tension of the whole parietes—bones and intervening membrane—then the note becomes clear, particularly as the density of the contents of such a case is low—the brain containing a considerable quantity of serous fluid. In the child whose fontanelles remain open, especially in delayed closure from serous over-distension, a clear drum-like note is elicited on percussion. . . .

. . . The author has found this clear percussion note in over forty children and young adolescents who have had distended ventricles arising from many different causes. In tumours of the cerebellum it is an aid to diagnosis. When present, along with abscess, it points to involvement of the cerebellar fossa. . . .

The cracked pot sound elicited on percussion of the head in extensive fractures of the skull, when large areas of bone are detached by fissures, the author has only been able to detect on three occasions in the adult. . . .

CASE XXVII. *Cerebral abscess in temporo-sphenoidal lobe; complicated with localized purulent meningitis of cerebellar fossa, both due primarily to chronic otitis media purulenta. Coming under observation seven days from onset of symptoms. Duration of illness sixteen days prior to evacuation of abscess. Operation. Complete recovery.*

H.M., aged 9 years, admitted into the Children's Hospital, Glasgow, on 26th January, 1893. Affected with purulent meningitis, accompanied by encephalitis terminating in cerebral abscess, involving the greater portion of the right temporo-sphenoidal lobe, due primarily to otitis media purulenta, an injury being probably the determining cause.

History.—*Heredity.*—Both parents are alive and well. Patient is one of a family of four, one of whom died when three months old from "inflammation of the brain." Other two are healthy.

Personal.—The parents believed patient to have been in good health previous to this illness. Though they had never observed discharge from his ears, yet on admission his right external ear was found to contain foetid inspissated pus.

Present Illness.—Fourteen days before admission the patient fell head first down a flight of stone stairs. He rose immediately, apparently uninjured, and went about as usual. A week afterwards he complained of a severe pain in his head in and around the right ear, which compelled him to remain in bed. Since then he has had complete anorexia. Three days previous to admission, the pain extended to the frontal region. On the following day he vomited repeatedly, and a swelling was observed over the right mastoid. He has had constipation of bowels for several days, and has urinated involuntarily.

Condition on Admission.—Patient was in an irritable state, semi-insensible and delirious, but could be occasionally roused to realize his surroundings. He frequently cried out and tossed about, and was evidently suffering pain, referred to his right ear and corresponding side of the head. His pupils were equal, contracted, and sluggish. The movements of the eyeballs were free, and there was occasionally a slight transient convergent squint of right eyeball. There was a degree of congestion of both retinae. A fluctuating swelling was observed behind the right ear over the mastoid. The right external auditory meatus contained foul smelling pus, and the membrana tympani was perforated. With the exception of the paresis of the right external rectus, there was no observable paralysis. There were very slight erratic twitchings of groups of muscles of limbs, mostly on the left, but also on the right side of body, and equally on both sides of the face. There was an herpetic labial eruption. His temperature was high, and his pulse rapid. On admission an incision was made to relieve the sub-periosteal mastoid abscess, and vent was given to about three drachms of foetid pus.

Operation for Meningitis (28th January).—Two days after admission, the temperature having remained high, the pulse rapid, and the meningeal symptoms persisting, along with an increasing and now marked retraction of the head, delirium and other indications of brain involvement, the following operation was performed.

The mastoid antrum was opened. It was found to be enlarged, filled with cholesteatomatous masses and pus. The cerebellar fossa was then opened. The sigmoid sinus was covered with pus and a mass of granulation tissue, varying from $\frac{1}{8}$ inch to $\frac{1}{4}$ inch in thickness. Though its lumen was markedly encroached on, it was still patent. Granulation tissue also covered the dura behind the sinus in the cerebellar fossa, and several drachms of pus were evacuated from between the skull and that membrane. The pus from the cerebellar fossa was submitted to bacterial examination, and both by direct stained specimen and culture experiments the streptococci pyogenes were obtained. The tegmen tympani was carefully scrutinized, but no erosion was discovered.

Relief to all the meningeal symptoms followed this operation. The temperature, pulse, and respiration all became normal. The muscular tremors, the crying fits, and the delirium ceased, the pupils resumed their normal mobility, and on the third day the last evidence of the retraction of the head and neck disappeared. Following this improvement, it was observed that the pulse and temperature became subnormal. On the fifth day after the operation he became drowsy, disinclined to speak, and when both eyes were exposed to a light, the right pupil was a shade larger than its neighbour and distinctly more sluggish. All these symptoms increased until the ninth day after the operation when the evidence of pressure on the brain was marked. He was then extremely drowsy and difficult to rouse. There was a passivity over the left side of the face, and the left arm when lifted up dropped in a heap. The right arm, though feeble, the patient still controlled. Both lower limbs moved actively when the toes were pinched. An operation for the relief of cerebral abscess was resolved upon. The symptoms pointed to abscess in the temporo-sphenoidal lobe; but as there had existed so much purulent meningitis in the cerebellar fossa which the former operation had revealed, it was deemed expedient to first subject the exposed cerebellar area to a careful scrutiny.

Operation for Cerebral Abscess (6th February, 1893).—The already exposed sinus was first inspected, and as some pus still exuded from the granulation tissue covering the dura behind the sinus, a quarter inch disc of bone was removed from the occiput covering the cerebellar fossa. The anterior half of the aperture left by this disc was covered with granulation tissue, while the posterior half exposed normal and almost transparent membranes, through which the underlying brain was just perceptible. There was no haziness or milkiness of the membranes over this area, such as would have been expected had there been an extension of the meningitis in this direction. Attention was now directed to the temporo-sphenoidal lobe, and as a preliminary a fresh scrutiny of the tegmen tympani and tegmen antri was made, but no visible erosion was detected.

The incision which had previously exposed the mastoid antrum was extended upwards over the squamous plate of the temporal, and from it a half inch disc of bone was removed from a point half an inch above and a little behind the external auditory meatus. At this point the dura was healthy, and so transparent that a flake of plastic effusion $\frac{1}{8}$ inch in diameter was seen either overlying or within one of the compressed pial vessels. This speck of effusion could be altered in position by probe pressure applied from the external surface of the dura mater. The surface of the brain was markedly avascular, probably due to the pial vessels being flattened against the dura and skull from intracranial pressure, but possibly from thrombosis of some of the larger trunks. When the membranes were incised the avascular brain bulged into the trephine aperture. A hollow needle was introduced into the temporo-sphenoidal lobe in an inward and downward direction; when it had penetrated the brain substance for about half-an-inch, there was first the escape of some gas followed quickly by a jet of pus, greenish in colour and of foul odour. A pair of forceps were afterwards introduced through the healthy brain tissue and expanded, when the pus was given free vent, and with it there came a series of cerebral sloughs, some of considerable size. The amount of pus and disintegrated cerebral tissue, though not accurately measured, was approximately about three ounces. After this matter was removed and the brain tissue held aside, a large cavity was seen to exist. Its limit in the anterior and posterior directions was not visible from the trephine opening, its depth was fully an inch, and a probe could be passed backward for about two inches and forward for about one and a half inches before coming in contact with brain matter. Considering the size of the child's head and that of the cerebral cavity, the greater portion of the temporo-sphenoidal lobe must have been obliterated. The brain tissue exhibited very little tendency to fill the gap, which remained as a cavity of the above dimensions at the end of the operation. The cavity was not syringed, lest infective particles might be disseminated especially into the lateral ventricles; but it was evacuated as thoroughly as possible, the head being placed in several directions to facilitate complete evacuation by gravitation. Iodoform and boracic powder were then introduced into the cavity, a short decalcified drainage tube was fixed in it by means of a stitch, and a wood-wool dressing was applied.

The pulse, which ranged from 56 to 70 before operation and was 72 before the evacuation of pus, increased in rapidity immediately after the operation, and when the patient was removed to bed was to be found to be 104, and two hours afterwards 116; subsequently it subsided to normal. . . .

Course after Operation.—From this date the patient made an uninterrupted recovery. He was dressed for the first time two weeks after the operation, and again at the end of a month from the date of the operation. At the former dressing the brain cavity no longer existed, and only a minute portion of the drainage tube lay exposed on the granulating surface, the remainder having been absorbed. The external wound healed by granulation tissue. . . .

CASE XXXIX. *Case of cerebellar abscess with partial thrombosis of sigmoid sinus, arising from infective otitis media. Operation. Recovery. Coming under observation on the sixtieth day of illness. Duration of illness ninety days.*

J.R., aged 38 years, was seen in consultation with Drs. Wood Smith and Barr, on 13th February, 1892, suffering from cerebellar abscess, with partial thrombosis of sigmoid sinus.

History.—*Heredity.*—Family history good. *Personal.* —Patient has had left facial paralysis and deafness since early childhood, but for many years there has been no suppuration in the left ear. Otherwise he has been in good health.

Present Illness.—On 15th December, 1891, he got chilled; felt pain in the right ear. Six hours afterwards he awoke in great agony with pain in the right ear, shooting thence through his head. Some days later the pain had further extended to the vertex and back of head and right side of neck. Along with the pain he had deafness in that ear. After a fortnight's treatment in bed he felt stronger, but the pain and deafness persisted. He was however able to be taken to the country for a change of air, from which he benefitted, but was never free from pain in the head and back of right side of neck. He returned from the country on the 11th February, and the same night and next day the pains becoming much aggravated, the writer was asked to see him on 13th February.

Condition when First Observed.—He then complained of pain over right ear, vertex, and more especially over the back of head and right side of neck, and he had pain on pressure over the course of the upper third of the jugular vein and at the apex of the posterior cervical triangle, in both of which regions the tissues were thickened and contained several enlarged deep cervical glands. There were several small superficial submastoid glands likewise enlarged and painful to touch. The pain he described as persistent and throbbing.

The motor power (with exception of left facial paralysis), sensations, and reflexes, were normal.

A slight purulent discharge emanated from the right ear, and the membrana tympani had a wash-leather appearance. There was slight papillitis in both fundi, especially the right. The pulse was 55 per minute, and the temperature was 99°F. His lungs were free from evidence of infective invasion. These symptoms pointed toward thrombosis of the sigmoid sinus with cerebellar suppuration, and immediate operation was advised.

Operation (13th Feb., 1892).—The mastoid antrum was opened and found to contain granulation tissue and pus. The sigmoid groove was then exposed. Masses of granulation tissue, sprouting from the knee of the sigmoid sinus, projected through the groove into the mastoid cells. These granulation masses being removed, the dura of the cerebellar fossa was found thinned at the inner and anterior side of the sigmoid sinus, and a drop of pus exuded by the inner side of the sinus through a minute erosion in the cerebellar dura. The dura was

opened at this part, and this gave vent to about three drachms of pus, which issued from the cerebellar tissue, which was at that part softened. The sigmoid sinus, though distinctly thickened, was not opened, as the mass of granulation tissue surrounding it in all probability had acted as a protection against the entrance of infective organisms. The cavity was washed out with a weak carbolized solution, the antrum as well as the middle ear being cleansed. The ossicles and membrane were left intact.

From that time the pain previously experienced greatly diminished, and he was soon able to have refreshing sleeps and to awake feeling well. The pulse still continued slower than normal, 50 to 55, though his normal pulse and that of some other members of the family was about 60. His temperature was normal. At the termination of a week he was quite free from pain. The tumefaction of the tissues at the upper part of the neck had almost disappeared. A fortnight afterwards the enlarged glands had greatly subsided. The wound closed by granulation tissue from below upwards. He made an uninterrupted recovery and regained his former health and strength. . . .

Prognosis.—Cerebral abscess must always be regarded as a serious affection imminently dangerous to life. The great majority of cases not dealt with surgically end in death within a short period, generally a few weeks. On the other hand, there is no cerebral affection more amenable to surgical treatment, and none which offers better results. An uncomplicated cerebral abscess, whose position is clearly localized, if surgical measures are adopted for its relief at a sufficiently early period, is one of the most hopeful of all cerebral affections. It is much more so than suppurative leptomeningitis, or even than infective thrombosis of the sigmoid sinus, unless the latter can be operated on before the disintegration and dissemination of the infective contents of the vein take place. After aseptic evacuation of the abscess, not only is the patient likely to recover, but in many instances it leaves no perceptible permanent mental or bodily damage. Within a few days, sometimes hours after the evacuation, the mind becomes bright and intelligent, the paralysis passes away, and within a few months the optic neuritis has disappeared, leaving the visual function unimpaired.

Occasionally, after evacuation of the abscess, there may be some soldering of the brain to the skull, or to the almost equally rigid dura mater or fibrous covering filling up the trephine aperture, though this is much less than what occurs after the removal of tumours. When this occurs the patient may be subject to occasional faintness on sudden exposure to great heat or on sudden exertion. One man, a blacksmith to trade, says that after he had been cured of his abscess he occasionally felt on sudden effort, especially when beside the furnace, a faintness coming over him, which caused him to drop what he held in his hands and to lie down for a moment. This occurred several times the first year, and seldom afterwards, as he carefully avoided exposure to great heat or *sudden* exertion. He was capable of strenuous and prolonged exertion provided it was not sudden.

The prognosis without operation will in some measure depend upon the size of the abscess, the smaller ones occasionally being absorbed, the larger ones usually ending in death. The position of the abscess in the brain will also affect the prognosis. If it be situated deeply, so as to involve the more vital parts, death will speedily follow. On the other hand, a superficial abscess not operated on may be evacuated, if a sufficient vent is formed for it by pathological processes through the dura and bone. This, however, is rare, and even those so connected with the exterior of the skull generally end fatally sooner or later.

Even an abscess which has become encysted, and has remained for a considerable period without evincing any signs of its presence, may be a source of danger. The encysted abscess may burst, or it may act as a foreign body round which fresh inflammation is set up . . . , and if situated in the cerebellum may cause death by oedema of the brain and serous distension of the ventricles. An encysted abscess may, however, become absorbed; but until it does so it is a menace to the patient's life, as it is still apt to have fresh suppuration induced in its vicinity whenever fresh organisms are introduced, probably gaining access by the original channel of infection. The source from which the abscess sprang remaining active is an additional element of danger, both by way of occasioning fresh suppuration round the abscess, and also by creating fresh foci of inflammatory disturbance, such as sinus thrombosis or lepto-meningitis.

The cure of cerebral abscess depends on its early detection, accurate localization, and speedy and efficient evacuation under aseptic precautions.

Course of cerebral abscess.—The time occupied by cerebral abscess in developing and pursuing its course when uninterrupted by treatment is variable. Acute abscess runs its course in from two to six weeks, whereas chronic cerebral abscess, when encapsulation takes place, may last for a very long period—months to many years. As a rule, abscess arising from infective otitis media runs a more rapid course than abscess arising from infective traumatism, without direct exposure of the brain. No doubt the nature of the specific organism introduced influences the duration of the course.

CHAPTER V. TREATMENT.

. . . Abscess in the brain, infective thrombosis of the intracranial sinuses, and lepto-meningitis originate in primary infective foci. The first step in prophylaxis is to prevent the occurrence of such foci, the second to eradicate them when present. . . .

When the skull is bruised, indented, and ingrained with dirt without fracture, great care is necessary in order to remove the whole of the infective matter. . . .

If fracture exists, the edges of the fractured bone ought to be inspected, and if impregnated with foreign matter, they ought to be refreshed with a chisel. . . .

. . . When the dura has been penetrated, and the inner membranes, or the brain itself, inoculated with infective products, the dura ought to be freely opened, in order to expose for inspection the inner membranes, as well as the brain; also to facilitate the removal of foreign matter, and prevent the ultimate extension of deleterious products. When, in addition to the puncture of the brain and its membranes, the cerebral substance has been bruised, it is very difficult in the midst of disintegrating brain tissue and extravasated blood to ensure the removal of all extraneous matter. When doubt on this point exists, it is preferable to leave the wound open—exposed to the influence of iodoform gauze,—first to permit of the free escape of inflammatory products, should they unfortunately form; and secondly to secure the direct application of antiseptics.

All sources of suppuration or infective matter in the orbital, nasal, buccal, oral, and pharyngeal cavities, and in the maxillary and frontal sinuses ought to be removed, or, when this is not practicable, the discharges ought to be rendered and maintained aseptic. This is sometimes difficult without extensive operation in lesions of the nasal fossa or its annexa, but as long as an infective source remains it is an element of danger and a menace to the patient. Cario-necrosis of the skull should be similarly dealt with. The frontal and maxillary sinuses, when in a state of persistent suppuration, may require trephining to afford free vent to the pus, and for the purpose of removing from the walls infected granulation tissue and eroded bone. The proximity of the frontal sinuses to the brain render infective processes in them very hazardous, especially when accompanied by erosion of their posterior wall. When the frontal sinuses are involved, both ought to be exposed. The neglect of this precaution in one case, reported to author, led to a fatal issue from suppurative lepto-meningitis, originating in the opposite frontal sinus from that which was exposed. . . .

As chronic purulent otitis media and the extension of inflammatory processes to the mastoid antrum and cells is the primary focus which leads most often to intracranial inflammatory lesions, the eradication of the *otitis media* must be regarded as the most potent factor in the prophylaxis of inflammatory cerebral lesions. . . .

. . . When the patient has presented symptoms of infective meningitis, extradural abscess or abscess of the brain, the mastoid antrum and the tympanic attic having been fully exposed, the tympanum ought to be carefully scrutinized, granulation tissue growing from it removed, and any fistulous openings leading intracranially explored, and their position relative to the exterior of the cranium noted.

. . . By enlarging the opening in the tegmen, extradural abscess may be thoroughly evacuated. The extent of bone removed must be determined by individual circumstances, but it ought to be sufficient to prevent re-accumulation of fluid between the dura and the bone. No pockets or crevices are to be left, and all granulation tissue should be removed. It is safe to open the tegmen freely in an outward direction from the seat of the perforation. Before injecting fluid—if such be deemed necessary—between the skull and the dura ascertain the limits of the extradural space, and whether there be an opening through the dura into the inner membranes or the brain. If no such opening exist, then the extradural cavity may be washed out with safety, and dressed with iodoform ·and boracic acid powder and iodoform gauze. . . .

. . . When pus issues through an aperture in the dura mater from the intradural structures, after the tegmen has been opened sufficiently and the extradural surface cleansed, the dura is opened freely. If the pus be found gathered in the arachnoid or pial meshes, or if it issues from ulceration of the brain surface, it may be thoroughly dealt with from the opening in the tegmen. The inner membranes ought to be opened, and the cerebral surface washed with a stream of antiseptic solution, and dusted with antiseptic powder. No drainage tube is required if the openings through the tegmen and dura have been sufficiently free.

. . . When pus is found to issue through the dura above the tegmen from a cerebral abscess in the temporo-sphenoidal lobe, the abscess may be evacuated by enlarging the aperture in the tegmen, and also extending the aperture outwards through the squamous portion of the temporal. Such an opening into the cerebrum suffices for temporary purposes, but though it always ought to be made in order to eradicate the source of the infection, it is not safe to trust to it alone, as in many cerebral abscesses there are sloughs of brain tissue which cannot be easily removed in this way, but require a larger opening in the skull for their evacuation. If these sloughs be allowed to remain in the brain, they retain infective matter, which maintains the irritation, and may give rise to fresh abscess formation.

. . . In abscess of the temporo-sphenoidal lobe, it has been proposed to make the opening through the skull at various points. It ought to be made as near to the seat of disease as possible. In the majority of cases the abscess in the temporal lobe originates in the tissues directly above the tegmen

tympani or antri, and therefore an opening in the squamous portion of the temporal above the tegmen will be the nearest point to the cerebral abscess.

When the mastoid antrum has already been opened, the incision in the soft parts made to expose the antrum is extended upwards for a couple of inches above the posterior zygomatic root. The soft tissues including the periosteum are reflected by the periosteal elevator, and a disc of bone half an inch in diameter is removed. The centre pin of the trephine is placed at a point in line with the posterior osseous wall of the external auditory meatus, and three quarters of an inch above the posterior root of the zygoma. . . .

When the dura is exposed, any purulent secretion which may exist extradurally is removed, and the colour and appearances of the dura are noted. . . . Before opening the dura, it is well to cover the exposed osseous surface and its cut edge with the iodoform and boracic acid powder, rubbing it into the cut osseous surface, in order to protect these parts from contamination by the infective pus about to be withdrawn. . . .

With the object of exploring for pus, and removing it when found, either of three instruments may be used—a cannula armed with a trocar, a hollow needle, or a pair of sinus forceps. The instrument ought to be inserted in an inward, downward, and slightly forward direction, so as to impinge, if it went far enough, against the cranial aspect of the tegmen tympani. While the instrument is being inserted, a *slight* to and fro lateral movement ought to be imparted to its point, with the view of ascertaining whether it has entered a cavity, inside which its extremity can move without resistance. When the sinus forceps are used the blades are several times gently expanded as they are introduced. . . .

. . . When the pus is found, its rate of flow from the cannula varies according to the amount of intracranial pressure, and when the abscess is becoming emptied the flow will be influenced by the respirations, increasing during expiration. Along with the pus, molecular debris and minute sloughs of brain tissue may be extruded through the cannula, but the larger sloughs, which are so frequently present in brain abscess, cannot escape in this way, they require a large opening for their removal. For this purpose, a quantity of brain tissue, existing between the abscess and the surface of the brain, may require removal, or the peripheral brain tissue may be turned aside. While the cannula is retained in the abscess cavity as a guide, the cerebral tissue may be removed by means of a Volkmann's spoon, or it may preferably be turned aside by introducing a pair of dressing forceps closed and opening them *in situ*. Frequently, when the forceps have thus been expanded, one or more of the sloughs flow between their blades and can at once be removed. Once the opening in the cerebral tissue has been sufficient, the sloughs are often extruded by the intracranial pressure, and are carried slowly to the surface of the brain. If the sloughs be too large to be thus extruded, they may be gently detached from the abscess wall, and assisted out by the forceps and the sharp spoon, it being necessary to discriminate carefully between the slough and the healthy brain tissue. It is of importance to remove these sloughs thoroughly, as if they remain they are apt to set up fresh irritation and abscess in their periphery by the infective matter which impregnates them, and which is contained in their interstices. The retention of such sloughs is one of the most fruitful sources of reproduction of abscess after evacuating the primary one, and is also a cause of delayed healing. It is true that were they rendered aseptic they could be absorbed, but this would be difficult to secure when they arise from an infected source. The leaving of cerebral sloughs is as dangerous as not eradicating the primary source of the infection or the channels by which it spreads to the brain.

. . . After removal of the sloughs, the cavity is washed out with a boracic or weak carbolized watery solution (1–100). In order to do this a second cannula is introduced by the side of that first inserted, the calibre of the second being at least a half greater than that of the former. A stream of antiseptic fluid is caused to flow gently through the cannula with the finer calibre, and allowed to find an exit by the larger tube. It need scarcely be added that the stream is to be gently introduced, and any resistance met with must not be overcome by forcing the fluid through, but by ascertaining that the tubes are not occluded by debris from the abscess cavity, and this applies especially to the exit tube. Fluid introduced with considerable force into the abscess cavity would burst it and disintegrate the brain tissue, and might inflict irreparable damage. The surgeon must be satisfied that the fluid is going into the abscess cavity and that it returns by the exit cannula, otherwise he must desist from injecting. . . .

After the stream of antiseptic fluid returns clear, before the removal of the cannulae, the head of the patient ought to be turned so as to allow the fluid to gravitate out. One ought to bear in mind that the fluid introduced may cause dispersion of the pus and dissemination of the infection, unless within a firmly formed capsule. In the absence of proper flushing arrangements instead of washing out the abscess cavity the introduction of the iodoform and boracic mixture is advisable.

. . . Where the abscess is seated near the floor of the middle fossa or has a direct communication with it, the opening in the tegmen ought to be enlarged so as to gain access to the abscess cavity

from below, if this has not already been done. The larger cannula inserted at this point serves to remove the fluid injected through the finer cannula introduced by way of the opening in the squamous, and more thorough washing of the abscess cavity is thereby secured. This aperture in the tegmen and membranes serves afterwards for drainage purposes, for which it is admirably situated, being at the lowest level of the abscess cavity when the head is raised on a pillow. When this method is adopted the Eustachian tube and the external ear are both shut off by filling the middle ear with iodoform and boracic powder. . . .

. . . After the evacuation of an acute abscess, drainage tubes are (for the reasons stated) of little value, provided the whole of the infective matter has been removed. If doubt exists on this point, a drainage tube is introduced. There can be no doubt that the pulsations of the brain cause, by striking against the tube, an irritation, which is increased if the tube be rigid. In chronic abscess the drainage tube may be required. An absorbable decalcified chicken-bone drainage tube is introduced into the abscess cavity and stitched to the skin so as to retain it in position. Its inner margin is made to project just within the outer wall of the abscess cavity.

When the abscess cavity is still foul and pus formation is likely to proceed, an india-rubber, glass, or other non-absorbable drain is preferable, but it ought to be removed as soon as possible— twenty-four to forty-eight hours. In the event of an opening having been made between the tegmen antri or tympani and the abscess cavity, then the drainage is best conducted through it, and the opening through the squamous bone is allowed to heal. . . .

Where the surgeon has succeeded in rendering the abscess cavity aseptic, the dressings are left for three weeks untouched, provided the temperature is normal and there is no stain through the dressings. At the expiry of that time they are removed, and the wound is either absolutely healed or there is a superficial granulating surface, according as the wound has been stitched or left open.

When the abscess cavity has been left infected, the dressings require to be changed daily and the cavity syringed out. In this case, boracic powder alone ought to be used instead of iodoform mixture, as the constant changing and renewing of the powder might induce the toxic effect of the iodoform. A great preventive against iodoform intoxication is the use of very large scales of iodoform instead of fine powder, as the latter is much more quickly absorbed. . . .

Abscess of the cerebellum, arising from otitis media, is usually secondary to suppuration in the vicinity of the sigmoid sinus, and is often accompanied by thrombosis of that vessel. It seldom

II. STATISTICAL TABLE OF INFECTIVE INTRACRANIAL LESIONS[6]

Disease	No. Cases	No. Operated on	No. Cured	No. Died
Pyogenic pachy-meningitis externa	17	17	17	0
Extradural abscess	5	5	5	0
Pyogenic cerebral lepto-meningitis	12	6	6	6
Pyogenic cerebro-spinal lepto-meningitis	6	5	1	5[1]
Superficial brain abscess and ulceration	4	4	4[2]	0
Cerebral abscess—				
Temporo-sphenoidal	10	9	8[3]	2
Frontal	2	1	1	1
Parietal	1	1	1	0
Cerebellar abscess	8	4	4	4[4]
Meningo-encephalitis of frontal lobe	1	1	0	1
Total necrosis of temporo-sphenoidal lobe	1	1	0	1
Thrombosis of longitudinal sinus	4	3	3	1
Thrombosis of cavernous sinus	5	0	0	5
Thrombosis of sigmoid sinus	18	17	13	5[5]
Total	94	74	63	31

[1] One of the fatal cases was not under author's care.

[2] One case died seven weeks after operation from tubercular enteritis.

[3] One of these successful cases, though under author's care, was first operated on by Dr. Clark.

[4] Two of the fatal cases were not under author's care, and the other two were not operated on.

[5] In all the fatal cases lung infection and systemic toxaemia were present before operation. Sigmoid sinus thrombosis occurred as a complication in ten of the cases above tabulated under various other headings, and of these seven recovered after operation.

[6] Out of twenty-three cases of pyogenic intracranial extension from otitis media here recorded the lesions were on the left side in seventeen and on the right in sixteen.

ensues from extension, by way of the internal auditory meatus, infective inflammation passing by this channel being much more frequently followed by lepto-meningitis. It is well to expose the sigmoid groove first, with the view of ascertaining the condition of the sinus. In such cases it is generally covered by granulation tissue, from which pus exudes. This ought to be removed along with the extradural pus. If there be an erosion in the dura at either side of the sigmoid, it would aid in indicating the locality of the fistula leading to the cerebellar abscess. Occasionally the pus from the cerebellum exudes by the inner side of the sinus, and it is possible, by extending the osseous incision inwards, to widen the aperture in the dura sufficiently to permit the free escape of discharge, and also to wash out the cavity. It is much better, however, to open the cerebellum from the outer and external aspect of the sinus as the abscess can always be reached in this way, while the facilities for evacuation and manipulation are greater and the subsequent drainage much more under control. The manner of evacuation, washing, and drainage is similar in detail to that given under treatment of temporo-sphenoidal abscess.

In operating upon cerebellar abscess cases, it occasionally happens that respiratory difficulties are experienced. When this occurs the operation ought to be proceeded with rapidly. Altering the position of patient's head relatively to the trunk sometimes effects an improvement in the breathing. The anaesthesia ought to be as light as is consistent with quietness of patient. In two cases reported the respiration was suspended during the operation, and was maintained by artificial respiration in one for twenty-four hours, in the other for six, the heart meanwhile acting rhythmically. The operation was abandoned when the respiratory difficulties ensued. It would have been much better to have finished the operation while maintaining the respiration, as the evacuation of the large abscess might have saved the patient's life by relieving the pressure on the respiratory centre.

Abscess of the frontal lobes.—These abscesses may be opened either from the front of the brow or from the temporal regions, the choice being determined by the precise locality of the abscess. From the brow any abscess in the frontal may be reached, though those situated in the back part of the frontal would be nearer the surface of the temporal fossa. The skull in front of the brow is thicker than in the temporal fossa, but, in the operations through the latter, the temporal muscle has to be divided and separated, and its planes of fasciae might be exposed to suppuration were they brought into contact with infective matter from the abscess. With proper precautions this ought to be avoided. The frontal sinus ought to be avoided in trephining from the brow, though in idiopathic frontal abscess the frontal sinus is frequently involved, and, if so, ought to be opened as a preliminary. Infection extending through the cribriform plate of the ethmoid may cause abscess near the mesial aspects of the frontal, and trephining through the frontal sinus and about the position of the middle line would suffice for the further search for pus. If the cribriform plate requires to be exposed, it is best done by removing a quarter-inch disc slightly above the glabella—remembering that the frontal lobes dip at this point to the level of the nasion. . . .

After the tongue and mouth have been cleansed, milk diet or fluid nutriment is given in small quantities, at first peptonized, as the patient's digestion and assimilation are weak. The light fluid nutriment is continued for a fortnight or three weeks, and until the temperature is normal. A week after the operation, if the bowels have not been moved, a purgative, which will not cause vomiting, and which will give an easy motion without straining, is administered. The patient is kept in bed for from four to six weeks after the operation, however well he may be. In no case is he allowed to rise before the wound is quite healed —which is generally at the end of a fortnight or three weeks. If there be secondary abscess formation, there will be further delay in healing the wound, and also in permitting the patient to rise. It is better to exceed the period of quiet rest in bed than allow accidents to occur by permitting the patient to rise too soon.

CHAPTER VI. RESULTS.

In the foregoing clinical record the cases which have been selected for publication are those which presented features of pathological or semiological interest, and they have for the most part been recorded *in extenso*, so as to form a contribution to the data from which conclusions may be ultimately formulated. This was felt to be especially necessary, as in consulting the scattered literature of the subject, the cases of intracranial pyogenic infective diseases recorded previously to the last few years were, for the most part, found to be fragmentary and defective. . . .

The following is a résumé of the results obtained by the author, and they present the data upon which the foregoing observations have, for the most part, been founded. In the first group of cases presented, there has been great difficulty experienced in keeping in touch with the majority of the patients after their recovery from simple ablation of the mastoid. While many had the goodness to present themselves regularly as asked, others did so on perhaps one or two occasions and then ceased to attend. The statistics of the ultimate results, to this extent, have been impaired. . . .

Of the twenty-five cases of abscess of the brain mentioned in the table, there were nineteen operated on, with eighteen recoveries. In these nineteen cases there were twenty-two abscesses evacuated, with twenty-one recoveries. One might almost conclude that in uncomplicated abscess of the brain, operated on at a fairly early period, recovery ought to be the rule.

Neurosurgical Classics—38, 39 and 40

Dᴜʀɪɴɢ the final two decades of the nineteenth century, a few general surgeons began the development of neurological surgery. Among the diseases that these surgeons sought to cure was tic douloureux, which had been resistant to all forms of treatment attempted previously. The independent efforts of four men—Victor Horsley, Frank Hartley, Fedor Krause, and Charles Frazier—were rewarded by the development of an excellent operation for the permanent relief of this condition.

By 1890, tic douloureux had been known as an entity for more than two centuries.[4,6-8,25,34] But even after its relationship to the trigeminal nerve had been discovered, no treatment of lasting value had been developed. Various medicines had been tried, systemically and locally, without effect.[4] Counterirritation had been proved worthless, and the destruction of the peripheral trigeminal branches by injection or operation had been shown to afford only temporary relief.[4,10,34] Numerous ingenious operations then had been devised for the interruption of the major trigeminal branches close to their initial exits from the skull.[4,10,16,30,34] However, none of these procedures gave lasting relief. For more than a century prior to 1890, many intelligent attempts at the cure of tic douloureux had been made, but all had been unsuccessful. The problem was solved by a combination of advances over the ensuing eleven years.

After it had been demonstrated that intracranial operations could be performed successfully, two related types of operations for tic douloureux were proposed. At first, extirpation of the gasserian ganglion was attempted.[1,26,29] William Rose, in 1890, developed a procedure for the piecemeal avulsion of the ganglion through an enlarged foramen ovale.[9,29] Because of poor exposure,

frequent hemorrhage, and incomplete removal of the ganglion, this operation proved unsatisfactory.[30] In 1891, Frank Hartley[12,13] devised an extradural temporal approach to the gasserian ganglion to facilitate intracranial neurotomy of the second and third trigeminal divisions. This approach proved to be the technical key that opened the way for later advances.[33,34] Six and a half months after Hartley's first operation, and unaware of it, Fedor Krause duplicated this operation.[18-20,22,24,30] However, Krause carried the operation a step further in 1893 when he first completely removed the gasserian ganglion successfully.[4,6,14,21] Two years later, he analyzed 51 gasserian ganglionectomies (performed by the Hartley-Krause approach) which had been reported in the medical literature.[23] The over-all mortality for these 51 cases was approximately 10 per cent.[30] Harvey Cushing[5] then modified the Hartley-Krause approach by minimizing traction on and subsequent hemorrhage from the middle meningeal artery. The result was a reduction in mortality to 5 per cent by 1905.[30] After this, extirpation of the gasserian ganglion was abandoned in favor of the second type of operation which had been developed for tic douloureux.

Foreseeing the probable difficulties of gasserian ganglionectomy, Victor Horsley proposed retrogasserian neurotomy instead. He and William Macewen worked independently to develop such a procedure.[3,15,16,34] After trial operations on monkeys and human cadavers, Horsley in 1890 attempted avulsion of the trigeminal root in a very ill woman who had had two previous extracranial operations for tic douloureux.[15,16] Because of the unfortunate operative death of this patient, and the simultaneous early successes with gasserian ganglionectomy, similar attempts at dividing the trigeminal root were abandoned temporarily.[34] David Ferrier (1890),[9] William Spiller (1898),[17] and Lewellys Barker (1900)[2] each proposed that section of the root might afford a permanent cure, but it was not until 1901 that this again was attempted. In that year, Charles Frazier performed such an operation, using the Hartley-Krause approach to the nerve.[31,32] His successes established retrogasserian neurotomy as the operation of choice, and later refinements minimized its morbidity and mortality.[4,6,11,14,27,28,30,33—36]

Victor Horsley's description of his first retrogasserian operation is reproduced below, followed by the report of the first extradural temporal approach to the gasserian ganglion by Frank Hartley, and the translation of the paper by Fedor Krause describing the first gasserian ganglionectomy by the Hartley-Krause approach. The classical paper by William G. Spiller and Charles H. Frazier in 1901, which established retrogasserian neurotomy, will be reproduced in a subsequent issue of the *Journal of Neurosurgery*.

References

1. ANDREWS, E. Cadaver studies on the removal of the semilunar ganglion through the floor of the skull. *J. Amer. med. Ass.*, 1891, *17:* 168–173.
2. BARKER, L. F. Protocols of microscopic examination of several Gasserian ganglia. *J. Amer. med. Ass.*, 1900, *34:* 1093–1094.
3. BROWDER, J. Advances in neurological surgery during the past fifty years. *Amer. J. Surg.*, 1941, *51:* 164–187.
4. CRAWFORD, J. V., and WALKER, A. E. Surgery for pain. In: *A history of neurological surgery.* A. E. Walker, Ed. Baltimore: Williams & Wilkins Co., 1951, xii, 583 pp. (see pp. 308–330).
5. CUSHING, H. A method of total extirpation of the Gasserian ganglion for trigeminal neuralgia. By a route through the temporal fossa and beneath the middle meningeal artery. *J. Amer. med. Ass.*, 1900, *34:* 1035–1041.
6. DANDY, W. E. An operation for the cure of tic douloureux. Partial section of the sensory root at the pons. *Arch. Surg., Chicago*, 1929, *18:* 687–734.
7. DANDY, W. E. The brain. In: *Lewis' practice of surgery.* Hagerstown, Md.: W. F. Prior Co., Inc., 1932, *12:* 671+17 pp. (see pp. 177–200).
8. DEWHURST, K. A symposium on trigeminal neuralgia. With contributions by Locke, Sydenham, and other eminent seventeenth century physicians. *J. Hist. Med.*, 1957, *12:* 21–36.
9. FERRIER, [D.] Excision of gasserian ganglion. *Lancet*, 1890, *2:* 925.

10. FOWLER, G. R. The operative treatment of facial neuralgia—a comparison of methods and results. *Ann. Surg.*, 1886, *3:* 269–320.
11. FRAZIER, C. H. Subtotal resection of sensory root for relief of major trigeminal neuralgia. *Arch. Neurol. Psychiat., Chicago*, 1925, *13:* 378–384.
12. HARTLEY, F. Intracranial neurectomy of the second and third divisions of the fifth nerve. A new method. *N.Y. med. J.*, 1892, *55:* 317–319.
13. HARTLEY, F. Intracranial neurectomy of the fifth nerve. *Ann. Surg.*, 1893, *17:* 511–526.
14. HORRAX, G. Neurosurgery. An historical sketch. *Springfield, Ill.: Charles C Thomas*, 1952, xi, 135 pp. (see pp. 76–80).
15. HORSLEY, V. An address on the surgical treatment of trigeminal neuralgia. *Practitioner*, 1900, *65:* 251–263.
16. HORSLEY, V., TAYLOR, J., and COLMAN, W. S. Remarks on the various surgical procedures devised for the relief or cure of trigeminal neuralgia (tic douloureux). *Brit. med. J.*, 1891, *2:* 1139–1143; 1191–1193; 1249–1252.
17. KEEN, W. W., and SPILLER, W. G. Remarks on resection of the Gasserian ganglion. *Amer. J. med. Sci.*, 1898, n.s. *116:* 503–532.
18. KRAUSE, F. Resection des Trigeminus innerhalb der Schädelhöhle. *Arch. klin. Chir.*, 1892, *44:* 821–832.
19. KRAUSE, F. Resection des Trigeminus innerhalb der Schädelhöhle. *Verh. dtsch. Ges. Chir.*, 1892, 199–210.
20. KRAUSE, F. Ueber Trigeminusresection innerhalb der Schädelhöhle mit Krankenvorstellung. *Berl. klin. Wschr.*, 1892, *29:* 734.
21. KRAUSE, F. Entfernung des Ganglion Gasseri und des central davon gelegenen Trigeminusstammes. *Dtsch. med. Wschr.*, 1893, *19:* 341–344.
22. KRAUSE, F. The question of priority in devising a method for the performance of intra-cranial neurectomy of the fifth nerve. *Ann. Surg.*, 1893, *18:* 362–364.
23. KRAUSE, F. Die Physiologie des Trigeminus nach Untersuchungen an Menschen, bei denen das Ganglion Gasseri entfernt worden ist. *Münch. med. Wschr.*, 1895, *42:* 577–581; 602–604; 628–631.
24. KRAUSE, F. Die Neuralgie des Trigeminus, nebst der Anatomie und Physiologie des Nerven. *Leipzig: F.C.W. Vogel*, 1896, xii, 260 pp.
25. LEWY, F. H. The first authentic case of major trigeminal neuralgia and some comments on the history of this disease. *Ann. med. Hist.*, 1938, n.s. *10:* 247–250.
26. MEARS, J. E. Study of the pathological changes occurring in trifacial neuralgia. With the report of a case in which three inches of the inferior dental nerve were excised. *Med. News, Philad.*, 1884, *45:* 58–63.
27. PEET, M. M. Tic douloureux and its treatment, with a review of the cases operated upon at the University Hospital in 1917. *J. Mich. med. Soc.*, 1918, *17:* 91–99.
28. PEET, M. M. The cranial nerves. In: *Lewis' practice of surgery.* Hagerstown, Md.: W. F. Prior Co., Inc., 1932, *12:* 106 pp. (see pp. 51–53).
29. ROSE, W. Removal of the Gasserian ganglion for severe neuralgia. *Lancet*, 1890, *2:* 914–915.

30. SCARFF, J. E. Fifty years of neurosurgery, 1905–1955. *Int. Abstr. Surg.*, 1955, *101*: 417–513.

31. SPILLER, W. G., and FRAZIER, C. H. The division of the sensory root of the trigeminus for the relief of tic douloureux: an experimental, pathological and clinical study, with a preliminary report of one surgically successful case. *Univ. Pa. med. Bull.*, 1901, *14*: 341–352.

32. SPILLER, W. G., and FRAZIER, C. H. The division of the sensory root of the trigeminus for the relief of tic douloureux; an experimental, pathological and clinical study, with a preliminary report of one surgically successful case. *Philad. med. J.*, 1901, *8*: 1039–1049.

33. STOOKEY, B. Early neurosurgery in New York: its origin in neurology and general surgery. *Bull. Hist. Med.*, 1952, *26*: 330–359.

34. STOOKEY, B., and RANSOHOFF, J. Trigeminal neuralgia. Its history and treatment. *Springfield, Ill.: Charles C Thomas*, 1959, xv, 366 pp. (see pp. 6–32; 166–183).

35. TIFFANY, L. McL. Intracranial neurectomy and removal of the Gasserian ganglion. *Ann. Surg.*, 1894, *19*: 47–57.

36. TIFFANY, L. McL. Intracranial operations for the cure of facial neuralgia. *Ann. Surg.*, 1896, *24*: 575–619; 736–748.

REMARKS ON THE VARIOUS SURGICAL
PROCEDURES DEVISED FOR THE
RELIEF OR CURE OF TRIGEM-
INAL NEURALGIA (TIC
DOULOUREUX).*

By VICTOR HORSLEY, F.R.S., F.R.C.S.,
Surgeon to the National Hospital for the Paralysed and Epileptic; Assistant-Surgeon
to University College Hospital, etc;

ASSISTED BY

JAMES TAYLOR, M.D.
Pathologist to the National Hospital for
the Paralysed and Epileptic;

AND

WALTER S. COLMAN, M.B.

(*Concluded from page 1193.*)

Operation for Removal of the Gasserian Ganglion and the Division of the Fifth Nerve behind the Latter.—In considering the possibility of relieving cases of inveterate neuralgia where recurrence of the pain had taken place, I thought one might be able to remove the Gasserian ganglion or divide the fifth nerve behind it, and I made, some years ago, dissections[38] to see how far the Gasserian ganglion could be separated from the cavernous sinus. On first exposing the ganglion from the

---

* Reprinted (pp. 1249–1252) from the *British Medical Journal*, 1891, *2:* 1139–1143; 1191–1193; 1249–1252, with the kind permission of the Editor.
[38] By the kind help of Drs. Savill, Lunn, and others.

pterygoid fossa and opening the middle fossa of the skull freely following up the inferior division of the fifth nerve, I found that one could raise the inferior division and so the lower half of the ganglion from its bed in the dura mater without damage to the carotid artery in the canal or to the cavernous sinus, but that when one attempted to strip up the upper half of the ganglion from the cavernous sinus it invariably tore the wall of that cavity. For this reason I believe that the operation of complete removal of the Gasserian ganglion is not possible, but that in the operation which Mr. Rose has subsequently described only a portion of it can be taken away.

Finding this to be the case, I then considered the possibility of dividing the fifth nerve behind the ganglion. It is well known that the fifth nerve enters the dura mater just beneath the edge of the tentorium, and that it runs afterwards in a small but roomy canal in the dura mater, joining the Gasserian ganglion, which lies in a similar cleft on the upper surface of the petrous bone and on the roof of the carotid canal. Some experiments on the monkey to expose the crura had shown me that it was possible to expose the temporo-sphenoidal lobe, and then, by raising the brain carefully with a broad retractor, to lay bare the floor of the middle fossa of the skull. On trying this on the dead body I found that it was perfectly possible in man also, the only trouble being the small veins which come from the temporo-sphenoidal lobe and which enter the petrosal sinuses. If these be ruptured the hæmorrhage is very free, and, although not dangerous to life, nevertheless very effectually hinders the performance of the operation.

This exposure of the temporo-sphenoidal lobe in man I have carried out by making a large temporal flap, starting from the anterior extremity of the zygomatic process, and running upwards to the temporal ridge, following that line and descending along it to the asterion. The temporal muscle, after being separated from the bone, is then best removed, so far as its posterior half is concerned, and then the whole of the squamous portion of the temporal taken away by means of a trephined hole and suitable bone forceps. Anteriorly the middle meningeal artery may be dealt with where exposed, being simply ligatured in the dura mater. The dura mater is then to be opened along the full length of the area of bone removed, and the temporo-sphenoidal lobe thus laid bare. A broad copper retractor, with smooth and everted edges, is then gently slipped underneath the lobe and slowly but steadily raised. The lobe is partly moulded partly lifted upwards, and the floor of the skull is then easily seen and illuminated with the electric light. The guide to the fifth nerve now is the upper border of the petrous bone. The lobe being raised a little more, the edge

Table showing the Results of Removal of the Branches of the Fifth Nerve.

No.	Sex and Age	Duration.	Presumed Exciting Cause.	Nerve Distribution Affected.	Trophic Changes.	Previous Treatment.	Operative Treatment.	Mode of Healing.	Notes.	Result.
1	M., 60	7½ yrs.	Worry	Left 2nd division; pain also in supra-orbital region	None	Extraction of all teeth; usual drugs, and opium in large doses	Mar. 2, 1886. Removal of 2nd division through antrum	First intention	—	Pain in upper gum remained.
a*	—	—	—	Left upper gum	—	—	Aprl. 16, 1886. Removal of posterior palatine nerve	First intention	—	Complete relief for 7 months.
b	—	—	—	Left inferior dental	—	—	Dec. 21, 1887. Removal of inferior dental and lingual	First intention except where tube introduced	—	
c	—	—	—	Left 2nd and 3rd divisions	—	—	Nov. 15, 1888. Division of 2nd and 3rd divisions inside cranium	Cellulitis; necrosis; small piece of bone; sinus for one year	—	Relief 18 months; return from local abscess; relief when this opened, and complete so far.
2	M., 65	7 yrs.	Exposure to cold	Left 2nd division	None	All usual drugs	Nov. 19, 1886. Removal of 2nd division	First intention	—	Complete cure.
3	F., 55	3½ yrs.	Worry	Right inferior dental	—	Usual drugs	Dec. 14, 1886. 1 in. inferior dental removed	First intention	Collection of serum; aspiration 3 weeks after operation	Complete relief; slight temporary return during illness in 1890.
4	M., 61	4½ yrs.	None	3rd division; also supra-orbital pain	None	Teeth extracted	Aug. 24, 1887. Excision of 1 in. of 3rd division	First intention	—	Complete relief when last heard of.
5	F., 66	8 yrs.	Cold and cleaning teeth	Right 2nd and 3rd divisions	Swelling of right cheek and lower lip	Extraction of all teeth; usual drugs	May 24, 1887. Removal of inferior dental	First intention except for small salivary fistula closing in a few days	Fed by rectum for 1 month before operation	Complete relief for two years.
a	—	—	Cold	Right 2nd division	Swelling of right cheek & upper lip; herpetiform pustules; conjunctivitis	—	Nov. —, 1889. Removal of 2nd division at spheno-maxillary fissure	First intention	—	Disappearance of trophic change, and relief for 1 year.
b	—	—	—	Right auriculo-temporal, July, 1890	Herpes and swelling of lower lip	—	Dec. 11, 1890. Avulsion of 5th nerve from bulb	—	Liquid food 6 months before operation	Death from shock.
6	F., 55	27 yrs.	None	Right lingual inferior dental and auriculo-temporal	None	Various drugs; caustic to tongue	Jan. 13, 1888. Excision of part of inferior dental and lingual	First intention	—	Complete cure.
7	M., 38	6 yrs.	Exposure to cold	Right inferior dental and lingual; pain over vertex	None	Drugs; baths at Aix	Aug. 8, 1888. Removal of inferior dental and lingual	Partly granulation	—	Cure.
8	F., 58	2 yrs.	Movement excites pain	Infra-orbital	—	All teeth on affected side extracted	Aug. 7, 1888. Nerve cut in infra-orbital canal	First intention	—	Cure.
9	M., 64	7 yrs.	Cold	Left 3rd and 2nd divisions	—	Usual drugs	Aug. 21, 1888. Removal of inferior dental and lingual	First intention	Brother and sister melancholic	Relief for a year.
a	—	—	—	Left 2nd division	—	—	Aug. 13, 1889. Removal of infra-orbital	First intention	—	
b	—	—	—	Left 2nd and 3rd division; also supra-orbital	—	—	Jan. 6, 1890. Removal of 2nd and 3rd divisions inside cranium	First intention	—	Temporary relief: recurrence in 1st division; dementia.
10	M., 63	6 yrs.	Exposure to cold	Right inferior dental; lingual once in upper jaw	Swelling of lower lip	All drugs; some teeth removed	Nov. 22, 1888. 1 in. of inferior dental and lingual removed	First intention except small salivary fistula for three weeks	Herpes zoster 4 years before on right shoulder	Complete cure.
11	F., 68	15 yrs.	Getting wet	Right inferior division, right 2nd divison	Occasional swelling of right lower lip	Quinine, electricity etc.	Jan. 23, 1889. Removal of inferior dental and lingual	First intention	—	Temporary relief, *vide infra.*
a	—	—	—	Severe pain in 2nd division	—	—	March 26, 1890. Removal of infra-orbital	First intention	—	Relief so far.
b	—	—	—	Severe pain in inferior division; recovery of sensibility in this region, June, 1891	—	—	Aug. 10, 1891. Removal of inferior division at foramen ovale	First intention	—	Relief so far.
12	F., 54	5 yrs.	—	Right 2nd division	Swelling of right upper lip; unilateral furring of tongue	—	Jan. 15, 1889. Excision of part of right infra-orbital	First intention	—	Relief so far.
13	M., 69	12 yrs.	Pressure or movement excites pain	Left infra-orbital; pain supra-orbital	—	—	May 8, 1889. Removal of 2nd division at foramen rotundum; antrum opened	First intention	Sloughing of cornea from using strong carbolic	Cure.
14	F., 53	6 yrs.	—	Left infra-orbital, occasionally supra-orbital	—	Various drugs, relieving temporarily till 3 months ago	May 13th, 1889. Nerve twisted off at spheno-maxillary fissure from orbit	First intention	Blunting of smell, taste, and hearing on affected side	Cure.
15	M., 65	32 yrs.	Exposure to cold	Left 2nd division	None	All usual drugs	May 22, 1889. Removal of 2nd division	First intention	Marked emaciation	Complete cure.

* The letters *a*, *b*, and *c* signify second, third, and fourth operations respectively.

† At this operation a notable (pathological) bulging of the brain was observed when the skull was opened, and pressure thus relieved.

Table showing the Results of Removal of the Branches of the Fifth Nerve. (Continued)

No.	Sex and Age.	Dura- tion.	Presumed Exciting Cause.	Nerve Distribu- tion Affected.	Trophic Changes.	Previous Treat- ment.	Operative Treat- ment.	Mode of Healing.	Notes.	Result.
16	M., 55	13 yrs.	Wound of face with chisel four years pre- viously	All left side of face	None	Usual drugs; di- vision of nerve (buccal?) in cheek	Aug. 18, 1890. Remov- al of part of inferior dental	First intention	Free bleeding	Relief for month.
a	—	—	Pain began in scar	—	—	—	Feb. 6, 1891. Incom- plete operation for intracranial division of nerve	First intention	Diffuse ossifica- tion of petrous; operation aban- doned	Relief for months.†
b	—	—	—	—	—	—	Sep. 11, 1891. Modified Pancoast-Salzer op- eration	First intention ex- cept small point in front	Free bleeding	Relief so far.
17	M., 27	1 yr.	Influenza	Right side of cheek from socket of right lower 1st molar	None	Usual drugs	Jan. 15, 1891. Remov- al of parts of infer. dental and lingual	First intention	—	Relief so far.
18	M., 57	4 yrs.	Cold	Right supra-and infra-orbital	Scaling of right side of face; oc- casional swell- ing	Usual drugs	Aug. 6, 1891. Excision of supra- and infra- orbital from face; antrum opened	First intention	—	Complete relie
19	F., 46	10 yrs.	?	All right side of face.	None	Usual drugs, electricity, etc.	Jan. 26, 1891. Remov- al of parts of infer. dental and lingual	First intention	—	Complete rel in inferior di sion so far.
a	—	—	—	Right supra- and infra-orbital	—	—	Sept. 22, 1891. Exci- sion of supra-infra- orbital from face	First intention	Great quantity of chloroform re- quired.	Complete rel in whole face far.

of the tentorium will be defined and the point at which the fifth nerve passes beneath it could, in the first case I operated upon, be seen. The posi- tion of the canal in which the nerve is lying just above the ganglion must then be estimated, and a small puncturing incision made into it. As it is about a quarter of an inch in diameter, it can be recognised as soon as the puncturing instrument passes into it, and the dura forming its roof should then be further slit open. The nerve in this way is exposed, and is found to be freely lying in the little passage.

The first case on which I operated in this man- ner was the patient No. 5 in the table, in whom I had, as is shown there, previously removed a por- tion of the inferior dental and of the infraorbital. The recurrence of pain, for which she then desired further operative relief, began in the auriculo- temporal nerve, the only branch remaining of the inferior division which had not been cut. As the pain, however, also ultimately invaded appar- ently the stump of the middle division, I thought it best to attempt the operation of dividing the nerve behind the ganglion. The patient had not eaten any solid food for several months, and was not in a good condition to undergo the operation. However, as her state was a very desperate one, I agreed to perform the operation, warning the friends that there might be fatal collapse even on the table. As a matter of fact, the operation pre- sented no special difficulty beyond that of being very tedious. I resected the zygoma in order to have more room, but I feel sure now that that was a useless complication—that it was quite possible to have reached the nerve without it, and I regret having done it, because I think it of course aided in producing the shock which caused a fatal termi- nation to the case. On opening the dura mater the

brain bulged moderately into the opening, but as soon as the effect of the shock began to show itself it of course sank. On exposing the nerve in the canal behind the ganglion I passed a small blunt hook around it, and it then occurred to me that the small branch of the basilar artery which ac- companies the nerve might give some trouble. I therefore thought one might safely attempt avul- sion of the nerve from its attachment to the pons, and on gently drawing on it with a hook this was easily accomplished, and without even any note- worthy oozing. The wound was closed in the usual way. Unfortunately the patient never rallied from the operation, and died seven hours afterwards, obviously from shock.

At the *post-mortem* examination—which I ob- tained with some difficulty, and further details of which will be given in a paper on the pathology of the disease shortly to be published—I found that there was no cause of death except that already mentioned. There had been a slight amount of oozing into the subarachnoid space, but nothing to produce any compression at all, and of course of that there were no symptoms during life. At the moment when the fifth nerve was separated from the pons, although the patient was well under the anæsthetic, there was arrest of the respiration and the pulse could not be felt. This lasted for prob- ably not more than three to four seconds, and then the respiratory movements and the pulse became normal. On reviewing the result of this operation I am satisfied that the unfavourable termination was due to the special circumstances of the case, and the considerable series of experi- ments on the lower animals which have been made involving the division of the fifth nerve show clearly that the mere exposure and section of the nerve is not of itself dangerous to life.

It has been proposed by Mr. Rose to remove the Gasserian ganglion by removing a ring of bone around the foramen rotundum. I have already shown that the ganglion cannot be wholly removed from its bed, but only a small portion. This operation therefore resolves itself practically into section of the branches of the lower two divisions of the nerve just within the skull. In Mr. Rose's first operation the foramen rotundum was reached by resecting the upper jaw. It is quite easy, however, to reach the parts by the Pancoast-Salzer method without resorting to this procedure, and, moreover, in Mr. Rose's case the eye was lost—a grave consequence, which is avoided by the method I carried out in 1888 of trephining the middle fossa through the pterygoid region.[39]

It may now be asked, do the results of the operation in those cases of inveterate facial neuralgia justify the procedure? This question presupposes a previous one, namely, what is the condition for which the operation is undertaken? In other words, how is the operation supposed to act? Bell long ago suggested that section of the nerve in these cases produced an alterative and tonic effect on the nervous system. Erb[40] agrees with Bell in thinking that the "strong peripheral stimulus of the operation is the cause of the disappearance of the neuralgia." Tripier[41] regards facial neuralgia as probably due to some central change, and that a temporary inhibition is caused by the operation. Some cases, he thinks, may be peripheral, and may disappear if the irritant be removed. Wagner[42] also believed that the mischief is central. Carnochan attaches great importance to Meckel's ganglion in the production of neuralgia, and an essential in his operation was the removal of this. And even with this idea as to the origin of the pain and the consequently less radical operations undertaken for its relief, the success has been so marked as to convince many surgeons of the usefulness of operative procedures. But I hold very strongly the opinion that epileptiform neuralgia is a purely peripheral malady, affecting principally the small subcutaneous branches of the nerve, or possibly the nerve endings, as well as the trunks of the fifth nerve, as they run in the bony canals of the facial bones, and that complete removal of the pain in any given division of the nerve may be obtained by ablation of the nerve from the base of the skull, unless the stump of the nerve become the seat of neuritis. (*Vide* Case 1 in the accompanying table.)

All other measures, for example, stretching, simple division, destruction of the nerve in a bony canal by the drill or trephining, may, and undoubtedly do, give relief for a varying period, but the disease is extremely likely to recur in the stump or trunk as soon as the paralysing effects of the operation have passed off. I do not believe there is such a thing as reflection of pain along other branches, and certainly no proof of its existence is to hand, although it is freely spoken of as occurring. If pain is felt in two branches, for example, infraorbital and inferior dental, that means, I believe, disease of both those nerves. It is true that after operation on the nerve most affected, drugs such as gelsemium, etc., may so reduce the irritation in the other nerve as to render life tolerable and efficient, but in the end the remaining nerve, so far as I have seen, usually has to be extracted before permanent relief is obtained.

In this opinion I am supported by several authorities, and the evidence which they offer I shall discuss in a subsequent paper in the *Practitioner* on the pathology of this condition, in which I also hope to advance fresh evidence from cases of my own. Holding then as I do this opinion, I believe that operative procedure in those cases is an imperative duty when all medical measures of relief have failed. It is true that in many cases operation is not followed by that permanent relief which is aimed at, and this no doubt arises from several causes. One of these I believe to be the excision of too short a piece, permitting reunion of the cut ends. It is stated by Hüter[43] that experiments show that not less than 5 inches must be removed to prevent reunion with certainty. Although I am inclined to think that this is an excessive length, there seems to be little doubt that a considerable gap between the divided ends can be bridged over, but I am convinced that in many of the cases in which a return of pain after neurectomy is ascribed to reunion, the result is in reality due to the occurrence of neuritis in the stump of the nerve, chiefly because the wound was not treated antiseptically. Another reason for a want of permanent relief after neurectomy is, I believe, because the nerve is not fully freed in the bony canal. If the neuritis does not frequently start in such a place, it is, I am sure, often very intense there, and the free removal of nerve in the canal, or the removal of bone so as to widen the aperture and prevent pressure, is essential. Then, too, if the neuralgia has persisted long, it is necessary to go far back, and a minor operation on the anterior portion of a nerve trunk may be followed by a recurrence of the pain within a short time. I believe it is necessary to divide the nerve as near its origin as possible, so as to sever it where it is still healthy.

[39] In Mr. Rose's second operation (*vide Lancet*, 1891) he employed the Pancoast-Salzer method and opened the foramen ovale.

[40] *Von Ziemssen's Cyclop.*, xi, p. 95.

[41] *Rev. de Chir.*, Paris, 1879.

[42] *Langenbeck's Archiv*, vol. xi.

[43] *Grundriss der Chir.*, i, 144.

It is exceedingly difficult to get statistics as to the duration of relief after operations for this affection. Many cases are reported as cured after a few weeks or months, but there is nothing to show that the relief lasted even for a year. In many cases it is known to recur within that time, but I think that if the principles I have laid down are followed, recurrence will occur far less often than it has hitherto.

The occasions on which I have obtained what may be regarded as absolute cure or have observed recurrence of pain are grouped together in the accompanying table, which has been constructed so as to exhibit at a glance not merely the direct effect of the operation, but also the surgical details of the procedure, and the success or failure of the same.

The conclusions I would draw from this table are, that as soon as drugs and electricity have definitely proved unequal to the task of controlling the pain, the branch of nerve affected should be excised. The rapidity with which the wound heals and the absence of a noticeable scar deprive the procedure of obvious drawbacks, while the genuine nature of the relief it affords, in contrast to other methods, is shown by the fact that patients once operated upon will hardly wait to hear of other treatment if some other branch becomes affected.

INTRACRANIAL NEURECTOMY OF THE SECOND AND THIRD DIVISIONS OF THE FIFTH NERVE.

A NEW METHOD.*†

By FRANK HARTLEY, M.D.

In my experience, Mr. President, one of the most difficult instances in which the surgeon is called upon to decide upon the feasibility of further operative interference exists in recurrences of pain following neurectomies or neurotomies for persistent neuralgia. It is not always possible to determine whether the seat of pain is situated beyond the seat of the previous operation, whether a new painful branch still uncut sends by irradiation the feeling of pain in the nerves operated on, or whether pressure or enlargement of the proximal end of the nerve is the cause of the recurrence.

With such uncertainty we can not be reasonably certain of a good prognosis until all branches of the trunk in which pain is present are cut.

In many of the operations for the relief of prosopalgia involving the second and third divi-

* Read before the New York Surgical Society, January 13, 1892.
† Reprinted from *New York Medical Journal*, 1892, *55*:317–319.

sions of the fifth nerve, the difficult technique, the small field of operation, the arteries requiring ligature to preserve a clear field for the neurectomy, are important considerations. Especially is this the case where previous neurectomies have been done in the field of the operation. The history of the case which I wish to present this evening is as follows:

J. D., aged forty-six years, married, England, salesman, admitted to Roosevelt Hospital on August 8, 1891. The patient's father died of pleurisy; in other respects his family history is negative.

Personal History.—Patient denies rheumatism and syphilis. He has had malarial disease, but in other respects has been perfectly healthy.

In December, 1882, he was seized with a sharp neuralgic pain, at first referred to a spot about two inches to the left of the symphysis menti. This pain radiated over the whole left side of the face and head, involving the temporal region as far as the temporal ridge, and the left side of the tongue and mouth over the upper and lower jaws. The left orbit was involved in this attack.

This attack lasted eighteen hours, and, after an interval of four days, during which time momentary attacks of pain were present in the same region, it reappeared. The second attack was more severe, and lasted two or three days. For the next two years he had constant pain over this region and was treated medicinally with aconitine and morphine.

In September, 1884, the infra-orbital nerve, with Meckel's ganglion, was removed.

From the scars left, one would judge that either Wagner's or Chavasse's operation was performed at this time.

For four or five weeks he had partial relief. The constant pain disappeared, but the spasmodic twitchings continued. It soon reappeared, however, and the patient was again treated with aconitine and morphine.

He had at this time thirty-one teeth drawn, thinking that the origin of the pain was located in them.

After eighteen months (1886), section of the inferior dental nerve was made by the same surgeon. The scars would lead one to think that Velpeau's operation was performed at this time.

On recovering from the ether he had an attack lasting seventeen days. From that time to the present he has had no change in his condition. The pain has been constant, except for an occasional period of one or two days. The contractions in the muscles of the face amount to forty in about thirty minutes.

Owing to the previous operations and the involvement of the lingual and auriculo-temporal nerves, I decided to attack the nerve at a point where I could divide the second and third divisions of the fifth nerve completely by one operation. The operation intended was to attack the nerve on the inner surface of the skull outside the dura mater, to isolate the second and third branches completely, to divide and resect as long a portion as possible. The advantages thought to exist in this method over Pancoast's, or its modifications by Krönlein, Credé, and Salzer, or Lücke's operation, were the easy access to the nerve, the comparatively large field for work, the rapidity with which the operation could be done, and the small amount of hæmorrhage. The disadvantage was the inability to resect as long a piece as could be done in some of the other methods. This disadvantage I am certain can be overcome in the future when the knowledge of the degree of adhesion of the fifth nerve and dura mater is better appreciated. It is not difficult to go beyond the Gasserian ganglion.

This I did not appreciate fully before doing the operation on August 15, 1891. The operation performed was one in which an omega-shaped incision was made, having its base at the zygoma and measuring a distance marked by a line drawn from the external angular process of the frontal bone to the tragus of the ear.

The curved and rounded portion of this incision reached as high as the supratemporal ridge, the diameter of said circle being three inches. The skin and deeper tissues were cut in the shape of the Greek capital letter omega, a method of incision I first saw recommended by Uhle two or three years ago. This incision was carried down to the periosteum of the skull in all portions of the incision, except in the straight part at the base; the tissues were then retracted and the periosteum divided upon the bone in the same direction and as far as the straight part at the base.

With a chisel a groove was cut in the bone corresponding to the divided periosteum. This groove went to the vitreous plate, except at the upper angle over the rounded portion where it included the vitreous plate.

A periosteum elevator was here inserted and used as a lever to snap the bone on a line between the ends of the circular portion of the incision. In this way the breakage occurs along the lower portion of the wound, and a flap, consisting of skin, muscle, periosteum, and bone is thrown down, exposing the dura mater over a circular area of three inches in diameter. The middle meningeal artery was then tied, the dura mater was then separated from the bone, and the floor of the middle fossa of the skull was exposed. Broad retractors were used to raise the dura mater with the brain and to expose the foramen rotundum and the foramen ovale. The hæmorrhage was stopped by sponge pressure. The exposure of the first, second, and third divisions of the fifth nerve, together with the carotid artery and cavernous sinus, was exceedingly good.

The second and third divisions were isolated at the foramen rotundum and the foramen ovale, and, by slight pressure upon the dura mater, it could be stripped from the nerves to beyond the Gasserian ganglion. These were divided with a tenotome at the foramen rotundum and the foramen ovale, and that part between these and a point beyond the Gasserian ganglion was excised. As this amount of nerve is not very great, the ends of the nerves were pushed through the two foramina so as, if possible, to interfere with any reunion. In the retraction of the dura mater, owing to imperfect instruments, the third, fourth, and sixth nerves were somewhat injured. As no bleeding was present, the brain was allowed to fill the fossa. The flap—consisting of bone, periosteum, muscle, and skin—was replaced. The irregular edge of the vitreous plate which remained attached to the bone not involved in the flap acted as a shelf on which the flap rested and prevented its falling in upon the dura mater. The periosteum was stitched, the muscle sutured in place, and the skin sewn with silk. One drainage-tube was inserted at the lower angle; an antiseptic dressing was applied. Time of operation, one hour and forty minutes; the patient was carried to

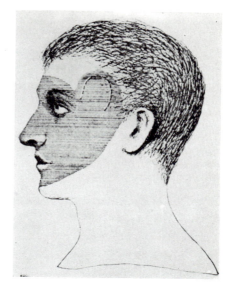

the ward in good condition. Following the operation, August 16th, ptosis of the left upper lid appeared, together with double vision and inability to move the eye. The patient was entirely free from pain and continued to do well for one week.

August 23d.—To-day a slight dermatitis appeared over the area of operation, which is treated with ichthyol (ten per cent.) and bichloride irrigation.

On August 24th Dr. W. Vought examined the patient for me, and reported as follows: "The area of anæsthesia may be seen upon the shaded portion of the drawing. The other areas were the left side of the mucous membrane of the mouth over the upper and lower jaws, of the soft palate, of the anterior two thirds of the left side of the tongue, of the left conjunctiva and cornea, and of the left nostril. Muscular paralysis, complete, of the left buccinator, the pterygoids, and the left occipito-frontalis (frontal portion); almost complete, of all the external muscles of the eye. Ptosis; pupil normal. Nerves divided: the second and third divisions of the fifth nerve, the branch of the seventh to the occipito-frontalis; injured, the third, fourth, and sixth nerves. The ophthalmoplegia externa I should give a fair prognosis for spontaneous recovery, as you will see by examining the patient that *slight* movement of all the eye muscles is present, which leads me to think the nerves have not been divided, but merely severely injured. The ptosis could be corrected at any time."

August 30th.—Patient is to-day discharged cured and returned to the Vanderbilt Clinic, Nervous Department.

September 30th.—Patient has recovered from his paresis in the third nerve; the double vision, ptosis, and inability to use the third nerve have entirely disappeared. The paralysis of the pterygoids, temporal, and masseter muscles produced by the division of the motor portion of the fifth seems to have incommoded him to a very slight extent. The false teeth worn in the lower jaw before the operation fit quite accurately their opponents in the upper. Protraction and retraction of the lower jaw seem to be diminished, but elevation and depression of the lower jaw seem good. As the patient has chewed since 1882 all his food on the side opposite to the present paralysis, he has not been distressed by the division of the motor portion of the fifth.

The patient informs me that he is at present entirely free from pain and has gained in weight sixteen pounds.

I wish to say in conclusion that this method of reaching the base of the skull I have employed in the posterior fossa in a case of suppurative meningitis following otitis media. Though the case had a fatal issue, the exposure of the posterior fossa was good.

January 13, 1892.

Excision of the Gasserian Ganglion and of the Trigeminal Trunk Situated Centrally from It*[1]

By Fedor Krause

Last year I was able to present to you a report concerning a new procedure, which in incurable cases of trigeminal neuralgia, when surgery has already been performed on the peripheral branches extracranially without any lasting effect, makes it possible to expose the nerves within the cranium itself and to resect them there. In the meantime I had to perform surgery in two additional cases and I was planning on presenting these two patients to you. But since the date of the lecture was postponed for two weeks, and one of the patients has returned to his home, I can only show you the pictures and give you his case history. The last case is the most difficult and most interesting and for this reason I shall present it.

Case 1. It concerns a woman of 68 years, Mrs. R. from Hamburg, with no history of previous illness. In the summer of 1873, she felt pains for the first time in the left side of her face, but these pains quickly subsided. Soon the pains returned in severe form and persisted for a longer period of time. Since the pain was getting more acute and all internal medicines were useless, in November 1880, the alveolar nerve was resected. At first the operation had a successful result, but within a year the pains reappeared in their old severity and in 1883 the third branch of the trigeminus at the base of the cranium had to be resected. This operation had no effect. From that time on, the attacks of pain were continuously more severe and often persisted for days and weeks, followed by tolerable intervals. But in the last year the painfulness increased still further and since in addition the patient greatly overtaxed her weakened strength in caring for her husband

who was ill with cholera, her condition was aggravated and the severe pains persisted without cessation from September 1892. The afflicted woman suffered continuously from insomnia, her nutrition was very poor, because pains made chewing impossible and for days she did not leave her bed because of weakness. This condition explains why the patient had suicidal thoughts.

When I saw her for the first time on January 24th of this year, I did not at first have the impression that this was a case of trigeminal neuralgia. Rather, the unbearably severe pains, according to the report of the patient, affected quite uniformly the entire left side of the face and head and radiated even in the nape and neck. The trigeminal branches were hardly more sensitive to touch than the greatly hyperesthetic skin of the face and head. Only the past history and the definite information of the family doctor, that the suffering began years ago as neuralgia in the third branch, provided a hope that repeated surgery might help the patient.

Nothing could be expected from other medications, as the family doctor had used the most varied internal medicines for years without any appreciable success. Since the third branch had been resected by a renowned surgeon, first in the individual branches with a temporary success, and later in toto at the base of the cranium without any success, only the intracranial procedure reported by me could be considered.

For the following reasons I decided in this case to extirpate the gasserian ganglion and the trigeminal trunk itself: first, the third branch is functionally the most important; beside the sensory branches to the skin it also has the lingual nerve and supplies the musculature of the lower jaw; but the functions of this branch had already been destroyed in the case of my patient, by previous operations. In addition, as mentioned above, the pains were distributed so regularly over all the trigeminal branches and even far out in the surrounding area that no definite successful results could be expected from the intracranial resection of the third branch itself, even though it was justified to consider some of the pains as radiating and based on radiation. When operating on my first patient more than a year ago, I was able to determine that the direct resection of the second trigeminal branch at the gasserian ganglion was not followed by even a slight disturbance in the nutrition of the eye or any inflammation. Finally, as far as the first branch is concerned, it is the least significant with regard to its physiological functions. Therefore in the case of this patient I considered the removal of the entire trigeminus completely justified and surgery was performed on January 31 of this year.

While in my first two cases, both involving the removal of the affected second branch only, I divided the operation into two stages, so that bleeding in the depth of the middle cranial fossa would not obstruct my view, in this case I de-

* Translation of Entfernung des Ganglion Gasseri und des central davon gelegenen Trigeminusstammes, by Fedor Krause, *Deutsche medizinische Wochenschrift,* 1893, *19:* 341–344, printed with the kind permission of Georg Thieme Verlag, Stuttgart, Germany.
[1] Address and presentation of patients before a meeting of the Hamburg Medical Society.

cided to perform the operation at one time, because I did not wish to expose the old lady, who had been weakened by severe pains for years, to the danger of narcosis and surgical intervention twice in quick succession. In addition, in the two previous operations I learned that when the brain is in the closed dural sac, it tolerates an upward displacement very well, and no disturbances of its function can be detected later. This finding was of great importance with regard to the left side, since the important speech centers are situated in the posterior section of the third frontal convolution and in the first temporal convolution. As the brain must be displaced upward during surgery, exactly in this region, and even in the most careful procedure a certain pressure from below cannot be avoided, only experience could provide in this respect the information concerning the harmlessness of surgical intervention.

Furthermore, I already stated in my first report that it necessarily makes an essential difference, whether the brain is displaced upward in its protective casing, the closed strong dural sac, or whether—as Victor Horsley* has done in one case in order to sever the trigeminal trunk behind the ganglion—the dura mater is removed in the entire area of the trephined opening and the exposed brain is lifted with a spatulated instrument. The pressure—even if very small—that the spatula must necessarily exert, is distributed in my procedure on a larger area and thus reduced, while the exposed brain is pressed only at the place corresponding to the width of the spatula. The patient of Horsley did not recover from operation but died in shock seven hours after the operation, while my three patients—two women, 47 and 68 years old, and a man, 64 years old—recovered and did not present any cerebral symptoms. My first case of operation concerned a right-sided neuralgia, the second case the left trigeminus; the course after these operations showed to me again that, as in the first case, no injuries with respect to the functions of the brain took place. Therefore, on the basis of these experiences, I was able to proceed in the last operation more rapidly with the detachment of the dura and elevation of the brain, than in my first two cases, in which I had to proceed more cautiously.

I tried to shorten the operation also in another respect, in order to be able to finish it at one time. In my first cases, in accordance with the Wagner-Wolff procedure, I left the bones united with the soft parts, i.e. formed a flap consisting of skin, muscle, periosteum and bone. Since the dura

* Victor Horsley, Remarks on the various surgical procedures devised for the relief or cure of trigeminal neuralgia. Brit. Med. Journ. 28, Nov. 5 and 12, Dec. 1891.

mater must not be injured, the chiseling must be very careful; that takes time. Therefore in my last case, because the patient was in very poor condition, I did not retain the bone, in order to spare time. The flap incision visible in Fig. 3 was made directly to the bone, then the periosteum in the entire area of the flap was torn off with the raspatory and bleeding was checked. Then I chiseled a hole in the skull in the center of the very thin squamous portion of the temporal bone, just large enough to be able to insert Luer's gouge forceps, and with them broke off the skull capsule in the entire area of the flap. As is known, this can be accomplished in a very short time. Then I advanced, not very slowly as in my first operation, but relatively quickly, with the blunt raspatory between the hard cerebral meninges and the upper surface of the base of the skull in the middle cranial fossa, and when I had enough room I used the raspatory and my finger alternately, until the trunk of the meningeal artery and the third and second branch of the trigeminus were visible in their entire lengths up to the gasserian ganglion. In addition, I was gratified to find that in this quick detachment of the dura mater from the bone, the bleeding was less extensive than with a slow procedure.

This part of the operation, starting from the first cut, did not last more than twelve minutes; therefore, I was able to proceed at once to the clearing of the second and third branch and the gasserian ganglion, after I pushed the brain in the closed dural sac upward with the spatulated instrument.

However, since the trunk of the median meningeal artery in this procedure is almost in front of the third trigeminal branch, i.e., it obstructs further work, I ligated it at two places and cut it between the ligatures. As evident from this, my procedure is also very suitable for ligation of the trunk of the median meningeal artery in cases of bleeding. Before proceeding further I checked the massive bleeding by pressure application of sponges.

Subsequently, first the third, and then the second branch situated farther medially, were exposed for their entire length from the gasserian ganglion to the foramina ovale and rotundum, with the elevator, i.e., the dura mater was pushed back from the nerves, and then it was detached from the underlying bone. The same was then tried with the gasserian ganglion. This attempt was completely successful. I wish to emphasize this fact, since in my first work on the basis of postmortem studies I maintained that the dura mater could be retracted only from the convex anterior margin of the ganglion, from which the three trigeminal branches project, and from the adjoining section, while in the upper section of the ganglion the dura was presumably so

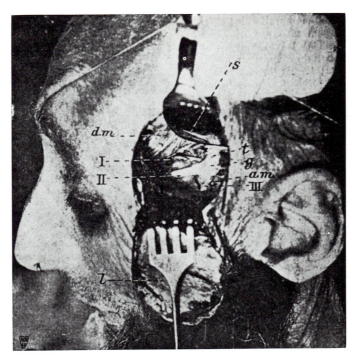

FIG. 1. Three-fifths of natural size. t = trigeminal trunk; underneath is placed a black needle, which indicates with its point the internal carotid. In front of it, i.e. between the carotid and the point of the needle, is the trochlear nerve. g = gasserian ganglion. a.m. = median meningeal artery, tied with black thread and cut. I, II, III = the first, second and third trigeminal branch. d.m. = dura mater. s = spatula, lifting upward the brain enclosed by the dura mater. Since it is highly polished it partly shows the mirror picture of the dissected nerves. i = inner surface of the bone of the flap consisting of skin, muscle, periosteum and bone.

closely fused with it that it could not be retracted with a blunt instrument. Additional postmortem findings showed me that this statement is not valid in such exclusiveness; rather, when some individual thin, but unusually strong bands of connective tissue are cut with scissors, the dura can be pushed back from the ganglion with a blunt instrument. The dural sac is not opened. In the case of the patient, the dura could be detached in this manner with the elevator without any difficulty in the entire length of the ganglion and retracted so far back that the trunk of the trigeminus could be seen. Finally, the ganglion was detached from the underlying bone. Now both the ganglion and the second and the third branches were completely exposed.

I intentionally exposed the first trigeminal branch only in the immediate proximity of the ganglion and no farther, for it extends in the wall of the cavernous sinus and although I verified in postmortem findings that it can be retracted from the latter, it must be kept in mind that the trochlear, abducens and, farther centrally, the oculomotor nerves are situated in its immediate proximity; and it is imperative that an injury or even laceration or bruising of these nerves be

avoided. How easily such a lesion can be produced when the procedure is not done with extreme care, is evident from a communication of Frank Hartley,* who performed the operation in the manner described. He resected the second and third trigeminal branches intracranially in the case of a 46-year-old man, who had already undergone repeated surgery without any lasting effect. As Hartley himself stated, during the retraction of the dura mater the oculomotor, trochlear and abducens nerves were apparently injured. ("In the retraction of the dura mater, owing to imperfect instruments, the third, fourth and sixth nerves were somewhat injured.") As a result, the patient had ptosis, double vision and inability to move the eye. Accurate examination nine days after operation revealed very weak movements of all muscles of the eye; consequently, the nerves could not have been cut. Six weeks later, the oculomotor nerve was again functioning; no special mention was made of the trochlear and abducens nerves, only a statement that the double vision disappeared.

* Frank Hartley, Intracranial neurectomy of the second and third divisions of the fifth nerve. New York Medical Journal, 1892, No. 12.

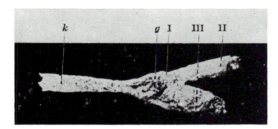

FIG. 2. Natural size. k = trigeminal trunk. g = gasserian ganglion, crushed in the center by the Thiersch forceps. The place where the first branch was torn off can be seen in the upper part. II = second trigeminal branch. III = third trigeminal branch.

I did not encounter a similar misfortune in my three cases and I believe that with a careful deep dissection it is completely avoidable. The wound can be surveyed easily, as shown in Fig. 1. In addition, an electric lamp is not needed for illuminating the deep-lying area. This is also evident from Fig. 1; if photography is possible under far worse lighting conditions of a morgue, the cavity of the wound would necessarily be easily visible in the operating room.

Since the illustration in my first report, which was made by a draftsman, who was not too proficient, did not give the correct relations, I performed the operation postmortem and photographed the preparation—with a very narrow lens opening and an exposure time of three minutes in order to show correctly the great depth of the wound in the picture. Consequently, the retractors could not be held, but were affixed to the head of the corpse itself by strings. A stereoscopic picture was passed around during the lecture, which demonstrates the spatial dimensions of the operative field far better, of course, than the simple photograph.

From the time of Thiersch's procedure we have been striving to accomplish the removal of the nerves in neuralgia to the greatest possible extent, and therefore I wanted to draw out in this case the peripheral branches with Thiersch's forceps, but did not succeed. This is understandable in the case of the third branch, because it had previously been resected in the periphery and held fast here by scar tissue. But the second branch also threatened to break off during the very careful rotating of the forceps, whereas normally, the ramifications of the peripheral nerves can be untwisted without any difficulty. Therefore I discontinued this maneuver and cut the two branches in the foramen ovale and rotundum as deep as possible with a sharp tenotome. Then I grasped the whole gasserian ganglion transversely in the Thiersch forceps and with a rotating motion pulled out the centrally (i.e., posteriorly, toward the pons varolii) situated trigeminal trunk in its

entire length of 22 mm. This procedure was performed in deep narcosis and no visible change could be observed either with regard to cardiac activity or respiration. After the trigeminal trunk was cut, Horsley* observed the cessation of breathing and disappearance of pulse; these disturbances lasted three to four seconds and then normal conditions returned. During the removal of the ganglion the first trigeminal branch close to the ganglion also broke off, and I did not have to cut it. Fig. 2, taken immediately after the operation, of the removed nerve sections in natural size, shows that the entire trunk of the trigeminus was removed up to its exit from the pons varolii. In addition to the photograph I am going to show you also the preparation hardened in osmic acid, from which only small pieces were removed for microscopic examination. The report of the histological findings will be given elsewhere.

The operation performed in this manner lasted no more than 55 minutes from the first skin incision to the completion of the nerve resection. The flap of skin, muscle, and periosteum was attached with interrupted sutures in its old place. A small strip of 10% iodoform gauze was placed between the dura mater and the base of the skull to guide out the oozing blood; it was removed the third day.

The course was completely undisturbed; in the evening after the operation the neuralgic pains had already gone and did not return in the nine weeks that have passed since that time. On the seventh day after operation, the patient felt strong enough to leave her bed for some time. Eighteen days after operation the patient returned to her home. The general condition, which because of the long suffering was so extremely poor, improved quickly and nervousness and insomnia also disappeared.

Dr. Nonne examined closely the important conditions in the area of the resected trigeminus on four different days (February 25 and 27 and March 2 and 6) and sent me the following report, which I greatly appreciate: [See Fig. 3.]

"In area a, complete anesthesia for all stimuli;
at b, sensitivity to all stimuli greatly reduced;
at c, less extensively, but still very considerably reduced for all stimuli;
at d and e, strong contacts were felt clearly—strong stimuli of pain (electric current, deep stabbing, etc.), felt as pain;
at f, only slight reduction of the sensitivity to all stimuli.

"At any place where the sensitivity is only reduced, but not completely abolished, the ability to localize the tactile impressions is, however, very strongly reduced.

"The ear has completely normal sensitivity (N.

* l.c.

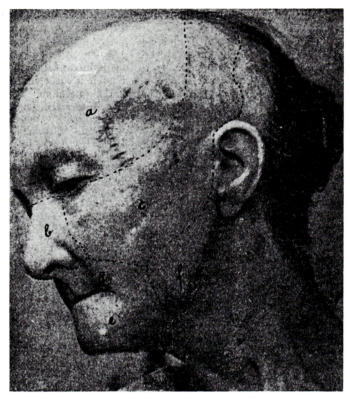

Fig. 3. See text for explanation.

auricularis magnus, even the trigeminal part, has intact sensitivity).

"Hearing: left slightly less than right.

"Smell: left = right.

"Taste: (sweet, sour, bitter, galvanic current) on the left—clearly present, but reduced. Sensitivity of the tongue (pricking, electric stimulus, heat, cold) on the left, weaker than on the right.

"Masticatory muscles: (temporalis, masseter) no action observed on the left. Degenerative reaction in masseter is not demonstrated.

"Bulbar and palpebral conjunctiva, as well as cornea, completely insensitive. Cornea completely clear, no conjunctivitis or keratitis. Movements of the eye, normal; sight as before.

"Sensitivity of the labial and buccal mucous membrane completely abolished on the left side.

"Vasomotor abnormalities of the skin of the face are absent, as well as trophic disorders of skin (glossy skin, etc.).

"In each of the four examinations an improvement of the sensitivity was observed."

In addition, I believe that I should emphasize that no ulcerative formations or trophic changes were found either on the tongue or the mucous membrane. If the patient happens to bite into her left side while chewing, she does not feel the bite. The movements of the jaw are completely free and she can again tolerate dentures, which in the first weeks produced unpleasant sensations.

The left eye no longer secretes more or less tears than the right one, and the nasal mucous membrane of the left side—except for anesthesia —does not differ in any way from the right side.

Unfortunately, it was not possible to perform an accurate examination of the nervous condition before operation; it would have been torture for the patient in her wretched condition and would not have provided any useful results.

Finally, as far as the formation of the flap in this case is concerned, I did not see any disadvantage resulting from the removal of the bone; anyhow, previously in each such trepanation, we were generally accustomed to break it. But in this case the dura mater was retained and the periosteum was supported by the muscular cushion. Brain pulsations are neither felt nor seen and the palpation of the upper part of the flap makes it highly probable that a new bone formed from the detached periosteum; the thick soft parts prevent us from determining this in the lower section of the flap. Nevertheless, in further cases, which would not require that the time of operation be limited as much as possible, I would prefer to retain the bone and include it together with the soft parts in the flap.

Case 2. Mr. C. Morris, aged 64, government employee from Washington, afflicted for 13 years with neuralgia in the region of the second trigeminal branch, in 1884 was operated on successfully by Agnew in Philadelphia with Langenbeck's method. But only a year later pains returned in their former severity. A new operation with partial removal of the upper jaw was performed in Washington, but without favorable outcome. In the spring of 1886 several surgeons were consulted even in Germany; they refused to do further operation. Injections in the lips, which were administered in Vienna, alleviated pains for some time. In recent years pains became more severe than before and in this condition the patient turned to me. It was a case of typical neuralgia of the second trigeminal branch of the left side; pains appeared three to four times a day and always lasted two hours. The attacks came only rarely at night.

The operation was performed on December 3 and 8, 1892, in two stages, in exactly the same manner as was described in my first report. The second trigeminal branch was excised from the gasserian ganglion to the foramen rotundum. In the first days after the second operation pains continued with diminished severity, then ceased and had not returned up to the day of his departure (March 8, 1893).

A HISTORY of the development of gasserian ganglionectomy and retrogasserian neurotomy was outlined in the November 1963 issue of the *Journal of Neurosurgery*, and papers relating to these two operations by Horsley, Hartley, and Krause were reprinted. To complete these early classics of trigeminal surgery, the important 1901 paper by William G. Spiller and Charles H. Frazier is reproduced below.

THE DIVISION OF THE SENSORY ROOT OF THE TRIGEMINUS FOR THE RELIEF OF TIC DOULOUREUX; AN EXPERIMENTAL, PATHOLOGICAL AND CLINICAL STUDY, WITH A PRELIMINARY REPORT OF ONE SURGICALLY SUCCESSFUL CASE.*†

By WILLIAM G. SPILLER, M.D.,
of Philadelphia

Assistant Clinical Professor of Nervous Diseases, University of Pennsylvania

AND CHARLES H. FRAZIER, M.D.,
of Philadelphia

Professor of Clinical Surgery, University of Pennsylvania

PART I

By WILLIAM G. SPILLER, M.D.,

From the William Pepper Laboratory of Clinical Medicine (Phoebe A. Hearst Foundation)

In a paper published in the November, 1898, number of the *American Journal of the Medical Sciences*, p. 532, I made use of these words: "If it could be shown that the sensory root of the Gasserian ganglion does not unite after its fibres are divided, we should have a fact of great importance. Division of this root would probably be a less serious operation than the removal of the entire ganglion, and might have the same effect in the relief of pain, but the surgical difficulties might be insurmountable. Experiments on animals to determine whether or not the sensory root of the Gasserian ganglion unites after section of

* Published synchronously with the University of Pennsylvania Medical Bulletin.
† Reprinted from *The Philadelphia Medical Journal*, 1901, *8:* 1039–1049.

its fibres might result in a lessening of the great mortality now existing in operations on the ganglion." Dr. C. H. Frazier has shown that the division of the sensory root may be performed in man, and probably with less danger than the removal of the Gasserian ganglion, as hemorrhage is not so likely to be severe. I should like to lay particular emphasis on the fact that in proposing this operation I did so with much caution. I believe that Horsley is the only one who before Dr. Frazier has divided the roots of the trigeminal nerve without removing the ganglion. Horsley avulsed them at their attachment to the pons, and his patient died seven hours after the operation.[1]

Frazier has cut the sensory root of the trigeminal nerve in a large number of dogs. Seven of these lived sufficiently long for a study of the nervous system by the method of Marchi. The results of my microscopical examination of the nervous systems from these seven dogs are as follows:

Dog No. 4.—Distinct degeneration by the Marchi method is found in the sensory root at its entrance into the pons, and this degeneration is much more intense in the external portion of the root than in the medial portion, although distinct degeneration is detected also in the latter. The motor root in its intracerebral portion shows slight degeneration. A few black dots are present in the mesencephalic root of the trigeminal nerve. In sections from the medulla oblongata the degeneration is especially intense in the dorsal portion of the spinal root, while comparatively few black masses are found in the ventral portion (see Fig. 1). The Gasserian ganglion and the nerve fibres at each end of this ganglion seem to be normal.

Dog No. 5.—The degeneration of the trigeminal nerve is similar to that in dog 4, only it is more intense in dog 5 (see Fig. 2). Both anterior pyramids show slight degeneration. Much degeneration is found in some of the fibres at one end of the Gasserian ganglion, while those at the other end of the ganglion are normal.

Dog No. 6.—The degeneration of the sensory root of the trigeminal nerve in this case is distinct, but is not very intense.

Dog No. 10.—The degeneration of the intracerebral portion of the sensory root of the trigeminal nerve in this case is very indistinct. The nerve fibres at the central end of the Gasserian

[1] Horsley: British Medical Journal, 1891, Vol. ii, p. 1249.

ganglion are much degenerated, while those at the peripheral end are not degenerated. This degeneration at the central end is probably the result of purulent meningitis.

Dog No. 11.—The degeneration of the sensory root of the trigeminal nerve in this case is present, but unimportant.

Dog No. 12.—The degeneration of the sensory root of the trigeminal nerve in this case is slight. Slight degeneration is detected in some of the fibres at one end of the Gasserian ganglion.

Dog No. 13.—Degeneration of the sensory root of the trigeminal nerve in this case is not distinct.

Two of these cases, dogs four and five, were especially satisfactory for microscopical study, while the others presented too little degeneration to permit valuable conclusions to be drawn. In dogs four and five it is evident that the lateral portion of the extracerebral sensory root of the trigeminal nerve was cut, while the median portion was only partially injured. In these cases the dorsal portion of the spinal root of the trigeminal nerve also was more degenerated than the ventral. I have not been able in these two cases to detect any attempt at regeneration of the sensory root of the trigeminal nerve, but these cases do not disprove the possibility of such a regeneration. The difficulties of technique in determining by micro-

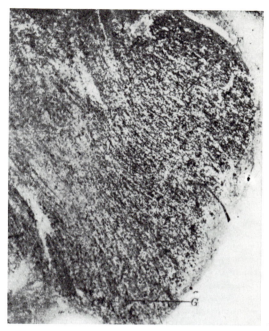

FIG. 2. The sensory root at its entrance into the pons, from dog 5. The lateral portion (F) is intensely degenerated, while the medial portion (G) is only slightly degenerated. The degenerated portion indicates the extent of the division of the sensory root. By comparing Figures 4 and 5 it will be seen that the fibres of the lateral portion of the sensory root at its entrance into the pons, in their further course occupy the dorsal part of the descending spinal root.

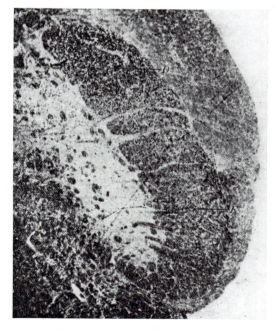

FIG. 1. Section of the medulla oblongata from dog 4, showing the descending spinal root. The dorsal portion of this root (D) is much more degenerated than the ventral portion (E), because only the lateral portion of the sensory root was completely divided between the pons and the Gasserian ganglion, as shown in Figure 2. The black dots represent the degenerated fibres.

scopical examination a regeneration of the cut sensory root of the trigeminal nerve are considerable. In removing the brains in dogs four and five the slight connection by means of the motor root between the Gasserian ganglion and the pons was destroyed.

It is important to determine whether regeneration of the central nervous system is possible, and with this object in view an examination of the literature is desirable.

Baer, Dawson and Marshall[2] state that, on the clinical side, so far as they were able to ascertain, no satisfactory cases are reported for man of regeneration and return of function after lesions causing the destruction of any part of the central nervous system. These authors do not discuss the histological evidence of regeneration. They conclude from a few experiments cited from the literature that in the lower vertebrates a certain amount of return of function seems to follow a lesion in the central nervous system, while it is not yet decided certainly whether any such return is

[2] Baer, Dawson, and Marshall: The Journal of Experimental Medicine, Vol. iv, 1899, p. 29.

possible among higher animals. They experimented on dogs by ligation of the roots of the second cervical nerve between the spinal ganglion and the cord, and from physiological results they conclude that after severance of the fibres of the dorsal roots of the spinal nerves between the ganglion and the cord, regeneration of the fibres into the cord will take place under proper conditions, so that normal reflexes through the respiratory, cardiac and vasomotor centres may be obtained. They do not venture to express a positive opinion as to the completeness of the regeneration and the average time necessary for the restoration of function, but their seven experiments showed that great individual differences existed in the rapidity of regeneration. In some cases the return of functional activity in the dorsal root fibres seemed to be nearly complete at the end of ninety days, while in one case the return was far from complete after an interval of 151 days. They conclude that if the posterior root fibres can thus be regenerated in the posterior columns of the cord, there seems reason to hope that the fibres in other tracts may possess the same property, and that therefore it is not impossible that with the proper technique a severed spinal cord might be made to regenerate its broken tracts, both the ascending and the descending. It is much to be regretted that the histological evidence of regeneration of the central nervous system obtained by these investigations of Baer, Dawson and Marshall has not been published.

I hesitate to criticise these carefully performed experiments, but it should be remembered that they do not afford satisfactory evidence that restoration of function after destruction of a part of the central nervous system in man will be complete.

It is presumable that if such restoration occurs in the dog it occurs also in man under similar conditions, but it is only presumable. In these experiments posterior roots were ligated; it would have been better if they had been resected. The divided ends would then have retracted from one another, and the bridge of degenerated tissue caused by ligation of the roots would not have existed. It is possible that such a bridge of tissue may guide the young nerve fibres to the spinal cord.

We know that where only a few sensory fibres exist these may be sufficient to convey impulses coming from the periphery of the body to the central nervous system. Fickler[3] states that in a case of his own, sensation was at one period fully lost but returned after a time to such a degree that almost all qualities became normal, only that warmth and cold sensations were somewhat impaired, and yet very few nerve fibres were found in the posterior and antero-lateral columns of the spinal cord at one level. These few fibres must

have been sufficient for the restoration of sensation. The motor tracts of the cord in this case contained more nerve fibres than the sensory tracts, but very little return of motion had occurred. It appears that more normal fibres are requisite for motor function than for sensory.

Fickler also states that Schiefferdecker, Kahler, Stroebe and others have not found any regeneration of nerve fibres worthy of the name after division of the spinal cord in vertebrates. He concludes that the nerve fibres he found within the pia of the spinal cord were regenerated fibres. This conclusion is hardly warranted. Dr. Dercum and I[4] have shown that such fibres may be present in the spinal pia when there is no reason for believing that they are regenerated fibres, and Bielschowsky[5] later has demonstrated the same fact. Bielschowsky also makes the statement that experiments have shown that the spinal cord is not capable of regeneration after it has been divided.

Stroebe's[6] article on regeneration of the spinal cord is especially praiseworthy. After a careful review of the literature on this subject he shows that the opinions of the investigators differ concerning the possibility of regeneration of the cord. Stroebe found from his experiments on rabbits that the nerve fibres of posterior roots that were injured at the level of the lesion in the cord, grow out again from the spinal ganglion toward the spinal cord, and push in a certain distance between the tissue of the scar formation. It was therefore evident that an attempt was made by the posterior roots to penetrate the scar tissue of the cord, but the attempt was not very successful.

The evidence of restoration of the spinal cord being so doubtful, it has seemed to me equally uncertain whether the normal relation of posterior roots to the spinal cord is re-established after these roots have been cut in man. The posterior columns of the spinal cord are largely composed of nerve fibres from the posterior roots, and if these fibres within the cord are not restored after they are divided, it seems probable that the portion outside of the cord, i.e., within the posterior roots, is not restored after these roots are divided. The chief difference between the structure of the intramedullary and extramedullary portions of these fibres, that I am aware of, is that sheaths of Schwann exist on the latter and not on the former, and yet this may possibly be an important difference.

The recent investigations of Bethe[7] may cause us to modify greatly our views regarding the regeneration of nerve fibres. Some investigators in

[3] Fickler: Deutsche Zeitschrift fuer Nervenheilkunde. Vol. xvi, Nos. 1 and 2.

[4] Dercum and Spiller: Revue Neurologique, March 15, 1901, No. 5, p. 222.
[5] Bielschowsky: Neurologisches Centralblatt, April 16, 1901, No. 8, p. 346.
[6] Stroebe: Zeigler's Beitraege, Vol. xv, 1894, p. 383.
[7] Bethe: Abstract in Centralblatt fuer Nervenheilkunde und Psychiatrie, July, 1901, p. 440.

the past have held that the nuclei of the sheath of Schwann have an important rôle in regeneration, but most authorities have taught that regeneration occurs by the outgrowth of axones from the old axones of the central stump of the divided nerve. Bethe has resected the sciatic nerve of the dog, and sewed the peripheral stump within the muscle to prevent union of the two ends. The peripheral end of the nerve degenerated below the point of division of the nerve, but later full regeneration of this peripheral portion occurred from the nuclei of the sheaths of Schwann. The nerve terminated at its proximal end blindly. Irritation of the newly formed nerve caused contraction of the muscles supplied by it, and the regenerated nerve differed in no way from a normal one, and yet it was not in continuity with nerve cell-bodies. If this regenerated nerve were cut, its peripheral portion below the line of division degenerated but the more central portion persisted, even though it were not in connection with nerve cell-bodies. These investigations of Bethe may possibly show that the presence of a sheath of Schwann is necessary for regeneration of a nerve fibre, and may compel us to accept the possibility of regeneration of posterior roots which are provided with sheaths of Schwann, and to deny the existence of regeneration of nerve fibres within the cord which have no sheaths of Schwann, even though they may be the continuation of posterior root fibres. These very experiments make it doubtful however whether the posterior roots would be restored beyond the point where the sheath of Schwann ceases, that is, at the entrance of the root into the spinal cord; they may possibly explain why peripheral nerves regenerate so readily while the spinal cord does not.

The nerve fibre of the posterior spinal root has apparently the same structure as the sensory fibre of the peripheral nerve, and yet the reaction of the cell-body in the spinal ganglion is very different according as its central or peripheral process is divided. Investigators (Lugaro, Mering, Fleming, van Gehuchten, Cassirer) have shown that division of the peripheral process of a spinal ganglion cell-body causes very distinct degeneration of this cell-body, or even complete destruction of the cell-body, while Lugaro[8] has demonstrated that the cell-bodies of the spinal ganglia belonging to the sciatic nerve undergo no distinct change when the posterior columns of the cord or the posterior roots belonging to these ganglia are divided. In advanced tabes dorsalis the posterior roots are intensely degenerated even close up to the spinal ganglia, and yet Schaffer, a very careful investigator, has found the cell-bodies of the spinal ganglia normal in tabes by the Nissl method, and I have confirmed his observations.

These findings seem to show that the peripheral process of the cell-body of the spinal ganglion has a different importance from that of the central process, and that although a peripheral nerve may be restored after it has been divided, it does not necessarily follow that the nerve fibres of the posterior root will also be restored after they have been divided. What is true of the spinal ganglion cell-body and its processes is probably true of the Gasserian ganglion cell-body and its processes.

We must, therefore, conclude that further study is necessary before we can be convinced that regeneration of sensory nerve roots in man occurs, and that full restoration of function is possible after division of sensory nerve roots. Even if a partial regeneration of these roots were possible, it does not follow that pain would return after division of the sensory root of the trigeminal nerve. There might be a partial return of sensation without pain. We must acknowledge that some evidence of partial return of function in injured posterior roots in animals exists, but no evidence of return of function in the trigeminus after the division of its sensory root is to be found in literature. It is a question whether the fibres of this root could penetrate through the thick bands of the middle cerebellar peduncle and pyramidal tract to the sensory terminal nucleus of the nerve within the pons.

In view of the uncertainty of regeneration of the sensory root of the trigeminal nerve, and of the great mortality in removal of the Gasserian ganglion, the division of the sensory root for the relief of tic douloureux is a justifiable procedure, and I trust we may be able to keep under observation for at least two or three years the patient on whom Dr. Frazier has performed this operation. We are not urging that division of the sensory root should at once replace removal of the Gasserian ganglion, and distinctly recognize that the former operation is on trial.

Frazier has shown by experimentation that the motor root of the trigeminus in the dog may be spared. The possibility of saving this root was present in my mind when I urged that this operation should be tried. The motor root has never been left intact when the Gasserian ganglion has been entirely removed, and it probably never can be. It seems to me a fortunate occurrence that in this first successful operation on the sensory root of the trigeminus Frazier divided the motor root as well as the sensory. All communication between the Gasserian ganglion and the pons was in this way fully destroyed and the best possible conditions were obtained for testing the possibility of regeneration of the sensory root. If this case should be as successful clinically[9] as it has been surgically we may be able hereafter to relieve the

[8] Lugaro, cited by Flatau: Fortschritte der Medicin, 1897, No. 15.

[9] Sufficient time to determine this has not yet elapsed; so far the case has been very successful clinically.

pain of tic douloureux without paralyzing the muscles of mastication, for Dr. Frazier's operation seems to indicate that he is able to save the motor root; and we may also be able to lessen the danger of loss of vision, inasmuch as by division of the sensory root the nerve cell-bodies of the Gasserian ganglion are left in normal relation with the peripheral distribution of the trigeminus, and changes in the cornea may be less likely to occur. It is not improbable that these cell-bodies exert a trophic influence on the peripheral branches of this nerve. If this operation should be done again, it would be well to resect the sensory and motor roots, instead of merely dividing them. If it should be fully established that the sensory root will not regenerate after it is cut, the motor root should be spared.

There are some other conclusions to be drawn from the microscopical study of the nervous system of the dogs operated on by Frazier.

Bregman[10] has obtained results from experiments on the rabbit very similar to my results obtained from the dog. In his cases, where the descending spinal root of the fifth nerve was fully degenerated, the sensory root at its outward entrance into the pons was also completely degenerated; but where only the ventral portion of the spinal root was degenerated, only the medial portion of the sensory root at its entrance into the pons was degenerated; and where only the dorsal portion of the spinal root was degenerated, only the lateral portion of the sensory root at its entrance into the pons was degenerated. Bregman also found degeneration in the intracerebral portion of the motor root of the fifth nerve after this root was divided, and this was an ascending degeneration in motor fibres. He found also the mesencephalic root of the fifth nerve degenerated.

From the results obtained by Bregman and from mine, we may conclude that the nerve fibres of the sensory root of the fifth nerve, in both its intracerebral and extracerebral portions, maintain the same relative positions throughout the course of this root. This is an important fact, because we may conclude that if the nerve fibres of the sensory root do not mingle freely without regard to order, the nerve fibres of the Gasserian ganglion also probably preserve a definite order of arrangement. The nerve fibres passing distally from the ganglion separate into three distinct divisions at the peripheral end of the ganglion. We can hardly suppose that the nerve fibres within the ganglion are arranged without definite order if in both the sensory root and the peripheral divisions a very definite arrangement exists. Tiffany's suggestion to spare the inner third of the ganglion in order to preserve vision seems, therefore, to have an ana-

tomical basis, although it is not improbable that if this inner third of the ganglion were removed, the relief of pain would not be permanent.

PART II
By Charles H. Frazier, M.D.

The surgery of the Gasserian ganglion has received a great impetus during the past few years, largely through the efforts of those who by the most careful study of the anatomical relationship of the structures in and about the field of operation have been successful in surmounting many of the operative difficulties. All the improvements in technique, for a practical consideration of the subject, may be grouped under two headings: (1) those which render the ganglion easier of approach, and (2) those which suggest means, not of controlling, but of preventing hemorrhage. The pterygoid route of Rose and the temporosphenoidal route of Doyen have practically been abandoned in favor of the temporal route first advocated independently by Hartley and Krause. In order to lessen the risk of injuring the middle meningeal vessel and to facilitate the exposure of the ganglion Cushing suggested a modification of the Hartley-Krause operation, which he has called the infra-arterial route. The base of the flap corresponds to the level of the zygoma and the trephining opening is sufficiently low to escape the sulcus arteriosus in the anterior inferior angle of the parietal bone, which lodges the middle meningeal vessel, and to give the maximum exposure with the minimum of cerebral compression. Sapejko (*Revue de Chirurgie*, September, 1901) goes so far as to recommend the removal of the great wing of the sphenoid up to and including the foramina rotundum and ovale.

No matter what the method of approach, each of these operations has for its object the removal or avulsion of the Gasserian ganglion and the adjacent portions of its first, second and third divisions. I am about to describe an operation for the relief of tic douloureux which depends for its success not upon the removal of all or part of the ganglion, but solely upon the division of its sensory root. This plan of operation, so radically different, was suggested to me by Dr. William G. Spiller almost three years ago. Granting for the time that from the operator's standpoint this measure could claim many points of advantage over those procedures which entail the removal of the ganglion itself, I withheld my endorsement until I was convinced that regeneration of the nerve fibres at the point of division was doubtful, and that in view of this uncertainty, therefore, this operation might be justified. In order to demonstrate experimentally that regeneration would not take place, I conducted, in connection with my colleague, Dr. Spiller, a series of experi-

[10] E. Bregman: Obersteiner's "Arbeiten," vol. 1, 1892, p. 73.

ments in which the proposed operation was practiced upon dogs. The interpretation of the results of these experiments and their significance from the standpoint of the neuropathologist is carefully considered in Dr. Spiller's contribution in this paper. Suffice it to say here that Dr. Spiller is of the opinion that the burden of evidence is still with those who would prove that regeneration of fibres with restoration of function does follow division of these sensory roots.

Operation

The following are the steps of the operation:

1. Reflection of a horseshoe-shaped flap of skin and subcutaneous tissue. The flap corresponds in width to the length of the zygoma; its base is on a level with the lower border of the zygoma, its convexity reaching a point 6 cm. above.

2. Division of the zygomatic processes of the malar and temporal bones. After reflection of the superficial flap of skin and subcutaneous tissue an incision is made in the periosteum over the middle of the zygoma throughout its length and the periosteum elevated sufficiently to allow of the introduction of the bone-cutting forceps and the division of the zygomatic processes of the malar and temporal bone.

In my operations upon dogs, where the field of operation was so much smaller than that of the human subject, and where the bellies of the temporal and masseter muscles were proportionally so much larger, I found it absolutely necessary to resect the zygoma in order to be able to retract the temporal muscle sufficiently to allow of a proper exposure of the field of operation and I determined to introduce this step into the technique of my next operation upon the human subject. It is better to practise a temporary rather than a permanent resection of the zygoma. At first thought one might think it inadvisable to replace the segment on the grounds that the bone might not become united owing to the difficulty of keeping it at rest. One will realize how unlikely it is that this will occur if one takes into consideration that the most likely cause of displacement, viz., muscular action, is not operative because the muscles attached to the fragment of bone and concerned in the act of mastication will have been deprived of their motor nervous supply, which is derived from the inframaxillary branch of the trigeminus, before the operation has been completed. (This assertion is based upon the assumption that the integrity of the motor root of the ganglion has in but very few instances been preserved.) One or two sutures introduced at either end of the fragment through the periosteum will suffice to insure fixation until union occurs. Necrosis of this fragment has been recorded as a possible unfavorable complication of temporary resection, but this can be avoided if one bears in mind that the bone receives a liberal blood supply through the periosteum and avoids stripping this structure from the bone except at the points where the bone-cutting forceps have to be applied.

3. Reflection of a horseshoe-shaped flap, composed of temporal fascia, muscle, zygoma and pericranium, corresponding in shape to the superficial one but of somewhat smaller dimensions. This flap is reflected sufficiently to expose to view the temporal fossa; during the operation it will be subjected to considerable traumatism consequent to the constant traction and pressure and will be swollen and tender for a short time. Owing to the contractile character of the tissues of which it is composed the flap will shrink at least one-third before the operation is completed, so that some little traction will have to be made in order to approximate the edges upon closure of the wound.

4. Removal with the trephine of a button of bone at a point corresponding to the middle of area exposed and enlargement of the opening with the rongeur forceps until its diameter measures three to four centimetres. The usual precaution must be taken in trephining here, as in any portion of the calvarium where the bone is of such variable thickness, in order to avoid injuring the dura; and additional precautions are necessary in this region owing to the fact that the middle meningeal artery lies immediately beneath the button of bone to be removed. With the rongeur forceps the trephine opening is enlarged about equally in all directions and should extend downwards to the level of the crista infratemporalis.

5. Separation of the dura and exposure of the ganglion and its sensory root. The adherent dura is separated by blunt dissection (the handle of a scalpel enveloped in a single layer of gauze will meet all indications) inwards and forwards until the foramen ovale or rotundum comes into view, either of which serve as a guide to the site of the ganglion. This is the most tedious stage of the operation and one which taxes the patience of the operator to the utmost. Hemorrhage now constitutes the great bugbear. Protracted and persistent oozing follows the separation of the dura from every point at which it is adherent to the skull; the older the patient the firmer the adhesion and the freer the hemorrhage. Hemostasis can be effected only by pressure and heat; small pledgets of gauze saturated with a hot saline solution are cautiously applied to the bleeding point and allowed to remain for periods of two to five minutes. In my series of operations upon dogs I tested the efficiency of gelatin in 5 per cent. solution as a hemostat in intracranial operations with practically negative results. The solution had no apparent effect. The dura is most adherent to the skull at the margins of the foramina so that the most troublesome bleeding is not experienced until one has arrived almost at the site of the ganglion.

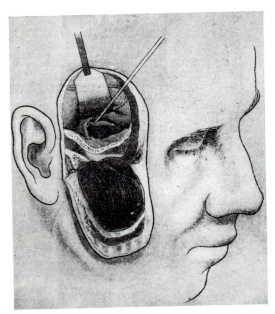

FIG. 3. Illustrating the final step of the operation. The sensory root is picked up on a blunt hook preparatory to its division. (This drawing made directly from a dissection upon the cadaver, shows the reflected dura propria and the relationship of the foramina rotundum, ovale and spinosum and the middle meningeal artery to the Gasserian ganglion and its sensory root.)

Second only to hemorrhage as a troublesome feature of this stage of the operation is the presence of large bony eminences on the floor of the middle fossa. As pointed out by Amyx these eminences are more commonly met with in heads not having a great transverse diameter between the ears, but whose external bony prominences are well marked rather than in those skulls with a large transverse width; these prominences are situated usually external to the foramina ovale and rotundum and, if very large, will have to be chiselled off in order to expose the foramina to view and remove the ganglion. In some cases the ganglion itself lies beneath a bony roof as though it were a continuation of the petrous portion of the temporal bone. While this is an anomaly in men, it is not so in the dog. Almost without exception in the series of dog's skulls which I had an opportunity to examine while carrying on the experimental work, the ganglion was covered by a thin shell of bone which had to be removed in order to bring to view the ganglion and its sensory root.

With hemorrhage well enough under control to enable one to recognize the anatomical landmarks, the operator makes an incision into the dura and dura propria between the foramen ovale and spinosum and with a blunt dissector separates the dural envelope from the upper surface of the ganglion as far back as may be necessary to ex-

pose to view the sensory root. Up to this point the method of procedure has not differed essentially from those operations which have in view the extirpation of the ganglion. From now on the courses diverge; in the one the operator proceeds to liberate and extract the ganglion and its branches, in the other to liberate and divide the sensory root. The division of the root is not a difficult performance. When fully exposed it is picked up on a blunt hook [Fig. 3] which is passed around the nerve from without inwards. The nerve is divided either by making traction with the hook or cutting directly upon the hook with knife or scissors. It would be a better plan, however, and I will carry it out in future cases, after elevation of the nerve upon the hook to grasp it with a pair of forceps, hemostatic or dissecting, and remove a small section with knife or scissors. This slight modification will add nothing to the dangers and little to the difficulties of the operation and will serve a two-fold purpose, on the one hand furnishing a specimen for a pathologic examination, and on the other leaving a defect in the continuity of the nerve which would render regeneration a possibility still more remote.

In connection with this step of the operation, there is one point which will naturally come up for discussion. Can the sensory root be isolated from the motor root so that the integrity of the latter may be preserved? This question may be answered in the affirmative if certain reservations be made. That it is possible upon the living subject to separate the motor from the sensory root was proven by my own case. I had practically concluded the operation and was about to close the wound; in order to assure myself that none of the fibres of the sensory root had been left undivided, I repeated the last step of the operation and in so doing picked up the motor root which up to this time had remained intact, and unintentionally divided it. It is *possible*, therefore, to divide the sensory without the motor root; whether we can attain sufficient dexterity to avoid the accident which happened in my case is a matter to be settled by future repeated observations.

6. Closure of the wound.—The section of zygoma is returned to its normal situation and secured in place by one periosteal suture at either end. While there is no danger of displacement as a result of muscular action, the fragment may be dislodged during the application, or the changing, or the pressure of the dressing and for this reason the introduction of a suture at either end is recommended. A narrow strip of gauze enveloped as it passes by the scalp in a cuff of rubber tissue is introduced for drainage. If the bleeding is free at the conclusion of the operation, it must be controlled by pressure with strips of gauze. The rubber tissue, by preventing the edges of the scalp wound adhering one to the other, will insure

perfect drainage. The wound in the temporal muscle and fascia is closed with buried interrupted catgut sutures, and the superficial wound with interrupted silk-worm gut sutures.

A special protective dressing is applied to the eye in order to prevent corneal ulceration.

Remarks

Whether this operation for the relief of tic douloureux will receive the endorsement of the surgical profession and take the place of the operation now in vogue, will depend altogether upon the acceptance without reservation of the facts embodied in the following two assertions: (1) Regeneration of the sensory root will not take place after its division, and (2) (a) Liberation and division of the sensory root, obviating many of the operative difficulties associated with the liberation and extraction of the ganglia, is easier of execution; (b) the integrity of the structures of the cavernous sinus is not endangered; (c) the operation should be attended with a lower mortality.

I will not enter into the discussion of the subject of the regeneration of the sensory roots of the cranial ganglion, as this is a problem which should be left to the neuropathologist for solution and in this paper has been very carefully and exhaustively treated by Spiller. It remains for me to substantiate the claims which have been advanced from the surgical aspect.

Every surgeon will frankly admit that hemorrhage is the greatest bugbear in operations upon the Gasserian ganglion and holds it accountable for many failures and many fatal issues. The bleeding that takes place during the operation in this field might be said to be either troublesome or alarming; troublesome when it follows division of the middle meningeal artery, the emissary veins; alarming when due to laceration of the cavernous sinus. Let us consider the various sources of hemorrhage separately. Hemorrhage from the middle meningeal artery, since the adoption of the infra-arterial route, will occur infrequently and when it does, may be controlled by plugging the foramen spinosum with gauze or, as Krause has suggested, with the end of a blunt hook (Krause has had constructed a series of hooks of various sizes which he keeps on hand to meet this emergency). If, in enlarging the opening in the skull, the operator should resect that portion of the skull containing the sulcus arteriosus, he runs the risk in the removal of that segment of bone of wounding the vessel. As it is not necessary, in order to expose the ganglion, to carry the resection so high, injury to the vessel at this stage of the operation should be regarded as a blunder. The vessel will most likely be injured at its other fixed point, namely the foramen spinosum. If too great traction be made upon the vessel at this point in elevating the brain, or if too great force be applied in

separating the dura in the neighborhood of the foramina where the attachments are firmest, the vessel is in imminent danger of being lacerated. Experience alone teaches one how much force can be applied to these structures without endangering their integrity. In so far as the middle meningeal artery is concerned, neither of the two operations under discussion can claim an advantage over the other. Hemorrhage will follow the separation of the dura from the various places at which it is attached to the skull; it is very variable in quantity, the degree of hemorrhage seeming to be in proportion to the number and firmness of the dural attachments. From this source bleeding is, to say the least, annoying but can always be controlled by pressure. The nearer one approaches the ganglion, the firmer the adherence of the dura, the correspondingly freer the bleeding. Inasmuch as the ganglion receives its largest blood supply from below, surgeons are advised in performing those operations which are designed to remove the ganglion, to put off the elevation of the ganglion till the latest moment in order, as Cushing says, to postpone what degree of hemorrhage is unavoidable as long as possible. In this particular, therefore, one can justly claim for the operation, which leaves undisturbed the attachments of the ganglion to its unyielding base, an advantage over one the execution of which invades this source of free and troublesome hemorrhage. The time required to separate the ganglion from its base and the additional time required to control or check the flow of blood before the operation can be proceeded with, must be taken into consideration and given due weight in the estimation of the relative merits of the operation under discussion.

The third source of hemorrhage is the cavernous sinus, and, as has been already said, should any injury happen this sinus bleeding may be so profuse as to give cause for alarm. The sinus is exposed to danger once the operator begins to free the internal aspect of the ganglion, and in this connection Cushing says "that it is well to conduct these manipulations *as near as possible to the sensory root, since that is the safest point*, and one at which there is less likelihood of injuring the cavernous sinus and sixth nerve." Therefore, in limiting our field of operation to the posterior aspect of the ganglion and its sensory root, we confine our manipulations to the point of greatest safety. So much stress would not be laid upon the superiority of one operation which is associated with less bleeding than another, because the amount of blood lost in either is not a menace to life and will not materially affect the ultimate results, but because the control of hemorrhage necessary to the continuance of the operative maneuvers is only effected after repeated application of pressure for various periods of time, which in the aggregate may rightly be considered as a factor unfavorably influencing the results. Patients of advanced years, and most of the sufferers of trifacial neuralgia that come to us for operation have reached that period of life, are not good subjects for prolonged general anesthesia, therefore any measure which will economize time should, other things being equal, carry some weight with it. Thus far I have aimed in drawing a comparison to throw the balance in favor of the operation requiring less time for its completion and attended with less hemorrhage. I now call your attention to the operative difficulties and dangers that are avoided by stopping short of the extraction of the ganglion. It goes without saying that the exposure of the ganglion is less difficult by far than its extraction. The ganglion and its three divisions are so firmly bound down to the base of the skull that the liberation of the structures is the step of the operation which, above all others, tests the skill, dexterity and patience of the operator. For the completion of this step of the operation one begins by exposing the superior surface (to quote Cushing again) "of the stellate structures well back on to the sensory root." Without going a step further, without exciting one whit more hemorrhage, without running any further risk of injuring adjacent structures, we have made all the preparation necessary for division of the sensory root. Thus one operation is practically complete before those difficulties, both serious and troublesome, common to the other operation have been encountered. Not only then do we obviate certain operative difficulties, but we are able as well to eliminate certain dangers to adjacent structures. In practically every operation in which the ganglion has been removed the motor root has been destroyed, but from what has already been said in discussing the last steps of the operation we not only believe it possible to divide the sensory without the motor root, but were able to demonstrate this on the living subject. Too much importance, it seems, has been attached to the question of the preservation of the motor root, since its division causes only the little annoyance to the patient that follows paralysis of the muscles of mastication on one side. The patient can chew his food only on the unaffected side. However, if it is possible to save the nerve, we are not justified in deliberately sacrificing it, and if the neuralgia involve both the right and left trigeminus, what is only an annoyance in a unilateral case becomes in the bilateral a serious complication.

As the motor root, so the sixth nerve is almost always injured during the extraction of the ganglion; its proximity to the ophthalmic division is such that division of one without the other is practically impossible.

Although a positive assertion cannot be made, there are some grounds for believing that trophic disturbances in the cornea, secondary to division of the first root of the ganglion itself, may not follow the division of sensory root because of the probable presence in the ganglion of trophic centres presiding over the peripheral nerve. In the case, which is reported in this paper, there was not a suspicion of a keratitis, although a very simple dressing, consisting of a compress saturated with boracic acid, was applied to the eye, and this for only one week following the operation.

On the assumption that we are recommending an operative procedure which obviates many difficulties and some dangers, which is easier of execution, comparatively speaking, and economical as to time, it is reasonable, at least, to prophesy a greater reduction in the mortality than that which has resulted from the improvements in technique which have within the past two years been suggested.

Conclusions

As a substitute for all operations which depend for their success upon removal of all or a part of the ganglion, I recommend an operation which depends for its success solely upon the division of the sensory root of the ganglion. Granting it will effect a radical and permanent cure, the advantages of this operation are the following:

1. It should be attended with a lower mortality.
2. It obviates a number of difficulties.
3. Its execution is, comparatively speaking, simple.
4. It is practically complete when the posterior aspect of the ganglion and its sensory root have been exposed; that is, it is practically complete before the difficulties most serious and troublesome common to other operations have been encountered.
5. The integrity of the cavernous sinus is never in danger.
6. The risk of injuring the sixth nerve is avoided.

The following is a brief history of the case upon which I performed this operation:

J.L., aged sixty-eight, was referred to my service in the University Hospital by Dr. D. J. McCarthy.

Family History.—Father and mother died from typhoid fever, one brother and sister living and well, two brothers died from unknown causes. His wife, four sons and one daughter are living. One son and one daughter are subject to attacks of supraorbital neuralgia, one son died from phthisis.

Previous History.—Had the usual diseases of childhood. About ten years ago had an attack of sciatica which lasted for some seven months, but did not confine him to bed.

Social History.—The patient was born in Ireland and came to the United States thirty-four years ago. Has been a hard worker ever since ten years of age. His occupation formerly was that of fireman, at present he is a watchman. Has never used alcohol excessively, occasionally taking a glass of liquor, which he found increased his neuralgic pains. No venereal history.

History of Present Illness.—About five years ago he first began to have sharp shooting pains referred to the course and distribution of the right supraorbital nerve, beginning at the supraorbital notch and extending up over the forehead as far back as the anterior edge of the parietal bone. These attacks were provoked by exposure to cold, dampness or wind. Four years ago a neurectomy of the supraorbital nerve was performed, after which he enjoyed a period of relief. Within a year of this operation the pains recurred with their former severity, when the second peripheral operation was performed. The latter afforded him relief for about six months; and since that time a third and fourth operation have been performed. Each succeeding operation seemed to afford him relief for a shorter period of time. The administration of large doses of salicylates had beneficial results for a while.

Condition on Admission.—Examination of the thoracic and abdominal organs negative.

Examination of the Head.—The area of tenderness extends on the right side of the head backward from the supraorbital margin a distance of 13 cm., and from the median line a distance of 8 cm. The area of anesthesia is 2 cm. wide anteriorly and 5 cm. wide posteriorly, and its inner margin is 1.5 cm. to the right of the median line.

Examination of the Eye.—Hypermetropia and astigmatism; no coarse changes.

Urine Analysis.—Clear, amber, acid, light flocculent precipitate, specific gravity 1019, urates and mucus, no albumin or sugar.

October 12, 1901. Operation. Division of sensory root of Gasserian ganglion.

October 17, 1901. Examination of patient under this date reveals complete anesthesia over the area corresponding to the distribution of the trifacial nerve (see Fig. 4).

November 2, 1901. Patient was discharged from the

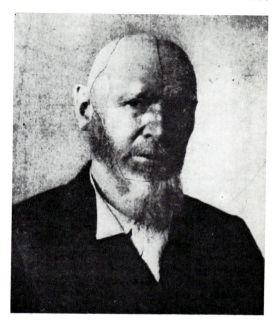

Fig. 4. Showing area of anesthesia one week after division of the sensory root of the trigeminus.

hospital to-day. During the post-operative period nothing occurred worthy of note.

Examination under present date reveals absence of the supraorbital reflex on the affected side. The area of anesthesia extends back from the supraorbital margin 18.5 cm. and 3.5 cm. to the right of the median line at this level. The zygoma has become firmly united. There are no corneal ulcers of the eye of the affected side.

Neurosurgical Classics—42 and 43

SIGNIFICANT medical advancements usually are based on preliminary observations and experiments made by various investigators over a period of many years. Frequently, though, the final steps in the process are not made until the introduction of a key idea or technique. An example of this is the development of the surgical treatment of intracranial arterial aneurysms. Procedures for the treatment of other arterial aneurysms were known for centuries, but because aneurysms of the intracranial arteries were hidden within the skull, these lesions were rarely diagnosed before the introduction of carotid arteriography in 1927. Since then, intracranial aneurysms have been diagnosed frequently, and a variety of operative procedures have been devised for their treatment.

Basic principles in the treatment of arterial aneurysms have been advanced since the time of the ancients. At first, attempts were made to empty or excise the aneurysmal sac after ligation of the artery, but during the Middle Ages conservative therapy by compression became popular. With the introduction of the tourniquet in 1674, treatment by arterial ligation again came into vogue.[28,29]

Arterial ligation for hemostasis was also practiced early in the history of surgery.[19] Exactly when the common carotid artery was first ligated is not clear because of the incomplete medical records of those times. This procedure has been credited to Ambrose Paré and to several surgeons of the late eighteenth and early nineteenth centuries.[18,22,33]

On November 1, 1805, Astley Cooper performed the first ligation of the common carotid artery for an aneurysm of that artery.[5] Hemiplegia developed on the eighth postoperative day and the patient died on the twenty-first day. Cooper's second operation of this type, on June 22, 1808, was successful.[6,7,22,33]

After it had been shown that the common carotid artery could be ligated for hemorrhage or aneurysm, the operation was applied injudiciously in the treatment of a variety of other conditions: epilepsy, exophthalmos, tumors of the head and neck, pain in the head, psychosis, etc.[4,33] The resulting operative mortality rates were so high that surgeons were stimulated to invent devices for the gradual occlusion of the artery.[33] George W. Crile[8] introduced a spring-end screw clamp, and William S. Halsted[16] recommended aluminum bands for this purpose. Rudolph Matas also emphasized the importance of testing and increasing the collateral circulation by the temporary occlusion of the carotid artery before its ligation.[22,24–26,33,34]

The history of man's experience with intracranial aneurysms, like his experience with carotid ligation, can also be traced back at least to the eighteenth century. Although it is difficult to be certain about previous observations, these lesions were definitely encountered at postmortem examination by Francisci Biumi in 1763 and John Hunter in 1792.[3] Surprisingly, aneurysms were not described by Fallopius, Casserius, Vesling, Wepfer, or Willis, whose studies during the sixteenth and seventeenth centuries established the anatomy of the circle of Willis.[3,14,20,27,30] By 1851, about 40 well authenticated cases of cerebral aneurysm had been reported, and in 1861 Jonathan Hutchinson became the first to clinically diagnose a saccular, nontraumatic intracranial aneurysm.[3,21,22]

Despite many later retrospective studies of the signs and symptoms associated with intracranial aneurysms, they were rarely diagnosed during life until the advent of carotid arteriography.[9,12,22,23,26,31,32,35] Surgeons therefore had few encounters with these lesions.

The following four operations are illustrative of the few attempts at surgical correction of intracranial aneurysms prior to 1933. At the turn of the present century, Victor Horsley accidentally found an aneurysm in the middle cranial fossa arising from the right internal carotid artery, and successfully treated it by ligating the common carotid artery in the neck.[17,22,26] In 1924, Wilfred Trotter performed the first planned operation for an intracranial aneurysm diagnosed preoperatively when he ligated the right internal and external carotid arteries for a traumatic aneurysm of the intracranial portion of the internal carotid artery.[2,22] Four years later a saccular aneurysm of the left middle cerebral artery in another patient was correctly diagnosed preoperatively, and treated by Walter Dandy by partial occlusion of the internal carotid artery in the neck.[1,22] Finally, in 1931 the first planned intracranial operation for aneurysm was performed when Norman Dott wrapped muscle around an aneurysm at the bifurcation of the left anterior and middle cerebral arteries.[13,22]

Then in 1933 Dott became the first to operate on an aneurysm previously demonstrated by carotid arteriography. With the use of this diagnostic technique, a new era in the treatment of intracranial aneurysms was initiated.[13,22] Many of the modern intracranial procedures for the correction of these aneurysms were developed during the following five years.

"The first intracranial operation involving the actual excision of an aneurysm was reported by German[15] to the Harvey Cushing Society in 1938. German excised a posterior cerebral aneurysm with recovery.

"The difficulty in ascribing credit to the first person to do a particular procedure is illustrated by the discussion which followed German's report to the Harvey Cushing Society. McKenzie mentioned excising an aneurysm; Wilkins described opening an aneurysm by error; Poppen stated that he preferred to surround an aneurysm with strips of muscle; Lyerly described a case in which he ligated the artery and removed the sac; and Fay related removing an aneurysm under the impression that it was a meningioma."[22]

Two other significant procedures for the treatment of intracranial aneurysms also were developed during those few years. Both can be attributed to Walter Dandy. In 1936 he began to treat aneurysms of the internal carotid artery in or near the cavernous sinus by ligating this artery in the neck and intracranially, thus trapping the aneurysm between the proximal and distal points of ligation.[11,22] Two years later Dandy also introduced the important technique of directly occluding the neck of a saccular aneurysm with a silver clip.[10,22,26]

The publications describing these two procedures mark the end of the period when several new techniques were rapidly introduced for the treatment of intracranial aneurysms. They also mark the beginning of the present comparative evaluation of these techniques in large numbers of patients.

References

1. ALBRIGHT, F. The syndrome produced by aneurysm at or near the junction of the internal carotid artery and the circle of Willis. *Johns Hopk. Hosp. Bull.*, 1929, *44:* 215–245.
2. BIRLEY, J. L. Traumatic aneurysm of the intracranial portion of the internal carotid artery. With a note by Wilfred Trotter. *Brain*, 1928, *51:* 184–208.
3. BULL, J. A short history of intracranial aneurysms. *Lond. clin. med. J.*, 1962, *3:* 47–61.
4. CHEVERS, N. Remarks on the effects of obliteration of the carotid arteries upon the cerebral circulation. *Lond. med. Gaz.*, 1845, n.s. *1:* 1140–1151.
5. COOPER, A. A case of aneurism of the carotid artery. *Med.-chir. Trans.*, 1809, *1:* 1–12.
6. COOPER, A. Second case of carotid aneurism. *Med.-chir. Trans.*, 1809, *1:* 222–233.
7. COOPER, A. Account of the first successful operation, performed on the common carotid artery, for aneurism, in the year 1808: with the post-mortem examination, in 1821. *Guy's Hosp. Rep.*, 1836, *1:* 53–58.
8. CRILE, G. W. An experimental and clinical research into certain problems relating to surgical operations. *Philadelphia: J. B. Lippincott Co.*, 1901, 200 pp.
9. CUSHING, H. Contributions to the clinical study of intracranial aneurysms. *Guy's Hosp. Rep.*, 1923, *73:* 159–163.
10. DANDY, W. E. Intracranial aneurysm of the internal carotid artery. Cured by operation. *Ann. Surg.*, 1938, *107:* 654–659.
11. DANDY, W. E. The treatment of internal carotid aneurysms within the cavernous sinus and the cranial chamber. Report of three cases. *Ann. Surg.*, 1939, *109:* 689–709.
12. DANDY, W. E. Intracranial arterial aneurysms. *Ithaca, N. Y.: Comstock Publishing Co., Inc.*, 1944, viii, 147 pp.
13. DOTT, N. M. Intracranial aneurysms: cerebral

arterio-radiography: surgical treatment. *Edinb. med. J.*, 1933, n.s. *40*: 219–234.

14. FEINDEL, W. Thomas Willis (1621–1675)—the founder of neurology. *Canad. med. Ass. J.*, 1962, *87*: 289–296.

15. GERMAN, W. J. Intracranial aneurysm: a surgical problem. *Zbl. Neurochir.*, 1938, *3*: 352.

16. HALSTED, W. S. Partial, progressive and complete occlusion of the aorta and other large arteries in the dog by means of the metal band. *J. exp. Med.*, 1909, *11*: 373–391.

17. HAMBY, W. B. Intracranial aneurysms. *Springfield, Ill.: Charles C Thomas*, 1952, xxi, 564 pp. (see pp. 45–49).

18. HAMBY, W. B., and WILSON, W. J. The exorcism of a surgical literary ghost. *Surg. Gynec. Obstet.*, 1955, *101*: 772–778.

19. HARVEY, S. C. The history of hemostasis. *New York: P. B. Hoeber, Inc.*, 1929, xv, 128 pp.

20. HIERONS, R., and MEYER, A. Some priority questions arising from Thomas Willis' work on the brain. *Proc. roy. Soc. Med.*, 1962, *55*: 287–292.

21. HUTCHINSON, J. Aneurism of the internal carotid within the skull diagnosed eleven years before the patient's death. Spontaneous cure. *Trans. clin. Soc. Lond.*, 1875, *8*: 127–131.

22. JOHNSON, H. C. Surgery of cerebral vascular anomalies. In: *A history of neurological surgery.* A. E. Walker, Ed. Baltimore: Williams & Wilkins Co., 1951, xii, 583 pp. (see pp. 250–269).

23. McDONALD, C. A., and KORB, M. Intracranial aneurysms. *Arch. Neurol. Psychiat.*, Chicago, 1939, *42*: 298–328.

24. MATAS, R. Testing the efficiency of the collateral circulation as a preliminary to the occlusion of the great surgical arteries. *Ann. Surg.*, 1911, *53*: 1–43.

25. MATAS, R. Testing the efficiency of the collateral circulation as a preliminary to the occlusion of the great surgical arteries. Further observations, with special reference to the author's methods, including a review of other tests thus far suggested. *J. Amer. med. Ass.*, 1914, *63*: 1441–1447.

26. MATAS, R. Aneurysms of the circle of Willis. A discussion of Dr. Dandy's intracranial occlusion of the internal carotid for aneurysms of the circle of Willis, with supplementary remarks. *Ann. Surg.*, 1938, *107*: 660–680.

27. MEYER, A., and HIERONS, R. Observations on the history of the 'Circle of Willis.' *Med. Hist.*, 1962, *6*: 119–1390.

28. DE MOULIN, D. Aneurysms in antiquity. *Arch. chir. neerl.*, 1961, *13*: 49–63.

29. DE MOULIN, D. Some more historical notes on aneurysm. *Arch. chir. neerl.*, 1961, *13*: 277–284.

30. ROLLESTON, H. Thomas Willis. *Med. Life*, 1934, *41*: 177–191.

31. SYMONDS, C. P. Contributions to the clinical study of intracranial aneurysms. *Guy's Hosp. Rep.*, 1923, *73*: 139–158.

32. WALTON, J. N. Subarachnoid haemorrhage. *London: E. & S. Livingstone Ltd.*, 1956, xv, 350 pp. (see pp. 1–6).

33. WATSON, W. L., and SILVERSTONE, S. M. Ligature of the common carotid artery in cancer of the head and neck. *Ann. Surg.*, 1939, *109*: 1–27.

34. WEBSTER, J. E., and GURDJIAN, E. S. Carotid

artery compression as employed both in the past and in the present. *J. Neurosurg.*, 1958, *15*: 372–384.

35. WILKINS, R. H. Neurosurgical classic—XVI. *J. Neurosurg.*, 1964, *21*: 144–156.

INTRACRANIAL ANEURYSMS: CEREBRAL ARTERIO-RADIOGRAPHY: SURGICAL TREATMENT.*†

By NORMAN M. DOTT, F.R.C.S. Ed.

THE subject of aneurysms of the basal cerebral arteries has a long and sustained association with Edinburgh Medicine, with this Society, and with the *Edinburgh Medical Journal*. In 1886 the late Sir Byrom Bramwell[1] gave the first clear description of the clinical features of spontaneous subarachnoid hæmorrhage and its association with rupture of an aneurysm of one of the basal cerebral arteries. He gave this clinical syndrome a place of its own among the various forms of apoplexies or strokes. He made important further contributions to the subject during the next decade. In his earlier years in Edinburgh, from 1911 onwards, Professor Drennan was collecting a series of cases, to which he added later in New Zealand, and produced his important contribution to the clinical and pathological aspects of the subject in 1921.[2] In 1931, the next important clinical advance was made by Professor Edwin Bramwell's paper[3] in which he defines the association of basal cerebral aneurysms with recurrent oculomotor paralysis. Thus the subject has been carried forward in Edinburgh, and I have now the honour to bring before you some further observations, more especially on accurate diagnostic definition by means of arterial radiography, and on some experiences and suggestions as to practical surgical treatment. I have a personal experience of seventeen cases of aneurysms of the basal cerebral arteries, and shall proceed to mention some of them which illustrate matter of interest.

CASE I.—An apparently healthy man (No. 234) of 36 developed quite suddenly, in 1920, an almost complete left oculomotor paralysis. Its sudden onset was accompanied by a sharp pain behind the left eye and some left frontal headache persisted for a few days. In the course of a few weeks the ptosis and external strabismus had gone, but some enlargement of the left pupil remained permanently. He remained perfectly well until ten years later when he had an apoplectic seizure. This struck him while sitting quietly in his office. He suddenly felt "queer in the head," sound seemed to fade away, an intense left frontal pain developed, and the right leg and foot felt temporarily numbed and weak. He was able to walk to his club a few hundred yards away. There he suddenly cried out with extreme pain in his head and

* Read at a Meeting of the Medico-Chirurgical Society of Edinburgh, on 28th June 1933.

† Reprinted from *Edinburgh Medical Journal*, 1933, n.s. *40*: 219–234.

collapsed. He was unconscious, pale, and almost pulse-less for half an hour and then gradually revived. For the next four days he was confused, noisy, and partially aphasic, and he complained of severe headache and pain right down the spine. The temperature was moderately elevated, the neck rigid and retracted, the Kernig sign positive, and the pulse slow and full. During the next week these symptoms improved. A lumbar puncture on the twelfth day after the apoplexy yielded strongly yellow fluid in which some remaining crenated red blood cells and active phagocytosis of blood pigment by endothelial cells were observed. In addition a strongly positive Wassermann reaction was obtained from the cerebrospinal fluid and blood. In a few weeks all symptoms, except the formerly dilated left pupil, had disappeared. Anti-syphilitic treatment was given and the patient continues to enjoy good health, now four years after his apoplectic seizure.

In the light of experience with other similar cases it is easy to reconstruct the events in this one. He had an aneurysm of the left internal carotid or middle cerebral artery near the circle of Willis, in the development of which syphilis may have been a factor. In 1920 there was a slight leakage from the aneurysm which ceased spontaneously, but local effusion from which caused pain and oculomotor paresis. As the clot was absorbed and organised these symptoms subsided. Not until ten years later did the second and more serious leakage occur. As the blood escaped he experienced pain, and as it spread up via the left Sylvian fissure, he recognised numbness and weakness of the right limbs. There was a lull for a few minutes and then a larger effusion occurred causing apoplexy. This was followed by a period in which meningeal irritation combined with cerebral compression were the prominent symptoms, both being due to the presence of the effused blood in the subarachnoid space, and subsiding as this was absorbed. Firm clot had formed around and almost certainly within the aneurysm; this has been partly absorbed and partly organised. He may be spontaneously permanently cured by these processes, and in any event it is unlikely that he will have further trouble from this thrombosed aneurysm for many years. Such, then, is the clinical picture of spontaneous subarachnoid hæmorrhage, and such is the probable prognosis when the event has been survived for some months without further evidence of hæmorrhage.

The next case I wish to refer to illustrates a similar clinical picture, but a different and no less characteristic course of events.

CASE II.—The patient was a married lady (No. 32) of 47. Four years before the fatal illness she had suffered from eclampsia, and during the next two years there were recurrences of raised blood pressure and signs of cardiac overload. However, for the two years preceding her death she had remained well and able for such activities as tennis, and the systolic blood pressure averaged about 150. Sixteen days before her death, after she had

retired to bed, she experienced a sudden severe pain in her head which rapidly radiated to the left frontal region, down the back of her neck and spine and legs. She vomited and felt as if she would die. She was unable to summon assistance and probably lost consciousness for a considerable period. During the next five days, headache, backache and neck stiffness were present, the pulse was slow and the temperature slightly elevated. On the tenth day before death she had another attack, more abrupt and more severe than the former. It occurred at the breakfast-table; she gave a sudden cry of pain, collapsed, and was unconscious for two hours. During this time she was pale and almost pulseless. As she slowly recovered, signs of cerebral compression and of meningeal irritation were again present, and this time a definite degree of right hemiparesis and aphasia suggested that the effused blood was mainly implicating the left cerebral hemisphere. Papilloedema developed. Lumbar puncture at this time yielded fluid under high pressure, yellow from the former hæmorrhage and heavily loaded with fresh blood from the latter one. On the twelfth day there was another similar attack with similar sequelæ. On the sixteenth day a final and rapidly fatal hæmorrhage occurred.

A post-mortem examination was obtained. There was slight cardiac hypertrophy, but the arteries generally, including those of the brain, appeared healthy. There was a large clotted subarachnoid hæmorrhage occupying the basal cisternæ and extending up the left Sylvian fissure. There was blood pigment staining in the minutest sulci over the entire cerebrum and cerebellum, in the leptomenix of the spinal cord and in the sheaths of the optic nerves. The most recent hæmorrhage, being confined by surrounding clot from the previous effusions, had forced its way along the path of the choroidal arteries and ruptured into the temporal horn of the left lateral ventricle, which was filled with recent blood clot. Clot had apparently impacted in the foramen of Monro and had prevented the effusion from extending into the third ventricle. The responsible lesion was found in a ruptured saccular aneurysm arising from the lateral aspect of the junction between the left internal carotid and unusually large posterior communicating arteries. Two smaller and unruptured saccular aneurysms were present, symmetrically situated on the upper aspect of the junction between internal carotid and posterior communicating arteries on each side. The larger ruptured aneurysm was about 5 mm. diameter, pedunculated, with a neck of attachment about 1 mm. The rupture was opposite this attachment, and in the form of a semi-detachment of the fundus of the sac. Around and within the sac was definite ante-mortem clot of considerable standing, and the recent hæmorrhage had pushed its way along one side of this. Elsewhere it was firmly adherent to the internal and external surfaces of the aneurysm. The two smaller aneurysms were sessile and their diameter was about 1–5 mm.

In this case I would emphasise the previous eclampsia, the sudden unprovoked onset of bleeding, the diagnosis from the character of the clinical picture, its confirmation by the finding of blood in the cerebrospinal fluid and the evidence of the approximate site of the aneurysm by the left-sided frontal pain and right hemiparesis and aphasia. It is especially important to note the recurrent attacks at intervals of ten to two days leading up to the fatal result of the fourth attack. The attempt at spontaneous healing by thrombosis is also noteworthy.

A third case (No. 338) illustrates a very similar train of events and I shall describe it in less detail.

CASE III.—The patient was a single lady of 56. She had not previously complained of associated symptoms but her systolic blood pressure was known to be in the neighbourhood of 190. Seventeen days before her death, while speaking at the telephone, she was struck with an intense pain in her head and immediately collapsed. In an hour she recovered and exhibited the characteristic signs of cerebral compression and meningeal irritation. Lumbar puncture three days later showed a spinal fluid pressure of 320 mm. of water, the fluid was yellow and contained crenated red blood cells. Gradually the patient improved, but on the fifteenth day she again suddenly collapsed. Again she m ide a partial recovery, but signs of cerebral compression and œdema were progressive and she died from thi cause two days later. In this case also there was fairly clear evid ·nce from the site of headache, from a degree of hemiparesis, and from cranial nerve involvements that the source of bleeding was to the right of the midline.

A post-mortem examination showed gross generalised arteriosclerosis, with extensive atheromatous disease of the cerebral arteries especially. There was an extensive subarachnoid hæmorrhage, filling every crevice of the subarachnoid spaces over the cerebrum, cerebellum, and in the spinal theca. The greatest mass of clotted blood was in the basal cisterns and in the right Sylvian fissure. The responsible lesion was found in a single small saccular aneurysm arising from the antero-inferior aspect of the junction of the right middle cerebral artery with its first large branch in the base of the right Sylvian fissure. The aneurysm was 1.5 mm. in diameter and was pedunculated in form, being attached to the artery by a neck about 0.5 mm. in diameter. The rupture affected the fundus of the sac which was semi-detached. Within and around the sac was ante-mortem clot of some standing, which was firmly adherent to the sac except along one side where the recent hæmorrhage had detached it.

In this case there was a previous high blood pressure from arterio-sclerosis. The general characters and diagnostic features of the attacks are similar to the preceding case. Again recurrent attacks at short intervals proved rapidly fatal. There was again evidence of an attempt at spontaneous thrombosis within and around the ruptured sac.

From observation of a number of cases with single attacks and spontaneous recovery and return to health, and of a number with recurrent bleedings at intervals of days or weeks which ended fatally, we began to appreciate the sinister significance of a recurrence and the possibility of satisfactory and indefinite survival in its absence. Also from post-mortem observations we saw how a leakage from one of these small aneurysms induces thrombosis within and around the sac, and inferred that if a hæmorrhage or series of hæmor-

rhages is not fatal it is likely to result in a fairly secure healing of the aneurysm by thrombosis and organisation into a solid mass. Thus we decided that if another patient should have recurrent hæmorrhages and there was evidence of the site of the aneurysm we should make some attempt to reinforce Nature's attempt at healing. We were accustomed to deal successfully with quite formidable intracranial hæmorrhages during operations by applying to the bleeding point a fragment of fresh muscle which formed a secure scaffolding for the clot, and became organised into fibrous tissue with it. Why not expose a bleeding aneurysm and deal with it after this fashion? It is surprising how few of these hæmorrhages from aneurysms on the large basal arteries are immediately fatal; the majority give sufficient warning to allow one to formulate a plan of treatment. A majority of these patients, moreover, are comparatively young, and many are perfectly healthy apart from this one small defect on a cerebral artery.

We had not long to wait in order to put these speculations to the test of practice, for, ten days after the death of the last recorded case, another presented, and began to run a similar course.

CASE IV.—The patient was a healthy active man (No. 345) of 53. For several years he had suffered from recurrent left frontal headaches with simultaneous drooping of the left eyelid. These symptoms are recognisable in the light of subsequent events as due to slight recurrent leakage from his basal aneurysm. Then he had a typical attack of spontaneous subarachnoid hæmorrhage with the characteristic sequelæ of meningeal irritation and cerebral compression. Lumbar puncture showed blood in the cerebrospinal fluid. The blood pressure was only 130, and the attack occurred as he re-entered his house after a quiet evening stroll. He was recovering well, when, eight days after this attack, there was a further hæmorrhage. Again he made a good recovery. On the fourteenth day, while at stool, he had a third and more serious hæmorrhage with collapse for some hours, and then recovery with a residual left oculomotor paresis and some degree of aphasia. These signs indicated the site of the aneurysm on the left side of the circle of Willis, and of its effusion of blood up the left Sylvian fissure. From former experiences we felt certain that the illness would end fatally from further bleeding, and decided to operate in the hope of averting this.

Accordingly, on the sixteenth day of illness, after three progressively severe attacks of hæmorrhage, the aneurysm was exposed by operation on 22.4.31. A left frontal approach was employed, and it was a difficult matter to elevate the tense and œdematous brain, and identify the basal structures which were blood-stained and largely embedded in clot. The left optic nerve was found, and the internal carotid artery was defined at its outer side. This vessel was closely followed upwards, outwards and backwards to its bifurcation into the middle and anterior cerebral arteries. As this point was being cleared of tenacious clot, a formidable arterial hæmorrhage filled the wound. With the aid of suction apparatus held close to the bleeding point, we were able to see the aneurysm. It sprang from the upper aspect of the bifurcation junction: it was about 3 mm. in diameter; blood spurted freely from its semi-detached fundus. Meanwhile a colleague was obtaining fresh muscle from the patient's leg. A small fragment of muscle was accurately applied to the bleeding point and held firmly in place so that it checked the bleeding and compressed the thin-walled aneurysmal sac. Thus it was steadily maintained for twelve minutes. As the retaining instrument was then cautiously withdrawn, no further bleeding occurred. The vessel was further cleared and thin strips of muscle were prepared and wound around it until a thick collar of muscle embedded the aneurysm and adjacent arterial trunks. A quantity of clot was removed from the left Sylvian fissure, and a small subtemporal decompression provided to relieve the considerable intracranial tension. It is now over two years since the operation. The patient has so fully recovered that he is able for the responsible legal and social duties on which he was formerly engaged, and he is able to indulge in shooting, mountaineering, etc. His old headaches have quite disappeared, and no trace of oculomotor paresis or aphasia remains. We believe that his aneurysm is tranformed into a solid nodule of fibrous tissue, and that the weak spot at his arterial junction is surrounded by a heavy collar of fibrous tissue organised from the muscle and clot.

The indications for carotid ligation in basal cerebral aneurysm will be considered later, but I should mention here that carotid ligation could not have benefited this man, for his aneurysm was situated on the collateral arterial channel via anterior communicating, anterior cerebral, and middle cerebral vessels, necessary to the adequate blood supply of his left cerebral hemisphere in the event of left carotid ligation. Thus the aneurysm would have remained with an active arterial circulation passing its mouth, and a normal blood pressure acting upon its walls. Nothing but an operation aiming at preserving and patching up the artery could meet the case.

In a second case (No. 562) we were successful in surgical treatment, by employing proximal carotid ligation.

CASE V.—The patient is a healthy woman of 26 years, a hospital nurse. Her systolic blood pressure is about 118. During two years before the more serious illness to be described she had had several attacks of severe left frontal headache with vomiting and elevation of temperature lasting for several days. The attacks are probably ascribable to slight premonitory leakage of blood from her basal cerebral aneurysm. Suddenly, while on duty, and without any particular physical exertion, she experienced pain in the head "as if something had given way." She felt faint and collapsed. She recovered, but was in bed with severe headache for two weeks. Papilloedema was noted at this time, and it persisted in a mild degree until her next attack.

The second major hæmorrhage occurred (rather exceptionally) four months after the first. It took place while she was standing in a shop. She was able to telephone for assistance, but then lost consciousness. She remained thus, pale and apparently dying, with a pulse rate of 50, and with Cheyne-Stokes' breathing for twelve

hours. Then she began to revive, and improved during the next four days. There was a left oculomotor paralysis, intense headaches, and gross papilloedema with unusually massive subretinal hæmorrhages. It now appeared likely that she would recover from the attack, but it was apparent that unless intracranial pressure were relieved, she would become blind. We decided to carry out a decompressive operation so that if she recovered she might retain some vision.

Accordingly, on the fifth day after the hæmorrhage, bilateral subtemporal decompression was carried out under local anæsthesia. On the left side I was surprised by encountering a large subdural clot. It was removed with marked relief of pressure. The pia arachnoid was quite free of blood. Evidently then the hæmorrhage had occurred into the subdural space, and not as usual into the subarachnoid space. It was inferred that the point of bleeding must be situated on the left internal carotid artery between the point where it penetrates the dura and the place of its entering within the subarachnoid space. This is just where the artery bends back under the optic nerve and gives off its ophthalmic branch. This aneurysm then was situated proximal to the anastomosing circle of Willis. Proximal ligation of the internal carotid artery in the neck would leave the carotid stagnant from the point of ligature up to the circle of Willis, and would almost certainly induce thrombosis in this segment of the vessel.

The decompression gave relief, but on the sixteenth day of the illness there was a sudden recurrence of headache, and the decompressions bulged ominously. Clearly there was further bleeding in progress. Accordingly, the left internal carotid artery was tied in the neck. The evidences of hæmorrhage subsided. On the third day after ligation there was a transient motor aphasia, which clearly indicated that a small embolus had lodged in one of the anterior branches of the left middle cerebral artery. The intravascular clot which furnished the embolus must have extended upwards at least to the junction of the posterior communicating artery. Thus we inferred that the part of the carotid artery carrying the aneurysm had become thrombosed, and that the dependent aneurysm must also be thrombosed and permanently cured. Fortunately, vision recovered unexpectedly well, and the patient is able to continue her work as a hospital nurse.

The point in this case is that by the unexpected discovery of a subdural clot we were able to infer the exact site of the aneurysm. The site was suitable for treatment by proximal ligation, and this treatment was apparently successful.

I would now refer to two cases in which the aneurysms simulated intracranial tumour.

CASE VI.—The first concerned a man (No. 181) of 58 years, who exhibited a marked degree of arteriosclerosis and a systolic blood pressure of 180. He complained of bad vision and headaches. He had a right homonymous upper quadrantic hemianopia, which was incongruous, and indicated a lesion at the junction of the left optic tract with the chiasm. He had a grossly enlarged sella turcica and evidence of long-standing hypopituitarism. The natural assumption was a tumour of the pituitary neighbourhood. At operation the optic nerves and chiasm appeared normal, and the large sella was empty except for cerebrospinal fluid. No tumour was found. The operative exploration did neither harm nor good, and the cause of his symptoms remained a mystery until his death eighteen months later. There had been no change in his symptoms, and he died from multiple cerebral softenings due to his arterial disease. At post mortem the cause of his chiasmal and pituitary symptoms was found in an aneurysm arising from the under surface of the junction of the right anterior cerebral artery with the anterior communicating artery. This aneurysm had undergone spontaneous thrombosis, fibrosis, and cure. It was a solid nodule of fibrous tissue about 5 mm. diameter. Evidently when filled with fluid blood it had been large enough to cause the symptoms of tumour described. There was no evidence that the aneurysm had ever become ruptured.

This case shows, then, that a basal aneurysm large enough to cause tumour symptoms may become spontaneously obliterated, and permanently healed. The cause of spontaneous thrombosis in this case was, no doubt, intimal degeneration of the sac wall from arteriosclerosis.

CASE VII.—The second tumour-like aneurysm I wish to refer to from the point of view of diagnosis and treatment. She was a married woman (No. 484), of 36 years, and was evidently a case of tumour in the pituitary neighbourhood. The left eye was blind from compression of its nerve, and the right visual field indicated that the optic chiasm was becoming involved at its junction with the left nerve. X-ray showed a shallow, wide depression in the bone between the two anterior clinoid processes. At operation a tumour was found underlying the left optic nerve, and presenting in the interval between the two nerves. Its bluish colour, even, rounded contour, and tense consistence, made us suspect aneurysm, and this was verified by aspirating arterial blood from it with a very fine needle. No direct treatment was attempted. We had in mind to tie the left internal carotid in the neck, but anticipated no harm from leaving this over for a few days. After an excellent primary recovery, this patient died suddenly twenty hours after operation from rupture of the sac. Evidently the removal of surrounding support occasioned by opening the skull had allowed this large sac to expand and burst.

In this case I wish to point out that although we could locate the swelling by perimetry and X-ray, we had no means of knowing that it was an aneurysm. Further, after learning at operation that it was an aneurysm suitable for treatment by proximal ligation, we made the error of not carrying this measure into effect at once, with disastrous consequences. I have no doubt that had the ligation been carried out immediately the rupture would not have occurred.

Arterial radiography has now come to our aid. By this means an intracranial aneurysm can be seen, together with the cerebral arteries, perfectly outlined on the X-ray film. Its size, connections, and relations can be seen as clearly as if it were exposed. Our earliest attempts at cerebral arterial radiography were made in 1927, when we used

sodium iodide as the opaque medium. More recently we have employed "Thorotrast"—a colloidal suspension of thorium dioxide. It seems to be quite harmless when injected into the internal carotid artery, and it gives very clear definition of the cerebral arteries. By this means any deviations of the vessels occasioned by distortion from adjacent tumours can be seen, and any vascular anomaly such as aneurysm or arterial angioma is clearly depicted. This method, then, has put into our hands a means of defining whether a basal intracranial tumour is an aneurysm or some other swelling. Similarly, in a case of suspected aneurysm giving signs of spontaneous subarachnoid hæmorrhage, an aneurysm may be detected and accurately located, and treatment planned accordingly. My next case exemplifies this eventuality.

CASE VIII.—The patient is a young married woman (No. 635) of 23 years. Her average systolic blood pressure is about 112. She had previously enjoyed good health. Five weeks prior to admission to hospital she had struck the vertex of her head forcibly against the mantelshelf in raising herself from bending over the fire. She experienced no immediate inconvenience beyond the pain of the blow, but an hour later she developed a severe left frontal headache, and she vomited. The headache gradually subsided in a period of about three weeks, and just about this time she developed a left oculomotor paralysis—external squint, ptosis and dilated pupil. The paralysis was at first incomplete, but increased progressively. At this time we saw her, and suspected an aneurysm of the intracranial portion of the left internal carotid artery. As the oculomotor paralysis continued to increase we suspected either that the aneurysmal sac was rapidly enlarging or that it was leaking and clot was accumulating around it progressively. In either event a serious rupture was an imminent danger, and if we could only determine its exact site, this might be averted by proximal ligation or muscle wrapping. We, therefore, made an arterial radiogram of the left internal carotid artery, and its branches. This showed a round aneurysmal sac, about 7 mm. in diameter, attached by a narrow neck to the inferior aspect of the junction of the left internal carotid artery with its posterior communicating branch. From this point the aneurysm projected in a backward and downward direction. It certainly was not large enough to press injuriously on the oculomotor nerve by its own volume, and the symptoms must, therefore, have been due to accumulating clot from progressive leakage of blood. With knowledge of this alarming state of affairs and of the site of the aneurysm just proximal to the circle of Willis, proximal ligation was decided on, and the left internal carotid artery was tied in the neck forthwith. The patient made an excellent recovery, and soon returned to her home. The oculomotor paresis gradually recovered. The treatment was carried out on 24th March 1933, and the patient remains entirely well to the date of writing.

It will be observed from the foregoing remarks that intracranial aneurysms may present three different clinical aspects. There are the ocular paretic type, the apoplectic type, and the tumour-like type. The ocular paretic varieties are usually characterised by an incomplete oculomotor paresis accompanied by homolateral frontal headache, and are due to small effusions of blood by limited leakage from an aneurysm near the circle of Willis. The apoplectic type is characterised by a more or less sudden "stroke"—with partial or complete loss of consciousness for a period, and subsequent signs of cerebral compression and meningeal irritation, with or without cranial nerve palsies and focal cerebral signs. These symptoms are provoked by a more extensive effusion of blood into the subarachnoid space or cerebral substance or both. There is blood in the cerebrospinal fluid obtained from lumbar puncture. The tumour-like variety is characterised by signs of compression of adjacent structures. The optic nerves and chiasm, the clinoid processes and adjacent bone are commonly involved.

In differential diagnosis the ocular paretic type offers little difficulty for the oculomotor nerve is not involved just in this way and with associated headache by any other disease process. Carcinomatous invasions of the base of the skull from the nasopharynx may simulate, but they involve the abducent before the oculomotor nerve. In the apoplectic cases the mode of onset and symptoms during recovery, and the fact that the patient is usually young and healthy, will serve to differentiate from cerebral thrombosis, intracerebral hæmorrhage and meningitis. The diagnosis is confirmed by finding gross blood in the fluid from lumbar puncture. An accurate localising diagnosis in both these types may be made from arterial radiography. In the tumour-like aneurysms the clinical diagnosis cannot be carried beyond the inference of a progressive swelling in a certain situation. In such a case the diagnosis that the swelling is an aneurysm can be made only by operative exploration or by arterial radiography. We have been employing arterial radiography in the diagnosis of doubtful tumours about the cerebral base, and, in addition to defining aneurysms, we have been able to gain information concerning tumours of other kinds by their effects in distorting the adjacent cerebral arteries.

The etiology of saccular aneurysms of or near the circle of Willis has been the subject of much speculation and dispute. There exists reliable evidence to show that aneurysms may develop here as elsewhere in consequence of infective emboli or by reason of adjacent pyogenic, tuberculous, or syphilitic inflammatory processes. These are instances of local disease damaging a presumably healthy vessel wall. They are rare eventualities. Aneurysms of the basal cerebral arteries, on the contrary, are relatively common. An average quotation of their incidence from available literature is about one in seven hundred consecutive post-mortem examinations, and in many instances the lesion has been symptomless and is not connected with the cause of death. They are much commoner in the absence of arteriosclerosis and of syphilis than in their presence. The average age for rupture of these aneurysms is about thirty-two years; instances of rupture at six and nine years of age are on record. It is evident enough that the primary factors both in formation and in rupture of an aneurysm are the pressure of the blood and a local weakness of the vessel wall.

Recent researches, and especially those of Forbus,[4] furnish us with an adequate explanation of the factor of local defect of the vessel wall. In the development of arteries the larger trunks acquire a muscular coat, while their smaller branches remain for a time as simple endothelial tubes. Later the branches acquire muscular coats, not as outgrowths from those of the larger trunks, but as independent developments. At the line of junction of branch with trunk the new and the old muscle coats meet and become fused, but the joint or fusion may be imperfect. In apparently normal arteries small developmental gaps are demonstrable along these lines. They constitute quite definite weak points of developmental origin in the vessel walls. In this connection it is significant that all the saccular aneurysms under discussion are found to arise along the line of juncture of arteries with their branches and never from the arterial walls between junctures. Cases are on record in which the "plumbing" of arterial joints has been generally effective, and in which small aneurysms were present at arterial junctions in many parts of the body. This is, however, quite rare; it is the basal cerebral arteries in particular which are affected with considerable frequency. Much remains to be learned about the cerebral arteries and their circulation, but it is true that they are peculiarly thin-walled, and that they are specially protected from the force of the pulse by obviously designed flexures or "baffles" on the main vertebral and carotid trunks just as they enter the skull. Why they are thin-walled and specially protected we do not know but only that they are so. Being much thinner in their walls than arteries elsewhere in the body, it is easy to understand why the developmental junction defects in the muscle coats should more readily give way in the cerebral arteries while they remain insignificant on the thicker-walled arteries elsewhere.

Lastly we come to the factor of the pressure of the blood in blowing out the arterial wall through such a defect to form a saccular aneurysm. It is evident from the clinical cases that this may be caused by a normal blood pressure, as in the cases occurring in children, and in most of the younger and some of the older adult subjects. There is, however, no doubt that an abnormally high arterial blood pressure may cause an arterial junction to give way which would have remained intact under a normal pressure. This is evidenced by the definite association of basal cerebral aneurysm with stenosis of the isthmus of the aortic arch. In such a case (No. 619) I have observed a blood pressure of 190 in the right arm and associated carotid arteries, while in the left arm and leg receiving blood distal to the stenosis it was 120. This man had had several attacks of sudden collapse associated with temporary oculomotor paralysis, headache, and neck rigidity, which left no doubt of the presence of an aneurysm on or close to the intracranial portion of his left internal carotid artery. The association is sufficiently frequent to make it clear that the abnormally high pressure thrown on the cerebral arteries by the stenosis is the essential cause of the formation of aneurysms in these cases.[5] In case No. 32, quoted above, who can doubt that it was the raised blood pressure of eclampsia which caused her multiple aneurysms to bulge through junctions which would have withstood normal pressures? Again in case No. 345 the third attack of bleeding was obviously precipitated by the rise in arterial pressure due to straining at stool.

It seems clear, then, that there is a developmental basis of weakness in the arterial walls at their junctions, and that this is accentuated in the thin-walled cerebral arteries. The developmental gap in the muscle coat may amount to a developmental defect or anomaly in such a degree that the vessel gives way, and an aneurysm forms under normal arterial blood pressure. In severe defects an aneurysm may form and burst even in childhood. In lesser defects the event may be delayed even until old age. On the other hand the arterial junctions may be normal, and capable of withstanding normal blood pressure, yet they remain the weak points in the vessel wall, containing minute gaps in the muscle coat which will give way and form aneurysms under conditions associated with abnormally high pressures in the cerebral arteries.

The commonest site of saccular aneurysmal formation is in relation to the termination of the internal carotid artery on one or other side. There is a preponderance in favour of the left side. These aneurysms are always at arterial junctions, and the junctions at the posterior communicating branch, the bifurcation into middle and anterior cerebral arteries, and the points of origin of the first considerable branch from the middle cerebral artery in the base of the Sylvian fissure are sites of election. These aneurysms are apt to manifest themselves by minor or major effusions of blood rather than as tumours, and are associated with recurrent ophthalmoplegia and with spontaneous gross subarachnoid hæmorrhage. The aneurysms arising from the junctions at the origin of the ophthalmic branch from the internal carotid artery and at the joining of anterior cerebral and anterior communicating arteries are rather less frequent in incidence and tend to manifest themselves as tumefactions rather than by the occurrence of bleeding from them. Of still lesser frequence are aneurysms arising at the junctions of vertebral and basilar arteries and at the bifurcation of the basilar into the posterior cerebral arteries. Aneurysms can occur at any arterial junction of the larger cerebral and cerebellar arteries.

In the practical treatment of these lesions a conservative line may be adopted, or proximal ligation of a carotid artery, or application of muscle fragments directly to the aneurysm. Each method has its indications. In the event of a minor hæmorrhage with associated ophthalmoplegia and headache, or of a major subarachnoid hæmorrhage, the presence of an aneurysm as its cause should be verified and the exact site of the aneurysm identified by arterial radiography on the internal carotid artery. If the aneurysm is found to be proximal to the circle of Willis (i.e., the posterior communicating branch), proximal ligation of the internal carotid artery in the neck should be practised. The procedure is not without risk of cerebral complications, but the advantage of diminishing the pressure on the aneurysm outweighs these risks. Similarly, in the event of an aneurysm being defined in this situation by radiography or operative exploration in cases exhibiting a basal tumour syndrome, proximal ligation should be employed. In the cases of operative exploration the ligation should follow immediately in order to minimise the danger of rupture.

If in a case of minor or major hæmorrhage from an aneurysm, the aneurysm is defined by clinical facts or arterial radiography as distal to or actually on the circle of Willis, I should advise conservative treatment in the first instance. Proximal ligation is obviously no use in such cases by reason of the relation of the anastomotic blood supply to the aneurysm. The only alternative to conservative treatment is direct operative exposure and application of muscle, which is necessarily a hazardous and difficult procedure. Experience teaches us that a considerable proportion of first bleedings settle down and remain quiescent for many years and perhaps permanently. It is felt that the patient's interests will be served best by relying on those chances of spontaneous healing rather than undergoing the risks incidental to direct operative exposure in the first instance. In the event of a repetition of bleeding, however, especially at an interval of a few days or weeks, the prognosis becomes extremely grave, the probability of spontaneous healing extremely low, and the risks of direct operation are then justified. At operation there is no question of ligation of a main arterial trunk distal to the circle of Willis.

The functional loss from this would be far too severe. The aim is to form a secure scaffolding for clot and fibrosis around the aneurysm by application of fragments of muscle, while the artery remains patent and intact.

In the case of an aneurysm giving a tumour syndrome and found to be distal to the circle of Willis, conservative measures should be adopted unless repeated hæmorrhages occur.

Conservative treatment by rest and morphia in the earlier days following a single subarachnoid hæmorrhage may be supplemented by lumbar puncture. I do not think that this is likely to promote further bleeding if the fluid is removed slowly, and so as not to reduce pressure below normal. By this means considerable quantities of irritating blood may be removed, and the symptoms of cerebral compression and meningeal irritation thereby relieved, and convalescence shortened. After recovery such patients should be warned against such activities as are likely to raise arterial blood pressure considerably, but with this reservation that they should be encouraged to live normal and active lives. No doubt they carry a potential source of danger in their heads, but, after all, any one of us may have such a latent lesion.

References.—[1] Bramwell, B., "Spontaneous Meningeal Hæmorrhage," *Edin. Med. Journ.*, 1886, vol. xxxii., p. 101. [2] Drennan, A. M., "Aneurysms of the Larger Cerebral Vessels," *New Zealand Med. Journ.*, 1921. [3] Bramwell, E., "A Case of Leaking Aneurysm of the Circle of Willis, and Two Cases of Recurrent Oculomotor Paralysis—a Clinical Comparison," *Edin. Med. Journ.*, 1931, vol. xxxviii., pp. 689–95. [4] Forbus, W. D., "On the Origin of Miliary Aneurysms of the Superficial Cerebral Arteries," *Bull. Johns Hopkins Hosp.*, 1930, vol. xlvii., pp. 239–84. [5] Woltman, H. W., and Shelden, W. D., "Neurologic Complications associated with Congenital Stenosis of the Isthmus of the Aorta," *Archiv. Neurol. and Psychiat.*, 1927, vol. xvii, pp. 303–16.

INTRACRANIAL ANEURYSM OF THE INTERNAL CAROTID ARTERY

CURED BY OPERATION*

Walter E. Dandy, M.D.

Baltimore, Md.

Case Report.—A rather frail, small, sallow man, age 43, applied at the Johns Hopkins Dispensary February 16, 1937, because of complete paralysis in the distribution of the right oculomotor (third) nerve. The family history was negative. His general health was good until last year when his stomach "went bad" from drinking. He was hospitalized from July to September, 1936, for

* Reprinted from *Annals of Surgery*, 1938, *107*: 654–659 with the kind permission of the Chairman of the Editorial and Advisory Board.

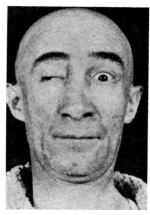

Fig. 1.—Photograph of patient taken before operation. Note the ptosis on the right, and the extreme pull of the eyeball outward due to paralysis of the 3rd nerve.

this gastric disorder which was pronounced "ulcer." He has been a very heavy drinker for the past 18 months.

Present History.—Six days ago he was awakened by a severe pain in the right frontal region. During the afternoon there was a very severe shooting pain in the right eye, but it lasted only a moment. He slept poorly that night because of the pain. On the following morning diplopia was first noted and in the evening the right eyelid drooped. The eye was completely closed the next morning. The pain became less severe but two days later became greatly intensified and prevented his sleeping. Since then the pain has been present but less severe. Examination at that time showed a complete paralysis of the right, third cranial nerve (Fig. 1). There were no other positive findings. The eyegrounds, visual fields and reflexes were normal. A diagnosis of aneurysm along the circle of Willis was made. A roentgenologic examination of the head revealed no abnormality. The patient returned to the dispensary from time to time until March 19, 1937—nearly five weeks after the onset of his trouble—when Dr. Frank Ford referred him to me with the thought that a surgical effort might be worth while. There had been no improvement in the local condition in the interim.

The following findings were reported by Dr. Frank Walsh, of the Ophthalmological Department, March 12, 1937;

"The upper lid is completely closed and can only be moved slightly by the frontalis muscle (Fig. 1). The globe is abducted to 45° and only moves laterally and slightly down when it rotates inward (Fig. 1). The pupil is $4\frac{1}{2}$ Mm. in diameter and one-fourth larger than the left. It reacts slightly to light, directly and consensually. Visual acuity 20/40 right and 20/25 left. Visual fields normal. Fourth and sixth nerves are functioning." The Wassermann reaction was negative.

Operation.—March 23, 1937: A small hypophyseal approach was made on the right side, using the concealed incision. There was marked cortical atrophy, evidenced by the pools of fluid in the subarachnoid spaces (doubtless the result of his heavy drinking). The removal of this fluid and that from the cisterna chiasmatis gave ample room for exposure of the chiasmal re-

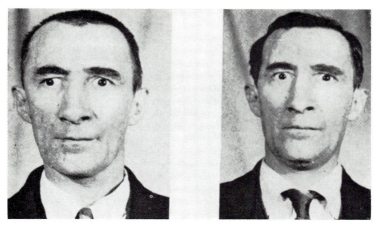

Fig. 2.—Photograph of patient taken 13 days after the operation, showing almost complete disappearance of the ptosis, and improvement in the abduction of the eyeball.

Fig. 3.—Photograph of patient taken seven months after the operation, showing complete return of all functions referable to the 3rd nerve.

gion upon retraction of the frontal and temporal lobes. A pea-sized aneurysm projected from the outer wall of the internal carotid artery and adjacent to the entry of the posterior communicating artery (Fig. 4). The aneurysm, however, did not involve this vessel, but arose from the internal carotid by a narrow neck beyond which it expanded to the size of a pea; therefore, it was quite a small aneurysm. Laterally it bridged the adjacent cerebral space and firmly attached itself to the free border of the dura which projects mesially from the middle cranial fossa; it spread out beneath the dura forming quite a broad attachment. At this site the covering of the aneurysm changed from the normal grayish-white, shiny covering, similar to that of the carotid artery, to a deep red color. Moreover, the surface was irregular, three or four tiny nodules projecting along the margin of the cavernous sinus. This change represented the false aneurysmal sac resulting from rupture of the aneurysmal sac. The third nerve passed obliquely backward in its normal course and was attached to the aneurysm at only one point—where it entered the cavernous sinus. Since it was quite evident that the red color of the aneurysmal wall indicated a reduction in its thickness, no attempt was made to dissect the attachment to the wall of the cavernous sinus. There was no evidence of subarachnoid bleeding; doubtless the growth into the wall of the cavernous sinus prevented this. Forceps placed upon the thick aneurysmal wall pulsated forcibly.

The small neck of the aneurysm afforded an easy surgical attack. An ordinary flat silver clip was placed over the neck of the sac and tightly compressed, obliterating it completely (Fig. 4). The clip was flush with the wall of the carotid artery (Figs. 5 and 6). The sac, lateral to the silver clip, was then picked up with the forceps and thrombosed by the electrocautery. It shriveled to a thin shred of tissue. It is worthy of note that the aneurysm became much softer after the silver clip had been applied; it also ceased to pulsate.

Postoperative Course.—Aside from an attack of delirium tremens which lasted three days, patient made an uneventful recovery and left the hospital April 5, 1937—two weeks after the operation. At that time there was a definite improvement in the function of the extra-ocular muscles (Fig. 2).

On April 8, 1937 (three days later), Doctor Walsh reports: (1) Improvement in the ptosis; (2) slight upward movement; and (3) the lateral movements of the eyeball are close to normal. The pupillary reaction is still a little less than the left. Seven months later there was complete return of all functions referable to the third nerve (Fig. 3).

Perhaps ten years ago I saw, with Dr. Fuller Albright, an aneurysm situated in a somewhat similar position, localized because of the paralysis of the third nerve and pain in the eye. An attempt was made to cure it by ligation of the internal carotid artery in the neck, but the patient died of cerebral softening as a result, probably from an extending thrombus. Such an indirect attack surely had little chance of curing the aneurysm but there then seemed no other rational effort indicated. The present case is a sequel to this unsuccessful attempt. The precise point of origin of this aneurysm could not be predetermined; it might have arisen from the carotid or the posterior communicating artery; the latter was our impression at the time of operation. If it had arisen from the posterior communicating artery it was hoped that a silver clip could be placed upon the artery on each side of the aneurysm if there was not a satisfactory neck by which the aneurysm could be attached directly.

A number of publications have appeared in recent years indicating that aneurysms of the circle of Willis are quite common. It is from them that most of the subarachnoid hemorrhages arise. Unfortunately, in most instances there are no localizing signs by which the position of the aneurysm or, indeed, the size of the aneurysm can be estimated. Those with paralysis of the third

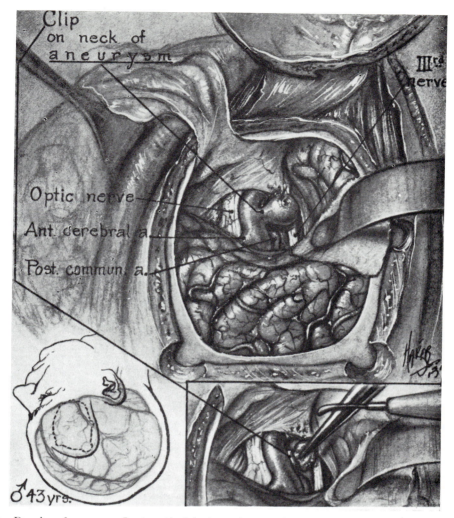

Clip on neck of aneurysm

IIIrd nerve

Optic nerve

Ant. cerebral a.

Post. commun. a.

♂ 43 yrs.

Fig. 4.—Drawing of aneurysm. Inset on the left shows the operative approach with the author's concealed incision. Inset on the right shows clip placed on the neck of the aneurysm and the cautery shrivelling the sac.

nerve, as in our case, are exceptional. Sands[4] makes the statement that 47 per cent of those along the posterior communicating artery produce signs referable to the third nerve. Certainly those with palsies of the third nerve may be given the chance of surgical cure. On the other hand, there is no assurance that the aneurysm after its disclosure may be amenable to surgical attack—the aneurysm may be too large, or it may be placed too far posteriorly on the posterior communicating artery. Under the latter condition perhaps a single clip anterior to the aneurysm might be effective; or the aneurysm, if arising from the carotid, may be less favored by a narrow neck by which it can be isolated and cured by the application of a silver clip. The present effort is but a beginning or a suggestion that an aneurysm at the

circle of Willis is not entirely hopeless. A word may be added concerning the cauterization of the aneurysm by which it is shriveled to a small shred. The silver clip, of course, added the same sense of security against an extending thrombus, which, I should think, would be quite likely if the cautery were used alone, but perhaps no more probable than by a spontaneous thrombosis, which may conceivably occur. At least I should be fearful of such an outcome without the intervening clip to prevent its spread. Should the outlook be hopeless one would, of course, be justified in this attempt, and it is not inconceivable that even then a cure might result from thrombosis of the aneurysm without extension into the main arterial trunk.

In general, the indications for operation on aneurysms at the circle of Willis and causing only

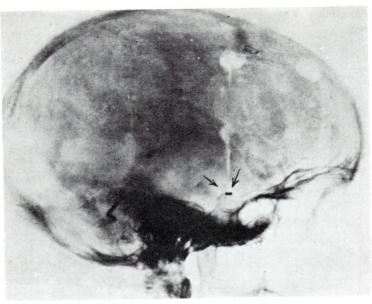

Fig. 5.—Roentgenogram showing the silver clip at the sella turcica.
It also shows the size and position of the bone flap.

subarachnoid hemorrhage, are none too clear. Certainly without a knowledge of the side of the circle of Willis upon which the aneurysm is located there would be no justification in exploring either side in search of the lesion. When a patient has had a subdural hemorrhage and has recovered, one is loath to suggest an operation, which certainly would be classed as hazardous, because another hemorrhage may never occur; at least many go for years with no further trouble, although this is not the usual story. During a subarachnoid

hemorrhage and the immediate period thereafter one would not dare operate because the intracranial room needed for operation would be occupied by blood—and one needs all the room obtainable for the operation. For cases with a third nerve palsy the indications are clear enough. And where subarachnoid hemorrhages are recurring and the eventual outlook seems hopeless I should feel inclined to advise operative attack if there is even a suggestion that the aneurysm may be on one side. Arteriography may here become an

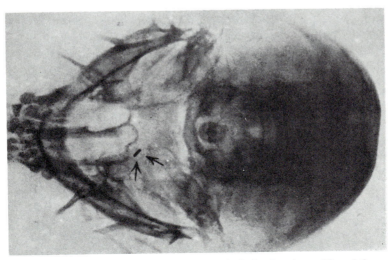

Fig. 6.—Roentgenogram of the base of the skull showing the position of the
silver clip placed upon the neck of the aneurysm.

important means of locating one of these aneurysms around the circle of Willis. Then, too, the frequency of multiple aneurysms, and under such circumstances the difficulty of locating the one that is at fault, make the problem of therapy an even more difficult one.

So far as I know, this is the first attempt to cure an aneurysm at the circle of Willis by direct attack upon the aneurysm.

REFERENCES

[1] Albright, Fuller: The Syndrome Produced by Aneurysm at or Near the Junction of the Internal Carotid Artery and the Circle of Willis. Johns Hopkins Hosp. Bull., **44**, 215, 1929.

[2] Dandy, Walter E.: Carotid-Cavernous Aneurysm (Pulsating Exophthalmos). Zentralbl. f. Neurochir., **2**, 77, 1937. Also ANNALS OF SURGERY, **102**, 916, 1935.

[3] Forbus, Von Wiley D.: Ueber den Ursprung gewisser Aneurysmen der basalen Hirnarterien. Centralbl. f. Allgemeine Pathologie und Pathologische Anatomie, **44**, 243, 1928–1929.

[4] Sands, I. J.: Aneurysms of Cerebral Vessels. Arch. Neurol. and Psychiat., **21**, 37, 1929.

[5] Symonds, C. P.: Contributions to the Clinical Study of Intracranial Aneurysms. Guy's Hosp. Rep., **73**, 39, 1923.

Neurosurgical Classic—44

PSYCHOSURGERY is essentially a contribution from the twentieth century. Although trephining for mental disturbance was performed for hundreds of years, serious efforts to understand the physical basis of behavior and to improve mental illnesses by surgery have been limited to relatively recent times.[19]

The controversy which raged during the nineteenth century about the cerebral representation of speech initiated an acute interest in patients with lesions of the frontal lobe.[43] Certain of these patients, however, were found to have changes in their behavior rather than in their speech. One such patient was Phineas P. Gage.[35] He sustained one of the most remarkable injuries in the history of medicine. In 1848, an iron tamping bar, 43 inches in length and $1\frac{1}{4}$ inches in diameter, was accidentally blown through the left frontal portion of his brain. Gage surprisingly recovered from his injury, but he suffered a marked change in personality. Before his injury he had been intelligent, honest, reliable and shrewd. However, from the time of his accident until his death 12 years later, Gage showed defective judgment, irreverent behavior, capriciousness, and lack of consideration for his fellows.[35]

Toward the end of the nineteenth century, when cerebral ablations were being performed in animals to prove or disprove the concept of cerebral localization,[41,44] changes in behavior were again noticed following injury to the frontal lobes.[40] Hitzig, Horsley and Schäfer, Ferrier, and Goltz all agreed that ablation of portions of the cortex anterior to the excitable motor area in the dog, cat, and monkey was frequently followed by definite behavioral changes.[40]

In 1891, G. Burckhardt, the superintendent of a mental hospital in Switzerland, reported the first operations on the brain designed to change mental functions.[4,26] He

" . . . argued that a mental disturbance could be relieved by removal of that portion of the brain which normally carried out the specific function involved. Thus, he believed that auditory hallucinations might be abolished by removing the cortical representation of audition, namely, the temporal cortex. He operated upon 6 patients, removing in several stages cortex from the postcentral, temporal, and frontal regions on the left side. His patients were benefited. One was said to be recovered, although she died about a month after the operation under suspicious circumstances, which suggested suicide. Another was less disturbed, less violent, and more amenable to supervision, although his dementia was unchanged. He did not seem to have so many hallucinations nor to react so violently to them as formerly. Burckhardt emphasized that his purpose was not so much to cure the patient as to change him from a dangerous, sick person to a harmless one. This pioneering work was laid in barren soil and remained buried beneath the accumulating earth of medical literature until recent archival research uncovered it.

"Puusepp[31] made the next attempt to solve the problem in 1910, but with so little success that he did not publish a report until the advent of prefrontal lobotomy. He transected the fibers between the parietal and frontal lobes unilaterally in 3 cases of mental disorder. These early attempts lacked the benefit of the exact neurophysiological studies of the functions of the frontal lobe, which were to be done in the next few decades."[39]

Because of the advances in neurosurgery between 1910 and 1935, patients with lesions in the frontal lobes began to survive for longer periods of time. The careful clinical analysis of these patients, combined with more sophisticated animal experiments, resulted in the gradual elucidation of the functions of the frontal lobes. The entire problem was of such fundamental importance that many of the world's foremost neurologists, neurophysiologists, and neurosurgeons became involved. Basic studies were performed by Vogt and Vogt, Foerster, Franz, Lashley, Bianchi, Penfield, Fulton, Jacobsen, Kennard, Bucy, German, Spurling, Brickner, and many others.[3,24,28,37]

At the Second International Neurological Congress in London in 1935, attention was given to this important problem. Brickner[1,2] gave a detailed account of the behavior of a patient whose frontal lobes had been removed by Dandy, and Fulton[5] and Jacobsen[25] described the changes in behavior which had occurred in two chimpanzees—"Becky" and "Lucy"—after bilateral ablation of their frontal association areas. Egas Moniz, a Portuguese neurologist who had come to the Congress to report on his own outstanding studies with carotid arteriography,[10,42] was especially impressed by the ideas presented at this symposium.[19,24,34]

" . . . He considered that certain mental states which appear to have no anatomical substrata were the result of a lack of the normal flux of psychic processes due to an inflexibility of certain neuronal relationships. He argued that if these could be altered or broken, the conduct of the individual would become normal, being no longer hampered by the fixed neural patterns. Since lesions of the frontal lobe modified behavior, he thought the abnormal neural fixation was probably in the connections of the prefrontal cortex. . . . "[39]

" . . . Egas Moniz returned to Lisbon with a plan of work which he placed in the clever hands of his neurosurgeon, Almeida Lima, who had returned to Portugal after his training in the London Hospital under the direction of Cairns. They initiated, on November 12 of that same year, a line of investigation that later became doctrine. In this way psychosurgery, already foreseen by Burckhardt, was born."[30]

Prudently, Egas Moniz also asked for the collaboration of two psychiatrists, Sobral Cid and Barahona Fernandez, and a clinician with neurologic experience, Caucela de Abreu.[30]

" . . . Moniz and the neurosurgeon Lima first tried injection of alcohol into the frontal association areas and later invented a leukotome, a trocar-like instrument from the end of which a wire loop or a cutting edge could be protruded. Rotation of this loop within the frontal lobes cut cores in the white matter. Moniz made a superior approach on either side, 3.0 cm. from the midline, and 1.5 cm. anterior to a vertical line passing through the base of the tragus. He advised cutting four to six cores in each frontal lobe located at various subcortical levels. . . . "[26]

" . . . His first statistical report, based upon his experience with 20 patients, presented the following results: 'None dead; none became worse after the operation.' The overall results were: 35 per cent were clinically cured; 35 per cent showed improvement; and in 30 per cent there were no results[11]. . . . "[30]

"In France, Germany, and England, where psychoanalysis and shock therapy were becoming fashionable, the procedure was practically ignored, but in Italy[6,32,38] it was enthusiastically received. In America, Freeman and Watts[21] introduced the operation and, in spite of emotional[8,29] and rational criticism, persisted in its practice until prefrontal lobotomy became recognized as a therapeutic method in psychiatric cases.[7,9,20]"[39]

Egas Moniz and Almeida Lima gained further experience with their method of leucotomy,[12–18] but modifications were soon made by Freeman and Watts, Lyerly, McKissock, Poppen, Fiamberti, Scoville, and others.[19,22–24,33,34] In addition, various other types of operations were also devised for the treatment of psychiatric disorders and later adapted to the control of pain: prefrontal lobectomy (Peyton et al.); gyrectomy (Penfield); topectomy (the Columbia-Greystone Associates); temporal lobotomy (Obrador); thalamotomy (Spiegel et al.); etc.[19,24,33,34,45] Though the initial enthusiasm for psychosurgery has waned, the evaluation of these procedures is still in progress.[27]

Egas Moniz was awarded a Nobel Prize in 1949 "for his discovery of the therapeutic value of prefrontal leucotomy in certain psychoses."[36] It was a fitting tribute to a man who persevered in the face of disappointments and criticism to develop two basic contributions to modern neurosurgery—carotid arteriography and psychosurgery.[30,42]

References

1. BRICKNER, R. M. An interpretation of frontal lobe function based upon the study of a case of partial bilateral frontal lobectomy. Res. Publ. Ass. nerv. ment. Dis., 1934, 13: 259–351.
2. BRICKNER, R. M. Modifications fonctionnelles constatées après intervention chirurgicale sur le lobe frontal. IInd int. neurol. Congr. (London, 1935). Rev. neurol., 1935, 64: 547.
3. BUCY, P. C. Frontal lobe of primates. Relation of cyto-architecture to functional activity. Arch. Neurol. Psychiat., Chicago, 1935, 33: 546–557.
4. BURCKHARDT, G. Ueber Rindenexcisionen, als Beitrag zur operativen Therapie der Psychosen. Allg. Z. Psychiat., 1891, 47: 463–548.
5. CRAWFORD, M. P., FULTON, J. F., JACOBSEN, C. F.,

and WOLFE, J. B. Frontal lobe ablation in chimpanzee: a résumé of 'Becky' and 'Lucy.' *Res. Publ. Ass. nerv. ment. Dis.*, 1948, *27*: 3–58.

6. DONAGGIO, A. In materia di discussione sulla neuropsicochirurgia. *G. Psichiat. Neuropat.*, 1939, *67*: 288–290.

7. EDITORIAL. Frontal lobotomy. *J. Amer. med. Ass.*, 1941, *117*: 534–535.

8. EDITORIAL. The lobotomy delusion. *Med. Rec.*, *N.Y.*, 1940, *151*: 335.

9. EDITORIAL. The surgical treatment of certain psychoses. *New Engl. J. Med.*, 1936, *215*: 1088.

10. EGAS MONIZ. L'angiographie dans le diagnostic des anévrismes et angiomes du cerveau. IInd int. neurol. Congr. (London, 1935). *Rev. neurol.*, 1935, *64*: 625–626.

11. EGAS MONIZ. Essai d'un traitement chirurgical de certaines psychoses. *Bull. Acad. Méd., Paris*, 1936, *115*: 385–392.

12. EGAS MONIZ. Essai d'un traitement chirurgical de certaines psychoses. *Strasbourg-méd.*, 1936, *96*: 113–116.

13. EGAS MONIZ. Les possibilités de la chirurgie dans le traitement de certaines psychoses. *Lisboa méd.*, 1936, *13*: 141–151.

14. EGAS MONIZ. Les premières tentatives opératoires dans le traitement de certaines psychoses. *Encéphale*, 1936, *31*: pt. 2: 1–29.

15. EGAS MONIZ. Tentatives opératoires dans le traitement de certaines psychoses. *Paris: Masson & Cie*, 1936, 248 pp.

16. EGAS MONIZ. Prefrontal leucotomy in the treatment of mental disorders. *Amer. J. Psychiat.*, 1937, *93*: 1379–1385.

17. EGAS MONIZ, and LIMA, A. Premiers essais de psycho-chirurgie. Technique et résultats. *Lisboa méd.*, 1936, *13*: 152–161.

18. EGAS MONIZ, and LIMA, A. Symptômes du lobe préfrontal. *Rev. neurol.*, 1936, *65*: 582–595.

19. FISHER, R. G. Psychosurgery. In: *A history of neurological surgery*. A. E. Walker, Ed. Baltimore: Williams & Wilkins Co., 1951, xii, 583 pp. (see pp. 272–285).

20. FREEMAN, W., TARUMIANZ, M. A., ERICKSON, T. C., LYERLY, J. G., PALMER, H. D., and GRINKER, R. R. Neurosurgical treatment of certain abnormal mental states. Panel discussion at Cleveland session. *J. Amer. med. Ass.*, 1941, *117*: 517–527.

21. FREEMAN, W., and WATTS, J. W. Prefrontal lobotomy in agitated depression. Report of a case. *Med. Ann. D.C.*, 1936, *5*: 326–328.

22. FREEMAN, W., and WATTS, J. W. Prefrontal lobotomy in the treatment of mental disorders. *South. med. J.*, 1937, *30*: 23–31.

23. FREEMAN, W., and WATTS, J. W. Psychosurgery in the treatment of mental disorders and intractable pain. *Springfield, Ill.: Charles C Thomas*, 1950, 2nd ed., xxviii, 598 pp.

24. FULTON, J. F. Frontal lobotomy and affective behavior. A neurophysiological analysis. *New York: W. W. Norton Co., Inc.*, 1951, 159 pp.

25. FULTON, J. F., and JACOBSEN, C. F. Fonctions des lobes frontaux; étude comparée chez l'homme, les singes et les chimpanzés. IInd int. neurol. Congr. (London, 1935). *Rev. neurol.*, 1935, *64*: 552.

26. GREENBLATT, M., and MYERSON, P. G. Psycho-

surgery. *New Engl. J. Med.*, 1949, *240*: 1006–1017.

27. GREENBLATT, M., and SOLOMON, H. C. Studies of lobotomy. *Res. Publ. Ass. nerv. ment. Dis.*, 1958, *36*: 19–34.

28. JACOBSEN, C. F. Functions of frontal association area in primates. *Arch. Neurol. Psychiat., Chicago*, 1935, *33*: 558–568.

29. KISKER, G. W. Remarks on the problem of psychosurgery. *Amer. J. Psychiat.*, 1943, *100*: 180–184.

30. PERINO, F. R. Egas Moniz. Founder of psychosurgery, creator of angiography, Nobel Prize winner. 1874–1958. *J. int. Coll. Surg.*, 1961, *36*: 261–271.

31. PUUSEPP, L. Alcune considerazioni sugli interventi chirurgici nelle malattie mentali. *G. Accad. Med. Torino*, 1937, *50*: pt. 2: 3–16.

32. RIZZATTI, E. Chirurgia delle psicosi. *G. Psichiat. Neuropat.*, 1939, *67*: 125–130.

33. SACHS, E. The history and development of neurological surgery. *New York: P. B. Hoeber, Inc.*, 1952, 158 pp. (see pp. 101–103).

34. SCARFF, J. E. Fifty years of neurosurgery, 1905–1955. *Int. Abstr. Surg.*, 1955, *101*: 417–513 (see pp. 487, 488, 493–497).

35. STEEGMANN, A. T. Dr. Harlow's famous case: the "impossible" accident of Phineas P. Gage. *Surgery*, 1962, *52*: 952–958.

36. STEVENSON, L. G. Nobel Prize winners in medicine and physiology, 1901–1950. *New York: H. Schuman, Inc.*, 1953, ix, 291 pp. (see pp. 264–271).

37. TIZARD, B. Theories of brain localization from Flourens to Lashley. *Med. Hist.*, 1959, *3*: 132–145.

38. TORSEGNO, M. E. La terapia violenta delle psicosi. *Note Psichiat., Pesaro*, 1938, *67*: 5–44.

39. WALKER, A. E. Psychosurgery. Collective review. *Int. Abstr. Surg.*, 1944, *78*: 1–11.

40. WALKER, A. E. The development of the concept of cerebral localization in the nineteenth century. *Bull. Hist. Med.*, 1957, *31*: 99–121.

41. WILKINS, R. H. Neurosurgical classic—XII. *J. Neurosurg.*, 1963, *20*: 904–916.

42. WILKINS, R. H. Neurosurgical classic—XVI. *J. Neurosurg.*, 1964, *21*: 144–156.

43. WILKINS, R. H. Neurosurgical classic—XIX. *J. Neurosurg.*, 1964, *21*: 424–431.

44. WILKINS, R. H. Neurosurgical classic—XXII. *J. Neurosurg.*, 1964, *21*: 724–733.

45. WILKINS, R. H. Neurosurgical classics—XXIII. *J. Neurosurg.*, 1964, *21*: 812–823.

Attempt at surgical treatment of certain psychoses*

By Egas Moniz

Psychiatric therapy is not very encouraging, with the exception of malarial treatment in general paralysis. All attempts to increase the possibilities of recovery in psychoses deserve, therefore, the attention of all who are devoted to the

* Translation of: Essai d'un traitement chirurgical de certaines psychoses, by Egas Moniz, *Bulletin de l'Académie de Médecine, Paris*, 1936, *115*: 385–392, with the kind permission of Masson & Cie.

thankless and difficult task of caring for the mentally ill. The concepts of pathogenesis and the new methods of treatment which we conceived may appear excessively daring; we hope, however, that the results which have already been attained will vindicate our audacity.

Furthermore, these surgical experiments only seem daring. We thought of excising or destroying portions of the centrum ovale in the prefrontal lobes. It is known, however, that one of these lobes can be cut without adverse consequences for the psychic life of the patient. More than that, in order to be able to extirpate a meningioma, Dandy excised both frontal lobes in a patient. This patient nevertheless retained a considerable part of his psychic functions. It is true that his character changed in some respects, that he became a little infantile; but to cite Richard Brickner, who observed him closely for a long time, the patient remained essentially the same "type of person" after the operation.

In summary, from the psychological viewpoint, this patient experienced difficulty in association and synthesis; Brickner considers this to be the primary phenomenon from which are derived all the other symptoms observed: puerility, change of character, loss of social and moral sense, instability, etc. But all these disorders are not total; a rather thorough examination is necessary before they are clearly revealed. The patient can still understand simple elements of intellectual material; Brickner believes that the psychic functions of this patient are altered more quantitatively than qualitatively.

In other words, even after the extirpation of the two frontal lobes, there remains a psychic life which, although deficient, is nevertheless appreciably better than that of the majority of the insane.

We did not perform surgical intervention in the mentally ill at random. We were guided by reasons of theory, which appear to prove that we were right.

It is difficult in a communication to give summaries of the various parts of our work: theoretical and surgical concepts, techniques, results obtained, etc. Nevertheless we shall attempt to do so by dealing with the subjects which we found to be most important.

The diseases in the field of neurology called "functional" have disappeared successively. The same will happen in psychiatry and the true progress of this science will be made with an organic orientation.

Psychic activity is a function of the nervous system as a whole. The sensitive and sensory perceptions, the memory, the intelligence, the will, the affectivity, the conscience, etc., are phenomena of cerebral activity, in which the peripheral nerves, the cranial nerves, the spinal cord, the medulla oblongata, the isthmus of the encephalon, the central nuclei, the cerebellum and neurovegetative system are involved. The whole organism, and, particularly the endocrine glands, the products of exogenous toxic disintegration and the autointoxications, are very important factors which influence the psychic life.

The latter, more or less concentrated in the central nervous system, depends on the activity of its cells under the action of blood that conveys the elements which nourish and stimulate them, of cerebrospinal fluid, and of stimuli which are brought to them by the connective pathways of other cells and which come from the whole nervous system.

The higher actions of the psyche are in our opinion the result of the activity of cellular groups and multiple connections established among them. The two elements, cellular bodies and connections, are indispensable; but the multiple intercommunications of cerebral cells, and their interdependence, are certainly very important.

The internal mechanism of the functioning of cerebral cells and of their connections is not known; the same lack of knowledge exists, however, with regard to the majority of cells which direct other organic functions when one wishes to define precisely the causes of the differences in the cellular activity of various organs. Since the brain is related to the physiology of the highest order of existence, one hesitates to admit simple deductions and satisfy himself with a biological explanation similar to that given for the activity of other organs.

It is said, for example, that the cerebral cells cannot function as glandular cells. The phrase "cerebral cells secrete ideas" is, in fact, not acceptable. Its meaning is indeed too glandular. We do not say that the muscles "secrete" the movements. The comparison of cerebral cells with those of the muscles is more comprehensible. The excitation of muscle fibers causes movements; the activity of cerebral cells also determines movements of a special order, which are expressed by manifestations of the psychic life.

The cellular elements of the brain, as a whole, govern the physical and psychic life. The latter, very frequently discussed in the field of philosophy since the most ancient times, is dependent on a number of phenomena quite similar to those that are observed in the physical life. In their development there exist only excitations similar to those that act on the other organs. The mechanism has the same characteristics.

The cellular body constitutes the central part of a neuron and is in relation with other elements of the nervous system by means of multiple connections. The body of the cell exists alone during a greater part of embryonic life and it is subsequently completed by the appearance of protoplasmic processes and the axon, which has collaterals and terminates in arborizations. These processes form the connections of a remarkable complexity, particularly in the brain. The axon appears to be the apparatus of transmission, the protoplasmic processes (the dendrites) the apparatus of reception, and the cellular body the center of functional activity. The psychic life is the result of this ensemble: nerve cells and their complex connections.

For a long time great importance has been attributed to the frontal lobes in psychic life, with the exception of the areas of motor localizations and of aphasia.

In effect, the frontal lobe is present only in the higher mammals and it undergoes a remarkable development in man. This phylogenetic evolution is an indication of its value in the psychic life of man. On the other hand, although the frontal lobe represents the most important mass of the brain, it is not possible to discover in it the localizations comparable to those that we know in the occipital, parietal or temporal lobes.

The functions of frontal lobes must be of a different category.

The frontal lobe, which we consider in this work, is the part of this lobe that is anterior to the motor region. The latter is formed by the areas of Brodmann: motor 4, and premotor 6 (1). Their functions are not identical. Bucy, who studied the motor functions in primates, wrote the following about functions of these areas: "The function of area 6, situated immediately anterior to area 4, was found to provide for the integration of voluntary motor activity and also for the coordination of postural adaptation."

Area 4 in man is smaller in comparison to that in primates. In the chimpanzee it represents 13.6 per cent of the total area of the brain, whereas in man it does not exceed 7.3 per cent. In contrast, the frontal lobe (we refer to it always without areas 4, 6 and 8) encompasses in man 29 per cent, whereas in the chimpanzee 16.9 per cent, in the dog 6.9 per cent and in the cat 3.4 per cent (Brodmann).

The frontal lobe is not only more developed in man than in the primates (almost twice that of the chimpanzee), but its cytoarchitectonic fields are more complex. The fields found in the monkey also exist in man, but in addition many others are found in the frontal lobe of man. The connections of the cells of these fields are certainly also more numerous and more complex in man.

The brain must have regions allotted specifically to psychic activity. Among these regions the frontal lobes probably have the most important mission to accomplish. They concentrate the majority of excitations and stimuli of the external and internal life. The majority of these stimuli do not arrive there, however, by direct paths; they traverse other centers or cellular groups.

The frontal lobes are probably not the single convergent station of all energies. There must be others and we must search for them in the silent zones of the brain, i.e., zones that do not correspond to known special functions. Thus the temporoparietal region is often cited.

It must be mentioned that we do not have in mind cellular centers related to the psychic life that are more or less comparable to those of motility, vision and sensitivity. These centers are not more isolated, but they present a particular individuality.

What is more, in the manifestations of the psychic life things are complex. There are no cellular areas in the brain that are assigned specifically to a determined psychic manifestation. These manifestations, even the simplest ones, originate from the activity of celluloconnective groups of the different parts of the central nervous system. These cortical, diencephalic, mesencephalic, isthmic, etc., cells, connected by multiple and interlaced connections, are excited by the stimuli brought by the blood in capillaries and the cerebrospinal fluid, and they themselves produce excitations which must be further concentrated in certain encephalic areas. We believe that the main areas of this type must be located in the frontal lobes. Lesions of these lobes, tumors of this region and surgical excisions have demonstrated a dominance of frontal lobes in the psychic life, but this does not mean that there exist psychic centers in the usual sense of this word.

It is not conceivable that we can discover a center of intelligence, of memory, of personality, of conscience, and of will. There are, however, psychic complexes related to the more or less extensive cellular groups, and all the elements that are differentiated by classical psychology certainly exist in them, sometimes in very different proportion, but forming a determined entity. There is no pathological state in which a single one of these elements can disappear while the others remain completely uninjured.

Those who recognize only anatomical ideas believe that a special and immutable function should correspond to each cellular element of the brain. In the nervous system, and particularly in the cortical cells, these conceptions can be defended in our opinion only in special sectors, probably those that are the oldest in the phylogenetic evolution (areas 4, 17, 18, etc.). In other sectors the cells can assume similar functions.

When a frontal lobe is cut, the cells of the other lobe assume the work that was performed by those that have disappeared; but it is not possible to as-

(1) And also area 8.

sert that the latter are replaced by the homologous cells only. Other cells, at least those that have similar activity, may also assume their functions.

In cases of certain destruction of cellular groups of frontal lobes, the substitutions may be effected in the opposite lobe or in the same lobe by the cellular groups which are more closely related to those that were affected.

There is a group of mental diseases in which the disappearance or the destruction of nerve cells is observed; this was verified by pathological anatomy. We can cite here idiocy, senile dementia, Pick's disease, Alzheimer's disease, etc.

The cellular bodies are destroyed in these diseases and with them the connections which originate in them. We shall not discuss this group of diseases which have well-known organic etiology and shall deal preferably with diseases of the psychofunctional type, in which remarkable sectors of the psychic life are left more or less intact. It even may be said that in the majority of these diseases there is a lucidity of conscience.

These patients have a fixed idea which not only dominates their psychic life but also directs their actions and can lead them to suicide or crime. The delusions of these patients constitute all that there is in their life; other things, even those which are of chief importance, are obscured in their mentality.

The normal psychic life depends on the functioning of celluloconnective systems; but the groups formed by the cells, the axons and the protoplasmic processes are not fixed physiologically; they change, they become complicated or simplified under the action of extraneural and intraneural stimuli. There is a relationship between these groups and mental elaboration, and they function in normal individuals so as to furnish the succession of diverse psychic manifestations of common life.

Since the mentally ill have delusions, there are no variations of thought; everything revolves around the delusional ideas. They constitute the path of their psychic life; nobody can divert the course of thought of these patients.

According to our psychopathogenic conceptions, like all psychic manifestations these delusions are related to the activity of certain celluloconnective groups of the brain.

These groups take on a special fixity in these cases. We termed them *established groups;* their functioning is more or less constant and their activity is related to the delusions and the dominant fixed ideas of the psychic life of these patients.

How is this physiological fixity of established groups produced?

The neurobiotaxis of Kappers may explain, at least in certain cases, the relative fixity of these celluloconnective groups.

If our theory is accepted, one important conclusion can be drawn from what we have just explained: *in order to be able to achieve recovery of these patients, we must destroy the celluloconnective arrangements and we think that the principal ones among them are those that are linked with the frontal lobes.*

For this purpose, at the beginning of our surgical experiments we injected a sclerosing agent (absolute alcohol) into the centrum ovale in the prefrontal lobes. Later on, we replaced the injections by sections and we now advise this operation.

The sections are made with a small instrument which we designed, the cerebral *leucotome* (1); it consists of a small probe, from which at a given moment a metallic loop is released, which, when the instrument is turned, cuts a spheroid of the white matter, about 1 cm. in diameter. In general, we make four sections in each prefrontal lobe, at different levels and in two directions—anterointernal and anteroexternal.

The operation is limited to the centrum ovale in the anterior portion of the frontal lobe, which corresponds almost to the anterior half of the frontal convolutions.

We have already obtained some positive results and it is this fact that lends a definite interest to the above exposition.

We operated on 20 patients, the majority of them considered chronic, from the "Manicomio Bombarda" asylum, thanks to the great kindness of our friend, Dr. Sobral Cid, renowned professor of psychiatry at the Medical School of Lisbon, who assisted us in the selection of the cases and provided us with excellent clinical observations from the asylum.

We performed 70 per cent of the operations on patients from the asylum and 30 per cent on patients from other sources.

Operations were performed on patients presenting various mental disorders, namely:

Involutional anxiety psychosis	1
Involutional melancholia	1
Anxiety melancholia	5
Anxiety neurosis	3
Mania	3
Paraphrenia and schizophrenia	7

The last named patients were agitated.

Briefly, the results obtained were as follows:

1. *No deaths. The intervention is harmless:* when the necessary care is taken.

2. None of the patients became worse after the intervention.

3. From all the cases, we obtained:

---

(1) Gentile and Company were in charge of the construction of this instrument.

Clinical recovery................. 35%
Ameliorations.................... 35%
No result........................ 30% (1)

The psychic symptoms that were improved by the treatment were anxiety, melancholic and hypochondriac delusions, psychomotor excitation, mania and secondary paranoid delusions.

From the total of 7 cases of anxiety melancholia, involutional melancholia and involutional anxiety psychoses we had 5 recoveries and 2 improvements. One of these improved patients had been very agitated and anxious, with a typical Cottard syndrome. She was in a state of great anxiety and intense psychomotor agitation. This

(1) In the volume which is now in press, entitled "Tentatives opératoires dans le traitement de certaines psychoses," we report all the clinical observations of the patients and the course after surgical intervention.

woman was treated by the sclerosing injections of alcohol (first phase of our work). She recovered from her anxiety and agitation, but the delusion of negation persists. The patient now manifests her delusional ideas in the tone of her usual conversation. In the other case, although there was much improvement, the operation appeared to us to be inadequate.

All the treated patients with melancholia recovered, even a patient with involutional melancholia who had been in the asylum for three and a half years.

We had recoveries also in cases of mania and anxiety neurosis, and improvements in psychomotor agitation in some cases of paraphrenia and schizophrenia. In these cases we achieved other improvements, although they were rather transitory (conduct, delusions, train of thoughts, etc.)

ACOUSTIC tumors have been observed at autopsy at least since the eighteenth century, and isolated clinical accounts of this condition began to appear during the first half of the nineteenth century.[7] During the second half of the nineteenth century, the clinical diagnosis of acoustic tumors was perfected as more cases were reported and as the mechanisms of cerebellar function were elucidated by experimental studies.[7,14] Ancillary techniques were soon developed to further perfect the diagnosis of these tumors.

"In 1912 the young Swedish pathologist, Folke Henschen, soon to become Professor and now one of the world's leading neuropathologists, added an important contribution. He was already well known as an authority on acoustic tumours. . . . In his communication Henschen gave an excellent up-to-date account[18] of the value and limitations of radiology in the diagnosis of brain tumours and went on to describe how he had found at autopsy that acoustic neuromas nearly always widened the internal auditory meatus. He felt convinced that this feature should be demonstrable radiographically in life and he sought the aid of his radiological colleague Dr. Forssell. . . .
"In February, 1910, Henschen had a case of suspected acoustic tumour which he submitted to radiography. Unfortunately only one side of the head was X-rayed and the patient was allowed to depart. Henschen had to wait just over a year for another case (March, 1911). On this occasion he obtained two radiographs, one of the normal and the other of the abnormal meatus. . . . The patient died in April and Henschen confirmed the radiographic findings at autopsy. . . . "[4]

By later modifications in radiological technique, Stenvers[25] and Towne[28] each increased the usefulness of Henschen's original observation.

Another significant contribution to the diagnosis of acoustic tumors was made by Robert Bárány when he originated the caloric tests of vestibular function.[1–3] Bárány had been born in Vienna in 1876, and after his formal medical training, he returned to that city to practice. He restricted his work

to otology and soon became widely recognized for his studies of vestibular function.[26]

" . . . In 1913–1914 he was awarded a number of international prizes, culminating in his selection as Nobel laureate. The confusion which accompanied the outbreak of the First World War caused postponement of the 1914 award until 1915. At that time Bárány was a Russian prisoner of war in Siberia. Through the intercession of the Swedish Red Cross, however, he was released, and the award presented to him through diplomatic channels. . . . "[26]

The operative treatment of acoustic tumors began during the last decade of the nineteenth century.[7,17]

" . . . However, in most cases, the results were poor. . . . At the International Congress of Medicine in 1913 in London, von Eiselsberg[15] reported 16 cases with 12 immediate fatalities, Krause[20] 31 cases with 26 deaths. Thus, the over all operative mortality in this condition was almost 80 per cent. These poor results were attributed by Cushing[7] to excessive emphasis on speed of execution and attempts to remove the tumor completely by finger enucleation. As was his custom, he proceeded in a much more painstaking manner, with the result that he was able to lower the operative mortality to 15 per cent by 1917. . . .
"Feeling that none of the originally used procedures provided enough room, and that the cerebellum and brain stem were traumatized by efforts to work in a restricted field, Cushing[7] utilized the cross-bow incision, and recommended that the entire operation, wherever possible, be carried out in one stage. After performing a bilateral craniectomy, and tapping the lateral ventricle, the dura was opened in stellate fashion, the cerebellar hemisphere retracted medially and the tumor exposed. Cushing[7] felt that attempts at total extirpation had led to the high mortality rate, and therefore suggested merely incising the capsule of the tumor and enucleating the tumor piecemeal from within, leaving the capsule in situ. . . . "[17]
"In November, 1920 Cushing,[8] in remarks at a meeting held at the Peter Bent Brigham Hospital, reported final statistics in 47 cases of acoustic nerve tumors with end results and pointed out that among the last 19 consecutive patients operated upon by him there was only one surgical death, bringing his operative mortality for this most difficult surgery down to 5.3 per cent! . . . .

"By a curious coincidence, in the very year (1917) that Cushing published his classic monograph 'Tumours of the Nervus Acusticus,' in which he made the following statement: 'I doubt very much, unless some more perfected method is devised, whether one of these tumors can safely be totally enucleated,' Dandy[9] presented before a local meeting of the Johns Hopkins Medical Society a patient from whom he had successfully extirpated in toto a tumor of the nervus acusticus while his surgical chief, Dr. Heuer, was out of town. This trick of fate seemed to fire Dandy with a special zeal to out-do Cushing in the latter's own special domain. . . .

"In 1922 Dandy[10] reported two more successful total removals of acoustic nerve tumors, and in 1925[11] he reported 17 cases in which the tumor had been totally removed, but with 7 deaths; however, in 12 of these cases the tumor had been shelled out with the finger and all of the 7 deaths occurred in this group; in the 5 cases in which the capsule had been carefully dissected away from the pons there were no deaths. In 1934 Dandy[12] described an operation for the removal of acoustic nerve tumors through a unilateral approach, but did not give any statistical results for this modification. . . ."24

Seven years later, Dandy13 supplied these results. There had been only 5 deaths in his series of 46 cases, a mortality of 10.9 per cent.

"The great disadvantage of the total excision method of treating acoustic tumors was the facial distortion resulting from the damage to the seventh nerve. Although surgeons had considered attempting to spare this nerve, it was not until 1931 that this was achieved. Cairns[5] in the course of removal of an acoustic tumor recognized the nerve and was able to complete the excision without sectioning or destroying it. Olivecrona[22] after 1937 attempted to save the nerve in every case. In 1940 he reported on 23 cases with anatomical preservation of the nerve in 15 cases. In 14 of the latter facial paralysis developed, but function returned in a few months to a year in almost all cases. . . ."17

The experience of other neurosurgeons with the techniques of Cushing and Dandy showed that the morbidity and mortality associated with the total removal of acoustic nerve tumors was consistently greater than the morbidity and mortality accompanying their partial, intracapsular removal.16,19,21,27

" . . . Survival after operation, however, is not the only consideration in evaluating the operative results. As reported by Cairns,[6] among 10 patients who had had intracapsular removal of the tumor by Cushing while Cairns was associated with Cushing, there were 8 survivors after an interval of 9 years, but only 3 were able to work, 2 had considerable disturbance of gait, and 3 were severely incapacitated. Givre and Olivecrona (1949) further pointed out that 50 per cent of their patients who had had the intracapsular operations had either died or had been reoperated upon within 3 to 4 years with a 50 per cent mortality attending the second operation."24

These experiences, combined with the development of techniques for restoring the function of the facial nerve, have resulted in the present emphasis on the total removal of acoustic tumors.23,24

References

1. Bárány, R. Über die vom Ohrlabyrinth ausgelöste Gegenrollung der Augen bei Normalhörenden, Ohrenkranken und Taubstummen. Arch. Ohrenheilk., 1906, 68: 1–30.

2. Bárány, R. Untersuchungen über den vom Vestibularapparat des Ohres reflektorisch ausgelösten rhythmischen Nystagmus und seine Begleiterscheinungen. (Ein Beitrag zur Physiologie und Pathologie des Bogengangapparates). Berlin: O. Coblentz, 1906, 106 pp.

3. Bárány, R. Physiologie und Pathologie (Funktions-Prüfung) des Bogengang-Apparates beim Menschen. Leipzig & Wien: F. Deuticke, 1907, x, 76 pp.

4. Bull, J. W. D. History of neuroradiology. Brit. J. Radiol., 1961, 34: 69–84.

5. Cairns, H. Acoustic neurinoma of right cerebello-pontine angle. Complete removal. Spontaneous recovery from post-operative facial palsy. Proc. roy. Soc. Med., 1931, 25: 35–40.

6. Cairns, H. The ultimate results of operations for intracranial tumours. A study of a series of cases after a nine-year interval. Yale J. Biol. Med., 1936, 8: 421–492.

7. Cushing, H. Tumors of the nervus acusticus and the syndrome of the cerebellopontile angle. Philadelphia & London: W. B. Saunders Co., 1917, viii, 296 pp.

8. Cushing, H. Further concerning the acoustic neuromas. Laryngoscope, St. Louis, 1921, 31: 209–228.

9. Dandy, W. E. Exhibition of cases. Johns Hopk. Hosp. Bull., 1917, 28: 96.

10. Dandy, W. E. An operation for the total extirpation of tumors in the cerebello-pontine angle. A preliminary report. Johns Hopk. Hosp. Bull., 1922, 33: 344–345.

11. Dandy, W. E. An operation for the total removal of cerebellopontile (acoustic) tumors. Surg. Gynec. Obstet., 1925, 41: 129–148.

12. Dandy, W. E. Removal of cerebellopontile (acoustic) tumors through a unilateral approach. Arch. Surg., Chicago, 1934, 29: 337–344.

13. Dandy, W. E. Results of removal of acoustic tumors by the unilateral approach. Arch. Surg., Chicago, 1941, 42: 1026–1033.

14. EDWARDS, C. H., AND PATERSON, J. H. A review of the symptoms and signs of acoustic neuro-fibromata. *Brain*, 1951, *74:* 144–190.

15. v. EISELSBERG, F. Ueber die chirurgische Behandlung der Hirntumoren. In: *XVIIth international congress of medicine (London, 1913)*. London: H. Frowde, 1914, sect. 7, pt. 2, viii, 362 pp. (see pp. 203–207).

16. GIVRÉ, A., AND OLIVECRONA, H. Surgical experiences with acoustic tumors. *J. Neurosurg.*, 1949, *6:* 396–407.

17. GREEN, R. E. Surgery of the posterior fossa. In: *A history of neurological surgery.* A. E. Walker, Ed. Baltimore: Williams & Wilkins Co., 1951, xii, 583 pp. (see pp. 114–133).

18. HENSCHEN, F. Die Akustikustumoren, eine neue Gruppe radiographisch darstellbarer Hirntumoren. *Fortschr. Röntgenstr.*, 1911–1912, *18:* 207–216.

19. HORRAX, G., AND POPPEN, J. L. Experiences with the total and intracapsular extirpation of acoustic neuromata. *Ann. Surg.*, 1939, *110:* 513–523.

20. KRAUSE, F. Discussion of v. Eiselsberg.[15] In: *XVIIth international congress of medicine (London, 1913)*. London: H. Frowde, 1914, sect. 7, pt. 2, viii, 362 pp. (see pp. 214–215).

21. OLIVECRONA, H. Technik und Ergebnisse der Radikaloperation bei Acusticustumoren. *Arch. klin. Chir.*, 1934, *180:* 445–448.

22. OLIVECRONA, H. Acoustic tumours. *J. Neurol. Psychiat.*, 1940, n.s. *3:* 141–146.

23. RANSOHOFF, J., POTANOS, J., BOSCHENSTEIN, F., AND POOL, J. L. Total removal of recurrent acoustic tumors. *J. Neurosurg.*, 1961, *18:* 804–810.

24. SCARFF, J. E. Fifty years of neurosurgery, 1905–1955. *Int. Abstr. Surg.*, 1955, *101:* 417–513 (see pp. 443–448).

25. STENVERS, H. W. Roentgenology of the os petrosum. *Arch. Radiol. Electrother.*, 1917, *22:* 97–112.

26. STEVENSON, L. G. Nobel Prize winners in medicine and physiology, 1901–1950. *New York: H. Schuman, Inc.*, 1953, ix, 291 pp. (see pp. 84–88).

27. TÖNNIS. Erfahrungen in der Erkennung und Behandlung der Geschwülste des Kleinhirnes, des Keilbeinflügels und des Chiasma. *Z. Hals- Nas.- u. Ohrenheilk.*, 1934, *36:* 225–227.

28. TOWNE, E. B. Erosion of the petrous bone by acoustic nerve tumor. Demonstration by roentgen ray. *Arch. Otolaryng., Chicago*, 1926, *4:* 515–519.

AN OPERATION FOR THE TOTAL REMOVAL OF CEREBELLOPONTILE (ACOUSTIC) TUMORS*

By WALTER E. DANDY, M.D., BALTIMORE
From the Department of Surgery, The Johns Hopkins Hospital and University

POTENTIALLY benign lesions, usually easy of recognition, not difficult of operative approach or even of enucleation, nevertheless tumors of the cerebellopontile angle[1] have presented surgical problems which have seemed well-nigh insuperable. Surely few lesions have enticed surgeons with more alluring prospects and have ultimately yielded so little reward for their best efforts for, with few chance exceptions, patients have succumbed following total or attempted total extirpation of the tumor. At the beginning of the twentieth century it seems probable that there had been but one tumor of this kind completely and successfully extirpated—one removed by Ballance (2) in 1894 and reported in 1907. Although there is some uncertainty as to the exact nature of this tumor (he terms it a fibrosarcoma), it seems highly probable that it was really one of the true cerebellopontile variety. It was clearly an encapsulated tumor in this region, shelling out readily with the finger, and the patient's survival for many years is alone sufficient evidence to preclude a sarcoma. Moreover, as most of these tumors in earlier years have been recorded as gliosarcomata—a classification well justified by the histological picture—such an entry is evidence in favor of the tumor being of the cerebellopontile variety.

At the beginning of the twentieth century cerebellopontile tumors were recognized by their more or less characteristic signs and symptoms and became a fairly well established clinical entity. Oppenheim of Berlin, Sternberg of Vienna, v. Monakow of Zurich, Hughlings Jackson and Gowers of London, Babinski of Paris, and Allan Starr of New York, were not only pioneers in the recognition of these tumors but they stimulated a group of surgeons to undertake their removal.

At the International Congress of Medicine in London in 1913, the three great European surgeons—Horsley of London, v. Eiselsberg of Vienna, and Krause of Berlin—who had in such large measure been responsible for the birth and

---

* Reprinted from *Surgery, Gynecology and Obstetrics*, 1925, *41:* 129–148, with the kind permission of the Editor.

[1] This group of tumors has long been recognized as a distinct clinical and pathological entity. Various other tumors in this region, whether encapsulated or infiltrating, have not been considered. I prefer the designation "tumors of the cerebellopontile angle"—the Kleinhirnbrueckenwinkeltumoren of the Germans—rather than "tumors of the acoustic nerve" for this well known group of encapsulated tumors because it does not include a theory of origin. Both appellations are defective—"cerebellopontile angle" because it merely denotes a location which is the abode of other tumors of varying types; and "acoustic" because the origin of the tumor is still in dispute and also because there are other tumors of the acoustic nerve which, both in structure and position, are entirely unlike those under consideration. Throughout the remainder of the paper the abbreviated term "cerebellopontile tumor" will be used. Though even less accurate, it has attained significance through general usage and has obviated the tendency to use the clumsy and grammatically incorrect expression, cerebellopontile "angle" tumor.

growth of brain surgery, presented their results on the extirpation of cerebellopontile tumors to that date. Horsley had 10 operative deaths in 15 cases (67 per cent), v. Eiselsberg 13 deaths in 17 cases (77 per cent), and Krause 26 deaths in 31 cases (84 per cent). Krause admitted they yielded the poorest results of all his brain tumors. There seems to have been no very great difference in the methods of attacking the tumor. Each used a unilateral cerebellar approach, often little more than an enlarged trephine opening, and the tumor was quickly shelled out with the index finger or spatula. Because of the disastrous results, the operation was often performed in two stages, particularly by v. Eiselsberg and Horsley. Sometimes Krause used suction to draw the tumor from its bed.

The conference ended with no prospect of better operative results in the future. In the hasty and necessarily blind extirpation of these tumors through a totally inadequate exposure, many of these tumors were broken and only partially removed, necropsy revealing more or less tumor undisturbed. Moreover, those few patients who survived were almost without exception badly crippled. So far as I am aware, the ultimate results of the few successes of Horsley, Krause, and v. Eiselsberg were never published, but a fortunately timed publication of Tooth (18) at the same International Congress in London, 1913, presents a comprehensive statistical study of the operative results in all brain tumors from the National Hospital of London to the date of this conference (1913), and appended thereto is a brief summary of each case together with the operator, operation, and, so far as known, the ultimate results. If not including all of Horsley's work, this report at least gives us a fair insight into his results. From this dismal story we learn much concerning the fortitude of these great pioneer brain surgeons who nevertheless persevered to blaze a trail through a forest which must have seemed utterly impenetrable. Looking back, it is clear that they were ill equipped for such a struggle; until the latter part of their work surgery was yet in its infancy. Cranial surgery offered technical problems foreign to those of other tissues; instruments of special character had to be devised; the control of haemorrhage from bone, the brain, and tumors, was unlike that elsewhere. A knowledge of the functions of the various parts of the brain and of the cerebrospinal fluid was only slowly accumulating. The effects on intracranial pressure of the immediate injury to cerebral tissues were at best imperfectly understood; and the avoidance of trauma continued to be almost impossible because technical difficulties prevented sufficient exposure of the desired field. Moreover, sepsis continued to exact a not inconsiderable toll. Though Horsley, v. Eiselsberg, and Krause were all firm adherents of the Listerian principles of combating infection, the avoidance of infection had not been mastered. And, last but not least, neurology was also just developing so that the diagnosis of tumors was usually made when the patient was blind and often *in extremis*. Cerebellopontile tumors, however, had one great advantage over all other brain tumors: not only could fair diagnosis and localization be made with fair accuracy, greater as time passed, but the tumor was known beforehand to be benign and encapsulated. The surgical problem, therefore, was direct.

With a minimum of scientific equipment, the struggle for solution of this surgical problem was necessarily in large part through trial and error, but the great Horsley early added to neurological surgery the far reaching and invaluable method of animal experimentation, but shortly before begun by Fritsch and Hitzig in Germany and by Ferrier in England.

One hardly knows whether to admire the indomitable courage of the surgeon or the persisting faith and hope of the neurologist the more. The story contained in these struggles differs only in degree from that of the pioneer efforts in advancing the frontiers of knowledge. It is, therefore, without possible taint of a critical attitude that the statistics of Sir Victor Horsley are studied. Without his contributions, both technical and physiological, to this field of surgery—his bone wax, his method of controlling haemorrhage with pieces of excised muscle, and his introduction of decompressions in order to combat acute postoperative intracranial pressure, etc.—it would not yet be possible to cope with the many problems of intracranial surgery.

Returning to Tooth's analysis of operations for tumor, we find under the heading "Extracerebellar Tumours—Removal of tumour, complete or partial," 12 cases of cerebellopontile tumor operated upon by Horsley.[2] From this group of cases, 5 (42 per cent) survived the operation for periods of 6 weeks, $2\frac{1}{2}$ months, 3 years, 3 years+ and 8 years

[2] In grouping these cases as cerebellopontile tumors, I have taken the liberty of disregarding Tooth's histological classification of tumors (glioma, fibroglioma and fibroma) and including those tumors which, from the history of the patient (early deafness with other symptoms appearing late) and even more the gross appearance of an encapsulated enucleable tumor in the angle, appeared to me probable tumors of this variety. For example, Case 222, entered as a glioma by Tooth, impressed me more as being a cerebellopontile tumor, and two cases of bilateral tumor classified by Tooth as fibroglioma, I have excluded, feeling that they were probably rather examples of Recklinghausen's tumors. I have also included four of Horsley's cases grouped under fibromata. As Horsley refers to fifteen cases at the same meeting, it is fair to assume that he and Tooth (who includes fourteen) refer to the same cases.

+; of these, 3 died of recurrence at the times stated, 1 had signs of recurrence at the end of 3 years (the wound was bulging and tight) and the last case was well and active 8 years after the operation. Of the 7 deaths (58 per cent), 2 were from meningitis on the sixth and seventeenth days. It is evident that Horsley has included in his own mortality statistics two deaths which occurred at 6 and 10 weeks, and included in his living cases one which lived 11 months after removal of a tumor on one side and died following extirpation of a second growth in the other angle, a case almost surely of Recklinghausen's disease and not of cerebellopontile tumor. But the most important result in Horsley's series is not his mortality rate but the report of the necropsy findings. Of six necropsies, in only one case had the tumor been totally extirpated, the remaining five showing more or less tumor still undisturbed. In two cases the cerebellar lobe had been very badly damaged.

Tooth's remarks on the results following extirpation of these tumors (including 5 cases operated upon by other surgeons at the National Hospital without a single recovery), well express the situation and faint degree of hope at that time. "The diagnosis of tumours in this region is so comparatively easy and accurate, and the surgical treatment at first sight so straightforward, that the results in this table are disappointing in the extreme. . . . No doubt the proximity to the vital centres is accountable for great shock, with respiratory and cardiac failure. If the danger of that period can, by any alteration in surgical procedure, be eliminated, there is no reason evident why these cases should not do well."

Nor had this impression of the surgical treatment of cerebellopontile tumors changed in England during the following 10 years, if we may judge correctly from the following quotation from Gordon Holmes (11), when discussing a case presented by Walshe (20) before the Royal Society of Medicine: "It was perhaps presumptuous on his part to refer to the surgical treatment, but so many of his cases had passed through the hands of surgeons that he had had some experience in the matter. He had seen one case recover only after gross removal of the tumour, a man upon whom Sir Victor Horsley operated many years ago, but though he lived for several years he was seriously crippled.[3] The danger seemed to be that total removal necessarily meant a disturbance of the vascular supply on the same side of the pons and medulla; the man to whom he referred had, after the operation, the characteristic symptoms of softening in the lateral side of the pons. He saw a few other cases which had survived operation for

[3] Doubtless this reference is to the same patient whom Tooth (1913) mentioned as living and well (with V and VII paralysis) 8 years after operation.

a week or so after total removal of the tumour, and all showed evidence of acute bulbar involvement."

The aggregate number of total extirpations of these tumors with recovery to date and freedom from recurrence, is impossible to estimate but with liberal allowance it will probably be less than half a dozen—and we are positive of only two. Foremost of these cases is the one removed by Ballance (2) in 1894. Apparently the only permanent sequelae of the operation many years later were palsies of the fifth and seventh nerves; the former had resulted in corneal ulceration and loss of vision in that eye. The second undoubted cured case is that of Horsley. From Eiselberg's series (9) of four recoveries (including one by his assistant, Clairmont) from the operation, one was able to resume work on the farm but there is no other record noting the ultimate results and freedom from recurrence. Leischner (13) collected from the literature eleven cases which had survived operation. Among these were four from Eiselsberg's Clinic, one of Horsley's (this was before Horsley's report (1913) of five recoveries), Krause (12) one, Poppert (16) one, Baisch (1) one, and Borchardt (3) three. This ensemble, however, is of little significance; they should not be confused with cures, for aside from the cases of Ballance and Horsley, and possibly the one of Eiselsberg's, the subsequent evidence of their cure has not appeared. In the light of the necropsy reports in Horsley's cases, in which but 1 of 6 cases was shown to be totally removed, it would appear fair to presume that few if any of these had been totally extirpated and the patients permanently cured. One of the best results reported in this group of tumors was by Willy Meyer of New York (14, 1912). In two stages, 4 weeks apart, this tumor was removed with a spoon. Three years later he was apparently well, but we have been unable to find subsequent notes on this patient's condition.

The operative method used by all operators was essentially the method of Horsley, v. Eiselsberg and Krause. A two-stage procedure came to be used almost universally and usually the dura was not opened in the first step. It seems probable, however, from Tooth's reports that Horsley always opened the dura and, toward the last at least, his decompression was bilateral. The unilateral exposure of the affected side of the cerebellum was used by Krause and v. Eiselsberg. Krause (12), it is true, suggested a bilateral cerebellar approach, but it was designed for exploration of the posterior fossa and was not intended to be used when the tumor was known to be in the cerebellopontile angle. It appears that in many instances the opening in the occipital bone was but little larger than necessary to insert the finger or spatula. The tumor was removed by sweeping the finger or spatula around the tumor and making the traction necessary to dislodge it. The finger was preferable for it could better detect the cleavage plane between tumor and brain stem. After such extirpations, furious bleeding must have been inevitable. Always the lobe of the cerebellum was injured, often much of it destroyed, and at times even deliberately removed. Not infrequently the tumor was extirpated through a transcerebellar defect which reached the upper surface of the tumor. Frazier (10, 1905) indeed urged deliberate resection of the outer part of the cerebellar hemisphere and, though a heroic procedure, it probably caused no greater damage to the lobe than that which customarily resulted from these extirpations.

Krause (12, 1903) introduced a very useful procedure to reduce the excessive pressure which was nearly always present with cerebellopontile tumors. A trocar was passed through the tentorium into the lateral ventricle permitting the evacuation of its fluid. This procedure (ventricular puncture), in much more refined form, has come to be a most important item in all operations for tumors below the tentorium

Perhaps the translabyrinthine approach suggested by the otologist Panse (15, 1904) should be mentioned in passing. At the time this method was proposed, attempts to remove cerebellopontile tumors appeared utterly futile and any suggestion might at least be tolerated. But it was a wholly impractical suggestion. After destroying much of the petrous bone, including the labyrinth and much of the mastoid bone and its contained air cells, and after passing through fields which could not be sterilized and might well harbor dormant infections, the resulting exposure must necessarily have been so meager that it would hardly be possible to do more than nibble at these great tumors. Quix (17, 1911) hastily reported the removal of a pea-sized tumor by this method but the patient died a few months later. The usual large recess tumor was present; its surface had only been scratched! The one prerequisite of any operative approach is adequate room to afford thorough inspection of the tumor during its attack in order to permit the deliberate control of haemorrhage. This exposure being lacking in the translabyrinthine approach, other consideration of the procedure is useless.

Inevitably a severe reaction must appear against attempts to remove cerebellopontile tumors, particularly as the gamut of possibilities, both of method and of individual skill, had apparently been run. All of the accumulated technical advances of a quarter of a century had made no improvement in the results. At any rate, the continuance of an operation carrying such an astounding mortality after such an exhaustive trial, was impossible.

The reaction came with the publication, in 1917, of Cushing's (5) important monograph on acoustic tumors, and with it a revolution in treatment. He accepts the only conclusion which the foregoing results and experiences of his own could justify, i.e., "I doubt very much, unless some more perfected method is devised, whether one of these tumors can with safety be totally enucleated." He no longer attempted to enucleate these tumors totally but was content to offer a method by which the tumor could be *partially* removed (intracapsular enucleation).

Cushing's contribution is the only important advance in the treatment of cerebellopontile tumors. For the first time the patient was offered a relatively safe surgical procedure with prospects of temporary relief and prolongation of life, in lieu of a hazardous and desperate effort carrying permanent disability in the wake of the very occasional chance recovery. In the first series of operations his mortality rate was reduced to 35 per cent, and in a subsequent series of about equal number to 11 per cent.

But intracapsular partial extirpation is far from satisfactory, for the growth must always recur. Partial removal of the tumor, even when the growth develops slowly, can never be considered a final operation for a potentially benign tumor.

THE DEVELOPMENT OF AN OPERATIVE PROCE-
DURE FOR THE TOTAL REMOVAL OF CERE-
BELLOPONTILE TUMORS

The purpose of this communication is to present an operative procedure by which it has been possible to remove the entire cerebellopontile tumor in a group of cases. Admittedly, it is a procedure of magnitude and carries potentialities of great danger. However, with care and attention to detail the mortality may not be greater, and not improbably even less, than Cushing's partial intracapsular enucleation. The method has been gradually evolved from the failures of other operative procedures. Finally it was forced upon us in an effort to avert an impending death several days following the partial (intracapsular) operation.

Our operations on cerebellopontile tumors cover the past 9 years. At the present writing the series consists of 23 tumors, the results of which are included in Table I under the various methods of operative attack. One case, apparently well on admission, died at stool a few hours before the time scheduled for operation. In a general way the order of the grouping is also chronological, though this is not strictly true. Our operations began at a time (1915) when the results of attempted enucleations were known, but our efforts were necessarily directed along the more or less generally recognized methods of operative attack. The initial attempts at a simple suboccipital decompression met a sharp and entirely unexpected reverse and dispelled at once our pre-existing im-

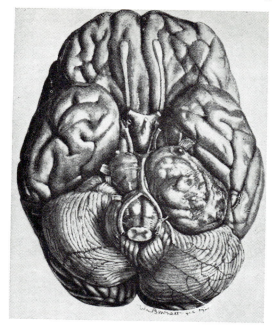

Fig. 1. An example of the characteristic cerebello-pontile tumor showing the extent to which the brainstem is excavated by the neoplasm. The intimate relationship with the medulla and pons explains the great danger which has attended all efforts at removal.

pressions of the value of this procedure as a palliative measure. Two cases so treated died within 12 hours, postmortem examinations revealing no haemorrhage or other cause in either instance. Al-

though the intracranial pressure was well advanced in both patients, each was conscious and in good physical condition at the time of operation. Disregarding for the moment the explanation of these deaths—now better understood—it is at least evident that this comparatively simple procedure has been accompanied by great danger and has in nowise helped to solve the problem of removing the tumors.

In desperation, our next effort, total extirpation with the finger at one stage, then seemed the only alternative. It was, of course, merely a reversion to the well tried and fruitless method of Horsley, Krause, Eiselsberg and others. Nor was there reason to expect better results. After two initial successes, four deaths in succession showed the futility of further attempts. It is of little concern that one case is well 5 years later, and the fate of the other after leaving the hospital is unknown. The results are of interest and importance only in that their careful analysis did explain the causes of death and therefore suggested methods of avoiding them.

At this time of despair, Cushing's method of intracapsular enucleation was introduced. Its great improvement over other procedures was at once obvious. Despite enthusiastic hopes, however, our first experiences with intracapsular enucleation were unfortunate in being less satisfactory than had been anticipated. Following an uneventful and quick recovery from the effects of the operation, the first patient 7 days later became listless and drowsy; vomiting, dysphagia and dysarthria appeared; and during the succeeding 3

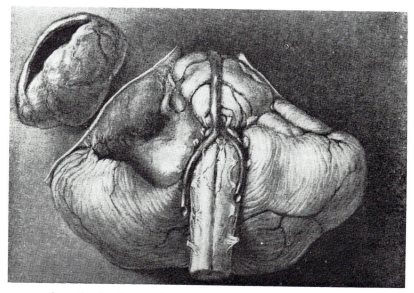

Fig. 2. Necropsy specimen showing the bed of the tumor after the capsule had been carefully removed. At operation the interior of the tumor had been removed and the patient died subsequently of meningitis. The marked excavation and destruction of the side of the pons and mid-brain is shown; also the fifth nerve intact.

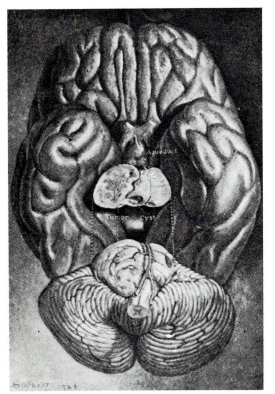

Fig. 3. Drawing of cross section of tumor and brain stem at the mid-brain level. The severe effect upon the brain stem is shown. Not only are the pons and the medulla markedly displaced to the opposite side, but the nodulations of the tumor have produced great loss of the brain stem. Such irregularities are doubtless responsible for focal disturbances which are at times associated with cerebellopontile tumors. Hydrocephalus, an inevitable sequence in the late stages, results from dislocation and obliteration of the aqueduct of Sylvius. This particular tumor shows a bridge of attachment to the brain stem, even as far anterior as the mid-brain, but the microscopic picture is identical with that of other tumors of this group. This patient died at stool a few hours before the time scheduled for operation.

days all symptoms became progressively worse and finally alarming. The late appearance of these symptoms seemed to exclude the postoperative complications which might have been expected, haemorrhage or infection, and suggested that in some way the reaction about the stump of tumor which remained was responsible for the condition. The wound was reopened and the shell of tumor extirpated with the index finger. There was surprisingly little haemorrhage, which was readily controlled. The patient's condition then steadily improved. Diminished drowsiness was at once apparent, the vomiting at once ceased, and 5 days later she was able to swallow. From the result of this case it seemed logical to infer that if the shell of the tumor could in some way be removed at the first operation, this stormy and dangerous course following subtotal removal might be avoided. In the succeeding cases in which the tumor has been

TABLE I.—KIND OF OPERATIONS AND RESULTS

Kind of Operation	Number of Cases	Recovery	Death	Cause of Death
No operation	1	0	1	Died at stool before time set for operation.
Patients in coma at time of operation (intracapsular enucleation and dissection of capsule)	2	0	2	Operation.
Suboccipital decompression. (Tumor not removed)	2	0	2	Operation.
Tumor shelled out with finger (interior not removed)	6	2	4	
Intracapsular enucleation	3	1	2	Both died of meningitis, one on the 46th, the other on the 4th day.
Intracapsular enucleation followed by finger enucleation of the tumor: 3 cases in 2 stages, and the fourth in one stage	4	3	1	Pneumonia, 8th day.
Intracapsular enucleation followed by deliberate, painstaking dissection of the capsule (all concluded in one stage)	5	5	0	

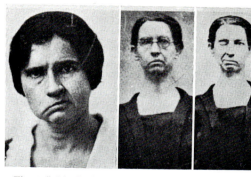

Fig. 4 (left). Patient 3½ years after total removal of cerebellopontile tumor. She has never been willing to have a spinofacial anastomosis performed to correct the facial paralysis.

Fig. 5. Patient one year after total extirpation of tumor. A spinofacial anastomosis performed shortly afterward has largely overcome the facial deformity. The tumor was on the right side. We see patient's ability to close the eyelids and draw the corner of the mouth after spinofacial anastomosis (right side).

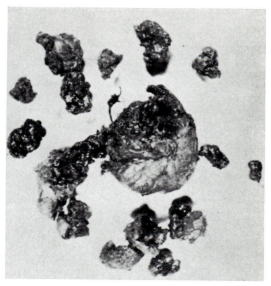

Fig. 8. Fragments of tumor removed by intracapsular method. The large mass is the upper pole which projected through the incisura tentorii. This is the most inaccessible and, from the standpoint of relief, the most important part of the tumor; upon its removal depends the release of the occluded aqueduct of Sylvius. In later cases the interior of this pole has been more thoroughly curetted, making the capsular removal easier and safer.

removed at one sitting, the results have amply supported this inference.

THE OPERATION (6)

Needless to say, the success of this procedure is dependant not only upon many technical advances which have been slowly accumulating, but also upon a clearer understanding of intracranial physiology and pathology. Without Horsley's bone wax or Cushing's silver "clips," without Horsley's principle of decompression to take care of post-operative traumatic oedema, without the bilateral cerebellar exposure (probably originated by Cotterill, 4) which allows more room for exposure and for decompression, and finally without Cushing's intracapsular method of removing the body of the tumor, the removal of the capsule of the tumor could hardly be accomplished.

A bilateral cerebellar approach, which has be-

come more or less a regular practice for all cerebellar lesions, is first made and the bony and dural defect extended laterally and superiorly on the side of the tumor as far as the transverse and lateral venous sinuses will allow (Fig. 11). Because of the great depth of the tumor, an ordinary bilateral cerebellar approach alone would not afford the direct inspection and lengthy manipulation which is necessary to dissect the growth from its bed. Indeed, in a survey of Cushing's cases, there are instances in which the tumor was missed at the first operation because of insufficient exposure, and there are other cases in which the tumors were found only by transecting the cerebellar lobe. Attempts to expose the tumor with an insufficient removal of bone causes serious injury to the brain from retraction. Always the mastoid cells are brought into view, but unless the easy exposure of the tumor makes imperative demand, their entrance is avoided. But when opened the cells are at once covered either with a sheet of wet cotton or by reflected dura (Fig. 12) which is sutured to the galea or trapezius muscle. The history of a mastoid infection would give great concern, and every other possibility of the tumor's exposure would be attempted before yielding to an easier approach which opening hitherto infected cells would provide. The anterior part of the bony extension is carried under the attachment of the trapezius muscle but the continuity of this

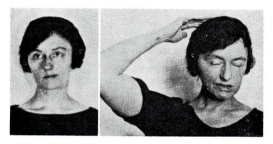

Fig. 6 (left). Another patient 18 months after extirpation of tumor, showing good return of facial function after spinofacial anastomosis.

Fig. 7. Showing the right facial movements which have returned after total removal of a right cerebellopontile tumor. Elevation of the shoulder brings out the maximum effect due to the associated movement.

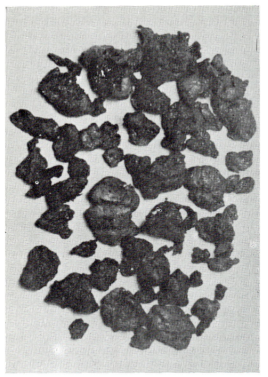

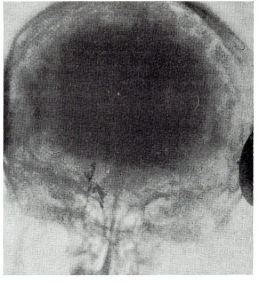

Fig. 10. Roentgenogram (anteroposterior view) showing cluster of silver clips, each representing a ligatured vessel. They also demonstrate how nearly the tumor approaches the midline.

Fig. 9. Grouping of fragments of the tumor removed by the curette. By drawing the capsule forward the interior of the tumor can be deliberately curetted for the brain stem is always exposed to view. The size of the extirpated fragments then becomes more uniform.

muscle with the galea is carefully preserved. A good exposure of the entire superior surface of the cerebellum is important in providing a good exposure of one large vein (Fig. 11) which bridges the space between the superior surface of the cerebellum and the tentorium which it enters en route

to the transverse sinus. Unless ligated and divided beforehand, this vessel may easily be stretched and torn in elevating the cerebellar hemisphere and in exposing the tumor. There is less danger of such injury to the contralateral symmetrical vein, and similar precautions against its injury are not necessary. Needless to say, special care is taken to avoid incising either the lateral or sigmoid sinuses, particularly the latter.

Almost without exception, the dura has been so tense that it has been necessary, or at least advisable, to relieve pressure in the dilated ventricles, tapping and withdrawing fluid from the posterior horn of a lateral ventricle. Hydrocephalus

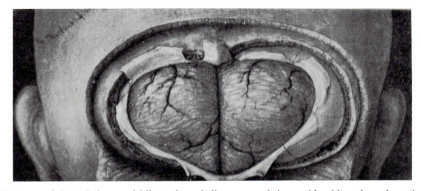

Fig. 11. The bony defect of the usual bilateral cerebellar approach is considerably enlarged on the side of the tumor, as far as the transverse and lateral sinuses. The exposed dura on the right indicates the additional bony removal obtained in this way. Incision of the dura along the dotted lines affords much additional room for exposure of the tumor.

invariably results when the tumor has occluded the iter (Fig. 3), and few tumors appear for operation before this phase of the tumor's progress is well established. Before removing the ventricular needle, gentle pressure can, if desired, be applied to the intact dura and additional relief of pressure which is exerted upon the posterior fossa will follow the further escape of fluid which is afforded by the upward push of the tentorium. In every case of hydrocephalus from cerebellar lesions, the intracranial pressure above the tentorium can be reduced to that of the atmosphere by this simple expedient and without danger of injury to the brain stem.

After this preliminary measure, gentle elevation of the cerebellar lobe quickly brings the tumor into view, though at a great depth (Fig. 12). Another invariable finding in all cases of cerebellopontile tumors is the partial or complete obliteration of the cisterna magna, the cerebellar tonsils projecting through the foramen magnum into the spinal canal (Figs. 11 and 12). If, however, the cisterna does still contain fluid, its release again contributes that much more room to the all-important exposure of the tumor. An encapsulated bed of fluid (having no communication with the subarachnoid spaces) may or may not crown the outer and superior surfaces of the tumor and, though largely or entirely obscuring the tumor, its presence is almost as characteristic of an underlying cerebellopontile tumor as the direct inspection of the neoplasm itself. Further elevation of the cerebellum brings the unattached outer surface of the tumor into full view and into a position where it can be subjected to an operative attack. Excepting the poles which have

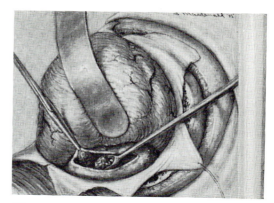

Fig. 13. Intracapsular removal of fragments of the tumor with a curette (after method of Cushing).

passed beyond the confines of the posterior cranial fossa (through the incisura tentorii and the foramen magnum), the entire longitudinal extent of the tumor is brought into full view. The capsule is then incised longitudinally from pole to pole (Fig. 12) and much of the outer contents removed piecemeal with a curette after the method of Cushing (Fig. 13). The capsule is then picked up at the margins of the opening in the tumor, drawn forward with forceps, and the attached surface of the capsule brought into view (Fig. 14). The contents of the tumor are then curetted with the brain stem and cerebellum always fully exposed. Continuing this method, the capsule gradually becomes thinner and when drawn forward permits inspection of the cleavage line between the brain stem and capsule of the tumor. When the poles of the tumor have invaded the middle cranial fossa and the spinal canal, removal of their interior allows them to be easily withdrawn into the posterior fossa; such polar extensions of the tumor are least adherent to the brain stem. Gradually in this way the entire capsule is separated from the brain stem. As the capsule is cautiously retracted, several small blood vessels crossing from the brain stem or cerebellum are brought into view and doubly "clipped" and the vessel divided. Practically all bleeding can be forestalled in this way (Fig. 10).

Removal of the capsule of the tumor in this way is necessarily very tedious and time consuming. The method employed is but the application of the fundamental surgical teachings of my former chief, the late Professor Halsted. By this great master every operation, whether unusual or commonplace, was performed with the utmost care. All tissues were handled with the greatest gentleness, the field unstained with blood, and a step was never taken blindly. Always his work was painstaking, the field of operation immaculate, and haemorrhage minimal. Time of operation was

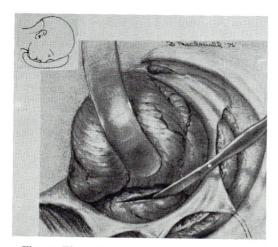

Fig. 12. The entire length of the tumor is exposed when the cerebellum is retracted. Throughout the operation this exposure is maintained. The outer surface of the capsule is incised almost from pole to pole.

always subordinate to accurate and thorough performance.

It is clear that as a measure preliminary to removal of the capsule, the intracapsular curettement must be carried out much more thoroughly than when this procedure is the end-result. When the tumor is curetted blindly, i.e., with only the outer aspect of the growth in view, the total amount of tumor removed, though seemingly great, will be relatively small, for the danger of penetrating the capsule and injuring the brain stem with the curette is always uppermost in the operator's mind, and in avoiding this possibility it is more probable that too little rather than too much will be removed. The more thoroughly the capsule is stripped of its solid contents (up to a certain limit), the easier becomes the final stage of its separation from the brain stem. It should not be inferred that the separation of the capsule is not attended by difficulties. It is always difficult and frequently for some time seems impossible. Only by persistently tugging at the capsule, often gaining but a millimeter at a step, does its attachment finally yield.

In one of the earlier cases the ultimate release of a fraction of the capsule seemed impossible of accomplishment and was given up. It is quite probable that with increasing experience and confidence this capsule could now be removed. On the other hand, only quite recently the capsule in another case was so delicate that at every attempt at traction it tore and when there seemed no way to overcome this difficulty in desperation the capsule was shelled out with the index finger. There is, however, a marked individual difference

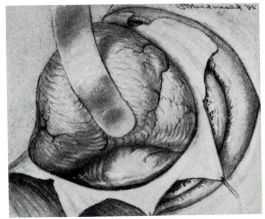

Fig. 15. Drawing made by Dr. Macdonald of the brain stem after the tumor had been completely removed. The several nerves (IX, X, XI, and XII) are intact posteriorly and the trigeminal nerve is compressed against the pons. In this particular case the largest vessel entering the tumor was ligated just dorsal to the origin of this nerve.

in the degree of attachment of the tumor to the brain stem, and there will probably always be instances in which a deliberate and painstaking removal will not be possible.

When the capsule is ultimately delivered, the denuded brain stem should and must be perfectly dry. A fatality will almost surely ensue if even the slightest ooze persists when closure is begun. Drainage has usually been avoided, though in two instances a rubber protective wick was placed in the lateral recess and removed in less than 24 hours.

The largest vessels encountered during the operation are the postero-inferior cerebellar and vertebral arteries which wind around the lower pole of the tumor and usually one and at times two branches to the tumor are given off from the former. These arteries are but loosely attached to the tumor and can easily be stripped from it after the branches have been divided. At the other pole of the tumor is a large venous branch of the inferior petrosal sinus. Closely applied to the tentorium and the tumor, from which it emerges, this vein may be very troublesome unless dissected free, ligatured and divided in the operation. Naturally the vessels causing greatest concern are the arteries which cross from the brain stem to the tumor. There are usually three to six of these vessels in addition to two or three from the inferior surface of the cerebellum. Though constituting probably the greatest danger of the operation, there is, however, no great difficulty either in exposing or ligating these vessels.

Removal of the tumor at a single stage is undoubtedly far preferable to two stages. Despite its

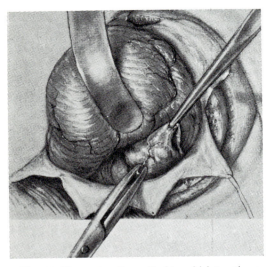

Fig. 14. Illustrating the method by which traction on the excavated capsule of the lower pole strips the remaining tumor from the brain stem and brings into view the vessels which cross from the brain stem.

great length (often 3 to 4 hours) the operation is usually well borne, and unless exceptionally difficult can be completed before lowering blood pressure or accelerating pulse gives warning of danger. Only once did the patient's condition necessitate abandoning operation and continuing at a second attempt. In three cases the capsule was intentionally left for a second stage (7 to 12 days later). In the interim the capsule had become so soft, swollen, and friable that the teeth of the forceps were no longer able to retain a grip and the capsule then had to be shelled out with the finger. If the capsule cannot be carefully extirpated at the first stage, its enucleation with the finger can undoubtedly be accomplished with greater safety at a second and not too distant stage, for the œdema of the tumor which remains, doubtless reduces the caliber of the small arteries supplying it and greatly modifies the bleeding.

It is not the purpose of this communication to commend finger enucleation for these tumors. However, in those exceptional cases in which the capsule of the tumor cannot be liberated, I believe the removal of the capsule at a second stage to be superior in the ultimate, and at times in the immediate results, to the subtotal intracapsular enucleation alone. An excellent example of this impression is given in the patient previously mentioned. When, several days after intracapsular enucleation, stupor, vomiting, dysphagia, and dysarthria appeared and progressively increased, not only did she promptly recover and the symptoms quickly disappear after enucleation of the capsule with the finger, but she has since remained as well as any of those patients in whom the operation was completed by careful dissection in one stage.

The bond between the brain stem and tumor may be solely by connective tissue, but in one case at least the tumor has been found at necropsy to be a direct outgrowth of the brain stem (Fig. 3). It can hardly be denied that when the tumor is actually continuous with and a direct outgrowth from the brain stem its origin must be from the brain stem and not from the region of the porus acusticus, as has been claimed. But the origin of these tumors is another story which we shall consider at another time. The capsule has always been most adherent at the pons; in the single case in which a line of cleavage could not be followed throughout, the fragment of tumor remained tightly adherent at the pons.

Cerebellopontile tumors are only slightly adherent to the dural covering of the base of the skull, but the separation of the capsule nearly always leaves an oozing, raw surface, and at times an even greater degree of bleeding. At the porus acusticus, however, the attachment is always firm for the auditory nerve is an integral part of the tumor. This attachment has usually been liberated after the tumor has been separated from the brain stem, but in one case the dissection was begun at the meatus and in so doing it was possible to pick up and follow the facial nerve in the capsule, in which it was superficially located, to the brain stem. But in liberating the capsule from the pons, the nerve was accidentally torn. Greatly elongated by its stretch around the tumor, the facial nerve in this case was a very delicate filament scarcely larger than an ordinary cambric sewing needle. In none of the other cases has the facial nerve been seen during dissection of the tumor. Should preservation of the facial nerve with total removal of the growth be ultimately possible, it could doubtless be more easily located at the internal auditory meatus. Its course is probably always, as in this case, on the under surface and toward the lower pole of the tumor.

The trigeminal nerve is always brought clearly in view during the dissection and throughout its intracranial course (Fig. 15). Usually it first appears when the upper pole of the tumor is withdrawn from the incisura tentorii or separated from the tentorium. But on one occasion when the dissection from the inferior pole proceeded with unusual ease, the nerve was first exposed at its junction with the pons; its exposure was then continued forward in the direction of the mid-brain. Being tightly squeezed between tumor and brain stem which it parallels (Fig. 2) the trigeminal nerve has been flattened like a ribbon. Its more distal course is determined by the upper pole of the tumor which pushes the nerve ahead, ofttimes into the middle cranial fossa, causing it to double back upon itself before entering the dural envelope surrounding the gasserian ganglion.

The remaining cranial nerves of the posterior cranial fossa (on the side of the tumor), though pushed aside and even somewhat elongated by the tumor, are much less seriously affected. Before the dissection is started, the spinal accessory nerve, most affected of this group, is often seen bending around the inferior pole of the tumor from behind, but in any case it is quickly brought into view when the inferior pole is drawn forward. The vagus and glossopharyngeal nerves appear in succession when the inferior pole is drawn a little farther forward. Never more than lightly attached to the growth, these nerves are pushed mesially and inferiorly, the distortion of each depending upon the size and configuration of this part of the tumor. In one case a tumor nodule projected between the spinal accessory and vagus nerves. The hypoglossal nerve, having a more mesially placed exit, is less disturbed by the tumor. This entire group of nerves fall away as the capsule of the inferior pole is dislodged (Fig. 14). Although the basilar artery has been exposed on two occasions, I have never recognized the abducens nerve.

We have carefully examined every porus acusticus after extirpation of the tumor, but in only two instances was there an appreciable widening of this opening. Not infrequently there was a rather diffuse concavity of the region surrounding the meatus, and in one instance a quite deep pit (about 1 by 1 centimeter and probably 3 millimeters deep) with fairly abrupt walls extended mesially from the porus and included its inner margin, but the outer margin remained unchanged. These findings explain the lack of positive changes in roentgenograms and they also constitute evidence against the theory of origin of the tumor in the internal auditory meatus. When the tumor has extended into the porus, its liberation has not been difficult. Only on one occasion was it necessary to chisel away the outer margin of this opening before this dissection could be completed.

With one exception the operations have been performed under ether anæsthesia. Novocain worked admirably in this exception until the brain stem was reached, when the pain became so severe that ether was given for the capsular dissection. The patients are maintained in the horizontal face-down position. Pulse and blood pressure readings have been the best criteria of the patient's condition and largely determined whether the operation could be concluded in one or two stages.

POSTOPERATIVE COURSE

Few brain tumor extirpations run a more uneventful and satisfactory course than these have done. Without exception, the patients have quickly become conscious, have remained so, and on the following day have appeared free of danger. That two of the series of total enucleations should have survived a superimposed purulent meningitis (streptococcus viridans and staphylococcus aureus), the symptoms of which appeared 48 hours after the operation, indicates the rapidity of recovery from the operation. The postoperative temperature curves of these patients are more or less uniform. The rectal temperature slowly rises to a maximum which is usually reached in 10 or 12 hours, and it almost as quickly descends to a level around 101 or lower the next morning. Usually the maximum temperature is about 103.6 to 104.2, though one case reached 104.8. At the end of the operation when the patient is coming out of ether, the quality of the pulse will be at its worst and the rate highest. Despite the gradual postoperative rise of temperature, the patient remains conscious and the pulse slowly falls, usually reaching 100 to 120 on the following morning.

Of the series of 5 cases in which the capsule was carefully removed (all in one stage), postoperative dysphagia was present in only one patient, and she had been unable to swallow for 36 hours before the operation. Five days later nasal feedings were discontinued. In all of the four cases in which the capsule was *enucleated with the finger*, nasal tube feeding was necessary, but in two of these patients inability to swallow had developed 7 and 10 days after a subtotal intracapsular enucleation (first stage) and was therefore not caused by the operation. The one death in this series was from pneumonia (eighth day) and was doubtless induced by aspiration during this period when swallowing was difficult. Surely this death could now be avoided. Fluids are now withheld from patients after operation until they are well able to swallow; in the interim the regular nasal feedings are substituted.

Each of the five cases was able to walk out of the hospital with support, and to some extent alone, the time of departure being 16, 18, 18, 25, and 76 days after operation. One patient was unable to walk when she entered the hospital because of a partial hemiplegia (there was also dysphagia) resulting from the tumor's indentation of the brain stem; 22 days after the operation she walked across the room without support. The protracted stay of the patient who remained in the hospital 76 days was due to a postoperative streptococcus viridans infection, which was cured by cisternal drainage. Fortunately this patient has retained no ill consequences of the infection.

SUBSEQUENT COURSE OF PATIENTS AFTER REMOVAL OF TUMOR

There has as yet been no recurrence, but the longest time since operation has been only $3\frac{1}{2}$ years. Every patient is well, free from headache, and has been able to return to work. The one outstanding sacrifice of the operation is the hemifacial paralysis (Fig. 4). It has as yet been impossible to preserve the facial nerve, though I am not so sure that this may not eventually be possible. The reason for this hope is that in one case (previously mentioned) the facial nerve was dissected from the porus to the pons but was finally inadvertently torn when the capsular dissection was continued. The patient is informed of the necessary loss of the facial nerve beforehand and is given the choice of an intracapsular curettement of the tumor. With a spinofacial or hypoglossofacial anastomosis, however, the degree of this deformity has been greatly modified (Figs. 5 and 6). Six of the 8 patients have had spinofacial anastomoses and all with returning function. Before attempting an anastomosis, the function of the spinal accessory or hypoglossal nerves must be tested in order to preclude union with a nerve trunk which may have been injured at the time of operation.

The auditory nerve, being incorporated in the tumor and totally paralyzed before the operation, is irretrievably lost. This, of course, holds equally true when intracapsular enucleation is performed.

The trigeminal nerve has been injured at operation in each of the 5 cases, but sensation has returned to a more or less degree in every instance. In the three finger enucleations, the trigeminal function has been destroyed in two and only injured in the third. Ulceration of the insensitive cornea is a danger which must be guarded against by shielding the eye. In one of the eight cases enucleation of the eyeball was finally necessary, and in another vision in the affected eye was lost following healing of the ulcer. The danger of this complication is the same as that following resection of the posterior root of this nerve for tic douloureux. With the improved methods of prevention now in vogue, corneal ulceration should become a less disturbing factor.

In every case there has been dizziness and consequently balance of the body has been disturbed, but always there has been a steady and progressive improvement. It is probable that this disturbance may be the result of retracting the cerebellum—a factor which should be lessened as our skill in removing the capsule improves. A very slight weakness and stiffness of the hand on the homolateral side has persisted in 6 cases, and in two recent cases (2 and 6 months) after finger enucleation of the capsule the affection is more pronounced. Soon after the operation there has at times been some slight subjective stiffness of the corresponding leg, but this has soon entirely disappeared except in the above two cases of finger enucleation. Doubtless this slight residual disturbance is the result of injury to the pyramidal tracts in the brain-stem, and for this reason the arm fibers presumably are situated more externally than the fibers for the leg.

Table II indicates in a general way the results obtained in these patients to date. While the time is too short to refer to the absence of recurrence, the encapsulated character of the tumor and its total removal should leave little doubt that they will not recur. It may again be emphasized that the determination of the total removal of the tumor is not by guesswork but by a careful inspection of the site of the growth at the end of the operation. It is at once evident that the results following finger enucleation are incomparable (excepting 1 case) to those following painstaking removal of the capsule.

EXPLANATIONS OF THE MORTALITY FROM VARIOUS PROCEDURES

At first glance it must seem incredible that the total removal of a cerebellopontile tumor can be accomplished with even less mortality than that following the relatively simple curettement of only part of the tumor's interior. It cannot be reasoned that because an operation is simpler, it is better and safer. The simplest operation for these tumors is a cerebellar decompression, but it has

been attended by the highest mortality in the hands of nearly every operator. The reason for these seemingly paradoxical results is the simple one of cause and effect. If the patient's condition will justify the additional effort, there is no relief so quick and so complete as that following removal of the cause. There are occasions when the effects of the cause can be relieved by a smaller and less dangerous palliative operation (decompression), but that is only true at times. There are many intracranial tumors which can never be even slightly benefited by any form of palliative procedures, and under such conditions the procedure itself becomes an insult added to an already overstrained intracranial pressure. Cerebellopontile tumors offer seemingly insuperable obstacles to the success of the customary palliative operations in the late stages of the tumor's effects.

The high mortality from the simple enucleation of cerebellopontile tumors with the finger or spatula is now readily understood. Death results from injury to the brain stem when the finger tears the tumor from the brain stem and from packing the denuded brain stem in the frantic efforts to check hæmorrhage. An examination of the brain after death in one of our cases showed the lateral margin of the brain stem softened and minute haemorrhages extending almost to the midline in the pons and medulla. This finding is not surprising since immediately after the tumor is shelled out there are always symptoms and signs which serve as telltale indicators that the medulla has been injured. At once respirations cease for many seconds (often a minute or more), after which they reappear irregularly and with serious embarrassment, and after several minutes they usually become more or less normal. However, after a severe injury the respirations may remain irregular, difficult, and ineffective, or apparently they may even fail to reappear, though it has never occurred in our cases. But even when the respirations seem to have become satisfactorily re-established, a secondary phase of embarrassment is almost sure to reappear 4 to 8 hours later. It seems probable that this may be a secondary reaction (œdema) of the tissues to the initial trauma. This phase of secondary reaction is characterized by harsh, slightly irregular, and more rapid respirations; the pulse rate accelerates and diminishes in volume, the temperature rises steadily, the reflexes diminish and the patient becomes progressively more difficult to arouse. Obviously precisely the same effects are produced when the brain-stem is compressed by hæmorrhage.

Why is there such a high mortality following a simple suboccipital decompression in the presence of cerebellopontile tumors? It would often be a great comfort to be able to do a simple bilateral suboccipital decompression and complete the re-

TABLE II.—END-RESULTS

CASES WITH RECOVERY AFTER CAREFUL REMOVAL OF CAPSULE

	Age	Time Since Operation	Gait	Balance	Arm and leg on affected side	Romberg	A-taxia	VN.	Head-aches	Wt.	Remarks
MRW I	49	1 yr.	Walks 1½ miles per day Feels safer with support	Still feels dizzy but is improving	Leg well. Arm and hand stiff	Slight	Neg.	Sensation felt but less acutely	None	+10	Postoperative meningitis (streptococcus viridans) Cisternal drainage.
TH II	56	1 yr.	Walks well	Slightly dizzy	Stiffness hand. Leg normal	Slight	Neg.	Not normal but present	None	−10	
EB III	44	1 yr.	Can walk 4 miles without support. Feels need of assistance only on rough ground and down steep grades	Still slightly affected but gradually disappearing	Hand still slightly affected	Neg.	Neg.	Patch of anæsthesia below eye	None	+8 to +15	Healed corneal ulcer. Little vision remains.
JM IV	29	2½ yrs.	Except narrow plank or down steep grade, can walk anywhere without support	Practically normal	Still slight weakness of arm; leg normal	Slight	+	Some loss but sensation present	None	−25	Was unable to walk before operation. Hemiplegia and difficulty swallowing.
IR V	36	1½ yrs.	Can walk a mile without support	Still feels slightly uncertain	Very slightly less than normal	Neg.	Neg.	Not quite normal	None	Same	

CASES WITH RECOVERY AFTER INTRACAPSULAR ENUCLEATION FOLLOWED BY FINGER EXTIRPATION OF CAPSULE

	Age	Time Since Operation	Gait	Balance	Arm and leg on affected side	Romberg	A-taxia	VN.	Head-aches	Wt.	Remarks
EL VI	25	3½ yrs.	Can walk any distance alone	Only occasional loss of balance	None	Very slight swaying	Neg.	Normal about lower face; diminished above	None	+15	Two-stage operation.
RLB VII	48	6 mos.	With support can walk briskly, but requires help except in house	Very marked difficulty in balancing	Good grip but quite shaky	Markedly positive	+	Sensation absent	None	+40	Ulcerated eye removed. Hearing much better. Smallest tumor of series but symptoms of 20 years.
WD VIII	23	2 mos.	On discharge from hospital can walk with support. Pt. has been 2 months recuperating from meningitis and a resultant hydrocephalus	Very marked difficulty in balancing	Markedly affected	Markedly positive	+	Sensation absent	None	−10	Postoperative meningitis (staphylococcus aureus); cisternal drainage; resulting hydrocephalus cured spontaneously. Largest tumor of series, wt. 46 gms. Two-stage operation.

NOTE.—As all of the patients live at a distance, this table is compiled from answers to letters of inquiry. Six of the eight cases have had spinofacial anastomoses with returning function in each instance.

moval of the tumor at a subsequent stage, but for reasons which are only now clear, the mortality is almost as high from this operation alone as from enucleation of the tumor. This danger is shown not only by our own two deaths (100 per cent), but by Tooth's reports which incorporate the results of Horsley's operations. From a series of 7 verified extracerebellar tumors, there were 4 deaths within 15 hours, a fifth died of respiratory distress on the sixteenth day, and the remaining two of meningitis. It is significant that only one of these tumors was actually disclosed at operation, but all were verified by necropsy. There was, therefore, no trauma to the tumor and the contiguous brain stem to account for the high death rate. More recently Trotter (19) has commented upon the dangers as well as the uselessness of sub-occipital decompressions for cerebellopontile tumors, a view also voiced by Gordon Holmes. Surely these figures are far too high but the results could never be reduced far enough to make this operation a commendable procedure. In Cushing's series the results following decompression were very much better; there was only 1 death in 10 cases in which a cerebellar decompression was done, but another patient survived only after a desperate struggle in which artificial respiration was maintained for an hour. The reasons for the excessive mortality in decompressing these tumors will be evident if the pathological changes which accompany the tumor's growth are understood, and again those alterations which must suddenly be induced by removal of the occipital bone and dura.

Cerebellopontile tumors not only deeply indent the brain stem (reducing its bulk as much as one-fourth or even more) but dislocate it to the opposite side causing its normal straight mid-axial line to become a pronounced curve. But this great defect and alteration in the brain stem are tolerated because the changes have been so gradual. It is even remarkable that no appreciable disturbance of function can usually be detected by our clinical tests.

Most cerebellopontile tumors are small in comparison with cerebral tumors or even with other tumors in the posterior cranial fossa. Although the posterior compartment is small, the actual bulk of the tumor is not difficult to compensation by (1) partial obliteration of the cisterna magna, the cisterna pontis, the cisterna beneath the mid-brain, and the fourth ventricle; (2) herniation of the tonsils of the cerebellar lobes into the spinal canal (through the foramen magnum); and (3) by pushing the tentorium cerebelli upward (7). Were it not for a new factor which inevitably supervenes as the tumor grows, life could doubtless be maintained for a much longer time by these adjustments,[4] This new factor is closure of the aqueduct of Sylvius. When this small channel becomes closed by the anterior extension of the tumor, hydrocephalus involving the third and both lateral ventricles inevitably results. It is only with the onset of hydrocephalus that the real intracranial pressure develops. The pressure caused by the hydrocephalus always develops rapidly and soon overcomes the space adaptations which had previously been consummated in the posterior cranial fossa; it also quickly reduces to a minimum nature's remaining reserves of space compensation. Though quite firm, tough, and inelastic, the tentorium cerebelli is gradually pushed backward reducing the space in the posterior cranial fossa.[5] These qualities of the membrane, however, must be of great service in temporarily protecting the contents of the posterior cranial fossa, and to the tentorium is doubtless due the preservation of life pending the advent of surgery. Without doubt the danger of cerebellar decompression is proportionate to the degree of hydrocephalus which is present at the time of operation.

What happens when the occipital bone is removed and the dura opened widely—cerebellar decompres-

sion? Removal of the occipital bone at once liberates the pressure in the posterior cranial fossa. But this benefit is at once countered, and may be greatly exceeded, by the injurious effects of the backward pressure on the tentorium (hydrocephalus) and its full force is now exerted without opposition upon the delicate brain stem jamming it backward. It would seem that this force must be exerted almost entirely through the incisura tentorii for the tentorium itself would hardly be sufficiently elastic to stretch so quickly as to produce these disastrous results.

It must not be inferred that the results following suboccipital decompression are the same for all tumors in the posterior cranial fossa. Variations result from differences in the character, position, and fixation of the tumor. Almost complete relief of all symptoms will at once follow suboccipital decompression when a cerebellar cyst is evacuated. And ofttimes even when a cyst has not been evacuated or an intracerebral tumor not removed, the same complete but temporary relief will be obtained, for the backward dislocation of the tumor may be great enough to relieve the obstruction at the aqueduct of Sylvius. But cerebellopontile tumors (and some other growths in the posterior fossa) are so firmly fixed to the floor of the skull that dislocation of the tumor cannot occur. Therefore, no relief of the hydrocephalus can be expected from decompression. Moreover, these tumors nearly always extend from one end of the posterior fossa to the other, and are closely attached to the brain stem throughout. Indeed, as noted before, they often extend posteriorly through the foramen magnum into the spinal canal and anteriorly through the incisura tentorii, even at times far enough anteriorly to destroy the posterior clinoid process. Not infrequently, however, a relatively small cerebellopontile tumor produces more severe and fulminating manifestations of intracranial pressure than larger growths because a small projecting nodule of the tumor imbeds itself deeply into the side of the midbrain, causing the aqueduct of Sylvius to be obstructed.

There can be no doubt that many obstructions of the aqueduct and fourth ventricle have a ball-valve action. This can be shown by the fact that at one time the intraventricular pressure will register very high, on a succeeding day it may be normal. In fact, one can easily be misled into assuming the absence of a neoplasm by finding a normal intraventricular pressure; the pressure may be low owing to the particular stage in the cycle of changes resulting from the ball-valve action of the tumor. Such vacillations in pressure are impossible in tumors which have infiltrated the aqueduct; they are most frequent in mobile non-infiltrating tumors; and are of intermediate frequency in fixed noninfiltrating tumors such as the cerebellopontile group. Periodical relief from

---

[4] The amazing adaptation of the central nervous system to the steady growth of the tumor is also shown in the trigeminal and facial nerves which become flattened, thinned, and elongated to several times their original intracranial span, and usually without any or at most only an insignificant depreciation of function.

[5] The extent to which the tentorium has been stretched can be roughly estimated by the quantity of fluid which can be recovered from a ventricular needle when pressure is gradually applied to the exposed cerebellar hemispheres.

pressure of this character is doubtless less frequent in occlusions of the aqueduct than of the fourth ventricle because the channel of the iter is so narrow.

It does not seem possible that the hydrocephalus could be relieved by any lateral dislocation of the brain stem away from the tumor in the tentorial opening, for usually the tumor has filled the superfluous space in the incisura tentorii, at least in the lateral aspect; and any anteroposterior dislocation of the brain stem can hardly have any effect other than to make any partial obstruction of the iter complete.

The injury resulting to the brain stem from the supratentorial pressure probably bears a close analogy to that following two other well recognized procedures, often erroneously considered harmless. Severe medullary embarrassment and even death are not rare sequels of a lumbar puncture performed in the presence of high intracranial pressure. Death or other injurious effect in these cases is surely due to the injury inflicted upon the brain stem when by the release of the intracranial pressure the cerebellar tonsils are suddenly driven more deeply through the foramen magnum into the spinal canal. One of the patients in our series was in coma from this ill-advised procedure.

The other example of the danger of disturbing established pressure relations is shown when lumbar punctures are performed in the presence of certain spinal cord tumors. In a not inconsiderable percentage of cases, sensory and motor function and sphincter control will be quickly affected, even lost, after lumbar puncture (8). In nature's effort again to equalize intraspinal pressure after lumbar puncture in the presence of a complete spinal block, the higher pressure above the tumor can only spend its force by jamming the spinal cord against the immobile tumor. Unless the tumor is situated in the high cervical region, these injuries to the spinal cord affect only function, whereas the analogous (though greater) effects of supratentorial pressure on the medulla in the presence of cerebellopontile tumors compromise life as well as function. We believe, therefore, that when the dural and bony support of the occiput is removed (suboccipital decompression), the supratentorial pressure pushes the brain stem backward through the incisura tentorii until its force is spent; also that this injury to the brain stem is probably augmented by the tug on the firmly fixed cerebellopontile tumor. The degree of this damage is probably proportionate to the grade of intracranial pressure and the size of the tentorial opening (the fixation of the tumor is probably fairly constant).

Why should a suboccipital decompression plus intracapsular removal (subtotal) of a cerebellopontile tumor be less dangerous than a suboccipital decompression alone? The fact that the mortality rate in

these tumors has been reduced only by the advent of Cushing's intracapsular method of enucleation is ample evidence for the assertion contained in this interrogation. When the interior of the tumor is sufficiently removed, the capsule will be freed of its rigid support, thereby permitting the obstruction of the aqueduct of Sylvius to be released. The supratentorial pressure (of hydrocephalus), which is the real dangerous factor in these operations, will be automatically relieved as effectually for the time being as if the tumor were removed. But one of the greatest defects of subtotal intracapsular enucleation is the difficulty of removing the proper amount of the contents of the tumor to permit this benefit to accrue. Unless the tumor is thoroughly removed so as to leave a fairly empty capsule, the remaining tumor will be essentially as rigid and immobile as the original tumor, and there would then be little if any relief either to the laterally deflected brain stem or to the hydrocephalus. During the removal of the contents of the tumor with a curette, only the outer surface of the growth is brought into view and one has great difficulty in knowing, indeed it is usually impossible to determine, the depth of tumor which still remains imbedded in or projecting beneath the brain stem. The importance of this determination we have learned from completely shelling out the interior of the tumors, as our deliberate total extirpations now necessitate. Curetting the interior of the tumor with the brain stem in the background, necessarily demands caution and, in playing safe, usually more tumor remains than seems possible from the apparent size of the exposed stump. In one of our two-stage extirpations 18 grams of tumor was curetted away and we thought but little was left with the capsule. The remainder of the tumor, when removed at the second stage, weighed 26 grams!

Since hydrocephalus results from occlusion of the iter, and since hydrocephalus is one of the chief factors in the operative mortality, it is safe to infer that the part of the tumor demanding urgent excavation is the upper pole. Otherwise, the hydrocephalus cannot be relieved. One of Cushing's necropsy specimens (Case xix) shows the upper pole of the tumor practically untouched by the intracapsular removal.

The configuration of the tumor also has something to do with the amount of tumor *in situ* after a subtotal removal. Nodules may project into the brain-stem from the inner side of the tumor. It has seemed that these deeply imbedded and invisible localized masses at times cause more symptoms referable to the brain stem and play a greater rôle in obstructing the aqueduct of Sylvius, than the big bulk of the tumor. The effect of the nodules will not be greatly, if at all, influenced by removal of the outer portion of the tumor with a curette.

Unless one is acquainted with the technical

steps in a bilateral cerebellar operation, it would be reasonable to question why the brain stem has not already been injured by the supratentorial pressure during the operation, when the dura is opened widely. This pressure, however, is always under control. Puncture of a posterior horn of a lateral ventricle is always utilized to reduce the supratentorial pressure to that of the atmosphere. The period of great danger to the patient when the hydrocephalus has not been relieved, is in the few hours succeeding the operation—when the intraventricular pressure is again re-established.

Why should there be less mortality after subtotal intracapsular enucleation of the tumor plus removal of the remainder of the tumor, than from the partial removal alone? From this series two deaths were surely impending about 2 weeks after partial intracapsular enucleation of the tumors and were finally prevented by removal of the remainder of the tumor at that critical period. The defects of the partial operation, therefore, really forced the total removal of the growth. In every case in which a subtotal intracapsular operation has been performed (6 in all, if those cases are included in which the intracapsular method was the first stage), the immediate postoperative course has been perfectly satisfactory. It has been several days later when the patient should have been out of danger that the alarming symptoms developed. In some way the stump of tumor caused the important functions located in the brain stem to be seriously compromised. We know from the gross appearance at the second operation that the stump of tumor which remained was swollen and friable—doubtless owing to nature's method of repair—but in all probability these same changes were also present in the contiguous brain tissue and were responsible for the symptoms. Whatever the exact explanation may be, complete subsidence of all symptoms at once followed extirpation of the residual tumor and capsule. No such complication has appeared in any of the cases (5) in which the entire tumor has been removed at one sitting.

A careful survey of the results after various operative attacks, brings us to one general conclusion: with proper care and attention to detail, that operation which at once removes the cause (other things being equal) not only carries the lowest mortality but at the same time offers incomparably the best immediate and permanent results.

OPERATIONS ON PATIENTS IN COMA FROM THE
EFFECTS OF CEREBELLOPONTILE TUMORS

There is one exception to the above generalization concerning the removal of the tumor, viz., patients in coma from this type of tumor.

I have excluded from the operative mortality of total extirpations, two patients who entered the hospital when totally unconscious and who were operated upon while in this state. One patient had been unconscious 8 hours, the other 3, when the operation began, and in each there was Cheyne-Stokes type of breathing. Furthermore, in the first instance the location of the growth was entirely unknown until determined by ventricular estimation. The treatment, if any, for such cases is, I believe, distinctly a different problem from that which obtains when patients are in coma from tumors situated elsewhere in the cranial chamber. When patients are comatose from intracranial pressure, it is often possible to restore consciousness by a palliative, properly placed decompression; and at times the tumor may even be safely removed while the patient is still unconscious, all of course depending on the depth and duration of coma and the location and character of the tumor. In many such cases it is incumbent and preferable only to relieve the intracranial pressure immediately and the removal of the tumor can await a second stage, if advisable.

But, as said before, coma from cerebellopontile tumors is not amenable to relief from any form of decompression. Even when the patient is quite conscious and in good condition, a suboccipital decompression is tantamount to a mortality in the advanced stages of intracranial pressure. The realization of the futility of operative palliation in these tumors urged the more radical attempt at removal of the tumor after first curetting the interior. Despite the fact that the extirpation was easy and bloodless in both instances, consciousness was not restored, there was no relief, and death followed within a few hours. In such cases we are dealing with a brain stem already severely injured before the operation began and any operation entailing even the slightest additional injury (such as the removal of the tumor must necessarily be exact), could not be tolerated, even with relief of the supratentorial pressure.

Whether the partial intracapsular procedure would ever be successful under such conditions, one can only conjecture. Realizing as we do now the underlying differences between the coma of these and other tumors, it would surely have been wiser to have desisted, though the results would hardly have been different. This particular phase of the problem seems very dismal from our present knowledge and experience. I fear some new and totally different line of attack must be evolved if any results are to be expected in such cases. One great difficulty in these comatose patients is the differentiation beforehand of the kind of tumor, though its location in the posterior fossa may be clear. For tumors other than the cerebellopontile variety (such as intracerebellar tumors), a cerebellar decompression would always be indicated and would frequently prove effective treatment. When the character of the tumor has been determined only by operation, one is faced with the problem of proceeding with operative treatment. And when patients in coma from the effects of cerebellopontile tumors have been subjected to operation, decompression alone will surely be fatal; one can hardly do less than perform the operation devised by Cushing, and surely not more.

SUMMARY

An operative procedure is presented by which cerebellopontile (acoustic) tumors can be completely removed. After a thorough and carefully guarded intracapsular enucleation, the capsule of the tumor is painstakingly dissected from the brain stem.

REFERENCES

1. BAISCH, B. Ueber Operationen in der hinteren Schaedelgrube. Beitr. z. klin. Chir., 1908, lx, 479.
2. BALLANCE, C. A. Some points in the Surgery of the Brain and Its Membranes. London: Macmillan Co., 1907.
3. BORCHARDT, M. Zur Operation der Tumoren des Kleinhirnbrueckenwinkels. Berl. klin. Wchnschr., 1905, xlii, 1033.
4. COTTERILL. Remarks on the surgical aspects of a case of cerebellopontine tumor by Bruce. Tr. Med.-Chir. Soc., Edinb., 1899, xviii, 215.
5. CUSHING, H. Tumors of the Nervus Acousticus. Philadelphia and London: W. B. Saunders Co., 1917.
6. DANDY, W. E. An operation for the total extirpation of tumors in the cerebello-pontine angle. A preliminary report. Johns Hopkins Hosp. Bull., 1922, xxxiii, 344.
7. Idem. The space-compensating function of the cerebrospinal fluid—its connection with cerebral lesions in epilepsy. Johns Hopkins Hosp. Bull., 1923, xxxiv, 245.
8. Idem. The diagnosis and localization of spinal cord tumors. Ann. Surg., 1925, lxxxi, 223.
9. EISELSBERG, A. VON, AND RANZI, E. Ueber die chirurgische Behandlung der Hirn- und Rueckenmarkstumoren. Verhandl. d. deutsch. Gesellsch. f. Chir., 1913, xliii, 514.
10. FRAZIER, C. H. Remarks upon the surgical aspects of tumors of the cerebellum. New York M. J., 1905, lxxxi, 272 and 332.
11. HOLMES, GORDON. Acoustic tumours. Proc. Roy. Soc. Med., Sect. Otol., 1923, xvi, pt. iii, p. 40.
12. KRAUSE, F. Zur Freilegung der hinteren Felsenbeinflaeche und des Kleinhirns. Beitr. z. klin. Chir., 1903, xxxvii, 728.
13. LEISCHNER, H. Zur Chirurgie der Kleinhirnbrueckenwinkeltumoren. Mitt. a. d. Grenzgeb. d. Med. u. Chir., 1911, xxii, 675.
14. MEYER, WILLY. Craniectomy for tumor of the acoustic nerve. Ann. Surg., 1909, xlix, 552; also 1912, lv, 323.
15. PANSE, R. Ein Gliom des Akustikus. Arch. f. Ohrenh. 1904, lxi, 251.
16. POPPERT. Exstirpation eines Tumors des Kleinhirnbrueckenwinkels. Deutsche med. Wchnschr., 1907, xxxiii, 613.
17. QUIX, F. Ein Acusticustumor. Arch. f. Ohrenh., 1911, lxxxiv, 252.
18. TOOTH, H. H. The treatment of tumours of the brain and the indications for operation. Tr. XVIIth Internat. Cong. Med., Lond., 1913, Sect. vii., Surg. p. 203.
19. TROTTER, W. Surgical treatment of eighth nerve tumours. Proc. Roy. Soc. Med., Sect. Otol., 1923, xvi, pt. iii, 37.
20. WALSHE, F. M. R. Acusticus tumours, Proc. Roy. Soc. Med., Sect. Otol., 1923, xvi, pt. iii, 32.

THE prognosis of patients with intracranial neoplasms has steadily improved since the first attempts at their removal were made in the nineteenth century.[50,51] Much of this progress has been attributed to the introduction of modern diagnostic procedures and the development of supportive techniques such as the transfusion of blood and the administration of antibiotics and intravenous fluids. But the greatest single contribution to the improvement in the prognosis of these patients was made by Harvey Cushing when he introduced the principles and standardized the techniques of meticulous cerebral surgery.[52,53]

The early operations for brain tumors

" . . . were all done by general surgeons who had no training or experience in brain surgery and no special interest in it; they simply felt compelled 'to do a brain case' and report it in order 'to keep up with Jones.' One unhappy experience usually sufficed to rid the general surgeon of his compulsion to be a 'brain surgeon,' and only the rare individuals let themselves in for another similar experience. A survey of the Surgeon General's Index Catalogue for the years 1886 to 1896 revealed the amazing fact that during the 10 year period immediately following the successful removal of a brain tumor by Horsley, more than 500 different general surgeons reported operations performed upon the brain! The fact that in the next 10 years from 1896 to 1906 the number of surgeons reporting cases had fallen to less than 80 reflected discouragement and a beginning return to sanity. . . . "[43]

Dr. Philip C. Knapp, a leading neurologist at the turn of the century, was one of several observers who collected the results of these early operations for brain tumors.[3—6,28,35—40, 42,44—46] By 1906,

" . . . he was able to see some improvement, due he says to the improvement in surgical technic, but even so the results were far from encouraging. In this final report Knapp was able to collect from the literature 828 cases of brain tumor which had been operated upon. Out of this number, 471 of the tumors were said to have been 'removed,' but as we now understand it, the removal in many in-

stances, even of the benign growths, was doubtless far from complete. In the remaining 357 cases the tumor was not removed, and there were 265 deaths in the series, a mortality of 32 per cent. . . .

"After the year 1906, when Knapp had collected his dreary operative statistics on brain tumors, a great deal of progress was made during the next decade. In 1913 Tooth[48] analyzed a series of 500 probable tumors from the National Hospital, Queen Square, and of these, 265 had been operated upon between 1902 and 1911, in the majority of instances unquestionably by Sir Victor Horsley. Out of the 265, there were 187 verified tumors and from this number there were at least 83 operative deaths, a mortality of 44 per cent. Nevertheless, there were 31 patients living at the time of Tooth's paper, a much better record than the figures Knapp had indicated in 1906. . . . "[33]

"Keen[34] in 1892 advised that cerebral tumors be enucleated, if possible, with the finger, but if this were impossible, then a knife, scissors, sharp spoon or ordinary teaspoon be used to remove the entire mass piecemeal. If the tumor were subcortical, then a tiny incision was made into the cortex and the tumor could be palpated and removed with the little finger.

"This rapid removal of tumors was common practice until the advent of Cushing with his slow careful technique. In his 1908 monograph[7] he stated, 'An encapsulated tumor may be shelled out of its bed, with but little bleeding, by careful manipulations and the proper use of cotton which I prefer to hot irrigations as a hemostatic. When the cortex is to be incised above a tumor which has not reached the surface, the individual cortical vessels radiating from it must be doubly ligated with delicate strands of split silk, and the cortex incised between ligatures. Below the cortex there is often surprisingly little bleeding. The brain must be carefully separated from the growth with smooth, fairly blunt dissectors, and if bleeding occurs, a pledget of cotton is placed in the gap while another side is worked upon. In this way, by slow dissection, the tumor can often be clearly outlined with but little loss of blood and the production of no shock. The attempt to hurriedly dislocate a tumor outward by plunging fingers into the brain is atrocious. There should be a legal penalty imposed for 'speeding' in brain surgery.' ([7], p. 240.)"[30]

"Tooth's figures of Horsley's tumor patients were . . . eclipsed . . . by the statistics offered by

Cushing [8] in 1915. In this report, which was an elaboration of his discussion of a paper by Professor Küttner on the operative treatment of brain tumors, Cushing reviewed the current operative mortality statistics pertaining to brain tumors as published at that time by the leading surgeons doing this type of work. Küttner's own mortality was 45 per cent; that of Krause about 50 per cent; and of Eiselsberg 38 per cent. We have seen that Horsley's mortality was in this general neighborhood. Cushing astounded his listeners by submitting a mortality figure of 6.6 per cent for supratentorial tumors, and of 17 per cent for those below the tentorium or a combined mortality of 8.4 per cent for all patients operated upon. A further feature of extreme importance in Cushing's report was the fact that he had lost but one patient from meningitis, whereas in the Vienna series 10.5 per cent, and in the London series 11.7 per cent, of the patients had succumbed from this type of infection. As Cushing pointed out, the reason for this absence of sepsis in his cases was due to his careful closure of the galea as well as of the skin, thus preventing the wounds from breaking down, with the resultant fungus and meningitis."[33]

During the ensuing years Dr. Cushing and his associates encountered a large number of intracranial tumors, which they classified, studied, and treated.[1,2,9-27,31,41,49,54] Our present knowledge of brain tumors is largely based on these experiences.

In 1931 Dr. Cushing performed an operation which

" . . . served to verify the 2000th brain tumor in his series. Without his knowledge the staff had made elaborate preparations for photographs, movies, and a gala tea party reminiscent of that held on his sixtieth birthday. . . .

"Louise Eisenhardt, fully prepared for the occasion, had all the tumor statistics available and was able to point to a steady lowering of Cushing's mortality rate during the previous ten years, save for a brief increase . . . immediately after the introduction of electrosurgical methods. Since there was no other comparable tumor series with which to compete, Cushing had become consumed with a desire to improve his own figures from year to year. He accordingly began in earnest to prepare on these lines for the 'paper' to be read at the International Neurological Congress in Berne —a paper which grew into a monograph and was later published by his friend, Charles Thomas[20-22] . . . ."[29]

At a meeting of the American Neurological Association on May 24, 1931, Dr. Cushing gave a preliminary account of

" . . . the mortality statistics pertaining to his large series of verified brain tumors, a grand total of 2,023 patients, 1,870 of whom were operated upon.[16,20] There were 382 postoperative deaths, namely, patients who died in the hospital from any cause whatever after operation, giving a case mortality of 20.4 per cent. This series, of course, included all of Dr. Cushing's brain tumor patients, starting with his earliest experiences in Baltimore in 1902. When the extremely high mortality of the early years is considered, it is indeed amazing that his total mortality was as low as it proved to be. As a contrast to the figures for the whole series, Cushing included the statistics for the three years previous to the communication. These showed that 412 patients with verified intracranial growths had been operated upon during that time, with 55 postoperative deaths, a case mortality of 13.3 per cent. . . . "[32]

A few months later Dr. Cushing presented a revised version of the same material at the First International Neurological Congress in Berne.[17-19] Twenty-five of his pupils attended, most of them to hear Dr. Cushing present his paper.

"Much of the life of the Congress centered about Dr. Cushing. He was returning after thirty years to the town where he grew up, as it were, and where he received the greatest inspiration for his life's work—and he was returning now to give an account of himself in the interval. . . .

"The Congress opened on Monday, 31 August, in the Municipal Casino. The high point of this session was the awarding (by the University of Berne) of honorary degrees to Cushing and Sir Charles Sherrington. That the degrees were to be given had been kept in the utmost secrecy and was to be a surprise to both of the recipients. Considerable difficulty was encountered in persuading Cushing that his presence at the session was imperative, for as usual he was belatedly putting the finishing touches on his paper for the afternoon session. . . .

"In the introduction to his paper, fourth on the program of the afternoon session, Cushing described his experiences in Berne in 1900–1901. At the beginning he spoke somewhat haltingly, but within a few minutes the hall was silent as he described the various factors which had led to the dramatic fall in his mortality rate in cerebral operations. 'Younger men,' he went on to say, 'picking up where I leave off, can reduce the mortality still further.' Then came the devastating and unexpected climax: 'Gentlemen, this will be the last report on the statistical results of brain tumors as a whole that I shall ever publish.' After a moment of complete silence there was a burst of prolonged applause. The Chairman, Ariëns Kappers of Amsterdam, broke the precedent of no votes of thanks for individual papers by expressing heartfelt gratitude to Cushing in the name of the Congress for placing before them in such an inspiring way the brilliant results of his life's work."[29]

Since Dr. Cushing's death in 1939, his patients have been followed through the Brain Tumor Registry at the Yale University School of Medicine. At the Second International Congress of Neurological Surgery held in Washington, D. C. in 1961, Dr. Eisenhardt reported that a large number of these patients were still living 30–50 years after the removal of a glioma.[27] Dr. Cushing's outstanding accomplishments in the treatment of brain tumors have remained a challenge for the neurosurgeons of today.

References

1. BAILEY, P. Intracranial tumors. *Springfield, Ill.: Charles C Thomas*, 1933, xxii, 475 pp. ·
2. BAILEY, P., and CUSHING, H. A classification of the tumors of the glioma group on a histogenetic basis with a correlated study of prognosis. *Philadelphia: J. B. Lippincott Co.*, 1926, 175 pp.
3. BALLANCE, C. A. Some points in the surgery of the brain and its membranes. *London: Macmillan & Co.*, 1907, xv, 405 pp.
4. VON BERGMANN, E. Die chirurgische Behandlung von Hirnkrankheiten. *Berlin: A. Hirschwald*, 1889, 2nd ed., 189 pp.
5. BRUNS, L. Die Geschwülste des Nervensystems. Hirngeschwülste.—Rückenmarks- und Wirbelgeschwülste. Geschwülste der peripheren Nerven. *Berlin: S. Karger*, 1908, 2nd ed., xvi, 480 pp.
6. CHIPAULT, A. Chirurgie opératoire du système nerveux. *Paris: Rueff & Cie*, 1894–1895, 2 vols.
7. CUSHING, H. Surgery of the head. In: *Surgery, its principles and practice*. W. W. Keen, Ed. Philadelphia: W. B. Saunders Co., 1908, *3:* 17–276.
8. CUSHING, H. Concerning the results of operations for brain tumor. *J. Amer. med. Ass.*, 1915, *64:* 189–195.
9. CUSHING, H. Tumors of the nervus acusticus and the syndrome of the cerebellopontile angle. *Philadelphia: W. B. Saunders Co.*, 1917, viii, 296 pp.
10. CUSHING, H. Brain tumor statistics. *Med. Rec., N.Y.*, 1920, *97:* 417–418.
11. CUSHING, H. Distortions of the visual fields in cases of brain tumour. (Sixth paper) The field defects produced by temporal lobe lesions. *Brain*, 1922, *44:* 341–396.
12. CUSHING, H. Notes on a series of intracranial tumors and conditions simulating them. Tumor suspects; tumors unverified; tumors verified. *Arch. Neurol. Psychiat., Chicago*, 1923, *10:* 605–668.
13. CUSHING, H. Studies in intracranial physiology and surgery. The third circulation. The hypophysis.

The gliomas. *London: Humphrey Milford*, 1926, xii, 146 pp.
14. CUSHING, H. Experiences with the cerebellar medulloblastomas. A critical review. *Acta path. microbiol. scand.*, 1930, *7:* 1–86.
15. CUSHING, H. Experiences with the cerebellar astrocytomas. A critical review of seventy-six cases. *Surg. Gynec. Obstet.*, 1931, *52:* 129–204.
16. CUSHING, H. The surgical mortality percentages pertaining to a series of two thousand verified intracranial tumors. Standards of computation. *Trans. Amer. neurol. Ass.*, 1931, 456–463. Also: *Arch. Neurol. Psychiat., Chicago*, 1932, *27:* 1273–1280.
17. CUSHING, H. Une série de deux mille cas de tumeurs intracraniennes vérifiées histologiquement. *Rev. neurol.*, 1931, *2:* 378.
18. CUSHING, H. The surgical-mortality percentages pertaining to a series of two thousand verified intracranial tumours. In: *Proceedings of the First International Neurological Congress (Berne, 1931)*. Berne: Stämpfli & Cie, 1932, xxv, 440 pp. (see pp. 73–78).
19. CUSHING, H. Bemerkungen über eine Serie von 2000 verifizierten Gehirntumoren mit der dazugehörigen chirurgischen Mortalitätsstatistik. *Chirurg*, 1932, *4:* 254–265.
20. CUSHING, H. Intracranial tumours. Notes upon a series of two thousand verified cases with surgical-mortality percentages pertaining thereto. *Springfield, Ill.: Charles C Thomas*, 1932, xii, 150 pp.
21. CUSHING, H. Intrakranielle Tumoren. Bericht über 2000 bestätigte Fälle mit der zugehörigen Mortalitätsstatistik. F. K. Kessel, Transl. *Berlin: J. Springer*, 1935, viii, 139 pp.
22. CUSHING, H. Tumeurs intracraniennes. Étude analytique de 2000 tumeurs vérifiées et de leur mortalité opératoire. J. Rossier, Transl. *Paris: Masson & Cie*, 1937, 194 pp.
23. CUSHING, H., and BAILEY, P. Tumors arising from the blood-vessels of the brain. Angiomatous malformations and hemangioblastomas. *Springfield, Ill.: Charles C Thomas*, 1928, x, 219 pp.
24. CUSHING, H., and EISENHARDT, L. Meningiomas. Their classification, regional behaviour, life history, and surgical end results. *Springfield, Ill.: Charles C Thomas*, 1938, xiv, 785 pp.
25. EISENHARDT, L. The operative mortality in a series of intracranial tumors. *Arch. Surg., Chicago*, 1929, *18:* 1927–1935.
26. EISENHARDT, L. Long postoperative survivals in cases of intracranial tumor. *Res. Publ. Ass. nerv. ment. Dis.*, 1935, *16:* 390–416.
27. EISENHARDT, L. Discussion of Tönnis.[47] IInd int. Congr. neurol. Surg. (Washington, D.C., 1961). *Excerpta med.*, 1961, No. 36, E10.
28. FRAZIER, C. H. Remarks upon the surgical aspects of tumors of the cerebellum. *N.Y. med. J.*, 1905, *81:* 272–280; 332–337.
29. FULTON, J. F. Harvey Cushing. A biography. *Springfield, Ill.: Charles C Thomas*, 1946, xii, 754 pp. (see pp. 604–608).
30. GREEN, R. E., and STERN, W. E. Techniques of intracranial surgery. In: *A history of neurological surgery*. A. E. Walker, Ed. Baltimore: Williams & Wilkins Co., 1951, xii, 583 pp. (see pp. 80–110).
31. HARVEY CUSHING SOCIETY. A bibliography of the

writings of Harvey Cushing. Prepared on the occasion of his seventieth birthday April 8, 1939 by the Harvey Cushing Society. *Springfield, Ill.: Charles C Thomas*, 1939, xv, 108 pp. (see pp. 59–89).

32. Horrax, G. Some of Harvey Cushing's contributions to neurological surgery. *J. Neurosurg.*, 1944, *1:* 3–22 (see p. 19).

33. Horrax, G. Neurosurgery. An historical sketch. *Springfield, Ill.: Charles C Thomas*, 1952, xi, 135 pp. (see pp. 70, 71, 86, 87).

34. Keen, W. W., and White, J. W. An American text-book of surgery, for practitioners and students. *Philadelphia: W. B. Saunders Co.*, 1892, xx, 1209 pp.

35. Knapp, P. C. The pathology, diagnosis and treatment of intra-cranial growths. *Boston: Rockwell & Churchill*, 1891, viii, 165 pp.

36. Knapp, P. C. The treatment of cerebral tumors. *Boston med. surg. J.*, 1899, *141:* 333–337; 359–363; 384–387.

37. Knapp, P. C. The results of operation for the removal of cerebral tumors. *Boston med. surg. J.*, 1906, *154:* 124–126.

38. Knapp, P. C., and Bradford, E. H. A case of tumor of the brain: removal; death. *Boston med. surg. J.*, 1889, *120:* 325–330; 353–359; 378–381; 386–388.

39. Kocher, T. Text-book of operative surgery. H. J. Stiles, Transl. *London: A. & C. Black*, 1903, xxv, 440 pp.

40. Krause, F. Surgery of the brain and spinal cord based on personal experiences. H. A. Haubold and M. Thorek, Transl. *New York: Rebman Co.*, 1909–1912, 3 vols.

41. Locke, C. E., Jr. A review of a year's series of intracranial tumors, June, 1920, to June, 1921. *Arch. Surg., Chicago*, 1921, *3:* 560–581.

42. Marion, G. Chirurgie du système nerveux. Crâne et encéphale. Rachis et moelle, nerfs. *Paris: G. Steinheil*, 1905, ii, 531 pp.

43. Scarff, J. E. Fifty years of neurosurgery, 1905–1955. *Int. Abstr. Surg.*, 1955, *101:* 417–513 (see pp. 419–421).

44. Starr, M. A. Brain surgery. *New York: William Wood & Co.*, 1893, xii, 295 pp.

45. Starr, M. A. A contribution to brain surgery, with special reference to brain tumors. *Med. Rec., N.Y.*, 1896, *49:* 145–150.

46. Starr, M. A. The results of surgical treatment of brain tumors. *J. nerv. ment. Dis.*, 1903, *30:* 398–407.

47. Tönnis, W. Gliomas. IInd int. Congr. neurol. Surg. (Washington, D.C., 1961). *Excerpta med.*, 1961, No. 36, E9–E10.

48. Tooth, H. H. The treatment of tumours of the brain, and the indications for operation. In: *Seventeenth international congress of medicine* (London, 1913). *London: H. Frowde*, 1913, Sect. 11, pt. 1, 279 pp. (see pp. 161–257).

49. Van Wagenen, W. P. Verified brain tumors. End results of one hundred and forty-nine cases eight years after operation. *J. Amer. med. Ass.*, 1934, *102:* 1454–1458.

50. Wilkins, R. H. Neurosurgical classic—I. *J. Neurosurg.*, 1962, *19:* 700–710.

51. Wilkins, R. H. Neurosurgical classics—II. *J. Neurosurg.*, 1962, *19:* 801–805.

52. Wilkins, R. H. Neurosurgical classic—V. *J. Neurosurg.*, 1963, *20:* 267–270.

53. Wilkins, R. H. Neurosurgical classics—VI. *J. Neurosurg.*, 1963, *20:* 366–369.

54. Wilkins, R. H. Neurosurgical classic—XVIII. *J. Neurosurg.*, 1964, *21:* 315–347.

19. The Surgical-Mortality Percentages pertaining to a Series of Two Thousand Verified Intracranial Tumours*[1]

by Prof. *Harvey Cushing*, Boston

Standards of computation. In calculating these mortality percentages the standard which we have set for ourselves is that *every death in hospital following an operation from any cause whatsoever, no matter how long the interval, is recorded as a postoperative fatality.* There is no possibility of any exception being made to this rule, however justifiable it might appear to be, for the record is automatically made by a secretary from the completed case record after the patient's hospital discharge, living or dead. Were this precaution not taken, those personally interested would, now and then, find the temptation to evade an admittedly severe standard well nigh irresistible.

But should one begin to make exceptions to the rule, there would be no end to them—a patient about to be discharged after a successful operation has a perforated gastric ulcer; another gets out of bed at night to go to the toilet, trips over an obstruction and dies in a few hours from a fracture of the base of the skull; another during an epidemic of influenzal pneumonia has a fatal infection; still another has a coronary thrombosis five weeks after making a perfect recovery from his tumour extirpation. Similar examples might be multiplied and were they not automatically recorded as postoperative deaths, the temptation to exclude fatalities from other complications more obviously postoperative, such as pulmonary embolism, postoperative pneumonia, tuberculous meningitis after the successful removal of a tuberculoma, and so on, would be difficult to re-

* Reprinted from *Proceedings of the First International Neurological Congress (Berne, 1931)*. Berne: Stämpfli & Cie, 1932, 73–78.

[1] This paper represents the last portion of the communication made at the International Neurological Congress in Berne, 1931. The mortality statistics for tumours of different kinds and situations, separately considered, which form the basis of these tables, has been published as a monograph: 'Intracranial Tumours,' by *Charles C Thomas*, Springfield (Illinois), 1932.

Has appeared in part in the Journal 'Der Chirurg' (Berlin), Band IV, Heft 7, April 1932; see also: 'Archives of Neurology and Psychiatry,' Vol. 27, June, 1932.

sist since no sharp line can be drawn between those due and those not due to the operation.

Having no convalescent home to which patients may be transferred and since a large proportion of them come from a distance, they are necessarily retained in hospital longer than would otherwise be necessary,[2] and there is ample time for intercurrent disorders to develop which bring additional risks. Another element which tends to increase the percentage of postoperative fatalities among histologically verified tumours is the high incidence (averaging over 90%) of postmortem examinations that are secured. Owing to this, many tumours are identified at autopsy which otherwise, owing to negative explorations, would have remained in the list of tumours unverified. What is more, we frequently retain in hospital for indefinite periods—five months in one instance— patients whose tumours we have failed surgically to verify with the understanding that in the end permission for an autopsy will be given.

Then, too, as was stated in another connection, the case mortality of all malignant gliomas, in the process of working out their life history, should theoretically be 100%; for if operations for recurrences are systematically pursued to the end, it is almost a certainty that the last of them will be followed by a postoperative fatality. With all these things to consider, it is obvious that the operative statistics of two surgeons with equal skill and experience may legitimately vary within wide limits.

In all calculations of operative-mortality percentages there is still another element to consider: viz., *What is and what is not to be recorded as 'an operation'?* Even though they may be attended with risk and lead to a fatality which permits postmortem verification of a tumour, we exclude, as all others would do, the simple punctures—lumbar, cisternal, transphenoidal or ventricular. Nor do we record as operations the minor surgical procedures necessary for the securing of muscle from the patient's leg, nor those for blood transfusions or those for ventriculography, even though the latter procedure may at times be hazardous and occasionally lead to a fatal issue. We do, however, record as separate operations those requiring

more than one session for their completion as they are almost invariably critical performances; and for the same reason we also record emergency re-elevations of osteoplastic flaps necessitated by postoperative clot formation.

Then there is a final point to be decided: viz., *When does the operation begin?* Does it begin with the ward preparations or with the anaesthetic or only after an incision has been made? In many patients with brain tumours having an advanced syndrome the condition at best is serious. Sudden respiratory failure may occur should a patient with a cerebellar tumour strain to expel a preparatory enema, or have the neck unduly twisted while the scalp is being shaved, or, in days when ether anaesthesia was employed, from the early effects of the anaesthetic. Many patients after such accidents have been immediately operated upon under artificial respiration and some few of them thus saved.

No surgeon would conceivably hesitate for a second to face emergencies of this kind though they are very bad for one's mortality percentages. In the last consecutive 50 operations for acoustic tumour, for example, one of the two recorded fatalities (cf. Table III) was that of a patient operated upon in an agonal state after a sudden respiratory failure. Had the surgeon been thinking of his score rather than of possibly saving a life, his mortality figures for this particular group of cases would have been cut in half. One must draw the line somewhere and it seems fair to do so with the incision of the scalp.

1. *Mortality percentages or the series as a whole.* The writer's experience in neuro-surgery may be divided into three decades; the first as a beginner at the Johns Hopkins Hospital, from 1901 to 1912; the second, with its lost ground difficult to regain, due to a two years' absence during the War; and the third, from 1922 to 1931, during which period detailed week-to-week statistical records with annual compilations of the intracranial tumours have been kept by Dr. *Eisenhardt*, who made a detailed report on the subject two years ago.[3] A highly condensed table (cf. Table IV) limited to the operative mortality percentages of the four major groups of verified

[2] The average hospital sojourn of the last 100 consecutive cases with surgically verified tumours has been 39 days.

[3] *Eisenhardt, L.* The operative mortality in a series of intracranial tumours. Arch. Surg., 1929, xviii; 1927–1935.

TABLE III. Showing Case-Mortality Percentages for Acoustic Tumours in Successive Groups of Fifty

Dates	Time Interval	Number Cases	Number Oper'ns	Number Deaths	Case Mortal.	Op'e Mortal.
Jan. 18, 1906—Oct. 5, 1915	9 years 9 mos.	21	32	6	28,6%	18,7%
Jan. 22, 1916—Feb. 13, 1923	7 years 1 mo.	50	64	10	20,0%	15,6%
Mar. 6, 1923—Sept. 6, 1927	4 years 6 mos.	50	62	7	14,0%	11,3%
Oct. 18, 1927—July 1, 1931	3 years 9 mos.	50	58	2	4,0%	3,4%

TABLE IV. Comparison of Operative Mortality Percentages for Verified Tumours of Four Major Groups Divided in Three Periods

	Hopkins Series to 1912	Brigham Series to 1929	July 1928 to July 1931
Gliomas (varia)	30,9%	17,8%	11,0%
Pituitary adenomas. . .	13,5%	5,3%	5,7%
Meningiomas	21,0%	10,3%	7,7%
Acoustic tumours. . . .	25,0%	11,5%	4,4%

tumours, as given in her paper, contrasted with the results the past three years, is appended.

2. *Mortality percentages year by year.* The preceding table shows, as would be expected, a progressive improvement in the figures that has come with the experience of later years. As a matter of fact, during each year of the last decade there has been a definite tendency to an annual lowering of the case and operative mortality as shown in Table V. This table gives the mortality figures for the cases discharged living or dead between May 1st and May 1st of each successive year. And were the figure included for the 549 patients admitted or readmitted with tumours unverified during these years, the percentages would be still lower in view of the relatively few fatalities (2,9% case mortality and 2,5% operative mortality) in the unverified group.[4]

This table points out, what the operating members of the neuro-surgical staff were themselves conscious of: namely, that in 1927 and 1928, on the introduction of electro-surgical methods, a number of patients, whose tumours when exposed had been regarded as inoperable, were called back and reoperated upon with a high mortality rate, partly because of the dangerous procedures undertaken and partly because of inexperience with electro-surgical principles.

[4] It should be clearly understood that the computations on which the figures in Table III are based represent each year's work taken by itself, including therefore both new and old patients, with primary operations as well as those for recurrences.

Apart from the figures for this particular 1927–1928 twelvemonth, there has been a slowly progressive decline in the mortality percentages with a pronounced drop during the last year, which came somewhat as a surprise even though we were aware that it has been a good year. This is all the more gratifying in view of the fact that as time goes on the clinic carries an ever increasing burden of patients readmitted for recurrence of symptoms; and though reoperations for medulloblastomas and glioblastomas are perhaps less readily undertaken than formerly, even the most conservative among us can hardly refuse to reoperate upon the less malignant lesions like meningiomas, neurinomas and astrocytomas when symptoms recur.

3. *Mortality percentages for the separate tumour groups.* These calculations are particularly illuminating in that they show how the percentages tumble so soon as the life history of any particular tumour has been thoroughly worked out. Of only a few tumours can it be said that this has been done with sufficient thoroughness to affect the operative results, but these few furnish striking illustrations. For example: The operative mortality of the once dreaded acoustic tumours (as shown in Table III) has fallen for each successive 50 cases from a 28% to 20% to 14% to 4% case mortality. The present operative mortality for the chromophobe adenomas, formerly *circa* 13%, has also dropped to slightly below 4 percent. The figures for the cerebellar astrocytomas, practically unknown ten years ago, have fallen from a 28% case mortality for the first 25 patients to 4% for the last 25 cases. Even the highly malignant glioblastomas of the cerebrum have shown a drop from 24% for the whole series to 14%; and now that the cerebellar medulloblastomas are better understood, even these—the most disheartening of all brain tumours—may be expected to show a great improvement in their operative percentages.

In Table VI, the mortality figures have been assembled, not only for the eleven major subdi-

TABLE V. Annual Statistics of Operations for Verified Tumours including New and Old Cases from 1922–1931

Successive May 1 to May 1	Number of patients	Patients operated on	Number of operations	Post-operative deaths	Case mortality (per cent)	Operative mortality (per cent)
1922–1923.	104	94	130	22	23,4	16,9
1923–1924.	156	140	190	26	18,6	13,7
1924–1925.	137	113	142	21	18,5	14,7
1925–1926.	155	133	172	25	18,8	14,5
1926–1927.	184	161	217	24	14,9	11,0
1927–1928.	185	149	183	28	18,7	15,3
1928–1929.	205	179	226	26	14,5	11,5
1929–1930.	178	147	191	24	16,3	12,5
1930–1931.	200	170	219	15	8,8	6,8
Total	1504	1286	1670	211	16,4	12,6

visions of the *verified tumours*, but separately for the *unverified tumours*. The table has been divided into two sections, the first giving the operative figures for the entire series which carries the heavy load of fatalities of the early years of inexperience. In the second section the figures are those only for the new cases that have first come under observation in the three-year period from July 1, 1928, to July 1, 1931.

This table, therefore, by the exclusion of old cases readmitted during the last three-year period because of the symptomatic recurrence of tumours imperfectly treated at an earlier day, gives a clearer idea of what results may reasonably be expected of those newcomers to neuro-surgery who can profit, not only by the present-day improvements in technique, but by the existing state of our knowledge regarding the life history of the various lesions. And should they take warning from the experience of others in avoiding over-radical attempts to remove large congenital craniopharyngiomas, in refraining from operating on obviously metastatic tumours, and in refusing all secondary operations for recurrences, they could easily attain a case mortality of four or five percent for the whole.

Factors influencing mortality percentages. These wholesale statistics, given in the last three tables, will serve, I hope, to give others who engage in like tasks something to play against. The more important figures are those which pertain to special tumours in special situations and they will be found in the body of the paper (to be published in another place) where the various lesions are separately considered. Had it not been for the industry of Dr. *Eisenhardt*, these calculations would never have been made; but now that they have been, they may well enough be published even though there is no reason for taking pride in what they show. The high mortality percentages of the early cases still cast their shadow over the figures for the complete series.

It has been erroneously assumed in some quarters that the improved results of recent years are due to earlier diagnoses rather than to greater skill and experience—in other words, that the neuro-surgeon of to-day deals with a selective list of relatively favourable lesions. This assumption is far from the actual facts. In reality, each year problems become more difficult than those of the year before. The proportion of patients admitted as «forlorn hopes» in the terminal stages of their malady, often after illjudged procedures at the hands of surgeons with little or no neuro-surgical training, is as large as it ever was. What is more, each succeeding year sees tumours surgically exposed, like tumours of the third ventricle, which formerly were regarded as hopelessly inaccessible. Hence, all things considered and in spite of the constant improvement in diagnosis and surgical technique, the operations as time passes become increasingly critical and difficult.

The principal steps which have made it possible not only to attack the more formidable problems of the present day but at the same time to lower the operative mortality may be chronologically enumerated: 1. the generally accepted methods of decompression to relieve tension; 2. such irre-

TABLE VI. Comparison of Mortality Percentages for Complete Series and Past Three Years

Verified tumours	Entire series (30 years)						New cases (past 3 years)				
	No. pts.	Pts. op. on	No. ops.	P. o. deaths	% Case mort.	% Op. mort.	No. pts.	No. ops.	P. o. deaths	% Case mort.	% Op. mort.
I. Gliomas (varia) . .	862	780	1173	202	25,9	17,2	198	282	31	15,7	11,0
II. Pituitary adenomas	360	349	403	25	7,1	6,2	59	70	4	6,8	5,7
III. Meningiomas . . .	271	260	489	54	20,8	11,0	69	103	8	11,6	7,7
IV. Acoustic tumours .	176	171	219	25	14,6	11,4	41	45	2	4,9	4,4
V. Congenital tumours (varia).	113	106	160	23	21,7	14,4	17	25	4	23,5	16,0
VI. Metastatic and invasive	85	63	80	18	28,6	22,5	10	11	4	40,0	36,4
VII. Tuberculomas and syphilomas . . .	45	40	49	15	37,5	30,6	4	5	0	0,0	0,0
VIII. Blood-vessel tumours	41	37	59	6	16,2	10,2	7	10	1	14,3	10,0
IX. Sarcomas (primary)	14	12	17	6	50,0	35,3	0	0	0	—	—
X. Papillomas	12	11	23	3	27,3	13,4	1	2	0	0,0	0,0
XI. Miscellaneous	44	41	63	5	12,2	7,9	6	9	1	16,6	11,1
Total	2023	1870	2735	382	20,4	13,9	412	562	55	13,3	9,8
Unverified tumours	859	496	557	12	2,4	2,2	66	73	0	0,0	0,0
Grand total	2886	2366	3292	394	16,6	11,9	478	635	55	11,5	8,7

proachable wound healing that secondary infections are practically unknown; 3. the separate closure of the galea by buried fine black silk sutures which has made the once dreaded fungus cerebri nigh forgotten; 4. in place of ether inhalation, the introduction by *de Martel* of local anaesthesia now supplemented when necessary by the rectal administration of tribromethanol; 5. the more precise tumour localisation which in obscure cases *Dandy's* ventriculography permits us to make; 6. the use of a motor-driven suction apparatus as an indispensable adjunct to every operation; and 7. the successive improvements in methods of haemostasis which since 1927 have been most advantageously supplemented by the introduction of electro-surgical devices.

But the operation itself is by no means the whole story. The after care is equally important for unsuspected complications may arise at any moment which if overlooked or neglected may wholly turn the scale. This has been well summarized in Dr. *Eisenhardt's* paper of two years ago:

Rarely is more than one major operation for tumour scheduled for one day. Most of the operations are carried through under local anaesthesia, and all are started in this way. Patients who have been subjected to a craniotomy are not moved from the operating suite until the danger of the formation of a postoperative extradural clot has passed. After critical cerebellar operations, particularly if inhalation narcosis has been necessitated, the patients are usually left on the table for several hours until they have fully recovered, and they are often kept in the operating suite for a number of days. Those with deglutitory difficulties must often be fed through the nares for prolonged periods. For charity patients who are in a critical condition, from this or some other cause, special nurses are provided and paid for out of a fund donated for the purpose.

Since this was written we have taken an additional safeguard: namely, in providing for the individed service of a highly trained nurse, who, while the surgeons are engaged in their time-consuming operations, can devote her attention to the more critically ill of the thirty or forty patients either awaiting operation or already operated upon whom we sometimes have under observation at one time. Unquestionably many lives have been saved in this way, for less experienced nurses or junior house officers can hardly be expected to appreciate the significance of symptoms which indicate that something is going wrong with a patient recently operated upon for a brain tumour; and a few hours' delay due to the misinterpretation or neglect of a warning signal may mean the difference between a fatality and a recovery.

Neurosurgical Classics—47 and 48

SINCE it was first performed in 1911, the operation of cordotomy has become a standard neurosurgical procedure. The background of this procedure is quoted from three authoritative sources, and the reports by Spiller and Martin,[15] and by Cadwalader and Sweet[3] are reprinted as they appeared in the *Journal of the American Medical Association* in 1912.

"From the time of the ancients, it was known that injury to the spinal cord produced a sensory and motor paralysis. It was a logical deduction that a surgical transection of the cord would eliminate all appreciation of pain below the cut but surgeons were loath to do this procedure because of the concomitant paralysis of motor function."[4]

"In 1910 Cushing[5] had suggested 'the deliberate transection, either of the entire cord or of the posterior columns alone, cephalad to the lesion' for intractable and excruciating pain from malignant spinal metastases. He performed such an operation in 1916, dividing the cord in the thoracic region with an entirely satisfactory result.[6] Previous to Cushing's operation, I had followed the same procedure in March, 1916."[1]

"In his work upon the anatomy and physiology of the human spinal cord, Müller[10] (1871) cited a case of stab wound involving one-half of the spinal cord and the opposite dorsal column, producing bilateral anesthesia for touch but causing analgesia only on the side opposite the lesion. A few years later Gowers[9] (1878) reported a case in which analgesia was complete but tactile sensation was unaffected following an antero-lateral injury of the cord, from which observation he concluded that it was this part of the cord that carried the fibers for the transmission of pain impulses. In 1889 Edinger[7] demonstrated the existence of the spinothalamic tract in new born cats and amphibians, and

Wallenberg in 1895[17] and 1901[18] contributed further to our knowledge of the spinothalamic tract in his studies of thrombosis of the posterior inferior cerebellar artery. It remained, however, for Spiller[13] (1905) to prove conclusively that it is the spinothalamic tract which carries pain and temperature impulses."[16]

"Spiller[13,14] reported, in 1905, a case in which pain and temperature appreciation was lost over the lower part of the body. As Spiller had diagnosed during life, bilateral tuberculomas of the lower thoracic spinal cord involving the anterolateral tracts were found at autopsy. In 1910 Petrén[11] came to a similar localization of the pain pathways in the anterolateral tracts on the basis of clinical studies. In 1910 Schüller[12] sectioned the anterolateral tracts in monkeys with the idea of ultimately using the procedure for the relief of spastic paralysis and tabetic crises. He named the operation 'chordotomie'."[4]

"The first cordotomy on man was made in January, 1911 by Martin at the instigation of Spiller[15]. . . . In 1912 Beer[2] cut the anterolateral tract for intolerable pain of metastases in the sacral plexus. The patient was walking, free of pain, in eleven days.

"Quite unaware of these operations Foerster[8] reported that he and Tietze sectioned the anterolateral tracts for tabetic pain in December, 1912 . . . Frazier developed the operation in America and Foerster in Europe."[4]

REFERENCES

1. ARMOUR, D. Lettsomian lecture on the surgery of the spinal cord and its membranes. *Lancet*, 1927, 1: 423–430; 533–537; 691–698.
2. BEER, E. The relief of intractable and persistent pain due to metastases pressing on nerve plexuses by section of the opposite anterolateral column of the spinal cord, above the entrance of the involved nerves. *J. Amer. med. Ass.*, 1913, 60: 267–269.
3. CADWALADER, W. B., and SWEET, J. E. Experimental work on the function of the anterolateral

column of the spinal cord. *J. Amer. med. Ass.*, 1912, *58:* 1490–1493.

4. CRAWFORD, J. V., and WALKER, A. E. Surgery for pain. In: *A history of neurological surgery.* A. E. Walker, Ed. Baltimore: Williams & Wilkins Co., 1951, xii, 583 pp. (see pp. 308–330).

5. CUSHING, H. The special field of neurological surgery: five years later. *Johns Hopk. Hosp. Bull.*, 1910, *21:* 325–339.

6. CUSHING, H. The special field of neurological surgery after another interval. *Arch. Neurol. Psychiat.*, Chicago, 1920, *4:* 603–637.

7. EDINGER, L. Vorlesungen über den Bau der nervösen Centralorgane des Menschen und der Thiere für Aerzte und Studirende. *Leipzig: F. C. W. Vogel*, 1900–1904, 2 vols.

8. FOERSTER, O. Vorderseitenstrangdurchschneidung im Rückenmark zur Beseitigung von Schmerzen. *Berl. klin. Wschr.*, 1913, *50:* 1499.

9. GOWERS, W. R. A case of unilateral gunshot injury to the spinal cord. *Trans. clin. Soc. Lond.*, 1878, *11:* 24–32.

10. MÜLLER, W. Beiträge zur pathologischen Anatomie und Physiologie des menschlichen Rückenmarks. *Leipzig: L. Voss*, 1871, 41 pp.

11. PETRÉN, K. Ueber die Bahnen der Sensibilität im Rückenmarke, besonders nach den Fällen von Stichverletzung studiert. *Arch. Psychiat. Nervenkr.*, 1910, *47:* 495–557. Also: *Upsala LäkFören. Forh.*, 1910, n.f. *15:* 211–285.

12. SCHÜLLER, A. Ueber operative Durchtrennung der Rückenmarksstränge (Chordotomie). *Wien. med. Wschr.*, 1910, *60:* 2292–2296.

13. SPILLER, W. G. The location within the spinal cord of the fibers for temperature and pain sensations. *J. nerv. ment. Dis.*, 1905, *32:* 318–320.

14. SPILLER, W. G. The occasional clinical resemblance between caries of the vertebrae and lumbothoracic syringomyelia, and the location within the spinal cord of the fibres for the sensations of pain and temperature. *Univ. Penn. med. Bull.*, 1905, *18:* 147–154.

15. SPILLER, W. G., and MARTIN, E. The treatment of persistent pain of organic origin in the lower part of the body by division of the anterolateral column of the spinal cord. *J. Amer. med. Ass.*, 1912, *58:* 1489–1490.

16. STOOKEY, B. The management of intractable pain by chordotomy. *Res. Publ. Ass. nerv. ment. Dis.*, 1943, *23:* 416–433.

17. WALLENBERG, A. Acute Bulbäraffection (Embolie der Art. cerebellar. post. inf. sinistr.?) *Arch. Psychiat. Nervenkr.*, 1895, *27:* 504–540.

18. WALLENBERG, A. Anatomischer Befund in einem als "acute Bulbäraffection (Embolie der Art. cerebellar. post. inf. sinistr.?)" beschriebenen Falle. *Arch. Psychiat. Nervenkr.*, 1901, *34:* 923–959.

THE TREATMENT OF PERSISTENT PAIN OF ORGANIC ORIGIN IN THE LOWER PART OF THE BODY BY DIVISION OF THE ANTEROLATERAL COLUMN OF THE SPINAL CORD*

WILLIAM G. SPILLER, M.D.

PROFESSOR OF NEUROPATHOLOGY IN THE UNIVERSITY OF PENNSYLVANIA

AND

EDWARD MARTIN, M.D.

JOHN RHEA BARTON PROFESSOR OF SURGERY IN THE UNIVERSITY OF PENNSYLVANIA

PHILADELPHIA

Remarks by Dr. Spiller

Occasionally the pain from tumor of the cauda equina is so intense that complete division of the spinal cord has been suggested for its relief, and it is only recently that I have seen a case in which this measure had been proposed. If division of the anterolateral columns alone will remove pain, it may be possible, if the other parts of the cord be left intact, to avoid paralysis of the lower limbs and of the bowels and bladder by this operation. It probably would produce ataxia. Such an operation may be considered only in extreme cases when life has become almost a burden because of severe suffering.

A. Schüller[1] has suggested that as a substitution operation partial division of the spinal cord might be employed instead of section of the posterior roots for spasticity and gastric crises. The posterior columns, he suggests, might be cut for spasticity either alone or with the direct cerebellar tracts; the anterolateral columns might be cut for gastric crises. He reported no cases in which this operation was performed, and he advised it for these two conditions.

I would suggest that the operation of division of the anterolateral columns is applicable for pain independent of gastric crises, and that it may be much more than an *Ersatzoperation* for division of the posterior roots. So far as I know, the case reported in this paper is the only one in which this operation has been done.

On what is this operation for the relief of persistent pain based? Are fibers of pain confined to one system within the spinal cord, and if so, can pain sensations be conveyed by other systems when the fibers usually employed for this purpose are destroyed? These are important questions.

Head and Holmes,[2] in their recent Croonian lectures, refer to the work of Rivers and Head, in which it was shown that beneath the skin, independent of all "touch" and "pain spots," lies an afferent system capable of a wide range of functions. Pressure which in ordinary life would be called a touch can be appreciated and localized with considerable accuracy. Increase of pressure, especially on bones and tendons, will cause pain.

---

* Reprinted from *The Journal of the American Medical Association*, 1912, *58:* 1489–1490, with the kind permission of the Editor.

[1] Schüller: Wien. med. Wchschr., 1910, p. 2292.

[2] Head and Holmes: Lancet, London, Jan. 6, 1912.

In the peripheral mechanism, therefore, there are two independent mechanisms for the initiation of pain. Within the spinal cord, however, the conditions are different. All impulses capable of generating pain become grouped together in the same path and can be disturbed simultaneously by an appropriate lesion of the spinal cord. In the same way, sensibility to heat or cold may be lost independently of one another, showing that all the impulses on which they are based have been sorted out into two functional groups, each of which passes by a separate system in the spinal cord. It should be possible, therefore, to divide the tracts for the conduction of pain sensation with little damage to the rest of the cord, except that the fibers of temperature sensation probably would be implicated. It is questionable whether objective disturbance of sensation would be produced by such an operation, and, if it were, whether it would be persistent.

Fabritius[3] recently has stated that little attention has been paid in neurology to the late results of interruption of the temperature and pain tracts in the spinal cord. It is in general assumed that the disturbance in these sensations gradually disappears, but if one attempts to determine on what this opinion depends he meets with difficulty. Fabritius was not able to find any extensive investigation of this subject, and he attempts to fill the gap by collecting cases from the literature. The summary of his findings is that after stab-wounds of the spinal cord no regularity exists in the restoration of pain and temperature sensations. In the majority of the cases (twenty-three out of thirty-five) temperature sensation seems to have been permanently lost. Pain sensation returned more frequently, but in diminished intensity, namely in eighteen out of thirty-eight cases, but was permanently lost in sixteen cases. It is questionable whether all the statements regarding sensation in these cases can be accepted as accurate.

Rothmann,[4] in a paper read at the recent meeting of the Gesellschaft deutscher Nervenärzte, gave as the results of his investigations that pain sensations are conducted essentially through the anterior part of the lateral column, and that the gray matter may be concerned in this function, but concerning the latter statement the report is not very definite.

The work of Petrén[5] and my own studies[6] of the location of pain fibers within the spinal cord lead to the conclusion that fibers for the conduction of pain are located in the anterolateral columns.

In order to make a test of this reasoning in a very severe case of tumor of the lower part of the cord, when pain was intolerable, I referred a patient to Dr. Edward Martin for division of the anterolateral column on each side. Dr. W. B. Cadwalader and Dr. J. E. Sweet later performed the same operation on dogs to further our knowledge in respect to the function of these columns.

Patient.—A man, aged 47, was admitted to the Philadelphia General Hospital, March 8, 1909, in my service, and came later under the care of my colleagues on the staff. He had had pain for two months in the knees

[3] Fabritius: Monatschr. f. Psychiat., u. Neurol., January, 1912.

[4] Rothmann: Monatschr. f. Psychiat. u. Neurol, January, 1912, p. 81.

[5] Petrén: Arch. f. Psychiat., xlvii, 495.

[6] Spiller: Univ. of Penn. Med. Bull., July and August, 1905.

and ankles, and at the time of admission had pain about the pelvis. The pain increased, and by August, 1909, he complained greatly of it and had almost complete flaccid paralysis of the lower limbs, with loss of tendon-reflexes, and paralysis of bladder and rectum. He had anesthesia over the buttocks and external genitalia and down the back of the thighs. The lower limbs were atrophied and faradic contractility was diminished.

Diagnosis.—In November, 1909, introduction of the finger into the rectum caused no contraction of the internal or external sphincter. Dr. W. P. Hearn operated and found a growth on the left side and lower part of the spinal cord about as large as a goose-egg, the cord being implicated by the tumor. It was regarded as malignant and irremovable.

In January, 1910, the man came again into my service and notes taken by me at that time record that he had very slight movement at each hip and in the left knee, and no movement elsewhere in the lower limbs. These limbs were greatly wasted. Sensations of touch, pain, heat and cold were lost in the back of each thigh and in all parts of the legs below the knees, although deep pin-prick seemed to be felt in the left calf and left foot. The tendon-reflexes were lost and the legs were contracted on the thighs and the thighs on the abdomen. Sensation in its various forms was preserved in the abdomen and front of the thighs. The man suffered greatly from pain in the lower limbs and required morphin every night for relief.

Operation.—The division of each anterolateral column was performed by Dr. Martin, Jan. 19, 1911. On January 22, there was great relief of pain in both lower limbs. The patient appeared very grateful for the relief from suffering and received only $\frac{1}{6}$ grain morphin on the day following the operation and a similar amount two days later, and this was given for the pain caused by the operation. The intern on the surgical service, who had the opportunity of observing the man constantly, believed that he was not suffering pain in the lower limbs. Sensation in its various forms objectively tested did not seem to be much impaired above the hip-joints. Pain was felt occasionally in the lower limbs during the three weeks following the operation, but the man was positive that it was less than before the operation.

Course.—In March, 1912, when he was again under my care, he lay in bed with his lower limbs greatly contracted and atrophied. Objective sensation was lost in the front of the thighs, but pain and pin-prick sensations were keen over the lower abdomen. His countenance expressed no pain and he never complained unless he was asked concerning his condition, when he would reply that he sometimes had pain. As he is a foreigner and not very intelligent, and his condition is pitiable, it is hard to judge whether he really has any pain from the tumor. The operation seems to have been successful in the diminution of pain. I should be unwilling to form an incorrect judgment regarding this case. When one remembers, however, that the pain from a malignant tumor of the lower part of the cord usually is excruciating and continues as the tumor implicates additional posterior roots, I think it may be said that the peaceful expression of this man's face is evidence that he has been greatly relieved by the operation. He has certainly not been made any worse, as his condition before the operation was very grave.

Remarks by Dr. Edward Martin

The problem presented by Dr. Spiller was the making of a transverse cut into the spinal cord, roughly 2 mm. in length, of a similar depth and with its posterior end 3 mm. anterior to the entrance of the posterior root, this cut to be bilateral. The only special instrument required was a small thin-bladed cataract knife, double-edged on its angled point, the latter being about 5 mm. long. Since in this individual case there was no need for conservation of the bone, the laminae and spinous processes of the sixth, seventh and eighth dorsal vertebrae were removed. The dura was split, retracted by threads, the cord was slightly lateralized by passing threads about the posterior roots and gently using them as tractors, and the cord incision was made on each side with very little bleeding. The wound was closed without drainage and, in so far as it was concerned, the aftercourse was uneventful.

The approach to the cord is greatly simplified and expedited—although it was not done in this case—by the use of the Hudson trephine and the Cryer bone-cutting instrument. By the help of these tools it is possible rapidly and safely to obtain, by unilateral resection, preserving the spinous processes, an exposure adequate for many forms of dural and cord intervention. It would certainly be so for a limited section, such as was practiced in this case, or for section of posterior roots. Such exposure leaves little or no subsequent crippling so far as the spinal column is concerned and is much simpler than an osteoplastic flap. In case of unilateral pain, uncontrollable by other means, cord section on the side opposite to that in which the pain is felt and sufficiently high to allow for the decussation of sensory fibers should be adequate.

2046 Chestnut Street.—1506 Locust Street.

EXPERIMENTAL WORK ON THE FUNCTION OF THE ANTERO-LATERAL COLUMN OF THE SPINAL CORD*

WILLIAMS B. CADWALADER, M.D.

INSTRUCTOR IN NEUROLOGY AND NEUROPATHOLOGY, UNIVERSITY OF PENNSYLVANIA

AND

J. E. SWEET, M.D.

ASSISTANT PROFESSOR OF SURGICAL RESEARCH, UNIVERSITY OF PENNSYLVANIA

PHILADELPHIA

The present investigation was undertaken at the suggestion of Dr. William G. Spiller, in order to determine what symptoms would be produced by destroying the anterolateral column, including Gowers' tract. In Gowers' original observation[1] he referred to a group of fibers situated in the anterolateral columns of the cord, which underwent degeneration from a lesion of the eleventh thoracic segment. He traced these degenerated fibers upward as far as the cervical region, and believed that they were concerned in the transmission of painful stimuli from the opposite side of the body.

Since that time innumerable clinical and pathologic studies seem to confirm Gowers' first impression. Experiments on animals, however, have not always lent support to this opinion, the results in some instances having been very confusing and even contradictory; indeed, Mott,[2] after cutting this tract in monkeys, concluded that its function was unknown. Bing,[3] experimenting on dogs, observed ataxia without disturbance of cutaneous sensation, but in his cases, as in Marburg's,[4] the area destroyed was chiefly the dorsal cerebellar tract or close to it. Bruce and Schäfer[5] conducted similar experiments on monkeys in which only the ventrolateral region was destroyed; they not only found sensation entirely normal, but, unlike Bing, could not demonstrate any sign of ataxia, though paralysis did occur. On the other hand, Lewandowsky,[6] Rothmann[7] and others rather positively state that section of Gowers' tract in dogs does produce a certain degree of analgesia.

In the following experiments our object was to completely destroy the anterolateral region, including Gowers' tract, and not to injure the area occupied by the dorsal cerebellar tract or any part of the gray matter. Dogs were chosen for purely extraneous reasons.

Under complete ether anesthesia an incision was made over two spinous processes and carried down directly to the bone; this incision was carried on as a subperiosteal resection of the processes and the laminae of the vertebrae, until the cord was exposed for about 3 cm. The dura was slit longitudinally in the midline and retracted on either side; the cord was then rolled over as gently as possible till the line of insertion of the ligamentum denticulatum was identified, believing this to correspond quite accurately to the posterior limits of the antero-lateral tract; a small knife was inserted immediately in front of that point and thrust obliquely forward, then cutting outward through the periphery of the cord. A similar incision was made at the corresponding point on the opposite side. There was little hemorrhage. The dura was closed with a fine silk suture and the wound repaired with catgut. Iodin and collodion were used for dressing. Wound healing was perfectly normal.

The dogs were carefully watched from day to day; generally the first observations recorded were made a day or two after operation, so that the effects of the operation itself might not be mistaken. Here we wish to point out one possible source of confusion. Any one at all familiar with animals, particularly the laboratory dog, should not lose sight of the fact that their general conduct and intelligence influences the manner in which they react to stimuli of any kind; even in health this

---

* Reprinted from *The Journal of the American Medical Association*, 1912, *58:* 1490–1493, with the kind permission of the Editor.

[1] Gowers: Diagnosis of the Diseases of the Cord, 1879.

[2] Mott: Brain, 1895, xviii, 1.

[3] Bing: Die Bedeutung der spinocerebellaren Systeme, Wiesbaden, 1907, Neurol. Centralbl., 1912, p. 270.

[4] Marburg: Arch. f. Physiol., suppl., 1904, p. 457.

[5] Bruce and Schäfer: Quart. Jour. Exper. Physiol., 1910, No. 3.

[6] Lewandowsky: Handbuch der Neurologie, pp. 773 and 779.

[7] Rothmann: Berl. klin. Wchnschr., 1906, No. 2, p. 47; ibid., 1901; Arch. f. Physiol., 1902, p. 154; Suppl., 1902, p. 440; Ztschr. f. klin. Med., 1902, xliv, 183; Neurol. Centralbl., 1911, p. 1207.

may differ very greatly. Each dog has his own peculiarity, and has a distinct individuality not unlike man. Many are extremely dull and apathetic and others highstrung, intelligent and active, and accustomed to responding quickly to the various stimuli originating through the association of friends and master. No doubt it was a thorough appreciation of these facts which led Lewandowsky and Kallisher to adopt their methods of training. Our dogs were not trained; nevertheless a careful estimate of individual traits and temperament was constantly kept in mind. In considering disturbances of sensation these facts are of the utmost importance and have therefore been referred to in detail.

After a period of time the dogs were killed and the brains and cords immediately removed and placed in Müller's fluid. The segment in which the incision had been made was mounted in celloidin and cut in serial sections in order to ascertain the exact limits of the area destroyed; sections were also made from each segment of the cord and parts of the medulla and pons, so that the course of degeneration could be followed.

In the following descriptions of cases the data have been given chronologically so as to show the course of the general symptomatology; then follows the microscopic study.

Dog 1.—Black and tan, short-haired male dog, weighing about 25 pounds. Operation Dec. 4, 1911. Cutting the anterolateral column of both sides in the seventh thoracic segment.

December 5: Incomplete weakness of both hind legs, more marked on right. Dog can stand but often falls behind. After falling it can rise on hind legs without evidence of weakness, but is awkward and can only stand a second or two before again falling. It frequently assumes curious positions as if kneeling, or may stand with right foot flexed so that dorsum of foot touches the floor; sometimes sits with weight on one leg which is crossed under rump. These positions do not seem to cause any discomfort, and appear to be from impairment of the sense of muscular position; it is very striking, and it even seems doubtful if there is any real motor weakness, the apparent weakness being due to uncertainty of ataxia. Sensation for pain tested with pin point and with hemostats shows definite impairment; dog reacts quickly in front legs and shoulders, and very slowly or not at all on hind legs. Extreme heat gives the same results.

December 8: Sensory tests gave same results. Ataxia seems definite and very striking, no motor palsy.

December 10: Sensory tests the same. Dog can stand on all four limbs without evidence of ataxia or of motor weakness. Ataxia very striking when in motion, trunk and rump involved, feet frequently crossed and seem to be misplaced so that dog often falls; curious positions when at rest as before, very striking. Both sides alike, possibly right side more ataxic.

Jan. 4, 1912: Bilateral ataxia of hind legs and rump very distinct in walking and running. Dog falls very frequently with hind leg. Curious position of legs seen less often than before. Painful faradic current causes slight or doubtful evidence of discomfort in hind legs and rump, but distinctly less marked than on front legs where it is positively painful. When applied to soles of feet, hind legs are drawn away but not promptly, while on soles of front feet legs are drawn away quickly and with vigor. Application of hemostats caudal to site of

operation is distinctly less painful than above operation-scar, though when attention is directed to the procedure, the dog seems to feel some discomfort very occasionally. For extreme heat the same holds true.

January 11: Ataxia is gradually recovering; no other change.

January 18: The same as on the 11th.

February 1: All sensory tests the same as before, but at times very confusing, depending very much on whether or not dog's attention is directed to what examiner is doing or to distant object. When attention is held by assistant then analgesia is very pronounced and unmistakable, but when attention is not diverted, sensation is affected, but not at all pronounced or even doubtful. Rapid examination might easily show that sensation was normal, but careful, frequent and prolonged examinations make it unquestionably correct that there is incomplete analgesia and thermo-anesthesia and pronounced bilateral ataxia of hind legs and no motor paralysis.

Dog 2.—Black and tan, long-haired male dog, weighing about 25 pounds. Operation Dec. 5, 1911; cutting the anterolateral column of both sides at seventh thoracic segment.

December 6: Dog cannot stand or walk on account of inability to use hind legs. Tendon-reflexes are equal and active. There is no spasticity nor do the hind legs feel exactly flaccid. Two sides are alike. Sphincters are not affected; no spontaneous pain. Application of hemostats over hind legs and also heated instrument seems to cause no discomfort; when it is applied to front legs dog reacts rather slowly so that conclusions are unreliable.

December 10: Ability to use hind legs voluntarily rapidly returning. Dog makes effort to stand and walk; can rise on hind legs but generally falls; muscular weakness very doubtful. Seems as if he had some loss of sense of muscular position; legs appear awkward. Pinching of skin over hind legs with hemostats does not seem to be appreciated; but when applied to front legs it is quickly recognized. Testing with heat perhaps the same but unreliable.

December 15: Loss of the sense of muscular position or ataxia very striking. No motor weakness. When standing at rest dog is inclined to lower head below line of shoulders, with hind legs somewhat further apart than normal and slightly rotated outward, vertebral column shows slight tendency to arching in lower thoracic and lumbar region; this varies from time to time; the tail is held in what may be a purposeful position, straight out from the body, varying in its angle as position of legs is changed, but generally curved, tip turned downward or laterally and more or less rigid at base. The general position is very like that assumed by a dog standing on a swing in motion, attempting to retain balance. In walking or running he repeatedly falls with hind legs, feet are often crossed but when moved are lifted clear of the floor, though not higher than normal. Rump sways a little. Dog often assumes unnatural positions, typical kneeling position, or stands on dorsum of foot, toes being in flexion, one or both hind legs may be crossed under rump when in sitting position. This does not seem to be in the least uncomfortable.

Pinching with hemostats and application of extreme heat over rump, hind legs and belly do not appear to be as distinctly or as quickly felt as when front legs are tested. At times there seems to be very decided analgesia but a few minutes later dog seems to feel quite well; although when compared to front legs there is a decided difference in reaction time. The tendon-reflexes are equal and active.

December 20: About the same as on the 15th.

December 29: Ataxia is somewhat less marked. Dog does not fall so often in walking and running. Sensation the same as before.

Jan. 4, 1912: Much the same as before. Application of painful faradic current gives exactly the same results as in first dog.

January 15: Sensory tests about the same. Analgesia seems definite at times while at another examination it seems very doubtful. Ataxia less marked; dog still falls when walking, but unnatural positions are assumed only very occasionally. In standing the position already described is still very striking.

January 24: Just the same.

February 6: Dog killed sixty-three days after the operation and the brain and cord removed for examination.

Conclusions: Ataxia very striking.

Impairment of sense of pain and for extreme heat and painful faradic current over lower half of body and lower extremities.

Microscopic examination showed that the anterior and lateral portions of the white columns of the cord had been destroyed on both sides. A line drawn through the posterior limits of this area would just bisect the central canal. Anteriorly it extended to a point which corresponded to the position of the most medially situated anterior root fibers. The ventral and dorsal cerebellar tracts were degenerated as far as the pons. In addition some of the degenerated fibers seen in the thoracic segments of the cord corresponded to the positions given by Edinger[8] for the spinotectal, spinothalamic, vestibulospinal and spinovestibular fibers. In segments below the area destroyed there were a few scattered degenerated fibers situated in the extreme lateral periphery. The pyramidal tract and von Monakow's bundles did not seem to be injured. The posterior columns were intact.

In both dogs motor paralysis was noted immediately following the operations, but it disappeared rapidly and was replaced by very marked ataxia. Why motor weakness should occur at all is difficult to explain, for we believe that Gowers' tract is sensory in function and the microscopic examination showed that the pyramidal and von Monakow's bundles were not injured. It may have been from temporarily disturbed vascular supply.

Rothmann has proved that when both the pyramidal tracts and von Monakow's bundles are destroyed, either in dogs or in monkeys, the resulting paralysis may not be permanent. He was forced therefore to conclude that volitional impulses might be conducted from the cortex by some other route. In this connection Schäfer's experiments are important. He cut Gowers' tract in monkeys and obtained motor weakness but without any evidence of ataxia or of cutaneous sensory disturbances. In order to explain the occurrence of paralysis he inclined to the opinion that voluntary impulses must be carried from the cortex down the cord by fibers which

arise in Deiter's nucleus, and pass through the ventral and anterolateral columns near the periphery, and represent therefore a subsidiary motor pathway. It does not seem possible to make a complete section of the anterolateral tracts without destroying these long descending fibers; in our cases they must have been destroyed, yet motor paralysis was not permanent. Microscopic examinations of the segments below the level of section did reveal some evidence of scattered descending degeneration; the great majority of degenerations, however, occurred above the area destroyed and extended in the ascending direction.

Consequently Schäfer's[9] explanation does not seem to us entirely satisfactory. The experiments of Mott and Sherrington,[10] on the other hand, are most suggestive. They divided the posterior roots of the nerves supplying the brachial plexus in a monkey and found that the arm was as much paralyzed for ordinary volitional movements as in other cases in which the motor nerves themselves were cut. This they attributed to the cutting off of sensory impulses which pass from the muscles to the cortex. Bastian, referring to these experiments, suggested that in consequence of dividing the posterior roots there must have been a loss of tone in the neuromuscular apparatus. This seems to us the most probable explanation, for we know that the fibers of Gowers' tract represent the secondary continuations of some of the posterior root fibers, and it is probable that the function of one is represented in part by the other. Furthermore, it is known that the fibers of Gowers' tract end chiefly in the cerebellum.

Inasmuch as our dogs did not show the ordinary signs of spastic paralysis and the apparent motor weakness gradually subsided, and ataxia became more and more apparent, and finally entirely replaced disturbance of voluntary motion, we believe that motor paralysis in the true sense never existed. But on account of a very profound derangement of the neuromuscular apparatus, together with impairment of cutaneous sensibility, a pseudoparalytic state or a true paralytic ataxia did occur, because sensory impressions which should pass through Gowers' tract had been cut off; and as the compensatory function of the remaining sensory tracts was being established the apparent paralysis gradually disappeared and ataxia which had previously been masked then became evident and remained permanent.

The character of the ataxia was similar to that described by Bing and Marburg and, according to them, should be expected, as the spinocerebellar tracts are essentially the afferent connections between the cerebellum and spinal cord. It seems to us that the rubrospinal and vestibulospinal fibers may, as Bing has lately indicated, repress efferent connections between the cerebellum and cord and their destruction might be partially responsible for the extreme incoordination; however, proof is lacking.

In regard to the occurrence of cutaneous sensory disturbances there is considerable difference of opinion. Schäfer, Bruce, Bing and others were unable to demonstrate definite cutaneous disturbances. On the other hand, Rothmann, Schuster,[11] Lewandowsky and others all agree that Gowers' tract in the dog does convey pain-

8 Edinger: Bau der nervosen Zentralorgane, Ed. 8, 1911.

9 Schäfer: Jour. Physiol., 1899, xxiv, 23.

10 Mott and Sherrington: Quoted in Schäfer's article.

11 Schuster: Monatschr. f. Psych., xx, No. 2.

ful sensations, though the posterior columns are also concerned. Why such contradictory views should be expressed we have no explanation to offer unless it is that the character of the dogs has not always been considered.

In concluding we feel certain that our dogs did have a definite, though incomplete, loss of cutaneous sensation for pain and for extreme heat, and very pronounced ataxia of the hind legs and rump. The fibers whose function it is to conduct painful sensations probably are connected with the thalamus and are situated close to the tractus spinocerebellaris ventralis, whose function is chiefly concerned in the regulation of purposive movements.

1710 Locust Street—301 St. Mark's Square.

To Victor Horsley belongs the credit for the first successful surgical removal of a neoplasm of the spinal cord.[1,2,4,13,15-18] This was not simply a feat of adroit excision of an uncommon lesion, but represented a significant advance in a new field of surgery.

The operation of laminectomy for spinal injuries had been known for more than a century, but it seldom had been performed because of the gravity of the operation, the danger of infection, and the probability that the cord was injured irreparably.[1,14,15] By 1887, despite the progress of antiseptic surgery, most medical authorities opposed laminectomy in humans.[12,15] In addition, antivivisectionists had created legal obstacles to the perfection of techniques of laminectomy in animals.[15] Horsley performed his operation in spite of these oppositions, and his fortunate success greatly stimulated the development of modern spinal surgery.

Prior to 1887, William Macewen had performed 3 successful decompressive laminectomies for "connective tissue tumors."[10-12] However, in none of these cases was a true neoplasm present.[17] On the other hand, at least 58 cases of verified tumors of the spinal membranes had been reported in the medical literature by 1888. Horsley[6] summarized their treatment and autopsy findings as follows:

"*Column 26. Treatment*

"For all the horrible sufferings of the fifty-eight cases in the Table, in only two was any treatment of avail, viz. Nos. 4 and 32. In the former case excision of a part of the growth relieved the pressure, and so the symptoms for a time.[8,9] In the second the complete removal of the growth has, it may be hoped, obtained permanent relief.[5-7] Unfortunately the condition of the patient, owing to the errors of diagnosis, has usually been made more hopelessly miserable by free use of the actual cautery, moxas and blisters, while in other instances the additional employment of mercury, iodide of potassium, &c., has been resorted to.

"*Column 27. Records of the Autopsy, especially with respect to the Presence or Absence of any other Lesion which, independently of the Tumour, would have caused Death.*

"The melancholy inspired by consideration of Column 26 is intensified by the facts of Column 27, for in no less than 74 per cent. of the extradural growths, and 83 per cent. of the intradural, the patient died simply from the direct effects of the tumour, *i.e.* from exhaustion (in a very large number of cases), owing to pain, &c., or from pyaemia owing to absorption from the bedsores, or from septic pneumonia, or from acute septic interstitial nephritis.

"Roughly speaking, therefore, about 80 per cent. of these miserable cases could have been relieved entirely by operation, and those which were hopeless might by relief of pressure have been granted a euthanasia.

"The simple effects of confinement and nerve exhaustion are seen in the four instances in which fatty degeneration is noted among the effects of the intradural growths."

Victor Horsley's experience as a neurophysiologist and brain surgeon had prepared him admirably for a pioneer role in the development of surgery of the spinal cord. His opportunity came in 1887 when William R. Gowers diagnosed a neoplasm of the spinal cord in a 42-year-old man and referred him to Horsley for treatment. The neoplasm was removed successfully on June 9, 1887, and the patient remained well up until the time of his death from another cause about 20 years later.[15]

The report of this case by Gowers and Horsley[6] together with discussion and conclusions is reprinted partially below. Horsley's review of 58 similar cases collected from the medical literature is omitted for the sake of brevity.

This operation opened the way to further successes in surgery of the spinal cord. Initially, however, Horsley's feat proved difficult to surpass. Of the 22 operations for tumors of the spinal cord reported by Starr 7 years later, there were 11 deaths, and only 6 patients showed improvement.[17] In fact, it was not until 1907 that an intramedullary neoplasm was removed successfully.[3,13,17]

References

1. ARMOUR, D. Lettsomian lecture on the surgery of the spinal cord and its membranes. *Lancet*, 1927, *1:* 423–430; 533–537; 691–698.
2. BALLANCE, C. Remarks and reminiscences. *Brit. med. J.*, 1927, *1:* 64–67.
3. v. EISELSBERG, A. F., and RANZI, E. Ueber die chirurgische Behandlung der Hirn- und Rückenmarkstumoren. *Arch. klin. Chir.*, 1913, *102:* 309–468.
4. ELSBERG, C. A. Tumors of the spinal cord & the symptoms of irritation & compression of the spinal cord & nerve roots. Pathology, symptomatology, diagnosis and treatment. *New York: P. B. Hoeber, Inc.*, 1925, viii, 421 pp. (see pp. 1–6).
5. GOWERS, W. R., and HORSLEY, V. Case of tumour of the spinal cord; removal; recovery. *Proc. roy. med. chir. Soc. Lond.*, 1885–1888, n.s. *2:* 406–409.
6. GOWERS, W. R., and HORSLEY, V. A case of tumour of the spinal cord. Removal; recovery. *Med.-chir. Trans.*, 1888, 2nd s. *53:* 377–428.
7. GOWERS, W. R., and HORSLEY, V. A case of tumour of the spinal cord: removal: recovery. *Brit. med. J.*, 1888, *1:* 1273.
8. JOHNSON, A. Fatty tumour from the sacrum of a child, connected with the spinal membranes. *Trans. path. Soc. Lond.*, 1857, *8:* 16–18.
9. JOHNSON, A. Fatty tumour connected with the interior of the spinal canal of the sacrum. *Trans. path. Soc. Lond.*, 1857, *8:* 28–29.
10. MACEWEN, W. Trephining of the spine for paraplegia. *Glasgow med. J.*, 1884, 4s. *22:* 55–58.
11. MACEWEN, W. Two cases in which excision of the laminae of portions of the spinal vertebrae had been performed in order to relieve pressure on the spinal cord causing paraplegia. *Glasgow med. J.*, 1885, 4s. *25:* 210–212.
12. MACEWEN, W. An address on the surgery of the brain and spinal cord. *Brit. med. J.*, 1888, *2:* 302–309.
13. MARKHAM, J. W. Surgery of the spinal cord and vertebral column. In: *A history of neurological surgery.* A. E. Walker, Ed. Baltimore: Williams & Wilkins Co., 1951, xii, 583 pp. (see pp. 364–392).
14. MARKHAM, J. W. The history of laminectomy prior to 1866. *Bull. Hist. Med.*, 1952, *26:* 375–384.
15. PAGET, S. Sir Victor Horsley. A study of his life and work. *London: Constable & Co. Ltd.*, 1919, xi, 358 pp. (see pp. 126–127).
16. ROGERS, L. The surgery of spinal tumours. *Lancet*, 1935, *1:* 187–191.
17. SCARFF, J. E. Fifty years of neurosurgery, 1905–1955. *Int. Abstr. Surg.*, 1955, *101:* 417–513.
18. THORWALD, J. The triumph of surgery. R. Winston and C. Winston, Transl. *New York: Pantheon Books, Inc.*, 1960, xi, 454 pp. (see pp. 162–190).

A CASE OF TUMOUR OF THE SPINAL CORD. REMOVAL; RECOVERY.*

BY W. R. GOWERS, M. D., F. R. S.,
AND
VICTOR HORSLEY, B.S., F.R.S.

Received March 8th—Read June 12th, 1888.

Medical History of the Case, by DR. GOWERS.

CAPT. G—, æt. 42, had good health until the year 1884. There was no history of syphilis. During 1883 and 1884 he endured much mental anxiety, and in the latter year he had a considerable mental shock—his wife was knocked down and run over in his presence, and he was able to save himself from a similar fate only by suddenly throwing himself backwards. Soon afterwards he began to suffer from a dull pain across the lower part of the back, which he thought was due to the strain of the accident. This pain passed away in the course of a few weeks and did not return. In June, 1884, he first felt a peculiar pain that was the most prominent symptom during the early part of his illness. It was localised in a spot beneath the lower part of the left scapula. This pain commenced suddenly one day while he was walking, and was continuous and severe for about a month. It was increased by active exertion and by the jolting of a carriage. Repeated examination failed to reveal any cause for it. After a time it became less, but was felt occasionally through the autumn and winter. By the spring it had all but ceased, and he was asked to go out to China on business. Before undertaking the journey he consulted a physician in London, who pronounced the pain to be an intercostal neuralgia and suggested that the voyage would probably do good. While Capt. G— was in the train, on the way to Brindisi, the pain returned in severe degree, at the same place, and of the same character. During the voyage it continued, varying in severity, but when he reached China it was so intense, and was so much increased by movement, that he could scarcely walk. A German doctor at Shanghai, after a course of Turkish baths had been tried without benefit, expressed the opinion that an aneurism was the cause of the pain. Digitalis and iodide of potassium were given, and the latter was increased to large doses by two English practitioners at Shanghai, who doubted, however, whether there was an aneurism. The pulse became curiously variable, changing from 120 in the morning to 75 in the afternoon. The pain continued, and some fainting attacks occurred, one of which was thought to be possibly epileptic in character. In October, 1885, still suffering much and very prostrate, he left China for England. During the voyage he improved in health, the faintings ceased, and the pain lessened, so that in December, 1885, he could walk a little. Walking had been interfered with only by the pain. Other physicians were consulted, and the rest of the winter was passed in the South of France. The improvement continued, and by the spring of 1886 he was so much better that he went on to Constantinople on business. While there the pain almost ceased. He returned to England in the middle of the summer, and, as the pain was still

* Reprinted in part from *Medico-chirurgical Transactions,* 1888, 2nd s. *53:* 377–428.

felt a little at times, he consulted other physicians and by them was sent to Aix-la-Chapelle. While he was there the pain returned in great severity and morphia was injected. In September, 1886, he returned to England, and the pain was then very severe, and, as before, was increased by movement so that he was again scarcely able to walk. The morphia was stopped and blisters applied. An aneurism was again suggested as the probable cause of the symptoms, and the use of morphia was resumed for a time, but was again discontinued at the wish of the patient himself. He became irritable; the continued pain seemed to lessen his power of self-control. So marked, indeed, was his mental state that the question was seriously raised whether he was quite sane, and whether this mysterious pain was anything like as severe as he described. He continued in this condition till the end of the year. In February, 1887, he again came to London for advice and consulted two physicians, who expressed the opinion that there was no organic disease and advised him to go abroad. During February and March there came on distinct loss of power in the legs. The left leg first became weak and a few weeks afterwards the right. In April he went abroad, and remained away from England for two months. During this time the weakness increased to complete loss of power, sensation became impaired, and the urine was retained in the bladder. Still the mental peculiarities were so conspicuous to those around him that fresh doubts were felt as to the reality of his symptoms, and it was suggested by someone that he should be put through a course of the Weir-Mitchell treatment. Before this step was taken another opinion was thought desirable, and the patient was brought to London for the purpose on June 4th. I saw him on the following day, in consultation with Dr. Percy Kidd, who was connected with the patient but had not had anything to do with the previous treatment.

The condition then presented by Captain G— was that characteristic of grave organic disease of the dorsal region of the spinal cord. There was absolute palsy of the legs, and cutaneous sensibility of all kinds was lost as high as the ensiform cartilage. At and just above this level, that is, in the region of the sixth and seventh intercostal nerves, he complained of severe pain around the chest, much more severe on the left side than on the right, and increased to evident agony on any movement. The legs from time to time became rigid in extensor spasm, and a clonus could be obtained with great readiness in the muscles of the calf and front of the thigh. The paroxysms of spasm involved also the muscles of the abdomen. The bladder was distended, and the urine that was drawn off contained pus. There was no irregularity of the vertebral column, nor could tenderness be discovered in any part. No trace of pulsation could be felt in its vicinity, and no murmur could be heard on auscultation. The thoracic organs seemed healthy, and both lungs were equally filled with air.

The development of complete paraplegia, which had taken place during the preceding four months, rendered the diagnosis, up to a certain point, a simple matter. The symptoms were those characteristic of a transverse lesion of the cord a little above the middle of the dorsal region. The gradual onset of the paralysis, the affection of one leg before the other, and the long-preceding signs of nerve irritation at the level of the lesion, made it practically certain that the spinal cord was damaged by compression and that the cause of the pressure was outside the cord itself. Caries of the spine was excluded by the absence of any irregularity of the spines or tenderness, taken in conjunction with the long duration of the symptoms. The diagnosis lay between an aneurism eroding the vertebrae and compressing the cord, a growth springing from the bones of the spine, and an intraspinal tumour within the canal, but outside the cord itself. Although aneurism could not be completely excluded, the absence of any of the characteristic physical signs of aneurism, and the absence of any indication of weakening of the spinal column, made this cause of compression far less probable than one of the two others. The distinction of a tumour of the bones from one within the canal can only be a matter of certainty when the enlargement of the bones, caused by the former, can be felt. In other cases the diagnosis can only be a matter of probability, and often of very low probability. A growth backwards from the bodies of the vertebræ may cause symptoms undistinguishable from those due to a tumour springing from the membranes. In this case, however, the symptom of longest duration, the pain, pointed to irritation of the posterior roots on the left side, and therefore to a lateral position of the growth, and the affection of the left leg before the right had the same significance. A growth from the bone on one side of the cord would be more likely to cause recognisable enlargement of the parts, than would one springing from the bodies of the vertebræ, and the absence of such enlargement in this case was therefore somewhat in favour of the growth being altogether within the canal.

The course of the symptoms, coupled with the inutility of iodide of potassium, precluded the supposition that the disease was syphilitic. The long duration of the symptoms in slight degree was in favour of the non-malignant character of any growth that might exist.

In a description of tumours within the spinal canal,.. I had previously suggested that the removal of spinal meningeal growths would be not only practicable but actually a less formidable operation than the removal of intracranial tumours. In this case the patient and his friends were exceedingly anxious that something should, if possible, be attempted. An operation gave a chance, the only chance, of cure. If the tumour should turn out to be one that could not be extirpated, it was possible that the removal of an arch, or the division of nerve-roots passing into the growth, might lessen the sufferings of the patient. If nothing were done, death after months of intense suffering was inevitable.

Sir William Jenner saw the patient with Dr. Percy Kidd and myself, and concurred in the probable diagnosis of a growth. The question of an operation was submitted to him and received his sanction, provided the patient himself clearly understood the nature of the operation and that a perfectly successful result was not more than a possibility. Capt. G— was, however, only too anxious to submit to anything that held out the faintest hope of relief. Accordingly Mr. Horsley was asked to see the patient, and, if he saw fit, to operate.

Surgical History of the Case, by MR. VICTOR HORSLEY.

I saw Captain G— on the 9th of June, 1887, at 1 p.m. The patient was half sitting up, complaining of paroxysms of very great pain in the lower limbs and abdomen, the former being completely paralysed and frequently flexed in clonic spasm, the pain accompanying which was so severe as to cause the patient to cry out. On careful examination of his spine, there appeared no undue prominence of any vertebra, and the only abnormality detected was tenderness on pressure to the left side of the sixth dorsal spine. This was very constant though slight; on movement the patient complained of a sensation of weakness (rather than pain) referred to the middle of the dorsal region, but such movement did not seem to start the spasm in the legs by interference with, or pressure upon, the spinal cord. He was very loth to move because it necessitated voluntary change of position of his legs, movement of any of the joints of which was liable to bring on a severe paroxysm of painful flexion. In addition to the complete loss of motor power just noted, there was loss of tactile sensibility as high as, and involving the destruction of, the fifth dorsal nerve. There was some doubtful diminution of sensibility in the left fourth intercostal space, but this could not be satisfactorily demonstrated when I saw the patient.[1] On the right side the insensibility was limited to the fifth interspace. The anæsthesia was complete for all kinds of stimulus.

There was complete loss of power over the bladder and rectum, and catheterisation had been found difficult with a metal instrument on account of the severity of the urethral spasm thus excited. (After the operation, when the spasmodic condition was equally severe, the passage of a soft rubber catheter was unattended by this trouble.)

The morning temperature during the week preceding the operation varied from 97.4° to 99.2°, and the evening temperature between 99° and 99.4°.

For the history and present state see the foregoing description by Dr. Gowers.

Operation.—June 9th, 3.30 p.m. Present: Drs. Gowers, Percy Kidd and Edmunds. Mr. White anæsthetised the patient with ether while he was lying in the semi-prone position on the right side, and I was

[1] This slight affection of the left fourth nerve was nevertheless of great diagnostic importance as the sequel of the operation shows.

kindly assisted by Mr. Stedman and Mr. Ballance. The skin was shaved and thoroughly cleaned with ether and 5 per cent. carbolic acid solution, the spray was used throughout the operation, and the instruments and sponges were kept in 5 per cent. carbolic solution. Free incision was then made in the middle line through the skin and the subcutaneous tissues extending from the third dorsal spine to the seventh. The deep fascia and tendinous attachments of the muscles were then cut from the spines and a transverse cut was carried outwards from the spines over the spinous muscles through the vertebral aponeurosis, so as to prevent all tension on the sides of the wound. (See Remarks.) Vessels bled freely by the sides of, and between, the spinous processes, and were secured with Wells's forceps. The muscles were then completely detached from the spinous processes, from the laminæ, and from the mesial aspect of the transverse processes. This was done in a way which I shall refer to later, namely by free use of the knife, and subsequently blocking the wound with sponges, while the same procedure was carried out on the other side of the spinal column. The sides of the wound being now strongly retracted and most of the vessels ligatured, the spines and laminæ could be seen perfectly.

The fourth, fifth, and sixth dorsal spines were then cut off close to their bases with powerful bone forceps, the laminal arch of the fifth vertebra was then trephined with a three quarters of an inch trephine, the pin being placed in the middle line. The bone was very hard and tough and one sixteenth of an inch thick. The rest of the laminæ were then removed with a bone forceps and knife, the ligamenta subflava giving much trouble owing to their toughness. The laminal arches of the fourth, fifth, and sixth vertebræ being thus cleared away, the dura mater was easily exposed by an incision in the middle line through the fat covering it. This fat, being pressed aside, shrank and showed the dura mater of a normal appearance, colour, and tension. Nothing very abnormal was then observed, save that on the left side the dura mater was distinctly pressed nearer to the bony wall of the neural canal. This, of course, was due to the fact that the tumour lay on the left side of the cord, and consequently pressed the dura mater on that side closer to the vertebræ. The wound being practically bloodless, the dura mater was slit open in the middle line with a knife and dissecting forceps. The cerebro-spinal fluid escaped freely, but not with any undue pressure to signify pathological tension. The spinal cord was now exposed for about two inches and appeared to be perfectly natural in colour and density; moreover, the vessels coursing on its surface were in every respect normal.

It will now be readily understood that the upper part of the roots of the sixth nerve and the whole course of the fifth nerve on each side from the spinal cord to the intravertebral foramen was completely exposed. Examination of the spinal cord on all sides with the finger and cautiously with an aneurism needle failed to reveal anything abnormal. Another lamina was removed at each end of the wound, the dura mater as before slit up, and the cord still further exposed, but still nothing pathological was discovered. At this juncture it appeared as if sufficient had been done, but I was very unwilling to leave the matter undecided, and my friend Mr. Ballance being strongly of the opinion that further exposure of the cord was indicated, I determined to go further if the state of the patient warranted me in so doing. Finding that his pulse was very strong, and that there would be no difficulty whatever in the anæsthetisation, I removed another lamina at the upper part of the incision. On opening the dura mater I saw on the left side of the subdural cavity a round, dark, bluish mass about three millimetres in diameter, resting upon the left lateral column and posterior root-zone of the spinal cord. I recognised it at once to be the lower end of a new growth, and therefore quickly cut away the major part of the lamina next above. This enabled me to see almost the whole extent of the tumour when the dura mater was divided. It was an oval or almond-shaped body of a dark, bluish-red colour, resting upon, and attached at its lower extremity to, the highest root of the left fourth dorsal nerve,[2] just where the posterior nerve-roots were gathered together in one trunk. On palpation the tumour markedly fluctuated. Above, it extended as far as the third dorsal nerve to which it appeared to be loosely attached by connective tissue, evidently a fold of the arachnoid. The tumour occupied exactly the position of the point of the ligamentum denticulatum, being jammed between the dura mater and the left side of the spinal cord. The pia mater and the arachnoidal sheath of the spinal cord evidently passed continuously from the cord over the surface of the tumour, forming a kind of capsule on its upper surface. At the same time it seemed as if the tumour could be pressed away from the spinal cord, so as to give the idea of its not actually invading the substance of the cord. I therefore made an incision through the pia matral sheath of the spinal cord, and then found that I could easily dissect the tumour from the surface of the cord, lifting it out of the deep bed which it had formed for itself in the lateral column of the cord. It was easily detached above by cutting through the loose tissue before described. Below, as it was firmly adherent to the fourth dorsal nerve, and as that nerve was of course of insignificant importance, I cut away the portion of nerve adherent to the growth. The outer border of the tumour was bathed in the cerebro-spinal fluid, and so required no dissection, but in removing the growth its inner surface, formerly of course in close contact with the cord, apparently gave way and some turbid serous fluid escaped, this reducing the volume of the tumour to about three fifths of its former size. (For description of the tumour *vide infra*.)

The cavity left by the removal of the growth was of course for the most part simply the subdural space, but the spinal cord was evidently greatly damaged by the pressure of the growth. The lateral column was so depressed or notched, so to speak, that the bottom of the groove in it nearly reached the middle line of the cord. It seemed likely, therefore, that most of the fibres in this column would be completely destroyed, moreover, there was evidently no resiliency in the damaged cord, for during the time that it was under observation the bottom of this pit showed no tendency whatever to rise. The surrounding adhesions of loose connective tissue oozed rather freely but gentle pressure with a fragment of sponge for a few minutes soon arrested this bleeding. The cord and subdural space was then carefully sponged with 5 per cent. carbolic acid solution and freed from

[2] The growth was found by measurement (at the operation) to be situated four inches above the level of complete anæsthesia.

blood-clot. The edges of the long incision in the dura mater were then approximated (incision fully four inches) and laid in position but not sutured at all. The few remaining vessels were ligatured, and the sides of the wound brought together by strong silk sutures passed vertically with curved needles through almost the whole thickness of the side of the wound, and at a distance of about half an inch from the border. These sutures were placed at distances of about one inch, and on being tied firmly were found to readily approximate the two sides of the cavity close to the dura mater. The edges of the skin were carefully approximated with numerous horsehair sutures, a small superficial drainage-tube was placed at the lower extremity of the wound and a long drainage-tube was placed vertically to the dura mater and reaching so far as that membrane at the upper end of the wound. The whole was then covered with a strip of carbolic gauze dipped in 5 per cent. carbolic solution, and a carbolic gauze dressing applied. The patient was put back to bed.

THE TUMOUR.—The growth, on microscopical examination, was found to be fibro-myxoma. It presents a nodular appearance, and the cavity referred to on p. 386 was found to be on the inferior and outer surface, being such a cystic space as might have resulted from a hæmorrhage. The wall of the cavity was found to be a false capsule derived from the pia mater and arachnoid. Unfortunately its contents were lost in the operation. The mass of the growth on section was pale and homogeneous, but indications of separation into nodular masses could be seen here and there. The tumour was enveloped, as already described, in a thin capsule, and consequently the parts will first be described under the headings of capsule and substance.

(1) *Capsule.*—The capsule was formed of very delicate connective tissue in which the ground substance was obviously mucinoid, and in which numerous corpuscles were embedded. The corpuscles were (*a*) leucocytes with darkly-staining round nuclei, (*b*) connective-tissue corpuscles with feebly-staining oval nuclei. Numerous large vessels with very thin walls (those of the veins in fact showing but one or two layers of muscle-fibres at the most) coursed through the exterior of the growth.

(2) *Substance.*—*Stroma.*—The stroma of the growth was composed of mucinoid ground substance and trabeculæ of spindle-shaped connective-tissue corpuscles closely applied to one another.

Parenchyma.—These trabeculæ marked off round spaces, which were entirely occupied by myxomatous connective tissue, *i.e.* mucinous ground substance which shrank greatly in alcohol, and in which were numerous corpuscles of varied shape. The nuclei of the corpuscles were (*a*) round and darkly staining, (*b*) oval and slightly staining, (*c* and *d*) ellipsoidal and spindle-shaped, darkly staining, and (*e*) very elongated, also darkly staining. These latter were as long and slender as the nuclei of involuntary muscle-corpuscles.

(3) *Vessels.*—A very few vessels were visible in the substance of the growth, and there were very small arterioles and venules with delicate walls of adventitia.

(4) *Pigment.*—In very many parts of the sections numerous collections of hæmatoidin granules were visible. In some instances these were obviously in corpuscles. No signs of any recent hæmorrhage, *i.e.*, within a year or two, could be found.

Further Course of the Case.[3]

June 10th, 1887, 1 a.m.—Patient restless, complaining greatly of painful spasm in the legs and bladder, with sensation of distension of latter. Urine drawn off with soft catheter. The flow of urine was of the kind characteristic of complete paralysis of the bladder. No further change. Gr. $\frac{1}{4}$ of morphia given hypodermically.

9 a.m., temperature 97.6° F. (It will be best stated here that the temperature throughout never reached 100° F., the highest recorded being 99.8° at 4 p.m. on June 11th, *i.e.* forty-eight hours after the operation. The temperature therefore will not be mentioned again, it being only needful to explain that its fluctuations were those of health, viz. low in the early morning and a little higher in the late afternoon.) Wound dressed, looked perfectly quiet. Tubes blocked with clot; cleared and replaced. Considerable amount of bloody serous discharge and cerebro-spinal fluid in the dressing.

On turning the patient over, a proceeding which was always difficult on account of the very severe pain in the abdomen and the left lower limb more especially, there was found an erythematous raised patch on the left side of the sacrum, but extending also across the middle line to the right side. The patch was about four inches broad and about three inches in vertical length on the left side, but only one inch on the right side. The nurse was positive that before the operation there was no such decubitus, and none was observed at the operation. This patch was immediately protected with boracic ointment spread on lint, and need not be again referred to, since it gradually disappeared, although on June 13th part of it in the centre of the gluteal fold appeared dusky, as though threatening necrosis of the skin. Fortunately it simply dried up.

11th.—Pulse 112. (The pulse varied very slightly after the operation, the rate gradually falling, thus on the 12th it was 108, on the 13th 95, and it varied between 90 and 100 till complete convalescence. Nothing was to be found to account for the high rate, except the pain. The patient still complained of much constant burning pain in abdomen, bladder, and limbs, in addition to which he suffered from violent painful spasm in the bladder and left leg especially. The left lower limb frequently flexed in spasm, but the right very rarely.

It need scarcely be stated that the indescribably excessive pain under which the patient laboured made examination of the limbs, &c., practically impossible, since the least touch excited the most violent clonic spasm, followed by tonic spasm, *i.e.* rigidity in extension, such spasm being agonisingly painful.

Urine.—Sp. gr. varied from 1024 to 1030. Strongly acid, no albumen or sugar. The urine never altered throughout, save a little in specific gravity, and therefore will also not be again referred to.

12th.—Wound dressed, uniting by first intention, though the edges looked reddish.[4] Discharge slightly serous, but enormous quantities of cerebro-spinal fluid escaped. The smaller (*i.e.* the lower) drainage-tube was

removed, the higher left in. (This was an error; the tube should always be left out on the second day, so as to prevent the formation of a sinus along which the cerebro-spinal fluid by escaping may cause serious annoyance.)

13th.—The patient still complained of the incessant pain keeping him without sleep. Hypodermic injections of morphia in half-grain doses only gave half-hour snatches of troubled sleep, therefore draughts of chloral and bromide of potassium were given (Hyd. Chlor. gr. xv, Pot. Brom. gr. xc in the twenty-four hours, and these were continued in gradually diminishing quantities during the succeeding weeks until about the end of September).

The bowels being constipated, an enema was given with result. The urine was drawn off whenever the patient felt it distend the bladder, *i.e.* about every six hours, and when the amount of urine was usually seven ounces. It is important to note that the patient said that the distension of the bladder increased the spasm of the abdominal muscles. This spasm was tonic and never (?) relaxed until some two months after the operation.

14th.—Wound dressed, union still perfect. Dressing soaked, but this was less marked than on the 12th inst. At 6 p.m. this day, *i.e.* on the fifth day after the operation, patient passed seven ounces of urine, and again at 9.30 p.m. six ounces. The micturition, however, was not "voluntary," but purely reflex action of the just recovered lumbar centre. The patient did not know when the urine escaped, although sensation was returning.

15th.—Sensation to touch is now rapidly recovering, only the left foot being still anæsthetic. On account of the severe pain of the spasms excited by touching the limbs no further observations were made, *i.e.* as to transmission of painful impressions, of heat and cold, &c., but there is little doubt that as regards tactile and painful stimuli, sensation had returned by about the tenth day after the operation. There remained for some time a subjective sensation of heat in the left lower limb especially. Wound dressed; the remaining (the upper) drainage-tube was removed. The last time the catheter was used was 5 p.m. this day, the patient passing urine afterwards about ten times in the twenty-four hours, and about four ounces on the average each time, the rare extremes being two ounces and eight ounces.

On the 23rd, *i.e.* fourteen days after the operation, the frequency had diminished to six times in the twenty-four hours, *i.e.* normal. The constant pain was very severe and at times became excruciating, in fact the patient thought it was worse than before the operation.

16th.—The spasms by this day had gradually become restricted to the left side and lower limb, except when very severe. The cerebro-spinal fluid continued to ooze in considerable quantity through the small track of the upper drainage-tube.

22nd.—The patient steadily improved, the appetite returning, &c. This day he for the first time distinctly moved the right lower limb at the hip by "voluntary effort." On this occasion and also when (see below) the patient moved his left lower limb for the first time, he regarded the movement as only a spasm and not purposive, the muscular sense from disuse (?) being apparently deficient. (I have noted the same phenomenon in a case recently under my care in which release by trephining of pressure on the spinal cord restored movement in

---

[3] Owing to the length of the case it will be best to give as far as possible succinct *résumés* of the course of each leading symptom, &c.

[4] The pain was always worse at night, and for some time before it disappeared had but very rarely occurred in the day.

the paralysed limbs.) The recovery of power spread down the limb to the foot.

At this time, however, the pain was still excessively severe at times, but was more paroxysmal, which was regarded, and rightly, as a favorable change.

July 20th.—About this date motor power returned in the left lower limb in the same manner as in the right limb, *i.e.* from the hip downwards. It is impossible to fix the date of this recovery as it was suspected for several days before the 20th, but the effort or initial spasm marred the observation, no aid forthcoming from the patient's sensations for the reason given above.

Further, the flow of cerebro-spinal fluid gradually diminished and ceased about six weeks after the operation. The arrest was aided by pressure with a pad of gauze and boracic acid over the sinus opening.

In this state, *i.e.* with recovered control of bladder and rectum, and with motion and sensation in the paralysed limbs, the patient was sent to the seaside on August 13th, 1887. The pain had gradually diminished and was confined to the left side.

A jacket consisting of a steel pelvic band from which shoulder crutches took origin, was applied to prevent possible kyphosis and to protect the cicatrix. .

Nov. 17th.—In answer to queries the patient wrote on this date, "I think I am making good progress. I take a daily turn in the garden with the aid of a couple of sticks, and also a daily drive for an hour. My back and legs are still very weak and at night I suffer a good bit of pain[5] and my sleep is broken, but I am in all respects much better. Though I walk with difficulty the movement of my legs is natural and tends to get better every day." At this time as from the end of July the legs had been passively moved and rubbed.

Jan. 24th, 1888.—This day the patient kindly allowed the members of the Society to inspect his back, &c. The only important point noticeable now in his condition was the character of the gait, which resembled that of a man rather stiff from fatigue. He could walk three miles with ease. The scar was very firm and indeed of almost bony hardness in the site of the fifth dorsal spine and arch. The patient was practically quite free from pain and discomfort and had very greatly increased in weight and muscular development.

Feb. 21st.—Seen again to-day; the patient's rapid progress continues, the gait is notably more free and natural than when last noted. Patient about to resume his professional work.

June 6th.—Letter received this day from patient states that he is in excellent health, of which the best evidence is that he recently did a sixteen hours day's work, including much standing and walking about.

Remarks.—This being the first case in which a tumour involving the spinal cord has been exposed and removed, it is very advisable that a full explanation should be given of the reasons which led to the adoption of the surgical procedure above described, and I think at the same time it is worth while to look back over the literature on the subject of tumours of the membranes of the spinal cord, and to see what light may thereby be thrown on this subject. . .

---

[5] I have noticed this reddish colour of the edges and suture holes in another case where the cerebro-spinal fluid rendered the wound sodden, but in which nevertheless union also occurred by the first intention.

Method of Operating.

The operation of trephining the spine has been of course known to surgery since it was suggested by Heister. It has, however, always hitherto been discussed with reference to cases of injuries of the spinal column. .

Since it was suggested, this operation has been performed, according to 'Erichsen's Surgery,' about thirty times. Before discussing its employment in these cases it must be stated that ever since it was proposed this operation has met with the greatest opposition from some surgeons for various reasons, principally no doubt because it was performed first in the prescientific epoch of surgery, *i.e.* before the introduction of antiseptic principles by Sir Joseph Lister, and consequently it obtained much of its evil reputation from the frequency with which septic infection followed the exposure of the dura mater and the subdural space. But it has also been discarded by some on account apparently of difficulties, &c., in its performance, and in fact it is regarded by some as a very difficult as well as dangerous operation. For instance, Mr. Herbert Page, in Heath's 'Directory of Surgery,' page 134, 1881, referring to the treatment of fractures of the spine, says, "The operation of trephining the spine, proposed many years ago and adopted several times, has made no progress in surgery, nor is it likely to do so . . . . It is an operation not within the range of practical surgery." In expressing this opinion Mr. Page has no doubt been influenced by the difficulties and dangers before referred to, but I would submit that they have no real existence.

Mr. Erichsen, in the last edition of his 'Surgery,' says, "The operation is not necessarily dangerous, it does not appear often to have hastened death, and has certainly in some cases afforded relief." With regard to the latter point I will discuss that when reviewing the cases I have succeeded in collecting, and I think a description of the mode of operating that I have adopted will show more briefly than anything else the way in which many of the so-called objections to the operation may be removed. In the first place the operation has been generally objected to on account of:

1. Hæmorrhage.

2. Difficulty in clearing the neural canal.

3. Physical difficulties of treating the fractured vertebræ.

4. The hopeless nature of the damage of the spinal cord.

5. Septic infection.

Of these objections we may with advantage consider Nos. 1, 2, and 3 together. In the course of some experiments upon the spinal cord, which are fully detailed in 'Brain,' vol. ix, 1886, I found that the mode of operating upon the spine for complete exposure of the bones as given in the text-books, namely, by removing the muscles from the bones by means of a blunt instrument, so far from being the best means for preventing hæmorrhage, is the easiest way of producing it. The knife must be freely and rapidly used while the soft parts are strongly retracted. It must be noted here that in every case I have found it necessary to divide the deep fascia, not only along the spinous processes, but also at right angles opposite the middle of the incision in order to prevent it resisting proper separation of the sides of the wound, indeed, it may in some extreme cases be found necessary to divide the vertebral aponeurosis at more places than one. It need hardly be added that this division of the fascia has no influence upon the rapid healing of the wound. The free bleeding which follows the separation of the muscles from the bone is best met by seizing what bleeding points can be seen with Wells's forceps and then tightly and quickly packing the incision on one side of the spine with dry sponges while the operation is proceeded with elsewhere. In this way very free oozing may be arrested in a few minutes, and the time spent in waiting for it to stop is certainly not lost, because the subsequent division of the bones can only be properly carried out when the wound is perfectly dry, as it is when the above-mentioned method has been followed. The periosteum is best reflected, without impairing its vitality, by scraping the bones with a suitably curved elevator after the mass of muscle has been turned aside.

Next with regard to the removal of the laminæ of the vertebræ. If, of course, there is a fracture of the laminæ or of the spine it will be detected at once by seizing the bones individually in strong forceps and shaking them (Erichsen), the fragment being easily extracted by dividing with a knife the ligamentous attachment, and no damage will be done to any important part if the edge be directed towards the bone. If now, however, the spine be perfectly uninjured, as in the foregoing case, it becomes a matter of great interest as to how we may most quickly remove the bones. From numerous experiments on dogs I have adopted the following method: The spinous processes of the vertebræ whose laminæ are to be removed are cut through close to their base by very powerful bone forceps. This is readily done in a few seconds and we then have the laminæ forming a continuous if irregular plate, and this can be perforated with a trephine with the usual precautions. The trephine should be almost as large as the diameter of the neural canal, this of course varying with the region operated on, the age of the patient, &c. If more than one arch is to be removed it will be better, by means of an angular saw, to partly cut through

the laminæ along the lines of the sides of the neural canal, and then the division of the bones can be completed with a bone forceps.

As in all these cases the wound cavity is necessarily deep, its walls steep, and relatively very unyielding, I have divised a form of bone forceps suitable for this stage of the operation. They simply consist of two ordinary bone forceps cutting blades set at an angle of about 120° to two short arms, which meet at the hinge and which are continuous with the ordinary long handles, the whole being bent at the hinge in a sharp curve, so that they can be employed to cut horizontally at the bottom of the cavity. More difficult than the incision of the bone is the removal of the ligamenta subflava. These can only be quickly and safely got rid of by steadily cutting with a sharp knife. After removal of the bone, as is well known, we find the dura mater covered with very vascular fat of a peculiar nature. This fat and loose connective tissue, if not treated in the way about to be described, may be very troublesome indeed in causing free oozing of blood, and at the same time owing to its elasticity in obscuring the proper view of the dura mater. The numerous vessels supplying it of course come from the spinal arteries and the vertebral plexus of veins. Consequently, these are best avoided by keeping the incision in the fat strictly to the middle line. When this is done there will be very little bleeding at all, but at the same time the dura mater is completely covered by the fat. It can, however, be practically completely got rid of from the field of operation if it be retracted with broad retractors, and pressed against the sides of the neural canal for a few minutes or seconds while the dura mater is opened. This fatty tissue being very spongy seems to shrink under the pressure and remains practically out of sight during the remainder of the operation.

The next point to be considered is the treatment of the dura mater, &c. The dura mater, if opened in the middle line, will be found to admit of quite sufficient retraction to either side to expose the whole spinal cord and the subdural space. If of course the longitudinal incision in it be very short, say less than half an inch, it will be necessary to make a transverse incision as well in order to expose the whole breadth of the subdural region. But, as in the present instance, if incision be at all long, it is quite sufficient to restrict it to the middle line.

The next practical point is the escape of the cerebral fluid since on the first opening of the dura mater the cerebro-spinal fluid wells up very freely indeed, fills the wound and prevents anything like accurate handling of the spinal cord. The best course to pursue is to keep mopping it out of the wound cavity with a sponge so long as it flows. If the patient be not moved and if the spine be horizontal and the head not raised, the flow of fluid will soon cease, and the spinal cord be then very freely visible. After inspection the spinal cord should be examined very gently by palpation, it being pressed against the bodies of the vertebrae in front, so as to reveal any change in its density. If it be suspected that some fragments of bone or a new growth may be pressing against the anterior surface of the cord from one of the vertebræ, it can best be detected by carefully passing an aneursim needle around the side of the cord, and exploring this aspect of it. In mentioning of course the opening of the dura mater, the escape of fluid, &c., due care will be taken to notice in the first place whether the dura mater is of normal appearance and whether there is any indication of its being inflamed or distended. It need hardly be stated here that of course if there is hæmorrhage beneath it it will appear dark, if pus yellow, &c. In cases where the theca is pressed backwards against the laminal arches, either from old traumatism or caries, &c., great care must be taken in perforating the laminæ with the trephine, but still more in raising the bone from the theca, for in such cases the dura is adherent to the anterior surface of the laminæ by firm fibrous adhesions, these requiring division with the knife.

A more difficult question, and one which requires experimental investigation at the present time, is the problem under what circumstances it is advisable to suture the incision in the dura mater or to leave it open. In the foregoing case, although the incision was relatively of very great extent, it was left open, but there can be little doubt that the union of the wound at the bottom of the uppermost drainage-tube canal would have been much more rapid if the dura mater had been even imperfectly closed by fine sutures.[6] There is another point which seems to me to be of practical interest, even if its existence be only theoretical. This is the possible cicatricial adhesion of the floor of the wound to the posterior surface of the dura and cord, and to the posterior roots of the nerves entering the same.

It has been long known to physiologists since the researches of Schiff in 1851, that the posterior columns of the cord are conductors of painful impressions, and this can be demonstrated on an animal which is completely narcotised with ether, so as to prevent the appreciation of pain, in the following manner. If in such an animal the various columns of the spinal cord be successively touched with a sharp point or other mechanical irritant, no reflex, i.e. involuntary, movements will result, except when the posterior columns are touched. This fact, as well as another mentioned

below, is worthy of notice, inasmuch as it makes a high degree of narcotisation necessary for the performance of the operation under the best possible conditions. The other fact I now refer to is the sensibility of the dura mater. It is not apparently generally known that the spinal dura mater is an exceedingly sensitive membrane. In the dog this is particularly noticeable, and even in an animal perfectly narcotised with ether, reflex movements will occasionally occur when this membrane, like the posterior columns of the spinal cord, is mechanically irritated. It is very necessary, therefore, that when the dura mater is about to be seized in forceps with the view of opening it, or when similarly any delicate incision is to be made in it or into the neighbourhood of the posterior column of the cord, that the patient should be very deeply under the influence of the anæsthetic to prevent any unconscious reflex start, which might lead to very unfortunate results.

To return, it will be readily understood now that possibly as before stated the wide cicatrisation together of the floor of the wound, the dura mater and the posterior roots of the nerves might produce adhesion which would cause pain if the spine were freely moved. This, however, after all may be purely imaginary since in the present case, where all these conditions must exist, the pain which occurred after the operation was not attributable to this condition, since in the first place it was merely a continuation of that which the patient endured before the operation and moreover has now (Jan., 1888) practically disappeared.

4. *The hopeless nature of the damage of the spinal cord.*

The consideration of this part of the subject is important of course only in those instances where the cord is diagnosed to be completely softened or where the operation is undertaken for the purpose of relieving the results of fracture of the spine, the whole bearing of which we may very properly now consider. I am the more anxious to do so since I can make my meaning clearer by referring to a case of Dr. Buzzard's, in which I performed the operation last summer. The patient had fallen down a quarry and was sent up from Derbyshire to the National Hospital for the Paralysed and Epileptic in a very critical condition. There was absolute paraplegia as regards movement and sensation together with complete loss of control over the bladder and rectum. The urine was already alkaline and contained mucopus. But the worst feature in the case was the existence of very severe and acute decubitus. Thus there was a large spreading sore over the whole breadth of the sacrum, extending especially deeply on the left side, sores over both heels, and a bleb on the left thigh.

---

[6] I have since sutured it with success.

It was very clear indeed to Dr. Buzzard and myself that unless the man was relieved from the most urgent symptoms he must speedily die. Examination of the spine showed that the spinous process of the eleventh dorsal vertebra was apparently broader than natural and a little more prominent, and at the same time very distinctly tender, in addition to which the patient very distinctly referred to this region as being the source of his weakness.

It was therefore decided to explore the seat of the fracture and if possible to remove any portion of the bone which might be pressing upon the spinal cord. The patient being placed in a prone position, and anæsthetised with chloroform, a longitudinal incision was made over the prominent vertebra. The soft parts, as before detailed, reflected, and then on grasping the spine of the eleventh dorsal vertebra it was found to be movable, but jammed forwards between the vertebræ above and below it. It was therefore seized in lion forceps and removed by cutting all the ligamentous bands attached to it. When it was extracted it was evident that the posterior surface of the dura-materal sheath was pressed backwards against the laminæ of the tenth vertebra. This therefore was also removed. The dura mater appeared perfectly normal. The theca therefore was not opened posteriorly, but on exploring its anterior surface and the bodies of the vertebræ with an aneurism needle a small puncture was made into it from which there escaped perfectly normal cerebro-spinal fluid. There was no evidence of any previous severe compression of the dura mater or its contents, and no evidence of hæmorrhage into the same. The wound was therefore closed and a drainage-tube placed opposite its middle; it was dressed strictly antiseptically. The further progress of the case was one of much interest; although the operation made no difference whatever in the motor paralysis and only slightly improved the sensory paralysis, it completely arrested the acute decubitus, the sores ultimately healing firmly, and what is still more interesting, from the time of the operation the urine became acid.

The drainage-tube was removed on the second day and the wound was completely healed at the end of seven days without a trace of suppuration.

In this case no doubt the spinal cord was momentarily jammed at the time of the accident so severely as to practically, *i.e.* functionally divide it. Though laminæ were found compressing it at the time of operation, nevertheless they did not do so so severely as to thereby alone cause the excessive degree of the symptoms, therefore it would seem that the cord, as suggested, must have been compressed at the time of the accident. Now, this is just a case in which if any attention had been paid to the ruling before quoted, the patient's life would have been lost, and indeed it

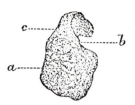

Photograph of the tumour, the natural size.

a. Points to the lobulated surface of the solid portion of the tumour, this producing the excavation of the cord.

b. Points to the open cavity in the tumour, this cavity being ruptured during the removal of the mass.

c. Shows the fibrous capsule forming part of the inner wall of the cystic cavity, and consisting of simple connective tissue, thus contrasting with the myxomatous tissue at *a.*

must be obvious that, considering the necessarily small amount of information on this subject, it should be our duty to operate in every case, since we may possibly do some good, and certainly, if proper antiseptic precautions be taken, we can, to use Mr. Erichsen's words, do no harm. This question of the damage to the spinal cord not appearing to discount the possible benefit of surgical interference so much as has been hitherto expected, gains additional illustration from the case which forms the subject of this paper, since nothing could well have appeared more hopeless than the indentation of the spinal cord produced by the tumour. This indentation appeared to divide the lateral column completely, and yet, owing doubtless to the gradual character of the compression, the restoration of motor and sensory function has been complete. I would repeat therefore that, so far from its being unjustifiable to operate on the spine owing to the possibility of the cord being hopelessly damaged, it seems to me to be criminal not to operate.[7]

5. Septic infection.

The possibility of septic infection following this operative procedure is of course exactly the same as that which attends any surgical interference, and needs only to be guarded against in precisely the same way, namely, by the Listerian principles of antiseptic surgery. No special liability to septic infection attends wounds in the region of the vertebræ, though of course the subdural space is undoubtedly an unusually favorable nidus for the organisms of putrefaction. As, however, I have

[7] Since this was written I have trephined the spine in two more instances, in both the wound healing without any complication whatever; one, a fracture: the other a case of complete paralysis of all four limbs, &c., from severe caries of the second and third cervical vertebræ is now rapidly regaining power, being able to move both legs on the eighth day after operation, and the upper limbs later.

repeatedly urged in discussing the surgery of the cranial cavity, this danger can be removed by the use of powerful disinfectants in a strong solution, *e.g.* 5 per cent. carbolic acid solution, &c., by irrigation of the wound during the operation, and this irrigation is afforded with the least inconvenience by the spray. The drainage of the wound is so extremely easy since the patient usually lies supine, that it can be completely provided for by a drainage-tube kept in for not more than forty-eight hours.

Summing up therefore, I think I have shown reason for regarding the operation of trephining the spine as a comparatively easy one, safe and justifiable, and that its reputed dangers are no more than those incidental to all wounds, the only peculiarity being the fact that septic meningitis is practically a fatal accident, the avoidance of which, however, is well understood and provided for in 999 cases out of 1000. . . .

Conclusions.

The lessons of the facts detailed in the foregoing pages are so extremely obvious that very few words are required to set them forth. They amount to this, that, granted the diagnosis is correctly made, there is but one treatment, viz. removal of the source of pressure by operation. It may at once be said, and rightly, that the question of diagnosis in the large majority of cases arises when only as yet one cardinal symptom is before us, most commonly pain, and that therefore a diagnosis of such certainty as to warrant exploration is not possible. To this nothing can be objected in view of the responsibility the surgeon takes upon himself, but at least absolution from the major part of such responsibility is obtained with the discovery of the first localising symptom independent of the constancy, the position, and the character of the pain. The differential diagnosis of the cause of painful paraplegias, material for which is given in the table, considered fully, would be quite beyond the object of the present paper, and must be reserved for another occasion. A close survey of the conditions under which tumours have been found will meanwhile afford the best aid to the recognition of the real nature of doubtful cases.

(For report of the discussion on this paper, see 'Proceedings of the Royal Medical and Chirurgical Society', New Series, vol. ii, p. 407.)

Rᴜᴘᴛᴜʀᴇ of the annulus fibrosus of the intervertebral disc with herniation of the nucleus pulposus is a common entity of disease which was not recognized as such until approximately 30 years ago. Consequently, the surgical treatment of this lesion has been a relatively recent development.

In contrast, the presence of the intervertebral disc and the occurrence of sciatic pain have been known for centuries.[13,16] Vesalius described the human intervertebral disc,[13] and the signs and symptoms of sciatica were mentioned in the works of Hippocrates.[18] The term sciatica, however, was used by the ancients to denote a syndrome produced by a variety of causes.[18] In 1764, sciatic pain finally was related to disease of the sciatic nerve by Cotugno.[16,37] Further characterizations of sciatica were made in the nineteenth and early twentieth centuries by Lazarevic, Lasègue, and Dejerine.[16,33,40]

The occasional occurrence of traumatic rupture of the intervertebral disc also has been recognized for many years. Single cases were reported by Virchow (1857),[38] Wilkins (1888),[42] Kocher (1896),[14] and Middleton and Teacher (1911).[19] Despite these observations, herniations of the nucleus pulposus usually were diagnosed and treated as extradural chondromas.[1,4,6,7,9–11,15,21,35,36,39]

The true nature of herniations of the nucleus pulposus gradually became apparent in the present century. Goldthwait[12] proposed in 1911 that herniations of the intervertebral disc might cause compression of the cauda equina, producing symptoms of sciatica and low-back pain. Between 1927 and 1934, important pathological observations were made by Schmorl,[26–32] Andrae,[5] and Mauric,[17] and clinical evidence in support of Goldthwait's hypothesis was provided by Petit-Dutaillis and Alajouanine,[2,3,23] Dandy,[8] Sashin,[24] Peet and Echols,[22] and others.[25]

However, it remained for William J. Mixter, neurological surgeon, and Joseph S. Barr, orthopedic surgeon, to definitely establish in 1934 the degenerative etiology of herniation of disc and its relation to sciatic pain.[20,33,34,41] Their classical work is reproduced below.

References

1. Adson, A. W. Diagnosis and treatment of tumors of the spinal cord. *Northw. Med., Seattle,* 1925, *24:* 309–317.
2. Alajouanine, T., and Petit-Dutaillis, D. Le nodule fibro-cartilagineux de la face postérieure des disques inter-vertébraux. I. Étude anatomique et pathogénique d'une variété nouvelle de compression radiculo-médullaire extra-durale. *Pr. méd.,* 1930, *38:* 1657–1662.
3. Alajouanine, T., and Petit-Dutaillis, D. Le nodule fibro-cartilagineux de la face postérieure des disques inter-vertébraux. II. Étude clinique et thérapeutique d'une variété nouvelle de compression radiculo-médullaire extra-durale. *Pr. méd.,* 1930, *38:* 1749–1751.
4. Alpers, B. J., Grant, F. C., and Yaskin, J. C. Chondroma of the intervertebral disks. *Ann. Surg.,* 1933, *97:* 10–18.
5. Andrae, R. Über Knorpelknötchen am hinteren Ende der Wirbelbandscheiben im Bereich des Spinalkanals. *Beitr. path. Anat.,* 1929, *82:* 464–474.
6. Bucy, P. C. Chondroma of intervertebral disk. *J. Amer. med. Ass.,* 1930, *94:* 1552–1554.
7. Clymer, G., Mixter, W. J., and Mella, H. Experience with spinal cord tumors during the past ten years. *Arch. Neurol. Psychiat., Chicago,* 1921, *5:* 213–215.
8. Dandy, W. E. Loose cartilage from intervertebral disk simulating tumor of the spinal cord. *Arch. Surg., Chicago,* 1929, *19:* 660–672.
9. Elsberg, C. A. Diagnosis and treatment of surgical diseases of the spinal cord and its membranes. *Philadelphia: W. B. Saunders Co.,* 1916, 330 pp. (see p. 238).
10. Elsberg, C. A. Extradural spinal tumors—primary, secondary, metastatic. *Surg. Gynec. Obstet.,* 1928, *46:* 1–20.
11. Elsberg, C. A. The extradural ventral chondromas (ecchondroses), their favorite sites, the spinal cord and root symptoms they produce, and their surgical treatment. *Bull. neurol. Inst. N.Y.,* 1931, *1:* 350–388.
12. Goldthwait, J. E. The lumbo-sacral articulation. An explanation of many cases of "lumbago," "sciatica" and paraplegia. *Boston med. surg. J.,* 1911, *164:* 365–372.
13. Keyes, D. C., and Compere, E. L. The normal

and pathological physiology of the nucleus pulposus of the intervertebral disc. An anatomical, clinical, and experimental study. *J. Bone Jt. Surg.*, 1932, n.s. *14:* 897–938.

14. KOCHER, T. Die Verletzungen der Wirbelsäule zugleich als Beitrag zur Physiologie des menschlichen Rückenmarks. *Mitt. Grenzgeb. Med. Chir.*, 1896, *1:* 415–480.

15. KRAUSE, F. Surgery of the brain and spinal cord based on personal experiences. H. A. Haubold and M. Thorek, Transl. *New York: Rebman Co.*, 1909–1912, 3 vols. (see *3:* pp. 1041–1047).

16. MARKHAM, J. W. Surgery of the spinal cord and vertebral column. In: *A history of neurological surgery.* A. E. Walker, Ed. Baltimore: Williams & Wilkins Co., 1951, xii, 583 pp. (see pp. 364–392).

17. MAURIC, G. Le disque intervertébral. Physiologie, pathologie et indications thérapeutiques. *Paris: Masson & Cie*, 1933, 195 pp.

18. METTLER, C. C. History of medicine. A correlative text, arranged according to subjects. F. A. Mettler, Ed. *Philadelphia: Blakiston Co.*, 1947, xxix, 1215 pp. (see pp. 493, 813–814).

19. MIDDLETON, G. S., and TEACHER, J. H. Injury of the spinal cord due to rupture of an intervertebral disc during muscular effort. *Glasgow med. J.*, 1911, *76:* 1–6.

20. MIXTER, W. J., and BARR, J. S. Rupture of the intervertebral disc with involvement of the spinal canal. *New Engl. J. Med.*, 1934, *211:* 210–214.

21. OPPENHEIM, H., and KRAUSE, F. Ueber Einklemmung bzw. Strangulation der Cauda equina. *Dtsch. med. Wschr.*, 1909, *35:* 697–700.

22. PEET, M. M., and ECHOLS, D. H. Herniation of the nucleus pulposus. A cause of compression of the spinal cord. *Arch. Neurol. Psychiat., Chicago*, 1934, *32:* 924–932.

23. PETIT-DUTAILLIS, D., and ALAJOUANINE, T. Syndrome unilatéral de la queue de cheval, laminectomie exploratrice et ablation d'un fibrome du disque intervertébral. *Bull. Soc. nat. Chir.*, 1928, *54:* 1452.

24. SASHIN, D. Intervertebral disk extensions into the vertebral bodies and the spinal canal. *Arch. Surg., Chicago*, 1931, *22:* 527–547.

25. SAUNDERS, J. B. DEC. M., and INMAN, V. T. The intervertebral disc. A critical and collective review. *Int. Abstr. Surg.*, 1939, *69:* 14–29.

26. SCHMORL, [G.] Die pathologische Anatomie der Wirbelsäule. *Verh. dtsch. orthop. Ges.*, 1927, *21:* 3–39.

27. SCHMORL, G. Über Chordareste in den Wirbelkörpern. *Zbl. Chir.*, 1928, *55:* 2305–2310.

28. SCHMORL, [G.] Über bisher nur wenig beachtete Eigentümlichkeiten ausgewachsener und kindlicher Wirbel. *Arch. klin. Chir.*, 1928, *150:* 420–442.

29. SCHMORL, G. Zur Kenntnis der Wirbelkörperepiphyse und der an ihr vorkommenden Verletzungen. *Arch. klin. Chir.*, 1928, *153:* 35–45.

30. SCHMORL, G. Zur pathologischen Anatomie der Wirbelsäule. *Klin. Wschr.*, 1929, *8:* 1243–1249.

31. SCHMORL, G. Die Pathogenese der juvenilen Kyphose. *Fortschr. Röntgenstr.*, 1930, *41:* 359–383.

32. SCHMORL, G., and JUNGHANNS, H. Die gesunde und kranke Wirbelsäule im Röntgenbild. Patho-

logisch-anatomische Untersuchungen. *Fortschr. Röntgenstr.*, 1932, suppl. 43, xi, 211 pp.

33. SPURLING, R. G. Lesions of the lumbar intervertebral disc. With special reference to rupture of the annulus fibrosus with herniation of the nucleus pulposus. *Springfield, Ill.: Charles C Thomas*, 1953, xi, 148 pp. (see pp. 3–8).

34. SPURLING, R. G. Lesions of the cervical intervertebral disc. *Springfield, Ill.: Charles C Thomas*, 1956, xi, 134 pp. (see pp. 3–8).

35. STEINKE, C. R. Spinal tumors: statistics on a series of 330 collected cases. *J. nerv. ment. Dis.*, 1918, *47:* 418–426.

36. STOOKEY, B. Compression of the spinal cord due to ventral extradural cervical chondromas. Diagnosis and surgical treatment. *Arch. Neurol. Psychiat., Chicago*, 1928, *20:* 275–290.

37. VIETS, H. R. Domenico Cotugno: his description of the cerebrospinal fluid, with a translation of part of his *De Ischiade Nervosa Commentarius* (1764) and a bibliography of his important works. *Bull. Inst. Hist. Med.*, 1935, *3:* 701–738.

38. VIRCHOW, R. Untersuchungen über die Entwickelung des Schädelgrundes im gesunden und krankhaften Zustande, und über den Einfluss derselben auf Schädelform, Gesichtsbildung und Gehirnbau. *Berlin: G. Reimer*, 1857, 128 pp.+6 pl.

39. WALTON, G. L., and PAUL, W. E. Contribution to the study of spinal surgery. One successful and one unsuccessful operation for removal of tumor. *Boston med. surg. J.*, 1905, *153:* 114–117.

40. WARTENBERG, R. On neurologic terminology, eponyms and the Lasègue sign. *Neurology*, 1956, *6:* 853–858.

41. WHITE J. C. Obituary. William Jason Mixter, 1880–1958. *J. Neurosurg.*, 1958, *15:* 581–584.

42. WILKINS, W. F. Separation of the vertebrae with protrusion of hernia between the same. Operation. Cure. *St. Louis med. surg. J.*, 1888, *54:* 340–341.

RUPTURE OF THE INTERVERTEBRAL DISC WITH INVOLVEMENT OF THE SPINAL CANAL*

BY WILLIAM JASON MIXTER, M.D.,† AND JOSEPH S. BARR, M.D.†‡

DURING the last few years there has been a good deal written and a large amount of clinical work done stimulated by Schmorl's[1] investigation of the condition of the intervertebral disc as found at autopsy. His work

* Read at the Annual Meeting of the New England Surgical Society, September 30, 1933, at Boston.

† Mixter, William Jason—Visiting Surgeon, Massachusetts General Hospital. Barr, Joseph S.—Orthopedic Surgeon to Out-Patients, Massachusetts General Hospital. For records and addresses of authors see "This Week's Issue," page 234.

‡ Reprinted from *The New England Journal of Medicine*, 1934, *211:* 210–214, with the kind permission of the Editor.

will stand as the most complete, painstaking and authoritative that has ever been done in this condition. This work, however, is purely pathological and it now remains for the clinician to correlate it with the clinical findings and apply it for the relief of those patients who are disabled by the lesion.

In the routine examination of spines from autopsy material he discovered that the intervertebral disc is often involved in pathological changes, the most common one being prolapse of the nucleus pulposus into an adjacent vertebral body. He found one or more such prolapses (Knorpelknochen) in about thirty-eight per cent of the spines examined. He also discovered that in about fifteen per cent of the spines there were small posterior prolapses beneath the posterior longitudinal ligament, but concluded that they rarely, if ever, produced clinical symptoms. He attributed their presence to weakening of the annulus fibrosus by degenerative changes, with mild trauma as a second factor, producing fissures in the annulus and escape of the semifluid nuclear material.

On the other hand, for a number of years clinicians have been reporting cases of spinal cord pressure from intervertebral disc lesions. In 1911 Goldthwait[2] reported a case of sciatica and paraplegia which he attributed to a posterior displacement of the intervertebral disc at the lumbosacral junction and suggested that such displacements might be the cause of many cases of lumbago, sciatica, etc. Middleton and Teacher[3] report a similar case confirmed at autopsy. Elsberg[4] in 1916 mentions chondroma of the vertebrae as causing compression of the cauda equina and states that Oppenheim has described a similar case. Mixter[5] in 1921 mentions a similar case and numerous other reports by Elsberg[6], Stookey[7], Bucy[8], Petit-Dutaillis and Alajouanine[9], and others have come into the literature. Thus the enchondroma, chondroma or ecchondroma arising from the intervertebral disc has become, to the neurosurgeon at least, a well-recognized lesion to be treated by excision and with a distinctly favorable prognosis. Dandy[10] in 1929 reported two cases from which he had removed loose cartilaginous fragments protruding extradurally into the spinal canal. He considered them "undoubtedly traumatic" in origin.

Our interest in this group of cases was stimulated particularly by a case seen by us two years ago in which the main symptoms were referable to root pain and in which the tumor was situated in the intervertebral foramen without cord or cauda equina compression of any moment.

Investigation of the cases of spinal cord tumor treated at the Massachusetts General Hospital and in our own private practice has shown a sur-

prisingly large number of these lesions, classified as chondromata, to be in truth not tumors of cartilage, but prolapses of the nucleus pulposus or fracture of the annulus. We have attempted to review these cases and differentiate true neoplasm and masses caused by rupture of the disc. We find as a result of this review that nineteen of our cases are rupture of the disc and six are true cartilaginous tumor or unclassified.

Clinically these cases of disc rupture, particularly the more recent ones, are of considerable interest. Diagnosis has been made difficult and operation has been delayed in them on account of the indefinite nature of the symptoms and signs and their similarity to those found in various conditions such as back strain, arthritis, sacroiliac disease, etc.

A summary of all cases of ruptured intervertebral disc is shown in table 1. For the purposes of this article abstracts of two cases will suffice.

CASE 4: On February 6, 1933 a white married chauffeur, aged 28, was admitted to the Massachusetts General Hospital. He gave a history of gradually increasing stiffness of his legs, noticed chiefly in walking, and of increasing numbness of the fourth and fifth fingers of each hand. The onset was insidious about six months before admission. He had been treated for cerebrospinal syphilis for three months.

P. H.: Essentially negative. There was no history of serious trauma.

P. E.: Showed definite hypesthesia over the ulnar distribution of each hand and very mild sensory disturbance of the trunk extending downward from the level of the nipples. There was definite spasticity of the legs with hyperactive knee and ankle jerks, bilateral ankle and patellar clonus, bilateral positive Babinski sign. Biceps and triceps reflexes were also increased.

Combined cistern and lumbar puncture was done. There was alteration in the dynamics in the lower needle indicative of a partial block. The total protein of the fluid from the cistern was 17, and of the lumbar fluid 52. If 40 milligrams be considered the upper limit of normal, then the lumbar fluid shows definite elevation in total protein. By injection of 2 cubic centimeters of iodized oil into the cisternal needle the block was localized at the level of the intervertebral disc between the fifth and sixth cervical vertebrae. Note that in the lateral view (fig. 4) the block is shown, and that the intervertebral disc is narrowed and there are hypertrophic changes present. After some delay the oil passed the point of obstruction and descended into the lower end of the dural sac. The patient was then placed on a fluoroscopic tilt table, head down. Another x-ray showed that the return of the iodized oil to the cistern was blocked at exactly the same point as on its descent.

Cervical laminectomy disclosed a spinal cord compression by an extradural encapsulated fibrocartilaginous mass 1.5×0.8×0.3 centimeters in size. The tumor lay in the midline in front of the cord and was exposed by rotating the cord and incising the anterior dura. It was easily removed from the underlying intervertebral disc.

TABLE 1

Case Number	Age Sex	Location of Lesion	History of Trauma	Symptoms	Signs
1 H.L.	37 M	C_3-C_4	Negative.	Bilateral paresthesias in ulnar distribution.	Stiff neck. Hypesthesia to pinprick from nipple line downward and in ulnar distribution of hands.
2 W.A.	39 M	C_4-C_5	Negative.	Numbness and stiffness in legs. Difficulty in urination and defecation. Pain in neck.	Mild spastic paraplegia. Hypesthesia to pinprick in ulnar distribution of both hands and from manubrium downward.
3 R.D.	50 M	C_5-C_6	Sudden onset while lifting a weight.	Numbness and tingling of fingers and legs. Stiffness of legs. Constipation.	Spasticity of legs. Increased reflexes. No definite sensory changes.
4 E.R.	28 M	C_5-C_6	Negative.	Stiffness of legs. Numbness of fourth and fifth fingers, bilateral.	Spasticity of legs. Increased reflexes. Positive Babinski. Ulnar hypesthesia.
5 M.P.	53 F	D_4-D_5	Negative.	Numbness and stiffness of legs. Incontinence.	Complete sensory and motor paraplegia.
6 A.N.	63 F	D_6-D_7	Negative.	Pain in legs and around abdomen. Inability to walk.	Hyperesthesia of legs and abdomen. Spasticity of legs. Increased reflexes.
7 M.M.	42 M	D_8-D_9	Negative.	Numbness of legs. Increasing difficulty in walking. Back pain.	Hypesthesia below umbilicus. Spasticity of legs. Increased reflexes in legs.
8 A.S.	56 M	D_{11}-D_{12}	Negative.	Pain in back, thighs and legs. Unsteady gait. Numbness of legs. Incontinence.	Spasticity of legs. Increased reflexes. Hypesthesia of feet and buttocks.
9 E.G.	24 M	L_2-L_3	Sudden onset while lifting a weight.	Pain and stiffness in back and legs. Weakness of legs.	Inability to walk. Flaccid paralysis (partial) of both feet. Hypesthesia of both legs over sciatic distribution.
10 J.D.	37 M	L_4-L_5	Fell fifteen feet at age of seventeen, landing on feet and buttocks. In hospital one month.	Pain in lower back. Numbness and weakness of legs.	Marked motor weakness of legs. Back motions markedly limited. Ankle jerks absent. Saddle anesthesia.
11 T.D.	29 M	L_4-L_5	Buried by shell explosion several years before entry.	Numbness of perineum. Severe back pain. Incontinence of urine and feces.	Generalized motor weakness of legs. Saddle anesthesia. Incontinence.
12 L.C.	20 M	L_4-L_5	Severe fall of seventy-five feet five years before present illness.	Low back-ache. Pain down right posterior thigh and calf.	Spine listed forward and to left. Lumbar kyphos. Sensation normal. Reflexes normal.
13 P.P.	44 M	L_4-L_5	Negative.	Pain in lower back. Pain down right posterior thigh and calf, worse on coughing.	Sensation normal. Weakness of muscles of both legs, right worse than left. Back motions markedly limited. Ankle jerks absent.
14 K.N.	25 M	L_5-S_1	Ski fall one month before present illness.	Pain in lower back, left posterior thigh and calf.	Lumbar kyphos, trunk listed forward. All motions of lower back limited. Left ankle jerk absent.
15 I.B.	36 F	L_5-S_1	Ether manipulation for "slipped sacro-iliac."	Urinary incontinence. Numbness of buttocks. Pain down left posterior thigh.	Saddle anesthesia. Sural anesthesia of left foot. Question of positive Babinski, left. Urinary and rectal incontinence.
16 A.V.	48 M	L_5-S_1	Negative.	Pain in lower back radiating down left leg laterally and posteriorly.	Tenderness over whole lower back. Trunk listed forward and to the right. Straight leg raising limited. Sensation and musculature normal.
17 J.A.	41 M	L_5-S_1	Twisted back by slipping off running board of car. Immediate pain.	Midlower back pain radiating down both posterior thighs.	Stands with knees flexed, spine stiff and lumbar kyphos. Tenderness at lumbosacral junction. Left ankle jerk absent.
18 B.R.	? F	L_5-S_1	Negative.	Low back pain radiating down left posterior thigh.	Sensory disturbance; hypesthesia of left side of vulva, thigh and lateral aspect of foot. Stiff back. Straight leg raising limited.
19 E.S.	35 F	S_1-S_2	Negative.	Pain in buttocks, anus, and vulva. Pain down left thigh posteriorly. Incontinence of urine and feces.	Saddle anesthesia of perineum and buttocks. Sphincter paralysis. Legs essentially normal.

TABLE 1—*Continued*

Spinal Fluid		X-Ray Examination		Operation	Histology of Tissue Removed	End Result
Evidence of Block	Total Protein	Local Changes	Lipiodol			
Partial at first examination; complete at second examination.	47 82	None of consequence.	Block.	Cervical laminectomy. Removal of extradural mass from disc between C_3 and C_4.	Annulus fibrosus.	Back at work. Much improved.
Partial.	74	None of consequence.	Block at C_5.	Cervical laminectomy. Removal of extradural mass from disc between C_4 and C_5.	Annulus fibrosus.	Much improved.
Partial?	33	Spur formation.	Not done.	Not done.		Died at home. Autopsy showed tumor arising from disc between C_5-C_6, compressing spinal cord and causing ascending and descending tract degeneration.
Partial.	52	Narrow disc. Spur formation.	Block at C_5-C_6.	Cervical laminectomy. Removal of extradural mass from disc between C_5 and C_6.	Annulus fibrosus.	Much improved.
Partial?	37	Calcification in disc between D_4 and D_5.	Not done.	Not done.	Nucleus pulposus.	Died of pernicious anemia. Autopsy revealed a small posterior prolapse of the disc between D_4 and D_5, which was degenerated and contained calcium.
Partial.	67	Hypertrophic changes. Narrow disc.	Block at D_6-D_7.	Dorsal laminectomy. Removal of extradural mass from intervertebral disc, compressing spinal cord.	Nucleus pulposus.	Complete motor and sensory paraplegia. Unrelieved.
Partial. (Complete?)	114	No films.	Not done.	Dorsal laminectomy. Piecemeal removal of mass from intervertebral disc, compressing spinal cord.	Annulus fibrosus and nucleus pulposus.	Complete paraplegia. Unrelieved.
Partial.	Increased. (Alcohol and ammonium sulphate tests.)	No films.	Not done.	Dorsolumbar laminectomy. Removal of tumor from disc between D_{11} and D_{12}, compressing cord.	Annulus fibrosus and nucleus pulposus.	Died seven months after operation; cause unknown. Slight postoperative improvement in symptoms.
Partial?	204	No films.	Block at L_2-L_3.	Lumbar laminectomy. Removal of extradural mass from intervertebral disc, pressing on cord.	Annulus fibrosus.	Improved. Motor and sensory changes are slowly disappearing.
None.	75	None?	Block at L_4-L_5.	Lumbar laminectomy. Removal of extradural intervertebral disc mass, compressing cauda equina.	Annulus fibrosus and nucleus pulposus.	Much improved. Slight residual motor and sensory changes.
Complete.	70	?	Block at L_4-L_5.	Lumbar laminectomy. Removal of extradural intervertebral disc mass, compressing cauda equina	Nucleus pulposus.	Much improved. Walks with a cane. Does light work.
Partial?	75	Biconcave L_4 and L_5 vertebral bodies.	Negative.	Lumbar laminectomy. Removal of extradural intervertebral disc mass pressing on right L_4 root.	Annulus fibrosus and nucleus pulposus.	Completely relieved.
None at L_3, first examination; almost complete at L_5, second examination.	174		Block at L_4-L_5.	Lumbar laminectomy. Free mass found extradurally removed. Probe could be passed into the middle of the disc.	Annulus fibrosus.	Relieved.
Partial.	108	None of consequence.	Not done.	Lumbar laminectomy. Extradural mass pressing on left L_5 root removed.	Annulus fibrosus.	Completely relieved.
			Block at L_5-S_1.	Lumbar laminectomy. Removal of mass compressing cauda equina, arising from the intervertebral disc.	Nucleus pulposus.	At first much relieved subjectively and objectively. Pyelitis followed by uremia and death five months after operation.
Partial.	67	None of consequence.	Negative.	Laminectomy with removal of pea-sized extradural tumor compressing left L_5 root.	Annulus fibrosus and nucleus pulposus.	Completely relieved.
None.	83	Narrowing of disc. "Lumbosacral arthritis."	Not done.	Laminectomy with removal of small tumor pressing on cauda equina. Spinal fusion.	Annulus fibrosus and nucleus pulposus.	Relieved.
Partial at first examination; complete at second examination.	62	?	Complete block at L_5-S_1.	Laminectomy. Removal of extradural mass compressing left L_5 and S_1 roots.	Annulus fibrosus?	Completely relieved.
None.	140	None of consequence.	Negative.	Lumbosacral laminectomy. Removal of tumor arising between S_1 and S_2, compressing lowest fibers of cauda equina.	Annulus fibrosus and nucleus pulposus.	Dead. Wound infection; septicemia; pyemia.

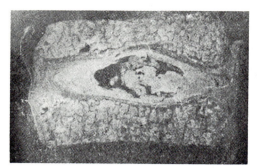

Fig. 1. A normal intervertebral disc. Note cartilage plate, anterior and posterior longitudinal ligament, annulus fibrosus, and the semifluid nucleus pulposus which bears the superincumbent body weight and is retained in place under pressure by the annulus.

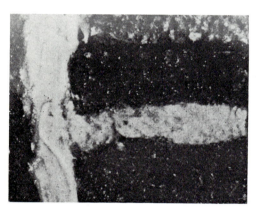

Fig. 2. Autopsy specimen. CASE 5. Note small posterior prolapse such as Schmorl describes.

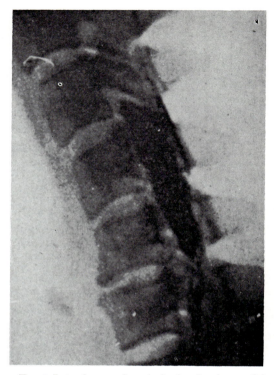

Fig. 4. Lateral x-ray of cervical spine showing partial lipiodol block at C 5–6 disc. CASE 4. Note the narrowed disc and early hypertrophic changes.

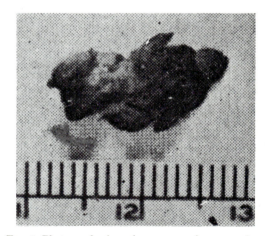

Fig. 5. Photograph of specimen removed at operation. CASE 4.

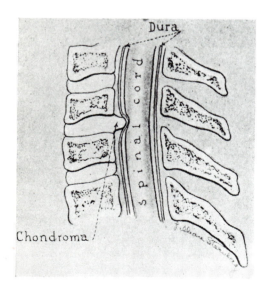

(FIG. 17. Showing the usual location of a ventral vertebral disc chondroma. [Legend in *Surgery, Gynecology and Obstetrics*].)

FIG. 3. Illustration taken from article by Elsberg, showing "chondroma" arising from intervertebral disc. (Elsberg: S. G. & O.; 46: 10: 1928.)

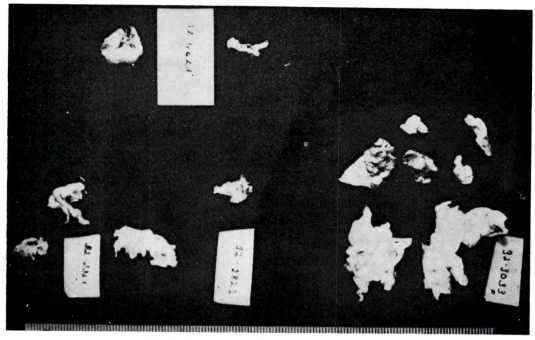

FIG. 6. A group of specimens taken from cases of this series.

Microscopic examination of the mass showed a homogeneous matrix containing elastic fibers and occasional cartilage cells. There was no evidence of malignancy.

CASE 14: A twenty-five year old white man was admitted to the Massachusetts General Hospital June 15, 1932 complaining of pain and stiffness in his left leg of two years' duration. A few months before the onset the patient sustained a severe ski fall, but had no immediate disability. He noticed at first only mild discomfort in his back and the posterior portion of his left thigh, but it increased gradually until he was unable to work. The pain radiated down the posterior thigh, calf and into the heel. There was a little discomfort in the other leg. He finally consulted one of us, who treated him with adhesive strapping and corset to support his back, with a tentative diagnosis of low back strain. He spent several months in absolute recumbency on a Bradford frame without relief. On account of lack of improvement it was decided to institute a complete neurological investigation.

On admission he presented the clinical picture of a man suffering from an extremely acute back strain. He stood with his knees flexed, the trunk listed forward and to the right. The motions of the lumbar spine were almost abolished by muscle spasm. Straight leg raising was limited to 25° on the left and 80° on the right. Neurological examination was negative except for absent ankle jerk on the left. There was tenderness along the course of the sciatic nerve, especially in the sciatic notch.

Lumbar puncture showed questionable partial block and a definite elevation in the total protein to 108 milligrams. Lipiodol examination was negative.

On June 29, 1932 an exploratory laminectomy from the second lumbar to the first sacral inclusive was done. After prolonged search a mass one centimeter in diameter was found in the intervertebral foramen pressing on the left fifth lumbar root and displacing the cauda equina to the right. It was removed piecemeal from the intervertebral disc and the wound was closed. Recovery was complete and uneventful. He had complete relief from pain immediately after the operation and has remained well since his recovery from the operation.

Pathological examination of the specimen showed it to be composed almost wholly of dense eosin staining fibrous connective tissue characteristic of annulus fibrosus. The original report classified this specimen as a chondroma.

The symptoms and signs of these so-called chondromata, which we believe in most instances represent rupture of the intervertebral disc, have been discussed at length by Elsberg and Stookey. The symptoms depend entirely on the location and size of the lesion. There is often a history of trauma not immediately related to the present condition. Numbness and tingling, anesthesia, partial or complete loss of power of locomotion, are usually present. Bladder and rectal sphincters may be involved. The condition of the reflexes varies with the level of the lesion. If it is compressing the cauda equina the tendon reflexes may be absent; if higher, compressing the cord, the legs may be spastic and the reflexes exaggerated with positive Babinski sign. If the lesion is low in the spine, the physical examination may be suggestive of low back strain or sacro-iliac strain. X-ray examination may be entirely negative, but nar-

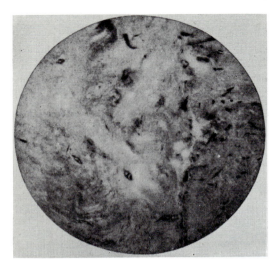

Fig. 7. Photomicrograph of specimen from Case 12 showing on the left, nucleus pulposus tissue; on the right, tissue characteristic of normal annulus fibrosus.

rowing of the intervertebral space is often present and is of significance, as it ordinarily means escape of the nucleus pulposus, not necessarily but possibly into the spinal canal. Lumbar or combined puncture and lipiodol examinations are of real value. If the mass is large, a partial or complete block is demonstrable at the level of the lesion. The spinal fluid rarely contains more than one or two cells, but the total protein in all of our cases was elevated moderately.

It so happens that most of the cases in this group have been operated on by one of us (W. J. M.) and not by a large number of surgeons; therefore we have developed certain ideas as to the operation when we suspect this lesion to be present. Exposure of the spine and laminectomy are performed as usual except that the laminectomy is narrow and on the side where the lesion is suspected, for we believe that a ruptured disc is a weakened disc and the strength of the spine should be preserved as much as possible. The dura is opened and the spinal canal carefully explored, particular attention being given to the intervertebral discs in front of the cord and the intervertebral foramina. If the lesion is found in the midline it is approached by incising the dura over it as suggested by Elsberg. If it is lateral, the dura is closed and the dissection carried out to the side between the dura and the bone. If a lesion is suspected in the intervertebral foramen it may be necessary to carry the removal of bone well out to the side, even taking in part of the pedicle. One must always remember that the tumor may be very small and extremely difficult to find on account of its position in the intervertebral foramen. After the tumor is exposed removal is a simple

matter. It frequently comes away without any dissection and if not, section across its base or removal with a curette is bloodless. Though we have done it in only two cases, we believe that it may be advisable to slip bone chips in between the stumps of the laminae before closing the wound, in order to facilitate fusion. After removal of the torn piece of the disc one frequently finds an opening through which a probe or half length may be passed into the nucleus pulposus. An interesting point is the appearance of the specimen before and after removal. The tumor in situ usually has the appearance of a half a pea with its flat side against the intervertebral disc, but as soon as it is removed it tends to unroll and can often be flattened out like a crumpled bit of wet blotting paper or a rolled up piece of fascia. The true chondromata on the other hand are rounded or lobulated masses of almost translucent cartilaginous tissue.

The microscopic picture of these chondromata is quite at variance with that of the normal disc. The chondroma is composed wholly of well-formed cartilage cells. The extruded portions of the intervertebral discs on the other hand may have occasional normal cartilage cells, but for the most part are made up of the different elements of the annulus fibrosus and nucleus pulposus, such as very poorly differentiated atypical cartilaginous

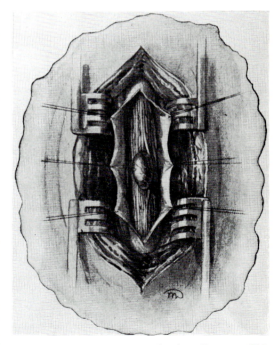

Fig. 8. Drawing of tumor in situ. Case 10. This illustration is taken from Lewis' Surgery (Prior & Company) in the report of a case of "enchondroma" of the intervertebral disc (W. J. M). Reëxamination shows the specimen to be normal intervertebral disc tissue.

cells scattered irregularly in a very granular and loose reticulum. The compactness of a true chondroma is not seen in this group.

We conclude from this study:

That herniation of the nucleus pulposus into the spinal canal, or as we prefer to call it, rupture of the intervertebral disc, is a not uncommon cause of symptoms.

That this lesion frequently has been mistaken for cartilaginous neoplasm arising from the intervertebral disc.

That in reality rupture of the disc is more common than neoplasm; in our series in the ratio of three to one.

That this lesion should be borne in mind in the study of certain orthopedic conditions, particularly in those cases which do not respond to appropriate treatment.

That a presumptive diagnosis may be made in many instances and that operation whether for this or for supposed spinal cord tumor should always be planned with the possibility of finding this lesion.

That the treatment of this disease is surgical and that the results obtained are very satisfactory if compression has not been too prolonged.

References

1. Schmorl, G., and Junghanns, H.: Archiv und Atlas der normalen und pathologischen Anatomie in typischen Röntgenbildern. Leipsig: Georg Thieme, 1932.
2. Goldthwait, J. E.: The lumbo-sacral articulation; An explanation of many cases of "lumbago," "sciatica" and paraplegia. Boston M. & S. J. 164: 365, 1911.
3. Middleton, G. S., and Teacher, J. H.: Injury of the spinal cord due to rupture of an intervertebral disk during muscular effort. Glasgow M. J. 76: 139, 1911.
4. Elsberg. C. A.: Diagnosis and Treatment of Surgical Diseases of the Spinal Cord and its Membranes. Philadelphia: W. B. Saunders Co. P. 238, 1916.
5. Clymer, G.: Mixter, W. J. and Mella, Hugo: Experience with spinal cord tumors during the past ten years. Arch. Neurol. & Psychiat. 5: 213, 1921.
6. Elsberg, C. A.: Extradural spinal tumors—primary, secondary, metastatic. Surg. Gynec. & Obst. 46: 1, 1928.
7. Stookey, B.: Compression of the spinal cord due to ventral extradural cervical chondromas. Arch. Neurol. & Psychiat. 20: 275, 1928.
8. Bucy, P. C.: Chondroma of intervertebral disk. J. A. M. A. 94: 1552, 1930.
9. Petit-Dutaillis, D., and Alajouanine, T.: Syndrome unilateral de la queue de cheval, laminectome exploratrice et ablation d'un fibrome du disque intervertebral. Bull. et Mem. Soc. Nat. de Chir. 54: 1452, 1928.
10. Dandy, W. E.: Loose cartilage from intervertebral disk simulating tumor of the spinal cord. Arch. Surg. 19: 660, 1929.

Note: Since the reading of this paper before the New England Surgical Society in September, 1933 we have obtained G. Mauric's monograph on the intervertebral disc published in Paris by Masson et Cie in 1933.

This monograph covers many of the points touched upon in this communication. It is a most complete and exhaustive study of the subject and includes a voluminous bibliography.

It is interesting to note that his deductions are drawn from exhaustive studies and review of the literature while ours are from a small group of personal cases. Notwithstanding this difference of attack, our conclusions are in substantial agreement. Anyone interested in this subject is advised to read this monograph which is too long and complete to be reviewed here.

Neurosurgical Classics—51 and 52

ADVANCEMENTS in scientific fields occasionally are made by two or more investigators working independently, each unaware of the other's efforts. An example of this in the field of neurological surgery is found in the simultaneous introduction of posterior rhizotomy for pain by William H. Bennett and Robert Abbe in 1888–1889.

During the early development of modern neurosurgery, operations for the treatment of neurological diseases were usually devised by neurologists, who then directed general surgeons in their performance.[26–30] In the case of posterior rhizotomy, Dr. Charles Dana, occupant of the first chair of neurology at the Cornell University Medical College, suggested that certain types of pain might be controlled by division of the posterior spinal roots,[4,8,18] and this operation was performed a short time later by Bennett in England and Abbe in the United States.

Mr. Bennett (later Sir Bennett), surgeon to St. George's Hospital in London, admitted a 45-year-old man to his service on August 29, 1888 for treatment of syphilitic osteitis of the left tibia. Various procedures, including amputation at the knee, failed to control the patient's pain, so on December 24, 1888, Bennett sectioned the first, third, fourth, and fifth lumbar and the first and second sacral posterior nerve roots on the left side. The patient was relieved of pain, but died of an intracranial hemorrhage on January 5, 1889.[6,7]

Within two weeks of Bennett's operation, Dr. Abbe, a pioneer in the surgical treatment of trigeminal neuralgia, spinal tumors, and syringomyelia, performed a similar operation. His patient, a 44-year-old man, was referred to him by Dana because of neuralgia of the right brachial plexus, which had been treated unsuccessfully by stretching of the posterior interosseous and ulnar nerves, amputation of the upper extremity, and excision of a neuroma of the musculo-spiral nerve. On December 31, 1888, Abbe sectioned the sixth and seventh cervical nerves extradurally on the right, and two days later he divided the seventh and eighth posterior nerve roots on the same side. At the same operations, Abbe also stimulated the exposed spinal nerves with faradic current to determine for the first time in a living human being the motor functions of these nerves.[1–3,19,22]

Following the reports by Abbe and Bennett, posterior rhizotomies were performed by a number of surgeons for the relief of peripheral pain. Mingazzini[17] suggested in 1899 that this operation should also be performed for the relief of the lightening pains of tabes dorsalis, and a decade later, at Foerster's request, Küttner successfully relieved the symptoms of a 47-year-old man suffering from gastric crises by dividing the seventh to tenth thoracic posterior nerve roots.[4,11,13]

Aside from adapting posterior rhizotomy to gastric crises and spastic paralysis,[10] Foerster made a far more significant contribution in this area. From his extensive experience with the operation during the following quarter of a century, he was able to carefully plot the dermatomes in man.[12,16,18]

Although posterior rhizotomy for pain aroused widespread interest after its introduction, the operation gradually lost favor because of its inherent disadvantages.[5,14,18,25] Because of the wide overlapping of sensory nerves, extensive laminectomies were required to achieve satisfactory relief of pain, and this led to a relatively high mortality rate in the patients debilitated by painful disease. In addition, the patients who survived the operation were found to be definitely handicapped by the loss of all forms of sensation in the involved area.

With the introduction of cordotomy,[28] higher spinothalamic tractotomy,[9,20,23] mesencephalotomy,[21,32] frontal leucotomy,[8,15,24,31] etc., the operation of posterior rhizotomy lost most of its original importance, but it still has historical significance as a major step in the development of modern techniques for the relief of pain.

References

1. ABBE, R. A contribution to the surgery of the spine. *Med. Rec., N. Y.*, 1889, *35:* 149–152.
2. ABBE, R. Intradural section of the spinal nerves for neuralgia. *Boston med. surg. J.*, 1896, *135:* 329–335.
3. ABBE, R. Resection of the posterior roots of spinal nerves to relieve pain, pain reflex, athetosis, and spastic paralysis—Dana's operation. *Med. Rec. N. Y.*, 1911, *79:* 377–381.
4. ARMOUR, D. Lettsomian lecture on the surgery of the spinal cord and its membranes. *Lancet*, 1927, *1:* 423–430; 533–537; 691–698.
5. BAILEY, P. Surgical trauma in treatment of neurologic disorders. *Texas St. J. Med.*, 1962, *58:* 625–632.
6. BENNETT, W. H. A case in which acute spasmodic pain in the left lower extremity was completely relieved by sub-dural division of the posterior roots of certain spinal nerves, all other treatment having proved useless. Death from sudden collapse and cerebral haemorrhage on the twelfth day after the operation, at the commencement of apparent convalescence. *Med.-chir. Trans.*, 1889, *72:* 329–348.
7. BENNETT, W. H. Subdural division of posterior roots of spinal nerves. *Lancet*, 1889, *1:* 839–840.
8. CRAWFORD, J. V., and WALKER, A. E. Surgery for pain. In: *A history of neurological surgery.* A. E. Walker, Ed. Baltimore: Williams & Wilkins Co., 1951, xii, 583 pp. (see pp. 308–330).
9. DOGLIOTTI, M. First surgical sections, in man, of the lemniscus lateralis (pain-temperature path) at the brain stem, for the treatment of diffuse rebellious pain. *Curr. Res. Anesth.*, 1938, *17:* 143–145.
10. FOERSTER, O. Resection of the posterior spinal nerve-roots in the treatment of gastric crises and spastic paralysis. *Proc. roy. Soc. Med.*, 1911, *4*, pt. 3: 226–246.
11. FOERSTER, O. Die Leitungsbahnen des Schmerzgefühls und die chirurgische Behandlung der Schmerzzustände. *Berlin: Urban & Schwarzenberg*, 1927, viii, 360 pp.
12. FOERSTER, O. The dermatomes in man. *Brain*, 1933, *56:* 1–39.
13. FOERSTER, O., and KÜTTNER, H. Ueber operative Behandlung gastrischer Krisen durch Resektion der 7.-10. hinteren Dorsalwurzel. *Beitr. klin. Chir.*, 1909, *63:* 245–256.
14. FRAZIER, C. H. Rhizotomy for the relief of pain. *J. nerv. ment. Dis.*, 1918, *47:* 343–362.
15. FREEMAN, W., and WATTS, J. W. Pain of organic disease relieved by prefrontal lobotomy. *Lancet*, 1946, *1:* 953–955.
16. JEFFERSON, G. Man as an experimental animal. *Lancet*, 1955, *1:* 59–61.
17. MINGAZZINI, G. Proposta di un atto operativo per la cura radicale della tabe inferiore. *Policlinico, Sez. prat.*, 1899, *5:* 750–751.
18. RAY, B. S. The management of intractable pain by posterior rhizotomy. *Res. Publ. Ass. nerv. ment. Dis.*, 1943, *23:* 391–407.
19. SCARFF, J. E. Fifty years of neurosurgery, 1905–1955. *Int. Abstr. Surg.*, 1955, *101:* 417–513 (see pp. 425–426).
20. SCHWARTZ, H. G., and O'LEARY, J. L. Section of the spinothalamic tract in the medulla with observations on the pathway for pain. *Surgery*, 1941, *9:* 183–193.
21. SPIEGEL, E. A., WYCIS, H. T., FREED, H., and LEE, A. J. Stereoencephalotomy. *Proc. Soc. Exp. Biol., N. Y.*, 1948, *69:* 175–177.
22. STOOKEY, B. Early neurosurgery in New York: its origin in neurology and general surgery. *Bull. Hist. Med.*, 1952, *26:* 330–359.
23. WALKER, A. E. Mesencephalic tractotomy. A method for the relief of unilateral intractable pain. *Arch. Surg., Chicago*, 1942, *44:* 953–962.
24. WHITE, J. C. Modifications of frontal leukotomy for relief of pain and suffering in terminal malignant disease. *Ann. Surg.*, 1962, *156:* 394–402.
25. WHITE, J. C., and SWEET, W. H. Pain. Its mechanisms and neurosurgical control. *Springfield, Ill.: Charles C Thomas*, 1955, xxiv, 736 pp. (see pp. 176–179).
26. WILKINS, R. H. Neurosurgical classic—I. *J. Neurosurg.*, 1962, *19:* 700–710.
27. WILKINS, R. H. Neurosurgical classics—II. *J. Neurosurg.*, 1962, *19:* 801–805.
28. WILKINS, R. H. Neurosurgical classics—III. *J. Neurosurg.*, 1962, *19:* 1007–1013.
29. WILKINS, R. H. Neurosurgical classic—XI. *J. Neurosurg.*, 1963, *20:* 814–824.
30. WILKINS, R. H. Neurosurgical classic—XIV. *J. Neurosurg.*, 1963, *20:* 1090–1099.
31. WOLFF, H. G. Some observations on pain. *Harvey Lect.*, 1944, 39–95.
32. WYCIS, H. T., and SPIEGEL, E. A. Long-range results in the treatment of intractable pain by stereotaxic midbrain surgery. *J. Neurosurg.*, 1962, *19:* 101–106

A CASE

IN WHICH

ACUTE SPASMODIC PAIN IN THE LEFT LOWER EXTREMITY

WAS

COMPLETELY RELIEVED BY SUB-DURAL DIVISION OF THE POSTERIOR ROOTS OF CERTAIN SPINAL NERVES, ALL OTHER TREATMENT HAVING PROVED USELESS.

DEATH FROM SUDDEN COLLAPSE AND CEREBRAL HAEMORRHAGE ON THE TWELFTH DAY AFTER THE OPERATION, AT THE COMMENCEMENT OF APPARENT CONVALESCENCE.*

BY

WILLIAM H. BENNETT, F.R.C.S.,

SURGEON TO ST. GEORGE'S HOSPITAL

Received February 12th—Read April 23rd, 1889.

THE following case is thought worthy of record, partly on account of its interest in relation to the

* Reprinted from *Medico-Chirurgical Transactions,* London, 1889, *72:* 329–348.

present position of the Surgery of the Nervous System, and especially as it is believed to be the first instance published in which the treatment described has been deliberately proposed and subsequently carried out.

History of the patient.—W.T—, æt. 45, a labourer, was admitted into St. George's Hospital under my care on August 29th, 1888, complaining of acute spasmodic pain in the left leg. Twenty-one years previously he had contracted chancres, which were followed by secondary symptoms and extensive ulcerations on various parts of the body. For nine years the left leg had been swollen and painful, the pain having during the past two years become more acute and persistent; whilst at times there had occurred violent spasms in the limb, during which his sufferings were described as agonising. In 1883 he had been in St. George's Hospital, under the care of Mr. Warrington Haward, with general thickening of the left tibia, for which he was treated with large doses of iodide of potassium, slight and transitory relief only being obtained. Since that time he had attended at several London hospitals, and had taken, he said, enormous quantities of iodide of potassium and mercury without feeling in any way the better for the medicine; on the contrary, the pain steadily increased in severity.

During the year prior to his coming under my care the man's sufferings were stated by his relations to have been terrible, so much so that they were compelled to move from lodging to lodging on account of the disturbance caused by his cries during the attacks of spasm. He was said to be of steady and sober habits, and there was no history of insanity or mental peculiarity in any of his family.

On admission, the patient was emaciated, pale, and anxious looking. He complained of acute pain in the left lower limb below the knee. This pain was persistent, but occasionally was greatly increased by spasms in the limb, during which he groaned, his face at the same time being expressive of extreme suffering. The anterior surface of the tibia was thickened and irregular, but the tenderness was less than seemed probable, and the increase of temperature locally was insignificant. Scattered over the body and limbs generally were many scars of old syphilitic origin. No visceral disease could be detected, and the urine was normal.

He was given large doses of iodide of potassium, but on September 4th the pain was so acute that I thought it wise to cut down upon the thickened bone, which I accordingly did, laying open the peritoneum, which in parts was a quarter of an inch in thickness, and subsequently trephining the somewhat sclerosed tibia above and below, afterwards connecting the trephine holes by an incision through the bone, which freely laid open the medullary cavity.

No benefit of any kind followed upon this treatment.

Gradually the spasms in the limb became more frequent and severe, especially at night, when they often awoke the patient in spite of large doses of narcotics, causing him to shriek loudly. At first these attacks could be rapidly controlled by antipyrin, of which he took large quantities, but a tolerance of the drug was soon established, and it became useless.

On September 29th, after consultation, it was decided to amputate through the knee-joint, a proceeding in which the man placed much faith. At the same time it was fully recognised that the pain was very probably due to some central lesion, and that the amputation might entirely fail to afford relief.

30th.—The leg was removed by Stephen Smith's method at the knee-joint, the operation being followed by no improvement.

On October 21st, as the patient attached some importance to a change into the country, he was sent to the Convalescent Hospital at Wimbledon, under the care of my colleague, Mr. Dent.

The spasms still continued to increase in frequency, and on November 10th Mr. Dent, with my concurrence, exposed and stretched the left sciatic nerve, removing also a small piece of the skin from the stump, over the spot from which the pain appeared to start. No benefit having been obtained from this treatment, Mr. Dent, on November 22nd, excised about two and a half inches of the sciatic nerve; but this again entirely failed to produce any effect upon the man's sufferings, which were now beginning to produce serious exhaustion.

On December 8th he returned to St. George's again to be under my care, when his condition was as follows:—The face was thin and hollow, and the expression was one of great distress; the body was extremely emaciated, the pulse weak and at times intermittent, the temperature was normal, and the urine free from albumen but full of phosphates. Referred to the whole of the leg, which had been removed by amputation, was continual pain, and at intervals varying in length from ten minutes to half an hour, there occurred in the stump and whole of the left thigh violent spasms, which caused the patient to clutch the part tightly and shriek with pain. These attacks lasted usually for five minutes or rather more, and then gradually subsided, leaving the man exhausted and bathed in profuse clammy sweats. The spasms were limited to the muscles of the left thigh, the left latissimus dorsi, and erector spinæ.

The affected thigh was wasted, the sensation was normal, and there was no loss of power beyond that which would naturally follow such extensive interference as the sciatic nerve had been subjected to by operation. Narcotics and anodynes, whether given by the mouth, rectum, or under the skin, had little effect, unless pushed to a dangerous extent; and even when so given the spasms occurred, causing the patient to groan and contract his facial muscles as if in pain.

By December 11th it appeared to me quite plain that the exhaustion was steadily increasing, from the combined effects of pain, want of sleep, and inability to take food; and must indeed, at no very distant period, end in death, unless something could be done to relieve the man's sufferings. I therefore thought that it would be justifiable to suggest any surgical proceeding, however severe, which was likely by any means to attain this end. Taking into consideration the character of the pain, as well as a certain weakness in the lower part of the spine, of which the patient sometimes complained, it seemed not impossible that there might exist some condition of the cord or its membranes, perhaps of syphilitic origin, within the area of the lumbar enlargement which might prove amenable to surgical interference, and further, that it would be almost certainly possible, in the absence of any such lesion, to relieve the pain in the manner to be presently described. I submitted the question therefore to my colleagues, who thought that before undertaking such a serious form of treatment a further trial of full doses of mercury should be made.

This was accordingly done, but by December 24th it was manifest that the patient was rapidly approaching the final stage of exhaustion. No good effect of any kind having resulted from the extended trial of mercury, I then made the following proposition:—First, to lay open the spinal canal and examine the membranes, or, if necessary, the cord itself, as high as the eighth dorsal vertebra, and, in the event of this exploration producing a negative result only, as seemed extremely probable, to proceed to the division of the posterior roots of those spinal nerves which seemed to correspond in their distribution to the area over which the pain was felt, leaving at least the fourth and fifth sacral nerves intact, in the hope that the control of the bladder and rectum may not be interfered with. By this operation it appeared to me that whatever may have been the cause of the symptoms I should, even if the spasms continued, at least render them painless. I also proposed to commence the exploration at the extreme lower end of the cord, in order that I might be enabled to at once divide the nerves mentioned, if, as was very likely, the condition of the patient's powers should at any moment render a rapid completion of the operation necessary, before I had been able to extend my examination as high as I hoped to do. The whole of this proposition was made with a full consciousness of the serious character of the treatment, as well as of the uncertainties which must necessarily be connected with a proceeding which, so far as I could ascertain, had not previously been adopted in the human subject.

Having received the consent of my colleagues, I carried out my intention at 1 p.m. on the same day.

The operation.—The patient having been anæsthetised, and placed on his left side with the thighs flexed, the vertebral canal was laid open in the manner indicated by Mr. Victor Horsley in the last volume of the Society's 'Transactions.' A vertical incision six inches long was made in the middle line of the back, having for its centre the spinous process of the eleventh dorsal vertebra. The muscular mass in each vertebral groove was then quickly separated from the sides of the spinous processes and posterior aspects of the laminæ by cutting freely with the knife. One vessel only was ligatured, and but three required to be clipped. The bleeding was insignificant, and rapidly ceased spontaneously. The spines of the first lumbar and of the eleventh and twelfth dorsal vertebrae were then removed with cutting forceps, and the posterior arch of the twelfth dorsal vertebra was taken away by means of a trephine one inch in diameter; the posterior arches of the eleventh dorsal and first lumbar vertebræ being then cut away with angular forceps. The extradural fat, for the most part, came away with the arches, and that which remained on the dura mater was easily pushed aside, giving no trouble of any kind. At the bottom of the wound, the sides of which could be widely retracted without any transverse incision, the dura mater was now freely exposed, and bulged backwards, not as a uniform tube, but at the lower part presented a circumscribed oval swelling corresponding to the area of the twelfth dorsal vertebra. There was no pulsation visible, but this could easily be felt by the finger upon gentle pressure being made. This irregular shape of the dura mater was so suggestive of the existence of some lesion beneath that it was decided to open it at once. A small puncture was therefore made, from which the clear cerebrospinal fluid immediately jetted forth to a height of about six inches. This fluid having been allowed to slowly drain away, the dura mater was laid open along the whole length of the wound. The cord exposed was now seen to be perfectly natural in every respect.

The posterior arches of the ninth and tenth dorsal vertebræ were then removed by the cutting forceps, and the cord further exposed by extension of the incision in the dura mater to the upper limit of the wound, nothing abnormal being detected, in spite of a very complete examination of the cord on all sides, by gently raising it on a blunt hook.

At this stage Mr. Haward, who was kindly watching the pulse, informed me that the patient's strength would probably stand no further exploration. I therefore, as quickly as possible, picked up, one by one, the left lumbar posterior nerve-roots, which were readily distinguished by their size and relation to the ligamentum denticulatum, and divided, as I supposed, the lower four of these with a pair of strabismus scissors. This proceeding resulted in the complete arrest of the pulse, which, however, almost immediately returned upon a little gentle pressure being made on the cord with a warm sponge. I then picked up what I supposed to be the two upper sacral nerves, and also divided their posterior roots, with the effect of again suddenly stopping the pulse which rapidly reappeared as before.

The patient had now become so exhausted that I dare not expend time in stitching up the wound in the dura mater, as I had intended to do, its edges were, therefore, merely adjusted as accurately as possible.

The wound in the soft parts was now closed by means of seven silk sutures, four deep, and three superficial. One drainage-tube having been placed at its lower end in contact with the dura mater, and a second at the upper extremity in the superficial parts. A moist sublimate dressing was then carefully applied, and the patient put to bed, the actual operation having lasted a little over one hour and a quarter.

In consequence of the haste with which the division of the nerve-roots had to be completed, there was some doubt as to whether I had not omitted to cut the second lumbar. This ultimately proved to be the case, but the immediate success of the treatment was fortunately not affected by the omission.

The most striking points noticed during the operation were the following:

1. The extreme comparative ease with which the spinal cord can be exposed even in its most inaccessible situation, as in this case, where it lay at its greatest depth from the surface.

2. The singular insignificance of the hæmorrhage, which was certainly less in quantity than is ordinarily lost during the removal of a mamma. The satisfactory result is undoubtedly due to the rapidity with which the muscular arterial branches retract and close after their division with a sharp knife.

3. The irregular shape of the dura mater, and the want of pulsation in it.

4. The absence of any sudden effect upon the pulse, either by the general severity of the proceedings, the escape of cerebro-spinal fluid, the free incision of the dura mater, or even the lifting of the cord from its bed for purposes of examination.

5. The sudden cessation of the pulse upon the division of the nerve-roots, and its rapid reappearance when slight pressure and warmth were applied to the exposed cord.

Subsequent progress of the case.—An hour after the operation the patient was sleeping, bathed in perspiration; but the pulse, although weak, was at least as strong as when he was first placed on the operating table.

At 9 p.m. on the same day the man was irritable and grumbling because his back felt so weak; he also complained of pain shooting down both thighs. The temperature was 100.6°, the pulse 104. He had taken nourishment.

A restless night followed, during which a good deal of discomfort was felt about the back. The spasms in the thigh occurred at intervals, and were distressing, because they shook the patient, rather than from any actual pain connected directly with them. Urine was voided naturally, although as a precaution it had been drawn off after the operation.

The next morning (December 25th) found the man still very irritable and discontented. There was considerable sweating. The pulse was rather stronger, the temperature 101°. Nourishment was taken freely.

The pain shooting down both thighs continued, but soon disappeared after the removal of the lower drainage-tube, which probably pressed a little on the theca as the patient lay on his back. The night following was better, with no pain worth mentioning.

On the 26th December the cerebro-spinal fluid, &c., had completely soaked the dressings again. The wound was therefore dressed. It was looking perfectly quiet, and was commencing to heal at the upper part, in spite of the violent twitches which frequently occurred in the mass of muscles forming its left side.

The temperature was 100.6°, the pulse distinctly fuller, perspiration less.

The bowels acted once naturally during the day. The urine was passed in the ordinary manner, and appeared normal.

27th.—The temperature was still rather high and irritable, fluctuating upon the least movement or excitement. The pulse was also very irritable, but, on the whole, not very weak. Nourishment was taken freely still, but towards night he was stated to have been slightly delirious once or twice. The next day, however, he was altogether better, and well pleased with his general condition.

29th.—The patient was comfortable, quite free from pain, and looking altogether better in the face. The spasms occurred at intervals, but were not painful; indeed, he had ceased to complain of them.

Some diarrhœa occurred during the morning, and unfortunately a portion of one of the loose motions passed up beneath the dressings, an accident, however, which was followed by no serious consequence.

The wound was dressed, and found to be almost

healed, the upper tube having been removed and two of the deep stitches taken out.

The flow of cerebro-spinal fluid was still free, but rapidly diminishing. In connection with this a rather curious fact was observed, viz. that whereas the irritation caused by this fluid on the right (sound) side of the wound was intense, on the left side, which was in great part insensitive, there was hardly any irritation at all. I at first thought that this was due to the fluid trickling more particularly over the right side; but it could hardly have been so, as the patient up to this time had been lying flat on his back; moreover, the moisture in the immediate neighbourhood of the wound was uniformly distributed over the dressings. It was further noticed that a small bedsore, situated over the left sacro-iliac joint, which had been quite inactive before the operation, rapidly healed after the part had become insensitive.

The notes of the case after this date need not be given in detail. The diarrhœa, which was very obstinate, ultimately subsided, the bowels acting twice daily. A small abscess, caused presumably by the passage of the loose motion into the dressings, formed along the tract of a suture, but was superficial, and gave rise to no serious inconvenience. The temperature gradually fell. The pulse varied considerably at different times, but on the whole steadily gained strength. The spasms occurred as before, but the pain did not return.

On the morning of January 3rd, 1889, the patient was comfortable and contented. The temperature was normal, the pulse 84 and regular, the appetite was good, the bowels had acted healthily. The wound, which was now dressed with boric ointment, had entirely healed, with the exception of a small sinus at the lower end, through which there drained in the twenty-four hours sufficient cerebro-spinal fluid to cause a mark on the dressings of about the size of a crown piece.

In the evening he complained of flatulence, and vomited some food which he had taken shortly before. A good night, however, was passed, and on the following morning (January 4th) at 10 o'clock, when I happened to be in the hospital, he was quite himself.

About 11 a.m. he said he felt "queer" in his head and placed both hands under his occiput. Almost directly he became suddenly collapsed, and vomited with violent straining. Copious cold sweats followed, and the vomiting recurred. All attempts to rally him from the collapse failed, he shortly became semi-comatose, and died on January 5th, at 2.30 a.m.

In the progress of the case nothing beyond the points incidentally alluded to in the notes requires special comment, excepting *the effect of the operation upon the sensation in the affected thigh*. This was in some respects remarkable. (See Diagrams, Fig. 1.)

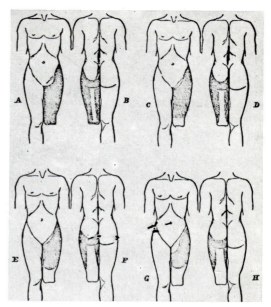

FIG. 1. Diagrams [to show effect of operation upon sensation in affected thigh].

On December 26th, at 1 p.m., the earliest time at which the patient's irritability would admit of the application of any reliable tests, the condition was as follows (Diagrams A,B):—The whole anterior aspect of the thigh was absolutely insensitive. The upper margin of this anæsthetic tract being abruptly marked by a line commencing just above the anterior superior iliac spine, and passing sinuously downwards to the point where the thigh joined the perinæum. Laterally this line of demarcation coursed downwards and backwards from a point about two inches behind the anterior superior spine, to the junction of the middle with the lower third of the buttock, from which, on the inner side, it curved upwards, passing close to the left sacro-iliac joint to terminate just below the middle of the operation wound, the left side of which at the lower part was quite insensitive.

The external, internal, and posterior aspects of the limb were insensitive, excepting along a narrow vertical tract, about one inch wide, which commenced suddenly at the lower border of the gluteal fold and passed down on to the back of the stump, fading away almost to nothing at its lower end.

Over an area extending downwards for about eight inches along the outer side of the thigh, from a point situated three fingers' breadth below the anterior superior spine of the ilium, the anæsthesia was less absolute than in the other parts.

The whole perinæum was normal in its sensation, and the external sphincter resented with its usual "grip" the introduction of the finger into the anus.

From the conditions just described it was clear that in dividing the nerve-roots I had not interrupted to any material extent the fibres passing to the small sciatic, that I had in no way interfered with the nerves supplying the parts about the perinæum, and that the nervous supply to the rectum and bladder had been left intact. It was also manifest that the genito-crural nerve had partly escaped injury, and that the external cutaneous had been only partly interrupted; these last two circumstances tending to strengthen the doubt which was felt as to my having divided the posterior root of the second lumbar nerve.

On January 3rd, 1889, the last occasion on which the sensation of the affected parts was tested, the condition was as follows (Diagrams G,H).

The whole circumference of the greater part of the lower half of the thigh was at least as sensitive as the corresponding part on the opposite limb. Over the upper half of the anterior surface there was an anæsthetic area, limited above by a line which, commencing one inch below the anterior superior iliac spine, passed with a double curve downwards and inwards, coursing round the inside of the thigh two and a half to three inches from its junction with the perinæum. Passing down the centre of the inner side of the thigh from the perinæum was a tongue-shaped sensitive tract, about five inches long, the base of which was three inches wide, or thereabouts. The posterior margin of this tongue passed upwards, and joined the gluteal fold at the outer end of its innermost fourth (Diagram H).

The superior half of the posterior aspect of the thigh was normal in its central (vertical) two fourths, this area of sensitiveness passing rather abruptly on each side into the anæsthetic parts.

The lowest third of the buttock was still insensitive, but above that level all the parts which had at first been deprived of sensation were now normal. The stages of transition from the condition of December 26th, 1888, to that of January 3rd, 1889, can be seen at a glance by reference to Diagrams C, D, E, F.

It is, I think, obvious that the rapidity with which sensation was recovered by the parts previously rendered insensitive by the operation, greatly exceeded anything of the kind commonly met with in surgical practice when a complete nerve-trunk (e.g. the median) has been divided. Moreover, this restoration, as was shown by the post-mortem examination, was quite independent of any attempt at union between the divided ends of the nerve-roots. Although it is, I understand, pretty generally accepted by physiological authorities, that complete restoration of sensation may follow, with remarkable rapidity after the division of the posterior root of a spinal nerve on the proximal side of its ganglion, there has been, so far as I can ascertain, no extensive corroboration

of this view in the human subject, until the occurrence of the case which I now record.

To whatever cause the return of function may be attributed, one very important contingency seems fairly certain in the case, viz. that had the patient lived sufficiently long the sensation over the whole of the affected part would have been regained, and further, that no danger of a recurrence of the pain need have been apprehended with the return of sensation, seeing that the restoration was independent of union between the cut ends of the nerve-roots.

Post-mortem examination.—The operation wound was soundly healed, excepting at its lower end, where a narrow channel led directly into the vertebral canal. On cutting down through the line of union a small abscess cavity was found between the muscular planes, following the course of two of the suture tracks; the abscess was, however, quite superficial to and unconnected with the spinal canal.

The posterior arches of the ninth, tenth, eleventh, twelfth dorsal and first lumbar vertebræ were wanting.

The wound in the dura mater was healed over its upper two thirds, but below the edges gaped, and were fringed with granulation tissue, lying upon which, on the right side, was a thin streak of organising lymph.

The spinal cord was perfectly normal as far down as the lower border of the sixth cervical vertebra. Below this point there were some minute recent blood extravasations in the subarachnoid space, and in the sub-dural space, about the level of the ninth dorsal vertebra, was also a small recent clot.

Opposite the seventh and eighth dorsal vertebræ there was a well-defined hardish thickening of the arachnoid on the left side, about a quarter of an inch wide and an inch long, somewhat spindle shaped, which apparently involved two of the posterior nerve-roots.

On the left side the first, third, fourth, and fifth lumbar and first and second sacral posterior nerve-roots had been divided, the proximal ends lying close to the cord, the distal extremities just appearing at the dural foramina. There was no attempt at union between the cut ends.

No lesion was found in any of the nerves forming the lumbar and sacral plexuses.

On opening the skull there was at once noticeable a relative smallness of the occipital lobes of the brain, especially on the left side, on which the surface was much discoloured by blood extravasation. On the upper surface of the tentorium, on each side of the falx, was a large patch of effused blood, and beyond this there was found, on the left side, another considerable blood-clot firmly adhering to the dura mater.

The occipital lobes, in addition to the peculiarity already alluded to, were distinctly harder to the touch than any other part of the brain. Scattered about the pia mater over the convexities of the two hemispheres, were a few well-marked opacities.

On section the whole brain with its vessels appeared healthy.

Microscopical examination.—Sections from the various regions of the spinal cord were prepared by Dr. Penrose, who has kindly provided the report which forms the appendix to this communication. As will be seen, the main point shown in the sections is a somewhat extensive *sclerosis* in the posterior root-zones and columns of Goll.

The sclerosed areas are more extensive in the left half of the cord than in the right, although the excess of sclerosis in the left side varies somewhat in different regions of the cord. Beyond the lesions noted in the cord itself nothing has been found which could in any way account for the pain from which the patient suffered.

As to whether the pain was in reality connected with the sclerosis I am unable to express any decided opinion, but the marked excess of the lesion in the left posterior region of the cord points to the possibility, at all events, of its having been the cause of the symptom. One point, however, seems quite clear, viz. that the perseverance in the administration of drugs could have effected no useful purpose, a circumstance which, in my mind, goes far to justify the treatment finally carried out, as I can conceive no other method by which the necessary relief to the sufferings could have been procured.

The cause of death.—On this point I am not quite clear. It is, of course, possible that the collapse which ushered in the fatal termination may have been in some way connected with the loss of cerebro-spinal fluid, but on the whole this seems unlikely when the length of time which had elapsed since the operation is considered, and also as the quantity of fluid draining away had become so small, and, indeed, was gradually growing less, there having been no sudden increase or diminution shortly before the onset of the fatal symptoms.

It is obvious that there was nothing whatever about the parts at the seat of operation to account for the symptoms, indeed, with the exception of the small abscess in relation with the track of the suture, which was of no consequence at all, the condition of the parts was quite satisfactory, the minute recent hæmorrhages being clearly due to the straining from the vomiting.

It is probable that the fatal issue may be attributed to one of two causes: (1) vomiting, possibly from flatulence with much straining, which produced the cerebral hæmorrhage and collapse; (2) apoplexy resulting in vomiting, collapse, and semi-coma.

Some slight evidence in favour of the former of these two causes is afforded by the fact that the patient was stated to have had on a previous occasion a similar attack of vomiting followed by collapse, from which he recovered slowly.

In conclusion little remains to be said. Cases in which a consideration of the treatment adopted in this case would be indicated must of necessity be rare. At the same time I can recall to mind certainly two patients who suffered from intractable pain of this kind, although hardly so severe, in each of whom repeated amputations were practised without any good result.

I venture to submit that in the case I now record the treatment was not only sound in theory, but was practically justified by the result, for the relief from pain was complete, and the patient lived not only long enough to survive the immediate effect of the operation, but also to commence what I think may, without any straining of terms, be called convalescence.

It is true that at the end of twelve days he died from a sudden and unexpected cause, but it is by no means clear that his death was even remotely connected with my operation; in fact, the inference seemed to be rather that the fatal issue was, as it were, accidental. Moreover, it was manifest to all who saw the patient before the operation, that he was certainly although slowly sinking, and that his survival for very many days was hardly possible. It was also quite plain that the attacks of exhaustion which followed the spasms might at any time end in fatal collapse.

Even if it be conceded for the moment that the issue was remotely contingent upon my operation, it seems extremely unlikely that life was shortened and it is certain that it was made comfortable.

Considering the remarkable way in which the man rallied, in spite of his previous state of extreme weakness, from the immediate shock of the operation, and the manner in which the strength was returning up to the time of the commencement of the fatal symptoms, I cannot help feeling that had I possessed the courage to propose and carry out the treatment earlier in the case, when the constitutional powers were comparatively good, instead of wasting valuable time by acquiescing in the patient's wish to go into the country, there is every probability that this paper, in the place of containing a description of a postmortem examination, would have been accompanied by a living specimen.

APPENDIX.

Result of Microscopical Examination by Dr. Penrose

No lesions other than the following have been detected in the contents of the spinal canal:

The pia mater sheath of the posterior root of the left sixth dorsal nerve is thickened by cicatricial deposit, which binds it down to the surface of the cord, forming an extra sheath completely sur-

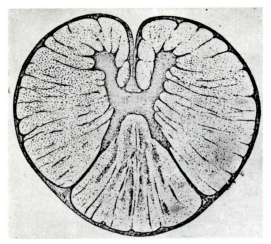

FIG. 2. Transverse section through spinal cord in lower dorsal region, showing distribution of sclerosis in posterior area.

rounding the fibres of the nerve, of which the endoneurium and perineurium are both increased. This sheath is apparently composed entirely of fibrous tissue, of tolerably recent though not of fresh origin, as is shown by the degree to which the fibrous tissue has been formed with the very small quantity of round-cells present. This condition may be taken as fairly clear evidence that the thickening had existed longer than twelve days (the period which had intervened between the date of the operation and the death of the patient). The nerve-fibres contained within this mass of tissue show signs of inflammation also in having lost their medullary sheaths. The axis cylinders are still for the most part, if not entirely, intact.

It is impossible, from the histological characters, to determine whether the mass is or is not gummatous in nature.

In the neighbourhood of the operation wound is a little recent granulation tissue tracking up the cord for a short distance along the pia mater.

The spinal cord.—Sections have been cut and prepared from the following regions:—Upper and middle cervical; upper, middle, and lower dorsal; upper, middle, and lower part of lumbar enlargement.

The sections have been stained by Pal's method (a modification of Weigert's); with aniline, blue-black; lithium carmine; and sections from all the regions have been stained by each of these methods.

Throughout the whole of the lower half of the dorsal portion of the cord there are small irregularly distributed areas of sclerosis in the posterior median (Goll's) columns and in the posterior root-zones.

The section shown in the drawing (Fig. 2) is from the lower dorsal region, and it shows fairly typically the condition of the whole of the lower half of the dorsal portion of the cord, although in the other parts the sclerosis is slightly different in position, and is apparently more irregular.

The sclerosed areas tend to gradually diminish towards the upper dorsal region, and finally disappear altogether, leaving the cord above the middle cervical portion quite normal in appearance.

The sclerosis throughout is distinctly more extensive in the left than in the right half of the cord, and tends to affect the posterior median columns proportionately more in the higher parts of the cord, although, as has been mentioned, the general area of the sclerosis is less in these regions.

In the posterior root-zones there is no one part in which the lesion can be said to be relatively more extensive than in another.

There are no changes in the vessels of the cord suggestive of syphilis.

The sections of the brain which have been examined show nothing abnormal.

(For report of the discussion on this paper, see 'Proceedings of the Royal Medical and Chirurgical Society,' Third Series, vol. i, p. 115.)

A CONTRIBUTION TO THE SURGERY OF THE SPINE.*

By ROBERT ABBE, M.D.

SURGEON TO ST. LUKE'S HOSPITAL, NEW YORK; CONSULTING SURGEON TO THE HOSPITAL FOR RUPTURED AND CRIPPLED; PROFESSOR OF SURGERY, POST-GRADUATE SCHOOL AND HOSPITAL, NEW YORK

THE surgery of the spine is one of the new chapters soon to be written, from which much may be expected. As yet, however, so little work has been done or published that statistical tables upon the subject are untimely and of little profit.

It should be a surgical axiom that every case of operative interference should be published, and I shall therefore present concisely, for our study, two cases that have recently come under my care, deducting such practical lessons as may be deemed important. I have the pleasure of showing you the patients themselves.

The second patient is one whose malady is more complicated, whose recovery is not yet so brilliant, but whose operation stands, as yet, quite unique. Intractable brachial neuralgia, nerve stretching, amputation, and finally, division of posterior roots of the sixth, seventh, and eighth cervical. Improvement.

* Reprinted in part from *Medical Record, New York*, 1889, 35: 149–152.

Mr. I. R. T——— is forty-four years of age, an iceman. He was referred to me three months ago by Dr. C. L. Dana, of New York, to see if I were willing to undertake an operation, conceived by him, to relieve the patient of one of the most intractable of neuralgias of the right brachial plexus, appearing in the arm and forearm. The essential features of the operation were carried out as planned from the first by Dr. Dana. The patient's history is as follows:

Prior to this trouble, he had no disease—rheumatism, malaria, or specific. During the war a shell explosion left a small piece of it in his left shoulder, which was extracted on the field, and left only a small flesh scar; never otherwise injured. One year ago last May, he spent a day putting a zinc lining in a large butcher's refrigerator, and on the night following he first had a throbbing pain, localized in a single spot on the posterior surface of the right forearm, above the middle. The pain kept him from sleep. It was continuous at that site, but about one week later, there was added a paroxysmal pain giving a peculiar twitching sensation in the thumb, index, and middle finger of the same hand. He was treated by electricity, blisters, counter-irritants, and internal medication, by excellent doctors, but his arm grew steadily worse. The pain still localized over the forearm, and supplemented by the paroxysms of painful twisting sensation. There seems to have been distinct muscular spasm with the sensation of pain.

During the spring of last year there had ensued a disablement of the hand. The fingers were not readily closed nor extended. The hand was kept in a stiff position, the fingers semi-flexed. The forearm and hand were slightly emaciated. There was atrophy of muscle in the interosseous spaces. Dr. Dana and others thus saw him, and a diagnosis of ascending neuritis was arrived at. At this time he came under the care of Dr. W. T. Bull, at the New York Hospital. After a week the patient begged an operation, and the doctor stretched the posterior interosseous and ulnar nerves. The pain was not improved. If anything, it was worse.

On July 16th, at the patient's earnest request, the arm was amputated by Dr. Bull above the humeral insertion of the deltoid, and above any site of local pain heretofore complained of. The wound healed by first intention. As far as the eye could judge, all nerves in the arm were in a normal condition. When the wound had healed it was found there was no abatement of pain. It still had a "drawing" character, and he could feel the fingers twist just as if they were on. He left the hospital August 1st, if anything, complaining of more pain than before. He then came under the care of Dr. William Kemp, of New York, who

again sought Dr. Dana's counsel. The patient had now got in the habit of taking morphine, one half grain every hour, to destroy the pain.

Of this interview Dr. Dana writes me thus:

"On September 25th I examined him again. The arm had been removed. The patient said he felt no better. There were twitchings and tonic contractions in the muscles of the stump. The patient had the Brauch-Romberg symptom, swayed in standing, and had a tendency to fall to the right when walking with eyes closed. Knee-jerks exaggerated and ankle clonus in right leg, all of which might be due to the morphine he was taking. There was much stiffness in the neck muscles. The patient could not rotate his head completely to the right, nor draw the head down to the right shoulder. The diagnosis, so far, had been neuritis—and of this there could be no doubt. The question was whether it might be due to a tumor or inflammatory process, either extra-spinal or extra-dural. An exploratory operation was advised with the idea, if no tumor was found, of cutting the posterior roots of the nerves transmitting pain. If it were a tumor, *that* could be removed. If it were ascending neuritis, cutting or resecting the nerve might stop it; while cutting the posterior roots would cause an ascending degeneration and destroy the sensory tract, even into the spinal cord."

At this juncture he went to Dr. Seguin for a month, and returning to Dr. Dana, was sent to me at St. Luke's Hospital. His condition then was as follows:

November 2d.—Had grown thin, was careworn and hollow under the eyes. Appetite fair, tongue coated. No fever. He gives evidence of sharp pain, every few minutes, in the stump of his right arm, and usually doubles over and grasps the stump with the other hand. When asked about it, says it jumps and the stump draws to his side when the pain shoots into the hands and fingers, as if they were still on, and he can feel them all drawn up. The pain seems to be genuine, and the recurrence every five or ten minutes. He says also that they keep up all night. Muscular atrophy is beginning to be marked about the shoulder, either from the disuse or degeneration. The deltoid, supra and infra spinati, and biceps are atrophied; while the lateral dorsi and pectoral major are short and thin, but still act strongly when called upon. A small, tender neuroma of the musculo-spiral nerve in the stump, can be felt, and on pressure gives the same pain as is generally complained of.

November 7th.—Dissected out the neuroma under cocaine.

November 24th.—Not relieved by the removal of the neuroma. Urine 1.024, no albumen or sugar. Some oxalates.

December 31st.—Operated under ether, Dr. Bangs assisting, in the presence of a number of prominent neurologists and surgeons.

The usual surgical precautions were carried out. An incision was made along the ligamentum nuchæ on the right side, from the third cervical spine to the first dorsal. The soft tissues were quickly separated from the spine, and the right half of all the laminæ well out on the articular processes. With rongeurs the laminæ were quickly gnawed away from the spine to articular processes —thus bringing into view the rather full pulsating dural membrane of the cord.

The seventh, sixth, fifth, and half the fourth nerves were thus treated. Severe venous bleeding from under the latter was only controlled by an aneurism-needle protected by cotton and hooked up beneath the bone. Over two inches of dura was exposed. It was soft and allowed the finger pressure to feel the cord. No tumor was thus detected, nor did a director passed up and down the canal feel anything like tumor. There was no inflammation or disease of the hard parts. With a heavy curved hook I then explored the intervertebral foramina, and drew back the sixth nerve by hooking under it and pulling gently, so that a short loop of it was raised on my hook outside its point of exit from the dura, but inside the vertebral canal. Upon this root, thus raised, I applied a small metal electrode, while the opposite pole (a sponge electrode) was held on the back. Dr. Dana noted the effect. The same was tried on the seventh nerve, with less effect. My own observations, as did those of Prof. Markoe and others, coincided with Dr. Dana's. He writes: "On the day of operation, a faradic battery of one cell, moderate current, was used. A sponge electrode on the back, a metal point electrode on the nerve. When applied to the sixth nerve just external to the dura, it caused contraction of the supra and infra spinati, rhomboid, latissimus dorsi, pectoralis major, teres, and deltoid. The results of electrizing the seventh nerve were not so satisfactory, it not being certain that the point reached that nerve alone (on account of fluid that collected around the electrode). It was impossible to drag out the fifth nerve without exciting more hemorrhage from the venous sinus." The eighth nerve also was hidden below the bone, and it was thought enough had been done. The sixth and seventh were then again dragged up from their beds and cut square across just outside the dura. Both motor and sensory roots lie together at this point, so that they must have been severed. The wound was packed, entirely open, with iodoform gauze covered by a voluminous gauze dressing. He bore the operation well, but soon found his old pain seemed much the same—still low down in the hand.

January 2d.—Forty-eight hours after operation

I felt that I ought to divide at least one more branch (the eighth), if I could do so, and if possible to examine the spinal cord, inasmuch as Horsley had not detected the tumor in his celebrated case until he had opened the dura. I therefore determined to do this, place the man prone, without ether, and open the dura, so as to get a clue to the sensations of the nerve-roots when handled. With the assistance again of Drs. Dana, W. T. Bull, and many others, I operated.

The patient was placed under a brilliant light, face downward, so as to maintain the operated part as the highest of the spinal axis. I carefully removed the packing, revealing a large, clean, dry wound, at the bottom of which lay the dura, throbbing and sound. Puncturing it with a knife, I slipped in a fine director and slowly let out the spinal fluid until it ceased to run. Then I slit up the dura for one and a half inch. The cord and membranes looked sound. The effect of evacuating two ounces of spinal fluid (carefully collected and measured) was practically nihil. The pulse did not change, and he experienced no sensations or pain. The dura was scarcely at all sensitive to cutting. I now picked up the roots of the eighth nerve within the dura at the level of the seventh nerve outside.

It looked normal, but I cut it close to the posterior spinal columns, and then snipped off a fourth-inch for microscopical examination. Handling this nerve-root gave him the greatest pain of anything I had done, and of a kind exactly corresponding with that which he constantly suffers. I had reason to hope, therefore, we had reached the offender. In addition I cut also the posterior roots of the seventh nerve close to the columns of the cord.

In two operations, therefore, I had cut the sixth nerve, both roots, outside. The seventh, both roots outside, and also the posterior root inside. The eighth posterior roots only inside the dura. It was observed that the contact of even a blunt soft instrument to the posterior columns gave a sharp agonizing pain over the entire body, the patient crying out, "Ah! I can't stand it."

We again tried the battery, and with regard to it Dr. Dana writes: "On the second trial, the patient being conscious, stimulation in the same way—of the peripheric end of the cut sixth nerve— caused contraction of the supra and infra spinati and rhomboid. Of the seventh nerve, contraction of the pectoral, latissimus dorsi, and adductors of the arm, with pains such as he usually suffers. Of the eighth nerve, similar contraction and intense 'drawing pain,' exactly such as is usually felt."

The slit in the dura was now sutured with fine catgut. A little cocaine had been injected along the cut wound half an hour before, and this allowed of painlessly suturing the entire length of the wound. Immediate union was thus obtained by second intention, and leaves a small linear scar. The patient had more or less of pain in the arm in the next ten days, but it changed in character. It no longer went down into the fingers. It was a "drawing of the stump," as he expressed it. It ceased to go up on the shoulder as it once did. He was allowed enough morphine to quiet pain for eleven days, when I deemed it best to let him sit up and stopped the drug entirely.

He missed it, but quickly got used to it, and since has had even less pain than when he was getting his morphine to quiet it. He walked freely at the end of the third week, and soon went in the open air. His gait is now as steady as for months past, and he can walk a crack in the ward any distance.

His temperature was 101° F. on the second day, and 102° F. on the fourth, but declined from that to normal on the tenth. The appearance of the upper arm and stump is one of increasing atrophy. There is no voluntary movement of the supra- or infra-spinatus, deltoid, or biceps, but there is of the latissimus and pectoral, though both are shrunken from disuse. There is anæsthesia of the skin of the entire outer side of the arm from the deltoid region downward, extending across the shoulder from the centre of the clavicle to the centre of the scapula. This area of the skin showed a short period of irritability, without sensation, from the fourth to the eighth day after the root section, as shown by getting quickly and persistently suffused when brushed over or handled; but when pinched retaining an extreme blanching at that point which did not recover for two or three minutes. This entire area is now, however, normal in appearance.

In considering the lessons drawn from these cases it is to be remembered that in any path of study knowledge never comes entire at once, but piecemeal. Truth presents herself in fragmentary form, and we put the pieces together; so that, while I do not present the case of cervical operation as a brilliant result as yet, so far as completely relieving the pain goes, I offer it as a unique case making a quick recovery from an operation, as conceived by Dr. Dana, at once simple and scientific.

. . . With regard to the case of neuralgia of the arm, no indisputable diagnosis had been made prior to my operation.

The man had neuralgia, but the cause of it, even such eminent neurologists as Drs. Dana, Seguin, Amidon, Starr, and others, were not united on.

It was believed to be ascending neuritis, but might be spinal tumor, or a delusional pain (Seguin) aggravated by morphine.

The language of pain is not at all times plain. If it were an ascending neuritis, could we expect to relieve it either by nerve-stretching, amputation, or neurectomy?

It has always been acknowledged difficult to get ahead of a neuritis of this type. The late Dr. Sands operated once on a similar case to this man's, by excision of the brachial plexus all the roots in the neck, but found it very hazardous and unavailing. It also left the arm powerless. It seems to me reasonable that the posterior roots should be severed alone, as they alone transmit sensation to the cerebrum.

The operation has endorsement from neurectomies of the sensory fifth nerve for the cure of tic douloureux.

There remains one point for consideration which this case of section of the sixth and seventh nerve will help to elucidate.

The exact supply of the nerve-roots to the muscles of the arm has been somewhat a matter of conjecture, and frequently subject to revision.

William Thorburn, of Manchester, has only very recently published the results of study of many cases of fractured cervical spines, in which nerve-roots were injured with varying paralyses. The conclusions from this attractive and well-observed series of cases seem to leave some gaps in testimony, and errors which further study will correct. My case gives some points of value.

Thorburn places the pectoralis major and latissimus dorsi muscles in the supply of the sixth root. Yet in my case these are not paralyzed, though I have cut the sixth and seventh. Therefore these must be largely innervated from the fifth.

That there was no error in identifying the sixth, is shown by the supra- and infra-spinati supply and the anæsthetic area.

Appendix of Additional References

A. Related to Specific Neurosurgical Classics

1. ZIMMERMAN, L. M. The beginnings of surgery and *the Edwin Smith papyrus*. *J. int. Coll. Surg.*, 1957, *27:* 14–21.

   ZIMMERMAN, L. M., and VEITH, I. Great ideas in the history of surgery. *Baltimore: Williams & Wilkins Co.*, 1961, xii, 587 pp. (see pp. 3–13).

2. BRODSKI, I. The trephiners of Blanche Bay, New Britain, their instruments and methods. *Brit. J. Surg.*, 1938, *26:* 1–9.

   CLARKE, E. The early history of the cerebral ventricles. *Trans. Coll. Phycns Philad.*, 1962, 4th s. *30:* 85–89.

   CLARKE, E. Aristotelian concepts of the form and function of the brain. *Bull. Hist. Med.*, 1963, *37:* 1–14.

   CLARKE, E. Apoplexy in the Hippocratic writings. *Bull. Hist. Med.*, 1963, *37:* 301–314.

   CLARKE, E., and STANNARD, J. Aristotle on the anatomy of the brain. *J. Hist. Med.*, 1963, *18:* 130–148.

   ELLIOTT, I. M. Z. A short history of surgical dressings. *London: Pharmaceutical Press*, 1964, x, 118 pp.

   KING, L. S. The growth of medical thought. *Chicago: Univ. of Chicago Press*, 1963, xi, 254 pp.

   MAJOR, R. H. Galen as a neurologist. *World Neurol.*, 1961, *2:* 372–380.

   MOODIE, R. L. Studies in paleopathology, XXIII. Surgery in pre-Columbian Peru. *Ann. med. Hist.*, 1929, 2nd s. *1:* 698–728.

   PENFIELD, W. Hippocrates comes to a symposium on epilepsy. In: *Epileptic seizures. A correlative study of historical, diagnostic, therapeutic, educational and employment aspects of epilepsy.* J. R. Green, and H. F. Steelman, Ed. Baltimore: Williams & Wilkins Co., 1956, xii, 165 pp. (see pp. 153–160).

   PENFIELD, W. The Aegean cradle of medicine. *Trans. Coll. Phycns Philad.*, 1956, 4th s. *24:* 20–30.

   PENFIELD, W. The Asclepiad physicians of Cnidus and Cos with a note on the probable site of the Triopion Temple of Apollo. *Proc. Amer. phil. Soc.*, 1957, *101:* 393–400.

   PENFIELD, W. From Hippocratic facts to fiction. Hippocratic foreword. *Clin. Neurosurg.*, 1957, *4:* 11–20.

   RYTEL, M. M. Trephinations in ancient Peru. *Bull. Pol. med. sci. Hist.*, 1962, *5:* 42–45.

   SINGER, C. Brain dissection before Vesalius. *J. Hist. Med.*, 1956, *11:* 261–274.

   SOLMSEN, F. Greek philosophy and the discovery of the nerves. *Mus. Helveticum*, 1961, *18:* 150–197.

   STEWART, T. D. Significance of osteitis in ancient Peruvian trephining. *Bull. Hist. Med.*, 1956, *30:* 293–320.

   TEMKIN, O. The doctrine of epilepsy in the Hippocratic writings. *Bull. Inst. Hist. Med.*, 1933, *1:* 277–322.

   TEMKIN, O. Galen's "Advice for an epileptic boy." *Bull. Inst. Hist. Med.*, 1934, *2:* 179–189.

   TEMKIN, O. Epilepsy in an anonymous Greek work on acute and chronic diseases. *Bull. Inst. Hist. Med.*, 1936, *4:* 137–144.

   TEMKIN, O. Research before Hughlings Jackson. *Res. Publ. Ass. nerv. ment. Dis.*, 1947, *26:* 3–7.

   TOOLE, H. Fractures of the skull. Diagnosis and treatment in ancient Greece. *J. int. Coll. Surg.*, 1964, *42:* 89–94.

   ULLRICH, H., and WEICKMANN, F. Prähistorische "Neurochirurgie" im mitteldeutschen Raum. *Zbl. Neurochir.*, 1963, *24:* 103–121.

3. BRAZIER, M. A. B. The history of the electrical activity of the brain as a method for localizing sensory function. *Med. Hist.*, 1963, *7:* 199–211.

   GRUNDFEST, H. The different careers of Gustav Fritsch (1838–1927). *J. Hist. Med.*, 1963, *18:* 125–129.

   KOSHTOYANTS, K. S. The history of the problem of brain cortex excitability. *Actes VIII Congrès int. d'Histoire des Sciences*, 1956, *2:* 862–864.

   LACHMAN, S. J. History and methods of physiological psychology. A brief overview. *Detroit: Hamilton Press*, 1963, 64 pp.

   SHEER, D. E. Brain and behavior: the background of interdisciplinary research. In: *Electrical stimulation of the brain. An interdisciplinary survey of neurobehavioral integrative systems.* D. E. Sheer, Ed. Austin: Univ. of Texas Press, 1961, xiv, 641 pp. (see pp. 3–21).

   WALKER, A. E. Stimulation and ablation. Their role in the history of cerebral physiology. *J. Neurophysiol.*, 1957, *20:* 435–449.

4. BAUMGARTNER, L. A note on the Fritzsche-Klebs description of acromegaly (1884). *Bull. Hist Med.*, 1940, *8:* 446–460.

   GERMAN, W. J., and FLANIGAN, S. Pituitary adenomas: a follow-up study of the Cushing series. *Clin. Neurosurg.*, 1964, *10:* 72–81.

   KELLY, E. C. Encyclopedia of medical sources. *Baltimore: Williams & Wilkins Co.*, 1948, v, 476 pp. (see p. 100).

   MAJOR, R. H. Classic descriptions of disease. With biographical sketches of the authors. *Springfield, Ill.: Charles C Thomas*, 1945, 3rd ed., xxxii, 679 pp. (see pp. 305–309).

   MONTGOMERY, D. A. D. Pituitary tumors in Cushing's syndrome. *Clin. Neurosurg.*, 1964, *10:* 169–187.

   PARDEE, I. Pituitary basophilism of Cushing—syndrome of the basophilic adenoma. *Res. Publ. Ass. nerv. ment. Dis.*, 1938, *17:* 590–608.

   ROBERTSON, J. D. Glinski and the aetiology of Simmonds's disease (hypopituitarism). *Brit. med. J.*, 1951, *1:* 921–923.

   SALVESEN, H. A. Case of Cushing's syndrome due to an adrenal tumour described in 1914 by Dr. Lucien Dedichen of Kristiania (Oslo). *Med. Hist.*, 1961, *5:* 283–285.

WEINBERG, S. J. Gigantism and acromegaly (hyperpituitarism). *Ann. med. Hist.*, 1931, 2nd s. *3*: 650–673.

5. BAY, E. The history of aphasia and the principles of cerebral localization. In: *Cerebral localization and organization*. G. Schaltenbrand and C. N. Woolsey, Ed. Madison: Univ. of Wisconsin Press, 1964, xii, 164 pp. (see pp. 43–52).

BENTON, A. L., and JOYNT, R. J. Early descriptions of aphasia. *Arch. Neurol., Chicago*, 1960, *3*: 205–222.

BENTON, A. L., and JOYNT, R. J. Three pioneers in the study of aphasia. *J. Hist. Med.*, 1963, *18*: 381–383.

CRITCHLEY, M. Broca's contribution to aphasia reviewed a century later. In: *Scientific aspects of neurology*. H. Garland, Ed. Baltimore: Williams & Wilkins Co., 1961, xi, 264 pp. (see pp. 131–141).

CRITCHLEY, M. The origins of aphasiology. *Scot. med. J.*, 1964, *9*: 231–242.

CROSBY, E. C., HUMPHREY, T., and LAUER, E. W. Correlative anatomy of the nervous system. *New York: Macmillan Co.*, 1962, x, 731 pp. (see pp. 514–518).

HÉCAEN, H. Clinical symptomatology in right and left hemispheric lesions. In: *Interhemispheric relations and cerebral dominance*. V. B. Mountcastle, Ed. Baltimore: Johns Hopkins Press, 1962, x, 294 pp. (see pp. 215–243).

JOYNT, R. J., and BENTON, A. L. The memoir of Marc Dax on aphasia. *Neurology*, 1964, *14*: 851–854.

NIELSEN, J. M. Agnosia, apraxia, aphasia. Their value in cerebral localization. *New York: P. B. Hoeber, Inc.*, 1946, 2nd ed., x, 292 pp. (see pp. 1–14).

RIESE, W. Hughlings Jackson's doctrine of aphasia and its significance today. *J. nerv. ment. Dis.*, 1955, *122*: 1–13.

WEISENBURG, T., and MCBRIDE, K. E. Aphasia. A clinical and psychological study. *New York: The Commonwealth Fund*, 1935, xvi, 634 pp. (see pp. 6–118).

ZANGWILL, O. L. The current status of cerebral dominance. *Res. Publ. Ass. nerv. ment. Dis.*, 1964, *42*: 103–113.

8. FULTON, J. F. A note on Francesco Gennari and the early history of cytoarchitectural studies of the cerebral cortex. *Bull. Inst. Hist. Med.*, 1937, *5*: 895–913.

HASSLER, R. Die Entwicklung der Architektonik seit Brodmann und ihre Bedeutung für die moderne Hirnforschung. *Dtsch. med. Wschr.*, 1962, *87*: 1180–1185.

JEFFERSON, G. Variations on a neurological theme —cortical localization. *Brit. med. J.*, 1955, *2*: 1405–1408.

LYONS, J. B. The advent of neurophysiology. *J. Irish med. Ass.*, 1963, *52*: 55–61.

OLMSTED, J. M. D. The aftermath of Charles Bell's famous "idea." *Bull. Hist. Med.*, 1943, *14*: 341–351.

SMITH, A. Ambiguities in concepts and studies of "brain damage" and "organicity." *J. nerv. ment. Dis.*, 1962, *135*: 311–326.

10. DAVIS, L. E. Decerebrate rigidity in man. *Arch. Neurol. Psychiat., Chicago*, 1925, *13*: 569–579.

DeJONG, R. N. The neurologic examination. Incorporating the fundamentals of neuroanatomy and neurophysiology. *New York: P. B. Hoeber Inc.*, 1950, xiii, 1079 pp. (see pp. 555–630).

FULTON, J. F., and KELLER, A. D. The sign of Babinski. A study of the evolution of cortical dominance in primates. *Springfield, Ill.: Charles C Thomas*, 1932, xi, 165 pp.

HOFF, H. E., and KELLAWAY, P. The early history of the reflex. *J. Hist. Med.*, 1952, *7*: 211–249.

WARTENBERG, R. Studies in reflexes. History, physiology, synthesis and nomenclature: Study I. *Arch Neurol. Psychiat., Chicago*, 1944, *51*: 113–133, 414.

WARTENBERG, R. Studies in reflexes. History, physiology, synthesis and nomenclature: Study II. *Arch. Neurol. Psychiat., Chicago*, 1944, *52*: 341–358.

WARTENBERG, R. Studies in reflexes. History, physiology, synthesis and nomenclature: Study III. *Arch. Neurol. Psychiat., Chicago*, 1944, *52*: 359–382.

11. CRITCHLEY, M. James Parkinson (1755–1824). A bicentenary volume of papers dealing with Parkinson's Disease, incorporating the original 'Essay on the Shaking Palsy'. *London: Macmillan & Co. Ltd.*, 1955, xvi, 268 pp.

DAVIS, R. A. Victorian physician-scholar and pioneer physiologist. *Surg. Gynec. Obstet.*, 1964, *119*: 1333–1340.

DAVIS, R. A., and BROOKS, F. P. Experimental peptic ulcer associated with lesions or stimulation of the central nervous system. *Int. Abstr. Surg.*, 1963, *116*: 307–320.

GREENFIELD, J. G. Historical landmarks in the pathology of involuntary movements. *J. Neuropath. exp. Neurol.*, 1956, *15*: 5–11.

LEWY, F. H. Historical introduction: The basal ganglia and their diseases. *Res. Publ. Ass. nerv. ment. Dis.*, 1942, *21*: 1–20.

MEYERS, R. Historical background and personal experiences in the surgical relief of hyperkinesia and hypertonus. In: *Pathogenesis and treatment of parkinsonism*. W. S. Fields, Ed. Springfield, Ill.: Charles C Thomas, 1958, x, 372 pp. (see pp. 229–270).

OSTHEIMER, A. J. An essay on the shaking palsy, by James Parkinson, M. D., member of the Royal College of Surgeons. With a bibliographic note thereon by Alfred J. Ostheimer. *Arch. Neurol. Psychiat., Chicago*, 1922, *7*: 681–710.

PARKINSON, J. An essay on the shaking palsy. *Med. Class.*, 1938, *2*: 964–997.

12. COURVILLE, C. B. Commotio cerebri. Cerebral concussion and the postconcussion syndrome in their medical and legal aspects. *Los Angeles: San Lucas Press*, 1953, xi, 161 pp.

COURVILLE, C. B. Development and use of helmets as a means of protection against craniocerebral injury. II. By the nations of antiquity. *Bull. Los Angeles neurol. Soc.*, 1954, *19*: 47–65.

COURVILLE, C. B. Trauma to the central nervous system and its envelopes. In: *Tice's Practice of medicine*. J. C. Harvey, Ed. Hagerstown, Md.: W. F. Prior Co., Inc., 1962, *10*: 139–223.

FORSTER, F. M. Benjamin Bell on traumatic

extracerebral hematomas. *Bull. Hist. Med.*, 1944, *15:* 289–305.

GROFF, R. A., and GRANT, F. C. Chronic subdural hematoma. Collective review. *Int. Abstr. Surg.*, 1942, *74:* 9–20.

JAVID, M., GILBOE, D., and CESARIO, T. The rebound phenomenon and hypertonic solutions. *J. Neurosurg.*, 1964, *21:* 1059–1066.

JEPPSSON, S., JÄRPE, S. E., and RABOW, L. The treatment of increased intracranial pressure in neurosurgery. A clinical report on the use of intravenous hypertonic urea in 174 craniotomies with an evaluation of this and other decompressive methods, alone and in combination. *Acta chir. scand.*, 1963, suppl. *312:* 3–26.

PICKLES, W. The treatment of head injuries in France in the early seventeen hundreds. With a note on Pierre Boudou and his recognition and treatment of subdural hematoma. *Bull. Hist. Med.*, 1950, *24:* 421–433.

PUTMAN, T. J. Chronic subdural hematoma. Its pathology, its relation to pachymeningitis hemorrhagica and its surgical treatment. With cases contributed by members of the Society of Neurological Surgeons and a prefatory note by Harvey Cushing, M. D. *Arch. Surg., Chicago*, 1925, *11:* 329–393.

SCHEINBERG, S. C., and SCHEINBERG, L. C. Early description of chronic subdural hematoma. Etiology, symptomatology, and treatment. *J. Neurosurg.*, 1964, *21:* 445–446.

STRAUSS, I., and SAVITSKY, N. Head injury. Neurologic and psychiatric aspects. *Arch. Neurol. Psychiat., Chicago*, 1934, *31:* 893–955.

STRAYER, L. M. Augustin Belloste and the treatment for avulsion of the scalp. The odd history of an operation in head surgery. *New Engl. J. Med.*, 1939, *220:* 901–905.

ZÜLCH, K. J. Störungen des intrakraniellen Druckes. Die Massenverschiebungen und Formveränderungen des Hirns bei raumfordernden und schrumpfenden Prozessen und ihre Bedeutung für die klinische und röntgenologische Diagnostik. *Olivecrona u. Tönnis Handb. Neurochir.*, 1959, *1,* pt. *1:* 208–303.

14. FALCONER, M. A., SERAFETINIDES, E. A., and CORSELLIS, J. A. N. Etiology and pathogenesis of temporal lobe epilepsy. *Arch. Neurol., Chicago*, 1964, *10:* 233–248.

FULTON, J. F. Clifford Allbutt's description of psychomotor seizures. *J. Hist. Med.*, 1957, *12:* 75–77.

GREEN, J. R., and SCHEETZ, D. G. Surgery of epileptogenic lesions of the temporal lobe. *Arch. Neurol., Chicago*, 1964, *10:* 135–148.

PENFIELD, W. L'écorce cérébrale chez l'homme. *Année psychol.*, 1938, *39:* 1–32.

PENFIELD, W., and PEROT, P. The brain's record of auditory and visual experience—a final summary and discussion. *Brain*, 1963, *86:* 595–696.

15. DANDY, W. E. Pneumoperitoneum. A method of detecting intestinal perforation—an aid in abdominal diagnosis. *Ann. Surg.*, 1919, *70:* 378–383.

17. DI CHIRO, G. and FISHER, R. L. Contrast radiography of the spinal cord. *Arch. Neurol., Chicago*, 1964, *11:* 125–143.

19. ABRAMS, H. L. Angiography. *Boston: Little, Brown & Co.*, 1961, 2 vols. (see *1:* 3–12).

DAVIS, L. Neurological surgery, so to speak, out of roentgenology. Hickey lecture, 1956. *Amer. J. Roentgenol.*, 1956, *76:* 217–225.

DI CHIRO, G. The reliability of neuroradiology. *Clin. Neurosurg.*, 1964, *10:* 151–168.

TAVERAS, J. M., and WOOD, E. H. Diagnostic neuroradiology. *Baltimore: Williams & Wilkins Co.*, 1964, x, 960 pp. (see pp. 469–471, 477–482, 485–490).

20. BARNERT, C. The determination of the systolic and diastolic pressure in the central artery of the retina (method of Magitot). Its value in the early recognition of increased intracranial pressure. *Res. Publ. Ass. nerv. ment. Dis.*, 1929, *8:* 245–255.

BEHRMAN, S. Pathology of papilledema. *Neurology*, 1964, *14:* 236–239.

RUCKER, C. W., and KEYS, T. E. The atlases of ophthalmoscopy, 1850–1950. (No publisher), 1950, 33 pp.

24. CLENDENING, L. Source book of medical history. *New York: Dover Publications, Inc.*, 1960, xiv, 685 pp. (see pp. 666–675).

DEWING, S. B. Modern radiology in historical perspective. *Springfield, Ill.: Charles C Thomas*, 1962, ix, 189 pp.

25. DOOLIN, W. The first hurdle: the arrest of haemorrhage. *J. Irish med. Ass.*, 1956, *38:* 92–98.

HARVEY, S. C. The history of hemostasis. *Ann. med. Hist.*, 1929, 2nd s. *1:* 127–154.

29. BUCY, P. C. Tumors of the brain. In: *Tice's Practice of medicine.* J. C. Harvey, Ed. Hagerstown, Md.: W. F. Prior Co., Inc., 1962, *9:* 565–746.

CUSHING, H., and EISENHARDT, L. Notes on the first reasonably successful removal of an intracranial tumor. *Bull. Los Angeles neurol. Soc.*, 1938, *3:* 95–98.

NETSKY, M. G., and LAPRESLE, J. The first account of a meningioma. *Bull. Hist. Med.*, 1956, *30:* 465–468.

37. RAND, C. W. The neurosurgical patient. His problems of diagnosis and care. *Springfield, Ill.: Charles C Thomas*, 1944, xii, 576 pp. (see pp. 442–453).

39. BETT, W. R. Frank Hartley (1856–1913) and the Hartley-Krause operation. *Med. Pr.*, 1956, *235:* 496.

BETT, W. R. Fedor Victor Krause (1857–1937) of "Krause's operation." *Med. Pr.*, 1957, *237:* 246–247.

MEYER, A. W. The Gasser of the Gasserian ganglion. *Ann. med. Hist.*, 1936, 2nd s. *8:* 118–123.

42. CUSHING, H., and BAILEY, P. Tumors arising from the blood-vessels of the brain. Angiomatous malformations and hemangioblastomas. *Springfield, Ill.: Charles C Thomas*, 1928, x, 219 pp.

DANDY, W. E. Arteriovenous aneurysm of the brain. *Arch. Surg., Chicago*, 1928, *17:* 190–243.

DANDY, W. E. Venous abnormalities and angiomas of the brain. *Arch. Surg., Chicago*, 1928, *17:* 715–793.

ELVIDGE, A. R., and FEINDEL, W. H. Surgical treatment of aneurysm of the anterior cerebral and of the anterior communicating arteries diagnosed by angiography and electroencephalography. *J. Neurosurg.*, 1950, *7:* 13–32.

MACKENZIE, I. The intracranial bruit. *Brain*, 1955, *78:* 350–368.

OLIVECRONA, H., and LADENHEIM, J. Congenital arteriovenous aneurysms of the carotid and vertebral arterial systems. *Berlin: Springer-Verlag*, 1957, iv, 91 pp.

SYMONDS, C. The circle of Willis. *Brit. med. J.*, 1955, *1:* 119–124.

44. BEEKMAN, F. A celebrated case of cerebral injury. *Bull. Hist. Med.*, 1945, *17:* 521–526.

BUSCH, E. Psychosurgery. *Olivecrona u. Tönnis Handb. Neurochir.*, 1957, *6:* 137–177.

HOFF, H. E. John Fulton's contribution to neurophysiology. *J. Hist. Med.*, 1962, *17:* 16–37.

RAMSEY, G. V. A short history of psychosurgery. *Amer. J. Psychiat.*, 1952, *108:* 813–816.

45. ATKINSON, M. Ménière's original papers, reprinted with an English translation together with commentaries and biographical sketch. *Acta otolaryng., Stockh.*, 1961, suppl. *162:* 1–78.

DAVEY, L. M., and GERMAN, W. J. Ménière's disease. A centennial historical note. *J. Neurosurg.*, 1962, *19:* 82–83.

HOUSE, H. P., and HOUSE, W. F. Historical review and problem of acoustic neuroma. *Arch. otolaryng., Chicago*, 1964, *80:* 601–604.

POOL, J. L., and PAVA, A. A. The early diagnosis and treatment of acoustic nerve tumors. *Springfield, Ill.: Charles C. Thomas*, 1957, viii, 161 pp.

46. GLOBUS, J. H. Brain tumor: Its contribution to neurology in the remote and recent past. *J. Neuropath. exp. Neurol.*, 1946, *5:* 85–105.

PATERSON, R., DE PASQUALE, N., and MANN, S. Pseudotumor cerebri. *Medicine, Baltimore*, 1961, *40:* 85–99.

VORIS, H. C. The evaluation of irradiation in the management of brain tumors. Collective review. *Int. Abstr. Surg.*, 1940, *71:* 307–313.

47. MEHLER, W. R., FEFERMAN, M. E., and NAUTA, W. J. H. Ascending axon degeneration following anterolateral cordotomy. An experimental study in the monkey. *Brain*, 1960, *83:* 718–750.

49. TURNBULL, F. Intramedullary tumors of the spinal cord. *Clin. Neurosurg.*, 1962, *8:* 237–246.

50. AUSTIN, G., and ROTH, J. G. The diagnosis and treatment of interveretebral disk disease. In: Austin, G. *The spinal cord. Basic aspects and surgical considerations.* Springfield, Ill.: Charles C Thomas, 1961, xiv, 532 pp. (see pp. 106–133).

BICK, E. M. Source book of orthopaedics. *Baltimore: Williams & Wilkins Co.*, 1948, 2nd ed., xii, 540 pp. (see pp. 202–206).

GRAY, C. The causes and treatment of sciatic pain. *Int. Abstr. Surg.*, 1947, *85:* 417–441.

HARMON, P. H. Indications for spinal fusion in lumbar diskopathy, instability and arthrosis. Part 1. Anatomic and functional pathology and review of literature. *Clin. Orthop.*, 1964, *34:* 73–91.

WARTENBERG, R. Neuritis, sensory neuritis, neuralgia. A clinical study with review of the literature. *New York: Oxford Univ. Press*, 1958, xii, 444 pp. (see pp. 107–137).

WOODHALL, B., and HAYES, G. J. The well-leg-raising test of Fajersztajn in the diagnosis of ruptured lumbar intervertebral disc. *J. Bone Jt. Surg.*, 1950, *32-A:* 786–792.

52. PARSONS, H. Robert Abbe: pioneer in neurosurgery. *Bull. N. Y. Acad. Med.*, 1956, *32:* 57–75.

B. Unrelated to Specific Neurosurgical Classics

Anesthesia for Neurosurgery

FULTON, J. F., and STANTON, M. E. The centennial of surgical anesthesia. An annotated catalogue of books and pamphlets bearing on the early history of surgical anesthesia. *New York: H. Schuman*, 1946, xv, 102 pp.

KEYS, T. E. The history of surgical anesthesia. *New York: Dover Publications*, 1963, xxx, 193 pp.

LAZORTHES, G., and CAMPAN, L. The evolution of anesthesiology in brain surgery. *J. int. Coll. Surg.*, 1954, *22:* 557–569.

SCHAPIRA, M. Evolution of anesthesia for neurosurgery. *N. Y. St. J. Med.*, 1964, *64:* 1301–1305.

Cranial and Dural Defects

GRANT, F. C., and NORCROSS, N. D. Repair of cranial defects by cranioplasty. *Ann. Surg.*, 1939, *110:* 488–510.

KEENER, E. B. Regeneration of dural defects. A review. *J. Neurosurg.*, 1959, *16:* 415–423.

REEVES, D. L. Cranioplasty. *Springfield, Ill.: Charles C Thomas*, 1950, x, 119 pp.

WOOLF, J. I., and WALKER, A. E. Cranioplasty. Collective review. *Int. Abstr. Surg.*, 1945, *81:* 1–23.

Electrodiagnosis

BRAZIER, M. A. B. Rise of neurophysiology in the 19th century. *J. Neurophysiol.*, 1957, *20:* 212–226.

BRAZIER, M. A. B. The development of concepts relating to the electrical activity of the brain. *J. nerv. ment. Dis.*, 1958, *126:* 303–321.

BRAZIER, M. A. B. A history of the electrical activity of the brain. The first half-century. *London: Pitman Medical Publishing Co.*, 1961, vii, 119 pp.

BRAZIER, M. A. B. Historical introduction. The discoverers of the steady potentials of the brain: Caton and Beck. In: *Brain function. Proceedings of the first conference, 1961. Cortical excitability and steady potentials. Relations of basic research to space biology.* M. A. B. Brazier, Ed. Berkeley and Los Angeles: Univ. of California Press, 1963, xviii, 394 pp. (see pp. 1–13).

GIBBS, F. A., and GIBBS, E. L. Atlas of electroencephalography. *Cambridge, Mass.: L. A. Cummings Co.*, 1941, 221 pp. (see pp. 2, 4, 6, 8).

LICHT, S. The history of electrodiagnosis. *Bull Hist. Med.*, 1944, *16:* 450–467.

LICHT, S. History of electrodiagnosis. In: *Electro-*

diagnosis and electromyography. S. Licht, Ed. New Haven, Conn.: E. Licht, 1961, 2nd ed., xiii, 470 pp. (see pp. 1–23).

WENZEL E. Luigi Galvani—Alexander von Humboldt—Hans Berger. (Aus der Geschichte der Elektroenzephalographie). *Münch. med. Wschr.,* 1962, *104:* 1146–1150.

General Neurosurgery

BAILEY, P. Anecdotes from the history of trephining. *J. int. Coll. Surg.,* 1961, *35:* 382–392.

BROWN, H. A. The Harvey Cushing Society. Past, present and future. *J. Neurosurg.,* 1958, *15:* 587–601.

BUCY, P. C. The Journal of Neurosurgery. Its origin and development. *J. Neurosurg.,* 1964, *21,* No. 7, pt. 2: 1–12.

CHRISTENSEN, J. C. History of neurosurgery in South America. *Acta neurol. latinoam.,* 1962, *8:* 63–76.

ELSBERG, C. A. The development of neurological surgery in New York City during the past twenty-five years. With remarks on advances due to experiences in the First World War. *Bull. N. Y. Acad. Med.,* 1942, *18:* 654–664.

FURLOW, L. T. The American Board of Neurological Surgery. *J. Neurosurg.,* 1962, *19:* 617–625.

GERMAN, W. J. Neurological surgery. Its past, present and future. *J. Neurosurg.,* 1953, *10:* 526–537.

GLOWACKI, J. The role of Jozef Babinski in the development of neurosurgery. *Bull. Pol. med. sci. Hist.,* 1962, *5:* 40–41.

JIRÁSEK, A. The priority of Czech surgeons in neurological surgery. *Rev. Czech. Med.,* 1956, *2:* 89–93.

LEONARDO, R. A. History of surgery. *New York: Froben Press,* 1943, xvii, 504 pp. (see pp. 459–464).

MILLER, D. Syme memorial lecture. The development of neurosurgery. *Med. J. Aust.,* 1963, *1:* 455–458.

MITCHELL-HEGGS, F., and DREW, H. G. R. The instruments of surgery. *Springfield, Ill: Charles C Thomas,* 1963, x, 526 pp. (see pp. 382–398).

MORTON, L. T. Garrison and Morton's medical bibliography. An annotated check-list of texts illustrating the history of medicine. *New York: Argosy Book Stores,* 1954, 2nd ed., xiii, 655 pp. (see pp. 424–429, 437, 438).

RAAF, J. Presidential address. Pacific Coast Surgical Association. *Amer. J. Surg.,* 1962, *104:* 129–134.

REEVES, D. L. "The Harvey Cushing Library." *J. Neurosurg.,* 1963, *20:* 545–556.

SHARPE, W. Brain surgeon. The autobiography of William Sharpe. *New York: Viking Press,* 1952, xvi, 271 pp.

SOROUR, O. The history of neurosurgery. *Kasr-El-Aini J. Surg.,* 1963, suppl. 4, 1–6.

STOOKEY, B. The Neurological Institute and early neurosurgery in New York. *J. Neurosurg.,* 1960, *17:* 801–814.

Hypothalamus and Autonomic Nervous System

ATKINSON, W. J. Surgery of the autonomic nervous system. In: *A history of neurological surgery.* A. E.

Walker, Ed. Baltimore: Williams & Wilkins Co., 1951, xii, 583 pp. (see pp. 428–450).

FULTON, J. F. Horner and the syndrome of paralysis of the cervical sympathetic. *Arch. Surg., Chicago,* 1929, *18:* 2025–2039.

FULTON, J. F. Introduction: Historical résumé. *Res. Pub. Ass. nerv. ment. Dis.,* 1940, *20:* xiii–xxx.

FULTON, J. F. Contemporary concepts of the hypothalamus and their origin. *Quart. Bull. Northw. Univ. med. Sch.,* 1954, *28:* 10–16.

GOETZ, R. H. The surgical physiology of the sympathetic nervous system with special reference to cardiovascular disorders. *Int. Abstr. Surg.,* 1948, *87:* 417–439.

HOFF, H. E. Vagal stimulation before the Webers. *Ann. med. Hist.,* 1936, 2nd s. *8:* 138–144.

HOFF, H. E. The history of vagal inhibition. *Bull. Hist. Med.,* 1940, *8:* 461–496.

KUNTZ, A. The autonomic nervous system. *Philadelphia: Lea & Febiger,* 1953, 4th ed., 605 pp. (see pp. 15–20, 491–543).

MACCARTY, C. S. Surgical procedures on the sympathetic nervous system for peripheral vascular disease. In: *Peripheral vascular diseases.* E. V. Allen, N. W. Barker, and E. A. Hines, Jr., Ed. Philadelphia: W. B. Saunders Co., 1955, 2nd ed., xiii, 825 pp. (see pp. 665–678).

MONRO, P. A. G. Sympathectomy. An anatomical and physiological study with clinical applications. *London: Oxford Univ. Press,* 1959, xx, 290 pp. (see pp. 3–9, 189–195).

SHEEHAN, D. Discovery of the autonomic nervous system. *Arch. Neurol. Psychiat., Chicago,* 1936, *35:* 1081–1115.

TIMME, W. The vegetative nervous system. Historical retrospect. *Res. Publ. Ass. nerv. ment. Dis.,* 1930, *9:* 1–11.

WHITE, J. C., and SMITHWICK, R. H. The autonomic nervous system. Anatomy, physiology, and surgical application. *New York: Macmillan Co.,* 1941, 2nd ed., xx, 469 pp. (see pp. 7–21).

Military Neurosurgery

COPE, Z. (Ed.) Surgery. *London: Her Majesty's Stationery Office,* 1953, xix, 772 pp. (see pp. 377–537).

CUSHING, H. A study of a series of wounds involving the brain and its enveloping structures. *Brit. J. Surg.,* 1918, *5:* 558–684.

DAVIS, L. Neurological surgery through the years of World War II. *Int. Abstr. Surg.,* 1949, *89:* 1–23.

LAFIA, D. J. S. Weir Mitchell on gunshot wounds and other injuries of nerves. *Neurology,* 1955, *5:* 468–471.

MEDICAL DEPARTMENT OF THE UNITED STATES ARMY IN THE WORLD WAR. M. W. Ireland, Ed. *Washington, D. C.: U. S. Government Printing Office,* 1921–1929, 15 vols. (see *11,* pt. 1: 749–1283).

MEDICAL DEPARTMENT, UNITED STATES ARMY. SURGERY IN WORLD WAR II. NEUROSURGERY, R. G. Spurling and B. Woodhall, Ed. *Washington, D. C.: U. S. Government Printing Office,* 1958–1959, 2 vols.

WALKER, A. E., and JABLON, S. A follow-up study of head wounds in World War II. *Washington, D. C.: U. S. Government Printing Office,* 1961, x, 202 pp.

Webster, J. E., and Gurdjian, E. S. Penetrating
cranial wounds. A summary of methods used in
management. *Int. Abstr. Surg.*,
1946, *82:* 353–380.

Woodhall, B., and Beebe, G. W. Peripheral nerve
regeneration. A follow-up study of 3,656 World
War II injuries. *Washington, D. C.: U. S. Government Printing Office*, 1956, xxiv, 671 pp.

Nerves

Browne, K. M. Surgery of the peripheral nerves.
In: *A history of neurological surgery.* A. E. Walker,
Ed. Baltimore: Williams & Wilkins Co., 1951, xii,
583 pp. (see pp. 396–424).

Holmes, W. The repair of nerves by suture. *J. Hist.
Med.*, 1951, *6:* 44–63.

Johnson, E. W., Jr. Brachial palsy at birth. *Int.
Abstr. Surg.*, 1960, *111:* 409–416.

Power, D'A. A mirror for surgeons. Selected readings in surgery. *Boston: Little, Brown & Co.*, 1939,
xii, 230 pp. (see pp. 128–132).

Thomas, K. B. Facial palsy before Bell. *Middlesex
Hosp. J.*, 1963, *63:* 254–256.

Upmalis, I. H. The scalenus anticus and related
syndromes. *Int. Abstr. Surg.*, 1958, *107:* 521–529.

Neurology, Neuropathology and Neurophysiology

Blackwood, W. The National Hospital, Queen
Square, and the development of neuropathology.
World Neurol., 1961, *2:* 331–335.

Brain, R. Neurology: past, present, and future.
Brit. med. J., 1958, *1:* 355–360.

Bruetsch, W. L. Neurosyphilis. In: *Clinical neurology.* A. B. Baker, Ed. New York: Hoeber-Harper,
1962, 2nd ed., *2:* 928–979.

DeJong, R. N. Migraine. Personal observations by
physicians subject to the disorder. *Ann. med. Hist.*,
1942, 3rd s. *4:* 276–283.

Hall, G. W. Neurologic signs and their discoverers.
J. Amer. med. Ass., 1930, *95:* 703–707.

Holmes, G. The National Hospital, Queen Square,
1860–1948. *Edinburgh: E. & S. Livingstone Ltd.*,
1954, xii, 98 pp.

Kesert, B. H. An historical review of neurology.
Proc. Inst. Med. Chicago, 1963, *24:* 284–290.

Keynes, G. The history of myasthenia gravis. *Med.
Hist.*, 1961, *5:* 313–326.

Mackay, R. P. The history of neurology in Chicago.
J. int. Coll. Surg., 1963, *40:* 191–205.

Mackay, R. P. The history of neurology in Chicago.
Illinois med. J., 1964, *125:* 51–58, 142–146, 256–
259, 341–344, 539–544, 636–640; *126:* 60–64.

McMenemey, W. H. Neurological investigation in
Britain from 1800 to the founding of the National
Hospital. *Proc. roy. Soc. Med.*, 1960, *53:* 605–612.

Pette, H. Stand und Entwicklung der Neurologie.
Internist, 1963, *4:* 258–266.

Riese, W. Dynamic aspects in the history of
neurology. In: *Problems of dynamic neurology.* L.
Halpern, Ed. Jerusalem: Hebrew Univ., 1963, xii,
509 pp. (see pp. 1–29).

Schumacher, G. A. The demyelinating diseases.
In: *Clinical neurology.* A. B. Baker, Ed. New York:
Hoeber-Harper, 1962, 2nd ed., *3:* 1226–1284.

Sherwin, A. L. Multiple sclerosis in historical perspective. *McGill med. J.*, 1957, *26:* 39–48.

Stookey, B. Historical background of the Neurological Institute and the neurological societies.
Bull. N. Y. Acad. Med., 1959, *35:* 707–729.

Viets, H. R. History of peripheral neuritis as a
clinical entity. *Arch. Neurol. Psychiat., Chicago*,
1934, *32:* 377–394.

Viets, H. R. A historical review of myasthenia
gravis from 1672 to 1900. *J. Amer. med. Ass.*, 1953,
153: 1273–1280.

Wechsler, I. S. Introduction to the history of neurology. In: *Clinical neurology. With an introduction
to the history of neurology.* Philadelphia: W. B.
Saunders Co., 1963, 9th ed., xviii, 719 pp. (see pp.
641–675).

Spine and Spinal Cord

Bors, E. Neurogenic bladder. *Urol Surv.*, 1957, *7:*
177–250.

Courville, C. B. Trauma to the central nervous
system and its envelopes. In: *Tice's Practice of
medicine.* J. C. Harvey, Ed. Hagerstown, Md.:
W. F. Prior Co., Inc., 1962, *10:* 139–223.

Delvin, D. G. Laminectomy in 1814. A report of a
manuscript discovered in the library of King's College Hospital Medical School. *King's Coll. Hosp.
Gaz.*, 1962, *41:* 68–71.

Gray, S. W., Romaine, C. B., and Skandalakis,
J. E. Congenital fusion of the cervical vertebrae.
Int. Abstr. Surg., 1964, *118:* 373–385.

Ingraham, F. D. Spina bifida and cranium bifidum.
Papers reprinted from the New England Journal
of Medicine with the addition of a comprehensive
bibliography. *Cambridge, Mass.: Harvard Univ.
Press*, 1943–1944, 216 pp.

Martin, J. The treatment of injuries of the spinal
cord. *Int. Abstr. Surg.*, 1947, *84:* 403–416.

Odom, G. L. Vascular lesions of the spinal cord:
malformations, spinal subarachnoid and extradural
hemorrhage. *Clin. Neurosurg.*, 1962, *8:* 196–234.

Rickham, P. P. Nicolaas Tulp and spina bifida.
Clin. Pediat., 1963, *2:* 40–42.

Schneider, R. C. Cervical traction, with evaluation of methods, and treatment of complications.
Int. Abstr. Surg., 1957, *104:* 521–530.

Seddon, H. J. Pott's disease. *St. Bart's Hosp. J.*,
1964, *68:* 14–15.

Thomas, K. B. Traumatic paraplegia treated by
operation in 1841. *Med. Hist.*, 1958, *2:* 228–230.

Index

ABBE, R., 512, 519
Ablation, experimental cerebral, 26, 119, 156, 226, 442, 516
Abnormalities, vascular, 347, 428, 518, 521
Abscess, brain, 317, 391, 518
Acromegaly, 28, 516
Adenoma, pituitary, 28, 474, 516
ALMEIDA LIMA, P., 264, 443
Anesthesia, for neurosurgery, vii, 335, 384, 519
Aneurysm, intracranial, 428, 518
Angle, cerebellopontile, 354, 449, 519
Antiquity, neurosurgery in, 1, 6, 516
Antisepsis, vii, 363, 374, 383, 400, 493
Antivivisectionists, 119, 484
Aphasia, 3, 6, 15, 61, 391, 516, 517
Apparatus, stereotaxic, 162, 517
Arteriography, carotid, 264, 429, 518
Artery, carotid, ligation of, 155, 341, 428

BAILEY, PERCIVAL, 202
BARR, J. S., 495
Basophilism, pituitary, 28, 516
BENNETT, A. H., 361, 372
BENNETT, W. H., 504
BERGER, H., vii, 520
BLACKFAN, K. D., 69
BOVIE, W. T., 329
BROCA, P., 61, 64, 517
BUCY, P. C., 202
BURCKHARDT, G., 442

CADWALADER, W. B., 480
Cautery, electric, 329, 363, 373, 374, 439, 518
Cerebellum, 158, 162, 351, 449, 519
Chondroma, spinal, 495
Cisterna magna, puncture of, 188, 299, 497
CLARKE, R. H., 162, 517
Clips, hemostatic, 319
COLMAN, W. S., 404
Compression, of the spinal cord, 1, 6, 261, 309, 488, 497, 516, 521
Concussion, cerebral, 517
Consciousness, 224, 518
Cordotomy, 477, 519
Craniectomy
    for decompression, 186, 387, 389, 465
    for infection, 399
    for psychosurgery, 442, 519
    for trauma, 10, 388, 516, 520
    for trigeminal neuralgia, 387, 404, 418, 518
    for tumor, 361, 372, 389, 449, 469, 518, 519
Cranioplasty, 519
Craniotomy
    for aneurysm, 428
    for tumor, 202, 469
    techniques, 318, 329, 377, 383, 387, 469
CUSHING, H., 28, 202, 319, 329, 383, 389, 449, 469, 516

DANA, C., 504
DANDY, W. E., 69, 242, 251, 437, 449
DARLING, A. P., 259
DAX, M., 62, 517
Decompression, subtemporal, 186, 387, 389
Defect, cranial, 1, 6, 377, 388, 399, 516, 517, 519, 520
Defect, dural, 7, 390, 488, 519
Dermatomes, 129, 504
Disc, choked, 205, 277, 301, 316, 337, 362, 398, 518

Disc, intervertebral, ruptured, 257, 495, 519
Disease, Cushing's, 28, 516
DOTT, N. M., 428
Dressings, 1, 7, 303, 363, 386, 397, 425, 488, 516
DUNGAN, C. E., 259
DURANTE, F., 375
Dyspituitarism, 28, 516

Edema, cerebral, 186, 463, 518, 519
EGAS MONIZ, 264, 442
Electrodiagnosis, 519
Electroencephalography, vii, 519
Electromyography, 519
Electrosurgery, 329, 474
Epilepsy, 6, 154, 224, 335, 516, 518
Estimation, ventricular, 243

FERRIER, D., 119, 373
Fluid, cerebrospinal, 1, 69, 186, 242, 251, 257, 298, 431, 491
FOERSTER, O., 129, 504
FORESTIER, J., 257
FRAZIER, C. H., 418, 477
FRITSCH, G., 15, 516
Function, vestibular, 449, 519
Fungus, cerebral, 364, 470
FURST, J. B., 259
Fusion, spinal, 519

Ganglion, gasserian, 387, 404, 418, 518
GIGLI, L., 380
Gliomas
    diagnosis, 242, 251, 257, 264, 277, 298, 313, 518
    pathology, 202, 469, 519
    treatment, 202, 318, 329, 361, 372, 377, 383, 387, 469, 484, 518, 519
GODLEE, R. J., 361, 372
GOLTZ, F., 119
GOWERS, W. R., 484
von GRÄFE, A., 293

HARTLEY, F., 410, 518
von HELMHOLTZ, H., 277
Hematoma, extradural, 377, 388, 517, 521
Hematoma, subdural, 433, 517
Hemorrhage, subarachnoid, 431, 521
Hemostasis, 318, 329, 363, 384, 387, 428, 459, 476, 490, 518
Herniation, cerebral, 186, 251, 364, 385, 465, 470
Hippocrates, 6, 15, 186, 298, 329, 516
HITZIG, E., 15
HORSLEY, V., 162, 318, 372, 404, 484
Hydrocephalus, 69, 242, 251, 298, 458
Hypertension, intracranial, 69, 186, 245, 251, 268, 277, 298, 385, 458, 517, 519
Hypophysis, 28, 474, 516
Hypothalamus, 520

Infection, intracranial, 6, 336, 364, 374, 391, 470, 518
Infection, intraspinal, 6, 306, 391, 493
Injury, craniocerebral, 1, 6, 154, 186, 377, 388, 391, 442, 516, 517, 519, 520
Injury, spinal, 1, 6, 492, 516, 520, 521

JACKSON, J. H., 154, 277, 372, 517

KRAUSE, F., 412, 518

Laminectomy, 129, 477, 484, 495, 504, 519, 521
Ligation, of aneurysm, 428
Ligation, of carotid artery, 155, 341, 428
Lipiodol, 257, 495, 518
Lobotomy, prefrontal, 442, 519
Localization, clinical, cerebral, 1, 6, 15, 61, 119, 154, 162, 224, 361, 372, 391, 442, 516, 517, 518, 519, 520
Localization, clinical, peripheral, 129, 404, 418, 504
Localization, clinical, spinal, 1, 477, 484, 516, 519

Macewen, W., 372, 391, 484
Malformation, arteriovenous, 347, 518, 521
Martin, E., 477
McKibben, P. S., 186
Memory, 224, 442, 518
Meningitis, 296, 306, 336, 366, 391, 470, 493
Meningocele, 521
Mixter, W. J., 495
Movements, involuntary, 162, 517
Myelography, 255, 257, 497, 518

Naffziger, H. C., 313
Nerves, cranial, 6, 277, 354, 387, 404, 418, 432, 449, 516, 518, 519, 521
Nerves, spinal, 129, 495, 504, 519, 521
Neuralgia, trigeminal, 387, 404, 418, 518
Neurinoma, acoustic, 354, 449, 473, 519
Neuritis, optic, 205, 277, 301, 316, 337, 362, 398, 518
Neurologists, initiation of operations by, 129, 361, 372, 418, 442, 477, 484, 504, 521
Neurology, history of, 521
Neuropathology, history of, 202, 521
Neurophysiology, history of, 15, 61, 69, 119, 154, 224, 442, 477, 516, 517, 518, 519, 520, 521
Neuroradiology, 202, 242, 251, 257, 264, 313, 428, 449, 495, 518
Neurosurgery, history of, 520
Neurosurgery, military, 6, 520
Neurotomy, retrogasserian, 387, 404, 418, 518
Nucleus pulposus, herniated, 257, 495, 519

Oligodendrogliomas, 202, 469
Operations, craniocerebral, 6, 69, 162, 202, 224, 318, 329, 361, 372, 377, 383, 387, 391, 404, 418, 428, 442, 449, 469, 516, 517, 518, 519, 520, 521
Operations, spinal, 129, 477, 484, 495, 504, 519, 521
Ophthalmoscope, 277, 518

Pain, operations for, 129, 162, 387, 404, 418, 442, 477, 504, 518, 519
Pantopaque, 259, 518
Papilledema, 205, 277, 301, 316, 337, 362, 398, 518
Papyrus, Edwin Smith, 1, 186, 516
Parkinsonism, 162, 517
Penfield, W., 224
Phrenology, 15, 61, 516, 517
Pineal, position of, 313, 518
Pituitary, 28, 474, 516
Plati, J. T., 259
Pneumocephalus, 242
Pneumoencephalography, 242, 251
Pressure, cerebrospinal fluid, increased, 69, 186, 245, 251, 268, 277, 298, 385, 458, 517, 519
Prize, Nobel, 154, 443, 449
Procedures, diagnostic, 242, 251, 257, 264, 277, 298, 313, 518
Psychosurgery, 162, 442, 519
Puncture, cisternal, 188, 299, 497
Puncture, lumbar, 77, 186, 242, 251, 257, 298, 431, 466
Puncture, ventricular, 89, 186, 242, 266, 298, 458

Queckenstedt, H. H. G., 309
Quincke, H., 298

Radiation therapy, 519
Radioisotopes, vii
Reflexes, 154, 517
Rhizotomy, posterior, 129, 504
Rigidity, decerebrate, 154, 517
Roentgenography, 202, 242, 251, 257, 264, 313, 428, 449, 495, 518

Saw, Gigli, 380, 385
Scan, brain, vii
Schüller, A., 313
Sciatica, 6, 495, 519
Seizures
    grand mal, 6, 516
    post-traumatic, 520
    psychomotor, 224, 518
    tonic, 154, 517
Sherrington, C. S., 154
Shift, pineal, 313, 518
Shunts, for hydrocephalus, 69
Sicard, J. A., 257
Smith, S. W., 259
Sound, cracked pot, 396
Spiller, W. G., 418, 477
Spina bifida, 521
Steinhausen, T. B., 259
Stimulation, electrical, of the brain, 15, 159, 172, 224, 335, 516, 517
Stimulation, electrical, of the peripheral nerves, 129, 159, 504
Strain, W. H., 259
Surgery, stereotaxic, 162, 443, 517
Sweet, J. E., 480
Sympathectomy, 520
Syndrome, Cushing's, 28, 516
Syndrome, Ménière's, 519
Syndrome, scalenus anticus, 314, 521
System, autonomic nervous, 129, 520

Tap, spinal, 77, 186, 242, 251, 257, 298, 431, 466
Taylor, J., 404
Test, caloric, for acoustic tumor, 449
Test, Queckenstedt, 309
Tic douloureux, 387, 404, 418, 518
Tract, spinothalamic, 477, 519
Traction, cervical, 521
Trauma, craniocerebral, 1, 6, 154, 186, 377, 388, 391, 442, 516, 517, 519, 520
Trauma, spinal, 1, 6, 492, 516, 521
Trephination, 1, 6, 186, 244, 361, 372, 377, 516
Tumor, intracranial, 28, 202, 242, 251, 264, 277, 313, 319, 329, 361, 372, 387, 449, 469, 516, 518, 519
Tumor, intraspinal, 255, 257, 309, 484, 518, 519

Ulcer, peptic, 517

Ventricle, puncture of, 89, 186, 242, 266, 298, 458
Ventriculocisternostomy, 69
Ventriculography, 242, 266, 476
Vivisection, 119, 484

Wagner, W., 377
Warren, S. L., 259
Wax, bone, 318
Weed, L. H., 186
Wolcott, E. C., Jr., 259